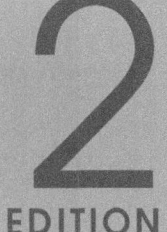

2
EDITION

Handbook of
Forensic
Neuropsychology

About the Editors

Arthur MacNeill Horton, Jr., EdD, ABPP, ABPN, received his EdD in Counselor Education from the University of Virginia in 1976. He also holds Diplomates in Clinical Psychology and Behavioral Psychology from the American Board of Professional Psychology and a Diplomate in Clinical Neuropsychology from the American Board of Professional Neuropsychology. Dr. Horton is the author or editor of over 15 books, more than 45 book chapters, and over 130 journal articles. He is a past president of the American Board of Professional Neuropsychology, the doctoral-level certification board in neuropsychology, and the National Academy of Neuropsychology (NAN). In addition, Dr. Horton was a member of the State of Maryland Board of Examiners of Psychologists for two terms. Previously, Dr. Horton was Program Officer with the National Institute of Drug Abuse (NIDA) of the National Institutes of Health (NIH) with responsibilities for neuropsychology. He has taught at the University of Virginia, The Citadel, The West Virginia University, The Johns Hopkins University, The University of Baltimore, Loyola College in Maryland, The Department of Psychiatry of the University of Maryland Medical School, and the Fielding Institute Graduate Program in Neuropsychology. Currently Dr. Horton is in independent practice as Director of the Neuropsychology Clinic at Psych Associates of Maryland in Towson, Columbia, and Bethesda, Maryland, and consults on clinical neuropsychology and drug-abuse research issues.

Lawrence C. Hartlage, PhD, ABPP, ABPN, has served as president of the National Academy of Neuropsychology, the American Psychological Association Division of Neuropsychology, and the American Board of Professional Neuropsychology. Elected to Fellow status by seven divisions of the American Psychological Association, he was a charter Fellow of the American Psychological Society and is listed in the inaugural issue of *Who's Who in Medicine and Healthcare*. He has served as consultant to the Canadian Research Council, the Centers for Disease Control, the North Atlantic Treaty Organization, the National Institutes of Health, and the U.S. Surgeon General.

Handbook of Forensic Neuropsychology

2 EDITION

Editors
Arthur MacNeill Horton, Jr., EdD, ABPP, ABPN
Lawrence C. Hartlage, PhD, ABPP, ABPN

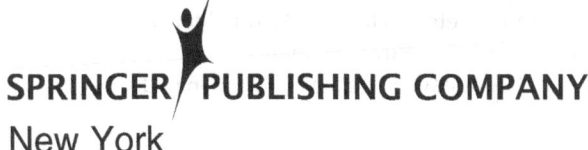

SPRINGER PUBLISHING COMPANY

New York

Springer Publishing Company, LLC
11 West 42nd Street
New York, NY 10036
www.springerpub.com

Acquisitions Editor: Philip Laughlin
Production Editor: Pamela Lankas
Cover design: David Levy
Composition: International Graphic Services

Ebook ISBN: 978-0-8261-1886-8

10 11 12 13 14 / 5 4 3 2 1

The author and the publisher of this Work have made every effort to use sources believed to be reliable to provide information that is accurate and compatible with the standards generally accepted at the time of publication. The author and publisher shall not be liable for any special, consequential, or exemplary damages resulting, in whole or in part, from the readers' use of, or reliance on, the information contained in this book. The publisher has no responsibility for the persistence or accuracy of URLs for external or third-party Internet Web sites referred to in this publication and does not guarantee that any content on such Web sites is, or will remain, accurate or appropriate.

Library of Congress Cataloging-in-Publication Data

Handbook of forensic neuropsychology / Arthur MacNeill Horton Jr., Lawrence C. Hartlage, editors.—2nd ed.
        p. ; cm.
    Includes bibliographical references and index.
    ISBN 978-0-8261-1885-1 (alk. paper)
    1. Forensic neuropsychology—Handbooks, manuals, etc. 2. Clinical neuropsychology—Handbooks, manuals, etc. I. Horton, Arthur MacNeill, 1947. II. Hartlage, Lawrence C. III. Title: Forensic neuropsychology.
    [DNLM: 1. Forensic Medicine. 2. Neuropsychology. W 700 H2365 2010]

    RA1147.5.H36 2010
    614'.1—dc22
                                2009050242

Printed in the United States of America by King Printing

To my wife, Mary, with all of my love,
and to my parents, who were both lawyers.

—Arthur MacNeill Horton, Jr.

To Ralph M. Reitan, PhD,
for inspiration over many years.

—Lawrence C. Hartlage

Contents

Contributors

Daniel Allen, PhD
Department of Psychology
University of Nevada Las Vegas
Las Vegas, NV

Thomas L. Bennett, PhD, ABN, ABPP, FACPN
Center for Neurorehabilitation Services
Fort Collins, CO

Shane S. Bush, PhD, ABN, ABPP, FACPN
Long Island Neuropsychology, P.C.
Lake Ronkonoma, NY

Christine L. Castillo, PhD
Children's Medical Center Dallas
Dallas, TX

Larry Cohen, JD, PhD
Cohen Law Firm
Phoenix, AZ

Barry M. Crown, PhD, ABN, FACPN
Independent Practice
South Miami, FL, and
Department of Psychology
Florida International University

Rik Carl D'Amato, PhD
Professor and Head
Department of Psychology
University of Macau
Taipa, Macau SAR China

Raymond S. Dean, PhD, ABN, ABPP, FACPN
Neuropsychology Laboratory
Ball State University
Muncie, IN

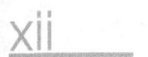
Robert L. Denney, PsyD, ABPP, FACPN
US Medical Center for Federal Prisoners
Springfield, MO, and the School of Professional Psychology at Forest Institute
Springfield, MO

Bradley C. Donohue, PhD
Department of Psychology
University of Nevada Las Vegas
Las Vegas, NV

Kevin Duff, PhD
University of Iowa
Department of Psychiatry
Iowa City, IA

Paul S. Ferber, Esq.
Director of Vermont Law School's General Practice Program
White River, VT

H. Scott Fingerhut, Esq.
Attorney at Law
College of Law
Florida International University

Ronald D. Franklin, PhD, ABPdN
Independent Practice
West Palm Beach, FL

Michael D. Franzen, PhD
Department of Psychiatry
Allegheny General Hospital
Pittsburgh, PA

Peter R. Giancola, PhD
Department of Psychology
University of Kentucky
Lexington, KY

Charles J. Golden, PhD, ABPP, ABN, ABAP, FACPN
Department of Psychology
Center for Psychological Studies
Nova Southeastern University
Fort Lauderdale, FL

Michael Haderlie, PhD
Department of Psychology
University of Nevada Las Vegas
Las Vegas, NV

Lindsay Hines, PhD
Department of Psychology
Center for Psychological Studies
Nova Southeastern University
Fort Lauderdale, FL

Laura L. Hoskins, PhD
Neuropsychology Program and Brain Imaging Laboratory
Department of Psychiatry
Dartmouth Medical School/DHMC
Lebanon, NH

Grant L. Iverson, PhD
Department of Psychiatry
University of British Columbia
Vancouver, BC

Sheryl J. Lowenthal, Esq.
Attorney at Law
Miami, FL

Thomas A. Martin, PsyD, ABPP
University of Missouri–Columbia
Columbia, MO

Robert J. McCaffrey, PhD, ABN, ABPdN, FACPN
SUNY/ Albany
Psychology Department
Albany, NY

Doris Shui Ying Mok, PhD
Department of Psychology
University of Macau
Taipa, Macau SAR China

Lisa A. Pass, PhD
Neuropsychology Laboratory
Ball State University
Muncie, IN

Dori Pelz-Sherman, PhD
School of Psychology
Fielding Graduate University
Santa Barbara, CA

Antonio E. Puente, PhD, ABN, FACPN
University of North Carolina at Wilmington
Wilmington, NC

Dorrie L. Rapp, PhD, ABN, ABPP, FACPN
Rehabilitation Psychologist
Private Practice
White River, VT

Michael J. Raymond, PhD, ABN, FACPN
Allied Services
John Heinz Institute of Rehabilitation Medicine
Wilkes Barre, PA

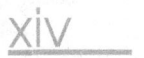

Cecil R. Reynolds, PhD, ABN, FACPN
Departments of Educational Psychology and Neuroscience
Texas A & M University
College Station, TX

Robert M. Roth, PhD
Brain Imaging Laboratory
Department of Psychiatry
Dartmouth Medical School / DHMC
Lebanon, NH

Robert J. Sbordone, PhD, ABPP, ABN, ABAP, FACPN
Independent Practice
Laguna Hills, CA

Raymond Singer, PhD, ABN, FACPN
Independent Practice
Santa Fe, NM

Henry V. Soper, PhD
School of Psychology
Fielding Graduate University
Santa Barbara, CA

Bruce H. Stern, Esq.
Stark & Stark, P. C.
Princeton, NJ

Griffin P. Sutton, PhD
Department of Psychology
University of Nevada Las Vegas
Las Vegas, NV

Elizabeth A. Tyner, PhD
US Medical Center for Federal Prisoners
Springfield, MO

Jana L. Vanderslice-Barr, PhD
SUNY/ Albany
Psychology Department
Albany, NY

Raquel Vilar-López, PhD
University of Granada and Neuroscience Institute "Federico Olóriz"
Granada, Spain

Betsy L. Williams, PhD, ABN, FACPN
Independent Practice
Albuquerque, NM

Deborah Witsken, PhD
University of Northern Colorado
Greeley, CO

Preface

The continued growth of forensic neuropsychology can be seen in a number of events. In the last decade, a large number of books dealing with forensic neuropsychology have been published for graduate, professional, and undergraduate markets. There are increasing numbers of requests from attorneys and judges for forensic neuropsychologists to provide services in the legal arena by quantifying the nature and extent of cortical brain damage in industrial or automobile accidents, or neurotoxin exposures. In addition, forensic neuropsychologists are increasingly being consulted on essentially legal questions such as competency to handle personal financial and legal matters, participate in research studies, and make major medical decisions, and capacity to participate in legal proceedings, dangerousness, and insanity. Research studies involving forensic neuropsychology have increased exponentially and are projected to continue to increase. New developments in addiction neuropsychology, child and adolescent psychopathology, medical neuropsychology, and neurotoxin exposure indicate continued strong growth in forensic neuropsychology.

To address the urgent need for an updated, contemporary, authoritative reference work for this rapidly growing field, the *Handbook of Forensic Neuropsychology, Second Edition* builds on the firm foundation of the previously published *Handbook of Forensic Neuropsychology, First Edition,* which was very well received by the academic, research, and professional communities. The *Handbook of Forensic Neuropsychology, Second Edition* will update the previous edition by including the multiple research and professional advances that have occurred in the decade since the first edition was published. In addition, there will be an increased emphasis in this edition on case examples and case materials that illustrate a variety of concepts and techniques of forensic neuropsychology.

The major areas that will be covered in the *Handbook of Forensic Neuropsychology, Second Edition* will include the foundations of forensic neuropsychology, ethical and legal issues, practice issues, and special areas and populations.

Foundations of forensic neuropsychology include the principles of brain structure and function, and the history of clinical neuropsychology, the neuropsychology of intelligence, normative and scaling issues, and symptom validity testing and neuroimaging. *Ethical and legal issues* will include security of test data, competency and civil commitment, criminal law, confidentiality, and conflicts of interest. *Practice issues* will include cross-cultural and multicultural considerations in forensic neuropsychology, measurement of change over time, dealing with depositions and courtroom testimony in the forensic arena, assessment of premorbid mental abilities, and the ecological validity of neuropsychological testing. *Special areas and populations* will include disability and fitness for duty evaluations, aging and dementia, children and adolescents,

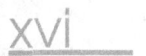

autism spectrum disorders, substance abuse, and neurotoxicology. A concluding section focuses on the future of forensic neuropsychology.

The *Handbook of Forensic Neuropsychology, Second Edition* provides an updated, contemporary, authoritative reference work intended for forensic neuropsychologists, psychiatrists, neurologists, neurosurgeons, pediatricians, attorneys, judges, law students, police officers, special educators, and clinical and school psychologists, among other professionals. All of these professionals, and possibly others, should find the *Handbook of Forensic Neuropsychology, Second Edition* to be of value. Our hope and expectation is that this new volume will be an important contribution toward promoting the very positive value that forensic neuropsychology brings to medical, educational, rehabilitation, and legal and forensic settings.

Acknowledgments

Many forensic neuropsychologists have indirectly contributed to the *Handbook of Forensic Neuropsychology, Second Edition* by their support and advice to the editors. These persons include Ralph M. Reitan, David E. Hartman, Tony Strickland, Arnold Purish, Robert W. Elliott, W. Drew Gouvier, Charles J. Long, Jim Hom, Paul Satz, Pat Pimental, Karen Steingarden, Sue Antell, Eric Zillmer, Joan W. Mayfield, Ralph Tarter, Gerald Goldstein, Deborah Wolfson, Francis J. Fishburne, J. Randall Price, Jeffrey T. Barth, Antonio E. Puente, and George W. Hynd.

Ira B. Gensemer, Daneen A. Milam, Danny Wedding, Randy W. Kamphaus, Robert L. Kane, Katleen Fitzhugh-Bell, Dennis L. Reeves, James A. Moses, Jr., Jeffrey J. Webster, Alan Gessner, John Blasé, John Meyers, Bradley Sewick, Francis J. Pirozzolo, John E. Obrzut, Richard Berg, Mark Goodman, Henry Soper, Marvin H. Podd, Martin Rohling, Barbara Uzzell, Greta N. Wilkening, Peggy Nichole McWhorter, Scott Sautter, Teri McHale, Art Williams, David Ranks, Denis McCarthy, Jose Vega, and Cindy K. Westergaard, among others too numerous to mention, have been most helpful.

A number of psychiatrists and neurologists have also been helpful, including Michael K. Spodak, Abdul Malik, Mahmood Jahromi, Daniel Drubach, Scott Spier, Mohammad Haerian, Francis J. Mwaisela, Marcella V. Mwaisela, and Maya R. Carter, among others too numerous to mention.

We also recognize the assistance of attorneys such as Tom Talbot, James Sullivan, Mitchell Blatt, Steve Van Grack, Patrick Donahue, Andrew Nichols, Eric Muller, Ralph Wilson, Andrew Connelly, Chris McNally, Allison Kohler, Suja M. Varghese, Lawrence Cohen, and Jeanie Garner, among others too numerous to mention.

Dr. Horton wishes to note that both of his deceased parents were attorneys and they provided him a unique, lifelong experience of dealing with the highest quality of legal reasoning and ethical decision making. Dr. Hartlage acknowledges the influence of Judges Bork, Borowiec, Quillian, and Williams, who called him to appear as an advisor in more than 3,000 cases over a 30-year period—and influenced his daughter, Mary Beth, to pursue a career in the field of law, graduating from Harvard Law School in 1993.

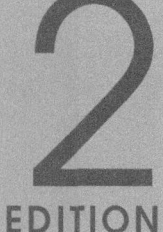

EDITION

Handbook of
Forensic
Neuropsychology

Part I

Foundations of Neuropsychology

Overview of Forensic Neuropsychology

1

Arthur MacNeill Horton, Jr.

Forensic neuropsychology is a fast-growing subspecialty of clinical neuropsychology in which the results of clinical neuropsychological assessments are used to address legal questions in the courtroom (Horton & Hartlage, 2003). The field of forensic neuropsychology is quite new and rests on an evolving research base. Moreover, the complex nature of forensic neuropsychology makes it a very difficult but rewarding area (Hartlage, 2003). The hope and expectation is that this and other chapters of this handbook will be helpful in terms of facilitating the delivery of forensic neuropsychological services to this needy population of brain-injured adults and children.

The history of forensic neuropsychology is short. The entry of psychology into the legal arena has been a relatively recent occurrence. Clinical neuropsychology only emerged as an area of scientific research in the 1940s (Ruff, 2004), so its entrance into the legal system was delayed. Clinical neuropsychology focuses on the clinical problems of assessment and treatment of disorders of the higher cortical functions in humans of all ages. Clinical neuropsychologists base their findings upon the results of objective psychological tests that meet recognized psychometric standards of validity and reliability (Jarvis & Barth, 1984). This clinical specialty area differs from, and yet is similar to, other areas of psychological or neurological practice, such as clinical psychology and behavioral neurology, to name but two related areas, in terms of the populations served, the neuropsychological problems addressed, and the procedures and techniques employed (American Academy of Neurology, 1996).

Since the emergence of clinical neuropsychology as a discipline, however, there have been a large number of examples of the cross-cultural validity of neuropsychological research findings, as well as very successful applications of neuropsychological assessment intervention methods with both adults and children (Horton, 1989, 1994; Horton & Miller, 1985; Horton & Puente, 1986; Hynd & Willis, 1988; Lawson-Kerr, Smith, & Beck, 1990). These remarkable demonstrations of the power of clinical neuropsychological methods have engendered great interest in forensic neuropsychology.

Neuropsychological Definitions

At this juncture it might be helpful to provide some basic definitions in neuropsychology. Neuropsychology was defined by Meier (1974) as "the scientific study of brain behavior relationships."

That definition was particularly apt and is as serviceable today, more than 35 years after it was proposed, as it was at that time. It is noted by Horton and Puente (1986) that neuropsychological performance may be influenced by both organic and environmental variables. The organic nature of neuropsychological variables has been clearly demonstrated through the work of famous neuropsychologists such as Ralph M. Reitan, Arthur L. Benton, and A. R. Luria, among others, over a number of decades. Attention to the environmental determinants of neuropsychological performance, however, is of more recent origin. As an example, it should be noted than in recent years, increased attention has been focused on the practice of behavioral therapy with brain-impaired adults and children (Horton, 1989, 1994; Horton & Sautter, 1986; Horton & Wedding, 1984).

A brief discussion of the concepts of "brain damage" and "cerebral dysfunction" is provided to clarify the neuropsychological context in which the concepts are applied. Very briefly, "brain damage" implies clear and substantial structural injury to the brain (Horton, 1994). Contemporary neurodiagnostic imaging methods such as positron emission tomography (PET) scanning and magnetic resonance imaging (MRI) can, in many cases, clearly identify structural brain lesions (Kertesz, 1994). Nonetheless, in some subtle cases, neuroimaging is totally inadequate to reflect changes in the physiological functioning of the brain that may result in behavioral abnormalities. At this point, it could be said that the behavioral correlates of neuroimaging are still poorly understood.

Although brain tumors or strokes often can be easily visualized, other neuropathological conditions such as sequelae of traumatic brain injury and neurotoxic conditions may produce clear neurocognitive, sensory-perceptual, and motor deficits without demonstrating clear structural brain changes under imaging (Horton, 1989). In situations of this sort where behavioral changes are clearly documented but structural lesions in the brain cannot be visualized, the term "cerebral dysfunction" is often used (Horton, 1994). The hope and expectation is that further research in neuroimaging and related procedures and methods will allow more precise detection of abnormalities in cerebral morphology.

The term "forensic neuropsychology" might be defined (Horton & Hartlage, 2003) as follows: "the application of the science of brain-behavior relationships to legal decision making."

This definition includes all of the science of clinical neuropsychology, but takes the clinical neuropsychologist out of the hospital or private practice office and places him or her in the courtroom. At the same time, the clear emphasis is upon the science of brain-behavior relationships (Jarvis & Barth, 1984) as the essential reason for bringing experts into the courtroom to assist judges and juries in legal decision making by providing objective scientific expertise. While attorneys are expected to be advocates for their clients, forensic neuropsychologists are expected to be objective experts who base their testimony on empirical scientific research findings (Bush & The NAN Policy and Planning Committee, 2005). If forensic neuropsychologists allow their objectivity to be compromised, then the rationale for their appearance in a courtroom is diminished.

In recent years, interest in forensic neuropsychology has increased at a tremendous rate and has included presentations at national meetings, and publications in relevant professional journals (Sweet, King, Malina, Bergman, & Simmons, 2002). Expectations are that the forensic emphasis in clinical neuropsychology will increase for both diagnostic and treatment aspects of clinical neuropsychology and the number of practitioners involved in forensic neuropsychology will accelerate dramatically (Hartlage, 2000).

When clinical neuropsychologists enter the forensic neuropsychology arena, however, there are important and difficult challenges to overcome. There are clear and important differences between clinical neuropsychology and forensic neuropsychology evaluations that must be understood by forensic neuropsychologists. These differences include relating neuropsychological findings to the relevant legal issues, the greater need for effort testing, and the importance of communicating neuropsychological implications for legal issues to judges and juries who may not have the necessary scientific backgrounds to comprehend and make legal decisions (Heilbrun et al., 2003). In the legal setting, forensic neuropsychologists must deal with the adversarial nature of legal proceedings and its implications for their forensic neuropsychological reports. Historically, contemporary courtroom procedures evolved from armed combat in the middle ages. In the forensic setting the legal issues to be decided are to be fought over and the forensic neuropsychologist will be treated as a weapon by lawyers (Zillmer & Green, 2006). This is very different from the typical clinical setting where a clinical neuropsychology report may be seen by other health care practitioners as authoritative knowledge. Still, the forensic neuropsychologist must present the implications of the neuropsychological findings for the legal questions at hand in an objective fashion in spite of the adversarial nature of the legal proceedings, but must not attempt to address the ultimate legal question, because that is the role of the attorneys, judge, and jury (Blau, 1998).

The greater need for effort testing arises from the fact that some individuals could profit greatly if the legal issues were decided in their favor, and that potential expected positive reinforcement may influence their forensic neuropsychological test performance (Iverson, 2003). Not all persons seen in the forensic setting will give poor effort on neuropsychological testing, but base rates of poor effort are higher in the forensic setting than in typical clinical settings (Mittenberg, Patton, Canyock, & Condit, 2002). Because of these higher base rates of poor effort, the forensic neuropsychologist must carefully evaluate the possibility of the patient giving poor effort and include effort testing measures as an essential portion of the forensic neuropsychological evaluation (Larrabee, 2005; Reynolds, 1998).

Similarly, clinical neuropsychologists typically present their findings in technical terms. While that behavior is appropriate for a clinical setting where other health care professionals are the intended audience, the forensic neuropsychology setting is different. Communication of forensic neuropsychological findings to a judge and jury, who most likely are not health care professionals, requires careful concern regarding the appropriate use of language.

As noted by Greiffenstein and Cohen (2005), forensic neuropsychological reports should be written in language that persons who are not technically trained can understand. Forensic neuropsychology reports are written to inform the attorneys, judges, and jury members about the scientific implications of the forensic neuropsychological findings for the legal questions to be decided. The forensic neuropsychology report should be written so that the jury members who have no scientific background can understand the conceptual reasoning and appreciate the legal implications of the forensic neuropsychological evaluation findings for the legal questions to be decided (Heilbrun et al., 2003).

Concepts

A crucial understanding for the forensic neuropsychologist is that the concepts involved in forensic neuropsychology are quite different from those found in clinical neuropsychology. Simply put, forensic neuropsychologists are practicing in the legal arena. The most important conceptual understanding in this arena is that the information desired from the forensic neuropsychologist must be objective scientific information that will assist judges and juries in making fair legal decisions. The forensic neuropsychologist must therefore be knowledgeable about the legal questions to be decided (Hartlage, 2003). Lack of knowledge or understanding of the legal questions posed can prevent the forensic neuropsychologist from being helpful to the court. There are specific legal standards for decision making, and it is essential for forensic neuropsychologists to know and understand those legal standards in order to best serve the court. For example, legal questions regarding competency to stand trial, criminal responsibility, capacity to make decisions or make a will, or to refuse medical treatment or participate in research studies all have specific forensic contexts that must be appreciated prior to conducting a forensic neuropsychological evaluation (Martell, 2005).

Populations

In the forensic neuropsychology context, services may be delivered in the outpatient setting, the courtroom, or in correctional institutions. Different populations may be associated with different settings. Similarly, legal matters may be related to civil or criminal issues. Individuals seen on death row are likely to be very different from persons seen in outpatient settings with regard to many clinical parameters. In addition, there may be demographic differences related to age, ethnicity, and gender that require careful consideration (Heaton, Grant, &

Mathews, 1991). Forensic neuropsychologists must understand the differences related to different populations and make adjustments in their practices in order to best serve the court (Hartlage, 2003).

Techniques

Test selection in forensic neuropsychology is frequently similar to a clinical neuro-psychological evaluation with the exception that there is a much greater reliance on the assessment of effort (Iverson, 2003). Most forensic neuropsychologists use a core fixed battery or group of neuropsychological tests that they administer to most patients, but augment the core battery depending on the specific legal questions that require the forensic neuropsychological evaluation, the patient's physical abilities, mental capabilities or fatigue level, the time available for evaluation, and the setting and circumstances under which the forensic neuropsychological evaluation is to be conducted (i.e., hospital, bedside, or jail) as well as the patient's particular educational, medical, neurological, and social characteristics. Such batteries of neuropsychological tests typically include measures to assess sensory-perceptual functioning, motor skills, language abilities, visual/spatial skills, executive functioning, attention and memory, emotional status, personality functioning, and effort (Horton & Wedding, 1984).

The crucial question with test selection, however, is the degree to which reliance can be placed on a neuropsychological test or various groupings of neuropsychological tests to answer specific legal questions (Horton, 1997). If a forensic neuropsychologist wishes to rely on a group of neuropsychological tests in a forensic neuropsychology setting, rather than on a single neuropsychological test, then the group of neuropsychological tests should have been empirically considered, as a group of tests, for the legal question being asked (Reitan & Wolfson, 1992, 1993, 2002). If a group of neuropsychological tests hasn't been considered as a group for the specific legal question being asked, then the established accuracy level would have to be considered to be equal to the best accuracy for any single neuropsychological test (Reitan, 1958) that has been empirically validated for the legal question being asked (Project on Scientific Knowledge and Public Policy, 2003). The importance of empirical validation is that there is always the possibility that an unethical forensic neuropsychologist could compose a battery of relatively insensitive neuropsychological tests to bias the neuropsychological findings. In short, forensic neuropsychological findings must have an empirical basis (Project on Scientific Knowledge and Public Policy, 2003).

Summary

In conclusion, forensic neuropsychology has the important purpose of providing the legal field with scientific neuropsychological evidence with which to assist judges and juries in making crucial legal decisions that affect both individuals and society (Horton & Hartlage, 2003). To the extent that forensic neuropsychology tests are seen as unbiased, based on empirical research findings, and able to assist in the fair dispensing of justice, the forensic neuropsychologist will be welcome in the forensic arena in the future (Zillmer, 2004). The hope and expectation is that this handbook chapter will be of value in explaining and understanding forensic neuropsychology, and will positively contribute to fair judicial decision making.

References

American Academy of Neurology. (1996). Assessment: Neuropsychological testing of adults: Considerations for neurologists. *Neurology, 47*, 592–599.

Blau, T. H. (1998). *The psychologist as an expert witness* (2nd ed.) New York: Wiley.

Bush, S. S., & The NAN Policy and Planning Committee. (2005). Independent and court-ordered forensic neuropsychological examinations: Official statement of the National Academy of Neuropsychology. *Archives of Clinical Neuropsychology, 20*(8), 997–1007.

Greiffenstein, M. F., & Cohen, L. (2005). Neuropsychology and the law: Principles of productive attorney–neuropsychologist relations. In G. Larrabee (Ed.), *Forensic neuropsychology: A scientific approach* (pp. 29–91). New York: Oxford.

Hartlage, L. C. (2000) Neuropsychology in the year 2000. *Psychotherapy in Private Practice, 8*(2), 139–142.

Hartlage, L. C. (2003). Neuropsychology in the courtroom. In A. M. Horton, Jr. & L. C. Hartlage (Eds.), *Handbook of forensic neuropsychology* (pp. 315–333). New York: Springer Publishing Company.

Heaton, R., Grant, I., & Mathews, C. (1991). *Comprehensive norms for an expanded Halstead-Reitan Battery.* Odessa, FL: Psychological Assessment Resources.

Heilbrun, K., Marczyk, G., DeMatteo, D., Zillmer, E., Harris, J., & Jennings, T. (2003). Principles of forensic mental health assessment: Implications for neuropsychological assessment in the forensic context. *Assessment, 10*, 329–343.

Horton, A. M., Jr. (1989). Child behavioral neuropsychology with children. In C. R. Reynolds & E. Fletcher-Janzen (Eds.), *Handbook of forensic child neuropsychology* (pp. 521–534). New York: Plenum.

Horton, A. M., Jr. (1994). *Behavioral interventions with brain injured children.* New York: Plenum.

Horton, A. M., Jr. (1997). Halstead-Reitan neuropsychology test battery. In A. M. Horton, Jr., & D. Wedding (Eds.), *The neuropsychology handbook* (2nd ed., pp. 251–278). New York: Springer Publishing Company.

Horton, A. M., Jr., & Hartlage, L. C. (Eds.). (2003). *Handbook of forensic neuropsychology* (pp. 137–177). New York: Springer Publishing Company.

Horton, A. M., Jr., & Miller, W. G. (1985). Neuropsychology and behavior theory. In M. Hersen, R. Eisler, & R. Miller (Eds.), *Progress in behavior modification* (pp. 1–55). New York: Academic Press.

Horton, A. M., Jr., & Puente, A. E. (1986). Behavioral neuropsychology for children. In G. Hynd & J. Obrzut (Eds.), *Child neuropsychology: Forensic practice* (Vol II, pp. 299–316). Orlando, FL: Academic Press.

Horton, A. M., Jr., & Sautter, W. (1986). Behavioral neuropsychology. In. D. Wedding, A. M. Horton, Jr., & J. S. Webster (Eds.), *Handbook of forensic and behavioral neuropsychology* (pp. 259–277). New York: Springer Publishing Company.

Horton, A. M., Jr., & Wedding, D. (1984). *Forensic and behavioral neuropsychology.* New York: Praeger.

Hynd, G. W., & Willis, W. G. (1988). *Pediatric neuropsychology.* Orlando, FL: Grune & Stratton.

Iverson, G. L. (2003). Detecting malingering in civil forensic evaluations. In A. M. Horton, Jr., & L. C. Hartlage (Eds.), *Handbook of forensic neuropsychology* (pp. 137–177). New York: Springer Publishing Company.

Jarvis, P. E., & Barth, J. T. (1984). *Halstead-Reitan Test Battery: An interpretive guide.* Odessa, FL: Psychological Assessment Resources.

Kertesz, A. (Ed.). (1994). *Localization and neuroimaging in neuropsychology.* New York: Academic Press.

Larrabee, G. L. (2005). Assessment of malingering. In G. Larrabee (Ed.), *Forensic neuropsychology: A scientific approach* (pp. 115–158). New York: Oxford.

Lawson-Kerr, K., Smith, S. S., & Beck, D. (1990). The interface between neuropsychology and behavior therapy. In A. M. Horton, Jr. (Ed.), *Neuropsychology across the life-span.* New York: Springer Publishing Company.

Martell, D. A. (2005). Forensic neuropsychology and the criminal law. *Law and Human Behavior. 16*(3), 313–336.

Meier, M. J. (1974). Some challenges for forensic neuropsychology. In R. M. Reitan & L. A. Davison (Eds.), *Forensic neuropsychology: Current status and application* (pp. 289–324). New York: John Wiley.

Mittenberg, W., Patton, C., Canyock, E. M., & Condit, D. C. (2002). Base rates of malingering and symptom exaggeration. *Journal of Clinical and Experimental Neuropsychology, 24,* 1094–1102.

Project on Scientific Knowledge and Public Policy. (2003). *Daubert: The most influential Supreme Court ruling you've never heard of.* Retrieved January 15, 2007, from http://www.defendingscience.org/courts/Daubert-report-excerpt.cfm

Reitan, R. M. (1958). Validity of the Trail Making Test as an indicator of brain damage. *Perceptual and Motor Skills, 8,* 271–276.

Reitan, R. M., & Wolfson, D. (1992). *Neuropsychological evaluation of older children.* Tucson, AZ: Neuropsychology Press.

Reitan, R. M., & Wolfson, D. (1993). *The Halstead-Reitan Neuropsychological Test Battery: Theory and clinical interpretation* (2nd ed.). Tucson, AZ: Neuropsychology Press.

Reitan, R. M., & Wolfson, D. (2002). *Mild head injury: Cognitive, intellectual and emotional consequences.* Tucson, AZ: Neuropsychology Press.

Reynolds, C. R. (1998). *Detection of malingering during head injury litigation.* New York: Plenum Press.

Ruff, R. M. (2004). A friendly critique of neuropsychology: Facing the challenges of our future. *Archives of Clinical Neuropsychology, 18*(8), 847–864.

Sweet, J. J., King, J. H., Malina, A. C., Bergman, M. A., & Simmons, A. (2002). Documenting the prominence of forensic neuropsychology at professional meetings and in relevant professional journals. *Clinical Neuropsychologist, 16*(4), 481–494.

Zillmer, E. A. (2004). The future of neuropsychology. *Archives of Clinical Neuropsychology, 19,* 713–724.

Zillmer, E. A., & Green, H. K. (2006). Neuropsychological assessment in the forensic setting. In R. P. Archer (Ed.), *Forensic uses of clinical assessment instruments* (pp. 209–227). Mahwah, NJ: Lawrence Erlbaum.

Principles of Brain Structure and Function

2

Lisa A. Pass
Raymond S. Dean

Clinical neuropsychologists work in concert with other health care professionals to diagnose and treat brain dysfunction. Patients' loss of functions secondary to trauma or other neuropathology is most often identified by an extensive battery of tests that are known as validity and reliability tests. The neuropsychologist provides an actuary-based prognosis and recommends physical treatment and medications that have the potential to maximize the patients' strengths and minimize weaknesses. Quantitative neuropsychological tests provide an empirically based description of brain functioning on a continuum ranging from severely impaired to within normal limits. Therefore, the neuropsychological battery is the most complete assessment of a patient's upper neurological/psychological status available (American Academy of Neurology, 1996).

As scientist-practitioners, clinical neuropsychologists have frequently been retained by attorneys or the courts to assist in the resolution of legal disputes. In most cases, neuropsychologists are asked to provide expert evidence based on their clinical observations, the results of neuropsychological testing, and the extant research relative to an individual's cognitive functioning and behavior that are consistent with a particular anatomical locus of the brain function, and the prognosis of the degree of permanent impairment.

With increasing litigious actions in the United States in general, and with regard to many neurological/psychiatric disorders specifically, and the importance of and ability to offer a quantitative basis for neuroanatomical functional loss, the need for clinical neuropsychologists who specialize in legal issues has been clear for some time. Indeed, forensic neuropsychology focuses on the interaction of legal questions and, therefore, is a rapidly growing specialty of clinical neuropsychology. Forensic neuropsychology is particularly well suited for this role. The conjunction of decision-making procedures using a hypothesis-testing model, with the practice of rigorous, data-based clinical procedures and assessment techniques, dovetails elegantly with the types of services required in a forensic setting. Calling on the wealth of comparative brain-behavior research that has accumulated over the past three decades, this chapter provides a research-based overview of normal and impaired neuroanatomical functions as they apply to forensic neuropsychology.

"The court" has long considered a scientist-practitioner as an "expert witness" based on education, knowledge, skill, and experience (Federal Rules of Evidence, Number 702 and 703), and evidence is based on generally accepted techniques and methods within the scientific field (*Frye v. United States*, 1923). As will be discussed later by Hartlage and Stern, expert testimony is founded in scientific methods that are empirical, relevant, reliable, normative, and valid. These issues will be discussed in greater detail in chapter 14. What has become known as the Daubert case (*Daubert v. Merrell Dow Pharmaceuticals*, 1993) has set a precedent for the administration and interpretation of formal neuropsychological assessments acceptable in federal courts. The wealth of comparative brain-behavior research accumulated over the past three decades, and the quantitative and objective neuropsychological assessment techniques to evaluate an individual's brain functioning, form a broad and multidisciplinary foundation for logical interpretive strategies for inferring neuropathology as well as cognitive behavioral patterns that explain specific acts and competencies (or lack thereof). Forensic neuropsychology, which focuses on legal questions, is a rapidly growing specialty of clinical neuropsychology (Denney, 2000). This chapter provides an overview of normal and impaired functions related to neuroanatomical areas of the brain as it applies to the field of forensic neuropsychology. In fact, forensic neuropsychology and the evidence required in the legal arena will ultimately affect the practice of clinical neuropsychology in general (Hom, 2003).

In criminal cases, the forensic neuropsychologist's role can include providing expertise regarding questions of competency, sanity, criminal intent, and the presence of neurologically based mitigating circumstances that might have bearing on the case (Denney & Wynkoop, 2000). Similarly, in civil cases, forensic neuropsychologists are often involved in providing their clinical expertise on questions of disability determination, child custody and guardianship rights, special education, due process, worker's compensation, and personal injury cases (Heilbronner, 2004). In such cases, the legal questions addressed by the forensic neuropsychologist often require documentation of the presence, nature, and extent of neurological deficits, recommendations for possible treatments, and the prospect of improvement and rehabilitation (Hom & Nici, 2004). Whether participating in criminal or civil cases, forensic neuropsychologists synthesize evidence clinically obtained from qualitative and quantitative data and gathered from formal assessments, clinical observation, interviews, and medical records to form educated opinions concerning the neurologically based questions raised by the details of a case (Horton & Hartlage, 2003).

Although the inclusion of neuropsychologists in criminal cases has gained in frequency in the past decade (Denney & Wynkoop, 2000), forensic neuropsychologists are more typically engaged in civil than in criminal cases (Hom & Nici, 2004). The relatively recent tradition of attorneys and neuropsychologists working in conjunction to inform legal decisions was established through case law precedent over 30 years ago (Puente, 1997). One of the first cases to allow the expert testimony of a neuropsychologist was a personal injury case in which Ralph M. Reitan, PhD, ABPP, ABN, testified as an expert witness (*Indianapolis Union Railway v. Walker*, 1974). Since the establishment of neuropsychologists as credible expert witnesses, forensic neuropsychologists have been involved primarily in personal injury litigation involving head trauma (Denney & Wynkoop, 2000; Hom, 2003; Hom & Nici, 2004).

Personal injury cases involving traumatic brain injury typically involve a plaintiff who claims acquired functional impairment as a direct consequence of a specific insult (i.e., motor vehicle accident, assault, fall, neurotoxin exposure) and is thus seeking compensation for redress. *Brain injury* typically is defined as substantial structural damage to the brain (see, for example, Horton & Wedding, 1984). The forensic neuropsychologist is often called to document the presence, nature, extent, and permanence of neurologically based sequelae caused by brain injuries incurred by a specific event. The forensic neuropsychologist must be able to directly link, with reasonable certainty, the neurological impairment to that particular incident. Moreover, differentiating symptoms caused by psychological trauma, malingering, and pre-existing conditions from symptoms that were acquired from the accident can be challenging (Purisch & Sbordone, 1997). A thorough understanding of the brain-behavior relationship is essential to accurately interpreting assessment data in the context of personal injury cases.

This chapter provides a general overview of functional neuroanatomy as it applies to the field of forensic neuropsychology. Based on the elevated rate of legal referrals for personal injury cases involving head trauma and the importance of functional neuroanatomy within this domain, a discussion of the brain-behavior relationship may best be served using a utilitarian framework focused primarily on the functional ramifications of brain injury.

Overview of Functional Neuroanatomy

The nervous system is divided into two principal systems: the central nervous system and the peripheral nervous system (see Table 2.1). The peripheral nervous system is composed of the spinal and cranial nerves, tracts that relay sensory information and motor commands between the brain and different areas of the body. However, this area of the nervous system tends to be of less focus for neuropsychologists. Therefore, for the purposes of this discussion, we will be focusing on the anatomy and function of the central nervous system.

Consisting of the brain and the spinal cord, the importance of the central nervous system (CNS) is reflected in the fact that the body provides extra protec-

2.1   Divisions of the Nervous System

Principal Divisions	Divisions	Subdivisions	Major Structures
Central Nervous System (CNS)			
	Brain		
	Forebrain	Telencephalon	Cerebral cortex Basal ganglia Amygdala Hippocampus Corpus callosum Lateral ventricles
		Diencephalon	Thalamus Hypothalamus Third ventricle
	Midbrain	Mesencephalon	Tectum Tegmentum Cerebral aqueduct
	Hindbrain	Metencephalon	Pons Cerebellum Fourth Ventricle
		Mylencephalon	Medulla oblongata Fourth Ventricle
	Spinal Cord		
Peripheral Nervous System (PNS)	Autonomic	Sympathetic	Sympathetic sensory and motor neurons
		Parasympathetic	Parasympathetic sensory and motor neurons
	Somatic		Cranial Nerves I-XII Spinal Nerves

Adapted from Zillmer and Spiers (2001); Dean (1985).

tion for it (Zillmer & Spiers, 2001). Encased in the bony structures of the skull and spine, the brain and the spinal cord float in a protective environment of cerebrospinal fluid (CSF), produced and circulated through the CNS by a system of interconnected, fluid-filled ventricular cavities. A complex network of arteries and blood vessels supplies the brain with nourishment and oxygen, while protecting it from potentially toxic substances via a blood-brain barrier. In addition, a thin set of three meningeal membranes cover the entire surface of the brain and spinal cord, effectively anchoring them in place and providing a protective buffer. Although not directly involved in cognitive functioning, these protective features are important to the overall health of the brain. Damage to these systems can lead to serious and life-threatening symptoms. A closer look at the structure and function of these systems is appropriate.

Overview of the Protective Features of the Central Nervous System

The central nervous system's primary protective features form an interconnected system of defense designed to effectively protect the brain and the spinal cord from damage by buffering them from insult and protecting them from potential neurotoxins in the body. The system is made up of three major anatomical divisions: the skull, the ventricular system, and the meninges.

The skull is the hard, rigid, bony structure that completely encases the brain. The part of the skull that encloses the brain and spinal cord, the neurocranium, is made up of a relatively few large bones connected by joints called sutures. The bones that make up the neurocranium are the frontal bone, two parietal bones, two temporal bones, the occipital bone, and the sphenoid bone (Zillmer & Spiers, 2001). The frontal bone underlies the front of the face and forehead and extends down to the top of the eye sockets. Just posterior to the frontal bone are the two parietal bones, one on each side of the head, which extend over most of the top and sides of the skull. The temporal bones are located on the sides of the head, located approximately above the ear and extending down behind the ear and toward the jaw. The sphenoid bone is located near the temple and eye orbit area, and forms part of the eye cavity. The lower posterior area of the skull is the occipital bone. The internal structure of the skull allows for blood vessels in the roof of the cranium, and orifices in the base of the skull provide an opening for nerves and blood vessels. Fossae, which are ridges in the base of the skull, hold the brain in place and protect it from moving within the skull.

In addition to the skull, the brain is protected from potential insult by being suspended in a bath of cerebrospinal fluid. This fluid is produced and circulated within and around the brain by a system of four interconnected cavities and canals called the ventricular system. The two largest ventricular cavities, the lateral ventricles, are relatively large, C-shaped structures located one in each hemisphere. The third ventricle, a narrow tube located deep in the brain between and below the two lateral ventricles, is connected to the lateral ventricles by a small opening called the foramen of Monro. The fourth ventricle is located in the brain stem, just beneath and anterior to the cerebellum. It is connected to the third ventricle through a narrow channel called the cerebral or Sylvian aqueduct.

A third protective feature located in the CNS is the meninges, a collection of three structurally supportive membranes. The pia mater, the innermost meningeal layer, is a thin network of blood vessels that directly covers the contours of the brain and the spinal cord. Just external to the pia mater is a delicate, web-like membrane called the arachnoid membrane. The pia mater and the arachnoid membrane are separated by a gap containing cerebrospinal fluid called the sub-arachnoid space. The uppermost layer of the meninges, the dura mater, is a thick, double-layered membrane that directly adheres to the surface of the skull.

The function of the skull, ventral system, and meninges is to protect the brain and spinal cord by acting as a buffer that shields them from any potentially harmful substances that might be present in the body. Choroid plexus tissue, a highly vascularized network of blood vessels that originate in the pia mater and extend into the ventricles, produces cerebrospinal fluid that flows from the upper to lower ventricles, and then around the spinal cord and brain. The cycle is completed with the reabsorption of the cerebrospinal fluid from the subarachnoid space. This fluid recirculates every six to seven hours.

Cerebrospinal fluid floats the central nervous system in a liquid buffer cushion that absorbs internal as well as external forces. The fluid also works to dispose of waste products from the brain, carrying the byproducts into the bloodstream to be processed by the rest of the body. Although the ventricles have no direct role in cognition, abnormal intracranial ventricular pressure may lead to general cognitive deficits. In terms of personal injury, outside force can cause damage to the intricate ventricular system, resulting in a change in the level of cerebrospinal fluid contained in the system. Ventricles can become enlarged with fluid, occupying a greater space than usual. This can result in brain swelling and an increase in intracranial pressure. The squeezing or displacing of brain tissue can lead to changes in behavior and cognition. This expansion of the ventricles with an increased intercranial pressure leads to a condition known as hydrocephalus, which may be caused by an imbalance in the rate of cerebrospinal fluid production or absorption, or by blockage of the circulation.

Typically, the brain and the spinal cord are well protected by the hard, protective barrier of the skull and spine. However, in cases of traumatic brain injury (TBI), the rigid features of the skull can contribute to the structural damage to the brain. Upon cranial impact, the gelatinous brain can shift violently within the skull and can bounce back and forth off of its walls in a coup-countercoup pattern. The internal contours of the skull are not smooth. Horny projections of bone in the front and sides of the skull can gouge into the surface of the brain, causing bruising and shearing of the brain, and tearing of the cranial nerves. The cerebral veins and large blood vessels found in the spaces between the dural layers, and between the dura mater and the arachnoid membrane of the meninges, are particularly sensitive to tearing and bleeding during traumatic brain injury. Subdural hematomas (bleeding between the brain tissue and the dura mater) and epidural hematomas (bleeding between the dura mater and the skull bone) can lead to inflammation, a condition that can compound the damage as the expanding brain is pushed against the rigid, sharp contours of the skull.

Symptoms of such damage can include the leakage of cerebrospinal fluid from the nose and bleeding from the ears. Loss of consciousness, irritability, seizures, numbness, headaches, disorientation, nausea and vomiting, slurred speech, difficulty walking, and blurred vision have all been documented as results of subdural hematomas.

The Principal Brain Divisions

The brain is divided into three principal parts, a designation with its origins in the early stages of fetal development. When the neural tube closes to produce what will eventually develop into the central nervous system, three prominent bulges form. These three bulges will eventually become the three major substructures of the brain: the forebrain, the midbrain, and the hindbrain. The remainder of the neural tube develops into the spinal cord. These three divisions eventually differentiate into five major subdivisions: (1) telencephalon, (2) diencephalon, (3) mesencephalon, (4) metencephalon, and (5) myelencephalon.

The Hindbrain: Lower Brain Stem and Cerebellum

From the standpoint of evolution, the oldest part of the brain, the lower regions of the brain stem and the hindbrain, are the most functionally primitive areas of the brain and are responsible for the basic functions of life. The lower brain stem is located at the base of the brain and connects the brain to the spinal cord. The parts of the brain stem included in the hindbrain are the medulla oblongata and the pons. The lower extension of the brain connects to the spinal cord. Neurological functions located in the brain stem include those necessary for survival (breathing, digestion, heart rate, blood pressure) and for arousal (being awake and alert). Most of the cranial nerves come from the brain stem. The brain stem is the pathway for all fiber tracts passing up and down from the peripheral nerves and spinal cord to the highest parts of the brain.

The medulla oblongata is immediately superior to the spinal cord, located just above the foramen magnum. It forms a transitional zone between the relatively uncomplicated neuronal organization of the spinal column and the intricate neural composition of the brain (Zillmer & Spiers, 2001). The medulla oblongata is made up of highly myelinated tracts designed to carry motor and sensory messages back and forth between the spinal cord and the brain. It is in the medulla that these tracts decussate, sending the transmissions of sensory and motor information from one side of the body to the opposite (contralateral) side of the brain. Therefore, for most of the brain-body relationship, the right side of the brain controls the left side of the body, and vice versa. Neuronal cell bodies in the medulla oblongata control blood pressure, heart rate, and breathing. Swallowing, coughing, and vomiting are also controlled from this area of the brain.

The pons can be identified by the two conspicuous bulges extending from the brain stem, located just superior and anterior to the medulla oblongata, and just inferior to the midbrain. One of the primary functions of the pons is as a message relay system, connecting neural pathways from the spinal cord to the higher areas of the brain, including an important connection between the brain and another hindbrain structure, the cerebellum.

The cerebellum, which literally means "little brain," is located posterior and superior to the pons and medulla, directly inferior to the posterior area of the cerebral hemisphere. The structure itself is composed of two large, oval hemispheres joined together by a central structure called the vermis. The cerebellum is particularly easy to locate on brain imaging maps based on its striking resemblance to the cortex of the brain with its own infolded cortex. The cerebellum is involved in the coordination of voluntary motor movement, in balance and equilibrium, and in muscle tone. It is relatively well protected from trauma compared with the frontal and temporal lobes and brain stem.

All of the information that passes between the body and the brain travels through the lower brain stem. As a whole, the lower brain stem is crucially involved in the conduction of information between the spinal cord and the brain. Ascending and descending tracts carry messages between the brain and the spinal cord, and play a crucial role in the production of reflexes. In addition, the lower brain stem is implicated in the mediation of arousal, in auditory processing, in visually guided movements, and in the smooth control of movement. Because the brain stem is located in an area in near proximity to bony protrusions inside the base of the skull, the brain stem area is susceptible to damage during an accident. The implication of these structures in basic survival processes means that damage to these areas can result in coma and death. Other observed symptoms of damage to this area include decreased capacity for breathing, which can affect the ability to speak. Dysphagia, difficulty swallowing food and water, is also a common symptom of lower brain stem damage. Vertigo, including dizziness and nausea, as well as sleeping difficulties, are also noted. Damage to the pons can result in problems with balance, vision, and auditory processing. Because the pons is the site for the transport of information among the spinal cord, the brain, the cerebellum, and the cranial nerves, damage to this site can interrupt these pathways, resulting in serious consequences for a variety of sensory and motor processes. The cerebellum has been implicated in coordination of motor and sensory information, motor coordination and postural control, body orientation, and muscle tone in voluntary movements. Damage to this area can result in a deterioration of motor control, characterized by irregular and jerky movements. Patients who have received damage to the cerebellum have been reported to experience tremors when trying to complete a voluntary task and static tremors while resting. Disturbances in gait and balance are also evident. Moving quickly and alternating movements becomes difficult.

The Midbrain

The midbrain lies anterior to and between the cerebrum and the pons, along with the hypothalamus and thalamus of the forebrain, and is the smallest portion of the brain stem. Although the structural boundaries of the midbrain are not well defined, it is divided into two major structures: the tectum in the dorsal part of the midbrain, and the tegmentum in the ventral region. The tectum consists of four small areas, a pair of inferior colliculi and a pair of superior colliculi. The inferior colliculi serve as an important relay center for the auditory pathway, influencing the movement of the neck and the head in response to auditory information. The superior colliculi contain important reflex centers for visual information and contain some retinal fibers feeding through the optic tracts and the visual cortex. The tegmentum surrounds the tiny cerebral aqueduct, which connects the third and fourth ventricles and plays an important role in motor control, in the regulation of awareness and attention, and in mediating of some autonomic functions.

Although the midbrain is a relatively small area of the brain, it is of particular importance in terms of attention. For example, the reticular activating system, a poorly-differentiated, netlike formation of neurons whose ascending and descending pathways run through the core of the brainstem, through the pons and medulla and up through the midbrain, is implicated in selective attention toward incoming stimuli (Horton & Wedding, 1984).

Together with structures in the hindbrain, the midbrain is made up of structures that play an important role in orienting visual and auditory information. Damage to the midbrain area often has serious ramifications and often is associated with poor outcomes, including coma and death (Rosenblum, Greenberg, Seelig, & Becker, 1981).

The Forebrain

The forebrain is the largest division of the brain, and is often considered of primary interest to neuropsychologists. It is made up of several important structures crucial to the cognitive, behavioral, and emotional health of the individual. These structures are often discussed in terms of their location within the two major subdivisions of the forebrain, the diencephalon and the telencephalon.

Diencephalon

The diencephalon is located along the midline of the brain, on the upper portion of the brain stem, and connects the cortex with the other, lower structures of the brain. The major structures of the diencephalon are the hypothalamus and the thalamus. Diencephalon dysfunction has been seen as "neurogenic storms" because control of many emotional features is lost.

Hypothalamus. The hypothalamus is a small, cone-shaped structure that forms the floor and part of the lateral wall of the third ventricle. Other adjacent structures are the optic chiasm and the mammillary bodies. Although small in size, the hypothalamus has a complex web of interconnections with other brain structure through a collection of complex nuclei. Through this system of neuronal connections, the hypothalamus can send and receive information directly from structures in the brain stem, from pre-optic and olfactory areas, and from the thalamus. In addition, the pituitary, the master gland of the brain, is controlled by neurons from the hypothalamus.

Clearly, the interconnectedness of the hypothalamus reflects its importance in a number of important brain functions. The hypothalamus plays an important role in the mediating of the peripheral autonomic process, endocrine activity, and somatic function. The regulation of body temperature, appetite and thirst, sexual activities, and circadian rhythms are all believed to be maintained by hypothalamic function. In addition, the interaction between the hypothalamus and the pituitary gland results in the hormonal regulation of digestion, sexual arousal, and circulation.

Based on the interconnectivity of the hypothalamus, injury to this area of the brain can have far-reaching implications. It has been proposed that hypothalamic damage during a traumatic brain injury often occurs secondarily to brain shearing or rising intercranial pressure due to swelling (Horton & Wedding, 1984). Because of the close proximity of the hypothalamus to the optic chiasm, swelling in this area can result in secondary damage that could affect vision (Horton & Wedding). Depending on the location and extent of hypothalamic damage, the symptoms can manifest as extreme somatic, sexual, and developmental disturbances. For example, damage to the ventromedial area of the hypothalamus can lead to excessive eating and eventual obesity, while damage to the lateral area of the hypothalamus can lead to the disruption of the processing of internal feeding signals (Kelley & Stinus, 1984). Likewise, disturbances of the medial hypothalamus may lead to severe behavioral disorders, primarily those associated with aggression. The hypothalamus is the integration center of the autonomic nervous system (ANS), which regulates body temperature and endocrine function. The anterior hypothalamus is involved in a number of maintenance functions, or parasympathetic activity. Conversely, the posterior hypothalamus regulates sympathetic activity, or stress response, often referred to as "fight or flight."

Thalamus. Located in the center of the brain, just superior to the hypothalamus, the thalamus is an ovoid structure of gray matter found deep in the white matter of cerebrum. The thalamus is made up of two large, symmetrical nuclei, with one nucleous situated on each side of the midline of the brain. The nuclei are situated around the third ventricle, and help to form its lateral walls. The thalamus contains a number of nerve endings and, like the hypothalamus, the nuclei of the thalamus are highly interconnected with most of the other parts of the central nervous system. Most information that reaches the cortex is processed at some point in the thalamus. Many pathways carrying information from the brain stem to the cortex relay their information through the thalamic nuclei. In addition, the thalamus is important as the pathway for primary sensory and motor impulses to and from the cerebral hemisphere. With the exception of the olfactory sense, axons from all other sensory systems use the thalamus as the last relay site before the information reaches the cerebral cortex.

As with the hypothalamus, damage to the thalamus can have various functional consequences. Common symptoms associated with brain injuries involving the thalamus include problems with short-term memory, attention, and concentration. Lesions to the thalamus also have been associated with areas that would be implicated in the interruption of the relay of essential information between the cerebral cortex and other areas of the brain, including marked deficits in gross areas of sensory or motor function, depressed scores on cognitive verbal tests, and problems associated with spatial ability, facial recognition, and perception of music. Symptoms in some thalamic lesions are relatively short lived, indicating that alternate pathways may be quickly formed after damage to the thalamus (Zillmer & Spiers, 2001). As the processing center of the cerebral cortex, the thalamus coordinates and regulates all functional activity of the cortex via the integration of the afferent input to the cortex (except olfaction). Its contribution to effectual expression is clear, as is its ability to alter levels of consciousness.

Damage to this area may affect the above, as well as cause the loss of perception and a relatively rare disorder known as thalamic syndrome, which is seen as an acute pain on the opposite side of the body.

Telencephalon

The telencephalon is the most anterior portion of the forebrain. It consists of the cerebral hemispheres, the limbic system, and the basal ganglia. The telencephalon (the cerebral hemispheres) is the largest of the divisions of the human brain, and it is what subserves language—at least those aspects of language that are of interest to linguistics. In fact, the same can be said of just the cerebral cortex, which is only one of the four parts of the telencephalon according to the traditional divisions given previously.

Of the subcortical and interior portions of the telencephalon, the basal ganglia, which partially surround the diencephalon, participate in motor functions, including articulation of speech, whereas the hippocampus and the amygdaloid nucleus, which lie deep within the lower part of the cortex, are very important in emotional expression. Present analyses of the telencephalon using a multiple approach have demonstrated, among other features, the presence of a ventral pallidal region, a striatopallidal subdivision in the basal ganglia, and three main components of the amygdaloid complex. Therefore, in spite of its apparently simple organization, within the telencephalon of urodeles it is possible to identify most of the features observed in amniotes and anurans that are only revealed with the use of combined modern techniques in neuroanatomy. The hippocampus is actually a paleocortical structure (thus part of the cortex) deeply embedded within the lower temporal lobe of either hemisphere. It is important for remembering events of one's personal history and other kinds of what are known as "declarative memory," and so it looms large in linguistic activity, as the linguistic system clearly has access to this kind of information. More than that, it appears that the hippocampus, since it plays an important role in declarative memory (along with higher cortical levels), is of great importance in language learning of the kind commonly done in high schools and colleges, which is quite different from that done by children, who automatically use lower levels of their cerebral cortices, acquiring their native language skills as procedural knowledge rather than declarative knowledge. That difference is directly correlated with the great skill and fluency of people using their native languages as opposed to the clumsiness with which they attempt to navigate their way in a foreign country with the aid of a school-taught second language. With recent research showing hitherto unthought-of subcortical features in cognitive functioning, this area of the brain has become of special interest.

The Limbic System

The structures most often associated with the limbic system include the fornix, the mammillary bodies of the hypothalamus, the cingulate cortex, the amygdala, the hippocampus, and the septum. As with the structures of the diencephalon, the complex associations of the limbic system with various areas of the nervous system comprise a maze of interconnectivity that makes a one-to-one, structure-function relationship difficult to outline. A good deal of data suggests that the limbic lobes are involved in sexual response, rage, fear, and emotions. Also, due to its placement, the limbic system plays a role in the integration of recent memory and control of biological rhythms.

Hippocampus

One of the most studied components of the limbic system is the hippocampus. In humans there are two hippocampal structures, one in each hemisphere of the brain. The hippocampal formation has been associated with memory acquisition and spatial navigation. Bilateral injury of the hippocampus often involves an inability to learn new, declarative memories. In contrast, memories for skills, such as riding a bicycle, or memories for procedures are often unaffected by hippocampal damage. Recent evidence implicates the hippocampus in the processing and storage of spatial information (Ekstrom et al., 2003). Damage to the hippocampus may lead to an inability to remember where one is or how to get to a destination. Losing one's way is a common symptom in amnesia, and may be related to hippocampal damage. In addition, the hippocampal function seems to be lateralized. While damage to the left hippocampal gyrus tends to cause problems with long-term verbal memory, right hippocampal damage tends to result in greater impairment of long-term spatial memory.

Other disorders are secondary with hormonal imbalances, such as malignant hypothermia and inability to control core temperature. Results also have resulted in agitation disorders, and loss of control of emotion and elements of recent memory. Patients report a loss of the sense of smell.

Amygdala

Another noteworthy element of the limbic system is the amygdala. The amygdalae are a pair of small, almond-shaped collections of nuclei located deep in the brain, adjacent to the hippocampus and medial to the hypothalamus. The amygdalae have both ascending and descending connections with the cerebral cortex, the thalamus, the hippocampus, and the spinal cord. At present, the amygdalae are believed to play an important role in the strength of stored memory, especially for episodic memories in which emotions play a role (Phelps, 2004). In addition, the amygdalae have been implicated as the center for the mediation of the autonomic fear response, a fundamental self-preservation mechanism that triggers the "fight or flight" response in circumstances of danger. Damage to the amygdala and its interconnections has been shown to have implications in severe emotional disturbances, including episodes of extreme violence and aggression. Humans with marked lesions in the amygdala lose the affective meaning of the perception of information, they are able to name a person, but unable to recall emotional features. In general, this limbic formation is responsible in part for emotions, sex, rage, and fear, as well as the integration of recent memory and biological rhythms.

Basal Ganglia

The basal ganglia, also termed the basal nuclei, are a collection of symmetric nuclei found deep in the telencephalon, and are enclosed by the cerebral cortex and white matter. These gray matter structures partially surround the thalamus.

The current understanding of the structure of the basal ganglia indicates three major, interconnected structures: the caudate nucleus, the putamen, and the globus pallidus. These structures are primarily connected to the cerebral cortex through the thalamus, the reticular formation, and the midbrain.

Researchers currently believe that the primary function of the basal ganglia is voluntary motor control, specifically related to the planning and initiating of motor behavior, maintaining muscular readiness to respond, and establishing posture. Together with the cerebral cortex in the midbrain and the cerebellum, the basal ganglia have been proposed as the area responsible for stereotyped postural and reflexive motor behavior (extrapyramidal motor system). In addition, the basal ganglia have been shown to play some role in language, specifically the motor planning and programming for speech (Horton & Wedding, 1984).

Damage to the basal ganglia, as in disorders such as Huntington disease or Wilson disease, often results in involuntary, jerking movements of the arm or leg and spasmodic movement of facial muscles. Patients with lesions in the basal ganglia may have difficulty initiating, sustaining, or ceasing motor movement, agitation, or loss of control of emotion and recent memory. Tremors, slowing of movement, facial and motor tics, difficulty walking, rigidity, and motor-related speech problems may all occur subsequent to head trauma affecting the basal ganglia. Comprising subcortical gray matter nuclei, the basal ganglia provide a processing link between thalamus and motor cortex and are responsible for the initiation and direction of voluntary movement, as well as balance (inhibitory movement) and postural reflexes that are part of the extrapyramidal system of regulation of automatic movement. Disorders of movement such as Parkinson's, chorea, tremors at rest and with initiation of movement, abnormal increases in muscle tone, and difficulty initiating movement reside in this area.

Cerebral Cortex

The cerebral cortex is the largest, most evolutionarily advanced part of the brain. This structure consists of two large cerebral hemispheres, separated by a deep longitudinal fissure. The two hemispheres are structurally and functionally coupled by a number of interconnections, most notably by the prominent bundle of intercerebral axons called the corpus callosum. The corpus callosum makes direct communication between the two hemispheres possible. The surface of the cerebrum, which is covered in gray matter consisting of neuronal cell bodies, dendrites, and interconnecting axons of neurons, is convoluted by both deep and shallow grooves (sulci and fissures, respectively) and ridges (gyri). Just underneath the cortex is white matter, millions of axonal pathways that link the neurons of the cortex with those found within the rest of the brain and central nervous system.

Three areas of the cerebral cortex receive information from sensory organs. Visual information is analyzed and processed in the primary visual cortex, an area located on the upper and lower banks of the calcarine fissure situated on the inner surfaces of the cerebral hemispheres. The primary auditory cortex is located on the lower surface of the lateral fissure, a deep groove that runs along the side of the brain. The primary somatosensory cortex, a vertical strip of cortex just caudal to the central sulcus, receives information from the body senses. Different regions of the primary somatosensory cortex receive information from different regions of the body. The base of the somatosensory cortex and a portion of the insular cortex, which is normally hidden from view by the frontal and temporal lobes, receive information concerning taste. The primary motor cortex, located just in front of the primary somatosensory cortex, is directly involved in the control of movement and directs the output through motor processing. Neurons in the primary motor cortex are connected to muscles in different parts of the body.

Other areas of the cerebral cortex are responsible for those elements of organization of higher cognitive functions, perceiving, learning, remembering, planning, and acting. These processes take place in the associated areas of the cerebral cortex. The central sulcus provides an important dividing line between the rostral and caudal regions of the cerebral cortex. The rostral region is involved in movement-related activities, such as planning and executive behaviors, whereas the caudal region is involved in perceiving and learning.

Localization of Cerebral Functions in Adulthood

The success over the past century in defining the behavioral effects of brain damage has allowed some appreciation for the functional correspondence of macroanatomical areas of the brain (Dean, 1985). Each hemisphere of the cerebrum is split into four divisions, or lobes: the frontal lobe, the parietal lobe, the temporal lobe, and the occipital lobe. These divisions are not only based on anatomical divisions, but also functional ones. It is the intent of the following section to provide a brief summary of the correspondence of neuropsychological functions to major subdivisions of the adult cerebral cortex. Although some structural divisions of the brain are somewhat arbitrary, an appreciation of the individual differences in neuropsychological functioning depends on sensitivity to such neuroanatomical relationships.

Frontal Lobe

The frontal lobe lies rostral to the central sulcus, and makes up approximately one-third of the entire cortical area (Horton & Wedding, 1984). Because of the frontal lobe's proximity to the sphenoid wing, a bony outcropping on the skull, the frontal lobe is extremely susceptible to injury. In fact, the frontal lobe has been described as the most common region of damage following mild to moderate traumatic brain injury (Horton & Wedding, 1984). As shown in Table 2.2, lesions in the frontal lobe have been implicated in a wide variety of symptoms. Impairments in motor function, problem solving, spontaneity, memory, language, initiation, judgment, impulse control, and social and sexual behavior have all been associated with frontal lobe lesions (Kolb & Whishaw, 1990). The frontal lobe is literally the front part of the brain; it is involved in planning, organizing, problem solving, selective attention, personality, and a variety of "higher cognitive functions" including behavior and emotion. The anterior (front) portion of the frontal lobe is called the prefrontal cortex. It is very important for the "higher cognitive functions" and the determination of the personality.

The posterior (back) of the frontal lobe consists of the premotor and motor areas. Nerve cells that produce movement are located in the motor areas. The premotor areas serve to modify movements. The frontal lobe is divided from the

2.2 Summary of Behavioral Effects Following Lesions to Either the Right or Left Hemisphere of the Frontal Lobe

Domain	Behaviors	Laterality
Cognitive		
	Recent-memory deficits	Both
	Memory impairment	Both
	Reduced ability to plan and follow through	Both
	Difficulty with serial order tasks	Left
	Weakened ability for mental abstraction	Both
	Distractibility	Both
	Impaired awareness of time	Left
	Problems with arithmetic & spelling, but not reading	Left
	Sequential and/or phonetically inaccurate spelling errors	Left
	Inability to respond consistently to tasks	Both
Personality		
	Impulsivity	Both
	Diminished concern for future	Left
	Mild euphoria	Both
	Lack of initiative	Both
	Lack of spontaneity	Both
	Distractibility	Both
	Alterations in personality	Both
	Anhedonia	Both
Perceptual		
	Figure ground difficulties	Left
	Misreproductions of figures	Right
	Disturbed body part identification when blindfolded	Both
	Difficulty with visual scanning of complex pictures and objects	Both
Motor Speech (Broca's area)		
	Dysgraphia	Left
	Difficulty with articulation/expression of spoken speech	Left
	Motor aphasia—can move lips and tongue but unable to carry out the coordinated movements required in speaking	Left
	Motor amusia (inability to sing or imitate a tune)	Right
	Articulation impairment	Left
	Dysrhythmia	Left
	Efferent-kinetic motor aphasia	Left
	Dysarthria	Left
	Slurred speech	Both
	Difficulty in spelling, reading, and writing	Left
Motor Control (motor strip)		
	Unstable feet	Both
	Poor eye–hand coordination	Both
	Reduced motor speed and accuracy (contralateral)	Both
	Reduced hand grip strength	Both
	Reduced finger tapping speed	Both
	Abnormal and involuntary facial expressions	Both
	Astereognosis	Both
	Apraxia	Both
	Localized paralysis of contralateral side of body	Both

For more information on behavioral symptoms related to frontal lobe damage, please refer to Afifi and Bergman (2005); Blumenfeld (2002); Clark, Boutros, and Mendez (2005); Silver, McAllister, and Yudofsky (2005).

parietal lobe by the central sulcus. Because the frontal region occupies the major portion of the cortex, it had been assumed to be primarily concerned with higher-level intellectual functioning unique to humans (see, for example, Morgan, 1943). However, numerous surgical resections of the frontal lobe have failed to produce obvious intellectual impairments, per se (Hebb, 1949; Teuber, 1972). More timely reports lead to the conclusion that the majority of the anterior regions of the frontal lobe (anterior prefrontal area) seem to be involved in functions more closely concerned with selective perception and sustained attention (see, for example, Horton & Wedding, 1984). In addition, established findings suggest that this formation in the frontal lobe is important in the inhibition of impulsive motor responses (Damasio, 1979). Damage restricted to this region in adults most often results in a considerable change in affective functioning that varies in severity with the nature and extent of the lesion (Valenstein, 1973). Generally, problems interpreting feedback from the environment are common characteristics of frontal lobe damage. Making cognitive shifts in attention, which are expressed behavior-ally in rigid cognitive styles or perseveration in applying strategies, have been linked with frontal lobe dysfunction (Dean, 1985; Horton & Wedding, 1984; Ochs, 1965). In addition, difficulties using external cues to guide behavior (Damasio, 1979), excessive risk taking, and noncompliance with rules (Dean, 1985) can arise after frontal lobe damage.

Because it is involved in the integration of sensory information from other regions of the brain, the motor strip, located on the posterior portion of the frontal lobe, is responsible for coordination of muscle movements. Its organization is such that the motor strip on one side of the frontal region serves functions of the contralateral side of the body. Early on, Penfield and Boldrey (1937) showed that the premotor areas (just anterior to the motor strip) coordinated intentional movements of the body, and damage in that area produced impairment of various motor skills. Generally, motor function disturbance is hallmarked by loss of fine movement and of strength in arms, hands, and fingers (Damasio, 1979). Patients with frontal lobe damage can exhibit difficulty in demonstrating spontaneous facial expressions (Damasio, 1979) and in executing complex chains of motor movement (Luria, 1966). See Table 2.2 for a summary of behavioral effects that result from damage to the frontal lobe.

Parietal Lobe

The parietal lobe lies between the central sulcus, with its posterior border at the parieto-occipital fissure. Functionally, it seems most clearly concerned with body sensations, notably kinesthetic and tactile perceptions (Ochs, 1965). Lesions in this area most frequently result in difficulty in identifying objects by touch or lack of tactile perception to one or both sides of the body (see Table 2.3). However, dysfunction here rarely occurs without some degree of language disturbance (Penfield, 1958). The left parietal lobe has been shown to mediate elements of verbal memory, calculation, and construction. This region of the left hemisphere is also involved, to various degrees, in the functions necessary for normal reading, writing, and other skills requiring the integration of stimuli (Penfield & Roberts, 1959). Examining localized right hemispheric lesions, Reitan (1964) showed dam-age in the parietal area to be expressed clinically in difficulties in constructing

2.3 Summary of Behavioral Effects Following Lesions to Either the Right or Left Hemisphere of the Parietal Lobe

Domain	Behaviors	Laterality
Cognitive		
	Defective association of abstract concepts and symbolic thinking	Left
	Poor memory	Left
Achievement		
	Acalculia (difficulty working with numbers)	Left
Language		
	Poor reading and spelling	Left
	Semantic aphasia	Left
	Difficulty understanding sentences	Left
	Agraphia (difficulty writing)	Left
	Spelling apraxia (can't spell written words)	Both
	Difficulty reading or counting	Left
Visual Perception		
	Difficulty with facial recognition	Right
	Topographic disorientation	Right
	Visual field defects, impaired visual perception	Both
	Impaired spatial abilities	Right
	Widened angles in drawing	Left
	Reduced angles in drawing	Right
	Constructional apraxia (difficulty in drawing/copying/constructing geometric designs)	Right
	Inability to trace a path or follow a route	Right
	Difficulty copying spelling words	Left
	Word blindness (inability to understand written words, although vision is not impaired)	Left
Tactical Perception		
	Apraxia—ideational and ideomotor	Both
	Graphesthesia	Both
	Tactile aphasia (name objects by sight, not by touch)	Both
	Poor judgement of weight or size of objects	Both
	Confusion in recognizing 2-points simultaneously	Both
	Finger agnosia	Both
	Poor finger localization	Both
	Suppression	Both
	Numbness or tingling	Both
	Inability to localize or measure intensity of pain and cutaneous perceptions	Both
	Kinesthetic sensation in face, lips, tongue	Both
	Neuromuscular coordination and control	Both
	Recognition of form by touch	Both
	Astereognosis	Both

(continued)

Table 2.3 *(continued)*

Domain	Behaviors	Laterality
Speech		
	Lacks functional speech	Left
	Fluent, rapid speech with paraphasis (misuse of words)	Left
	Impaired ability to name objects	Left
	Impaired oral and written comprehension	Left
	Echolalia	Left
Body Orientation		
	Poor body image	Both
	Right–left disturbance/disorientation	Both
	Tendency to omit left side of a figure	Right
	Neglect or inattention to body on left side	Right
	Muscular clumsiness	Both
Motor		
	Difficulty hitting a nail with a hammer	Both
	Difficulty carrying out manual tasks	Both

For more in-depth information on behavioral symptoms related to parietal lobe damage, please refer to Afifi and Bergman (2005); Blumenfeld (2002); Clark, Boutros, and Mendez (2005); Critchley (1953); and Silver, McAllister, and Yudofsky (2005).

puzzles, copying designs, and complex visual-spatial manipulations. In this same report, Reitan offered evidence that problems in full appreciation for the steps needed to construct a block pattern or puzzle were more likely to be expected in left parietal damage than in those of the right side. Damage in this area is often expressed clinically in the inability to discriminate between sensory stimuli, the inability to locate and recognize parts of the body or spatial neglect, an inability to write, or a construction dyspraxia. In severe injuries patients are unable to recognize themselves.

Occipital Region

The occipital lobe is located at the posterior pole of each hemisphere. As the primary visual region of the cerebral cortex, this area is responsible for the perception and, to a lesser extent, the comprehension, of visual stimuli. Areas of the occipital lobe are involved in visuospatial processing and discrimination of movement, and differentiation of color (Horton & Wedding, 1984). Damage in the occipital region produces disturbances that may range from visual field blindness (no visual perception in the left or right line of sight) to disability in the association of visually presented stimuli with corresponding verbal or nonverbal knowledge (visual agnosia) (Luria, 1965) (see Table 2.4). These visual associations of the more anterior occipital lobe seem less involved in visual perception than they are in the recognition of elements as familiar or naming them.

Temporal Region

The temporal lobe forms a flap that extends over portions of the frontal and parietal lobes. It lies rostral to the occipital lobe. As with the frontal lobes, the

2.4	Simplified Summary of Some Behavioral Effects Observed After the Occurrence of Lesions to Either the Right or Left Hemisphere of the Occipital Lobe	
Domain	**Behaviors**	**Laterality**
Visual Perception		
	Omissions	Both
	Rotations	Both
	Defective scanning	Both
	Perseverations	Both
	Difficulties in learning to spell and read	Left
	Vision process disruption and writing problems	Both
	Visual hallucinations: flashes of light, rainbows, brilliant stars, bright lines	Both
	Contralateral non-specific visual defects	Both
	Tactile agraphia (name by sight but not by touch)	Both
	Visual disorganization	Both
	Defective spatial orientation	Right
	Homonymous defects in visual fields without destruction of macular vision	Both
	Defective spatial orientation in homonymous halves of visual field	Both
	Alexia with ability to write	Left
	Alexia with agraphia	Left
	Dyspraxia—difficulty copying	Left

For more in-depth information on behavioral symptoms related to occipital lobe damage, please refer to Afifi and Bergman (2005); Blumenfeld (2002); Clark, Boutros, and Mendez (2005); Silver, McAllister, and Yudofsky (2005).

anterior temporal region is particularly vulnerable to injury due to its proximity to protrusions and cavities of the skull, especially in injuries involving rotational acceleration (Dean, 1985).

The temporal lobe is primarily involved in audition. Damage to the temporal lobes has been implicated in disturbances of auditory sensation and perception, as well as in selective attention of sensory input (Kolb & Wishaw, 1990). Cortical damage to the right temporal lobe is more likely than not to be expressed behaviorally in problems with comprehension and recognition of nonverbal sounds (Milner, 1962). Agitation, irritability, and childlike behavior have been reported with damage to this area of the brain. Although varying with premorbid language lateralization, patients rarely suffer language disorders following right temporal damage, but they apparently find it difficult to fully appreciate the subtleties of music or rhythmic patterns (Shankweiler, 1966) and often present problems in the integration of incomplete auditory presentations (Lansdell, 1970). Both are seen as auditory receptive areas and association areas of language and receptive speech. Impairment in this area is often referred to as receptive and/or sensory aphasia.

Milner (1962) offers rather convincing data that the functions of the left temporal lobe are closely tied to language comprehension and production. Damage here most often results in dysfunctions in verbal memory, comprehension, or the manipulation of abstract concepts, depending on the implicated area (Luria, 1965). Penfield and Roberts (1959) have shown that lesions near the temporal occipital juncture produce a devastating effect on the individual's ability to read, which varies with the individual and the extent or localization of the damage. The temporal area of the brain seems to be involved in information retrieval, triggering complex memories. A substantial amount of research has shown that ablation of the hippocampus affects the ability to consolidate memories or transfer them to long-term storage. Moreover, the bilateral sectioning of the hippocampus most often results in the inability to learn other than elementary motor functions (Barbizet, 1963). Because of its proximity to the hippocampus, the temporal area of the cortex appears to be closely involved in this process. Thus, it is involved in the intricate interplay between the cerebral cortices and the subcortical structures of the brain that relate to hearing deficits and receptive/sensory aphesis.

Summary

As scientist-practitioners, forensic neuropsychologists are particularly well suited to tender conclusions using empirical data, relying upon a hypothesis-testing model. Indeed, the practice of rigorous, data-based procedures and neuropsychological assessment techniques dovetails elegantly with the types of services required in a forensic setting.

Recognition by the court as an "expert" has long been based on education, knowledge, skill, and experience (Federal Rules of Evidence, Number 702 and 703), and evidence is based on accepted methods and techniques within the scientific field (*Frye v. United States*, 1923). As will be discussed by Hartlage and Stern (chapter 14), expert testimony is founded in scientific methods that are empirical, relevant, reliable, normative, and valid and that chapter speaks to this issue in greater detail. What has become known as the "Daubert" case (*Daubert v. Merrell Dow Pharmaceuticals*, 1993) has set legal precedent for the administration and interpretation of formal neuropsychological conclusions.

The wealth of comparative brain–behavior research accumulated over the past three decades, quantitative and objective neuropsychological assessment techniques to evaluate an individual's brain functioning and the interaction of the broad foundation of neuropsychology in conjunction with a databased method of interpretive and inferring neuropathology, offer cognitive behavioral patterns that explain specific behaviors and competencies (or lack thereof) (Clark, Boutros, & Mendez, 2005). Forensic neuropsychology and the evidence required in the legal arena must ultimately affect the practice of clinical neuropsychology in general.

Whether participating in criminal or civil cases, forensic neuropsychologists synthesize evidence obtained from qualitative and quantitative data gathered during standardized formal assessments, clinical observations, interviews, and medical records to form educated opinions concerning the neurologically based questions raised by a case (Hom & Nici, 2004).

References

American Academy of Neurology. (1996). Assessment: Neuropsychological testing of adults: Considerations for neurologists. Report of the Therapeutics and Technology Subcommittee. *Neurology, 47*, 592–599.

Barbizet, J. (1963). Defect of memorizing of hippocampal-mammillary origin: A review. *Journal of Neurology, Neurosurgery, and Psychiatry, 26*, 127–135.

Clark, D. L., Boutros, N. N., & Mendez, M. F. (2005). *The brain and behavior.* New York: Cambridge University Press.

Damasio, A. (1979). The frontal lobes. In K. M. Heilman & E. Valenstein (Eds.), *Clinical neuropsychology.* New York: Oxford University Press.

Daubert v. Merrell Dow Pharmaceuticals, Inc. 509 U.S. 529 (1993).

Dean, R. S. (1985). Foundation and rationale for neuropsychological bases of individual differences. In L. C. Hartlage & C. F. Telzrow (Eds.), *The neuropsychology of individual differences.* New York: Plenum Press.

Denney, R. L. (2000). Clinical neuropsychology in the criminal forensic setting. *Journal of Head Trauma Rehabilitation, 15*(2), 804–828.

Denney, R. L., & Wyncoop, T. F. (2000). Clinical neuropsychology in the criminal forensic setting. *Journal of Head Trauma Rehabilitation, 15*, 804–832.

Ekstrom, A. D., Kahana, M. J., Caplan, J. B., Fields, T. A., Isham, E. A., Newman, E. L., & Fried, I. (2003). Cellular networks underlying human spatial navigation. *Nature, 425*, 184–188.

Federal Rules of Evidence, 702 and 703.

Frye v. United States, 293 F. 1013 (D. C. Civ. 1923).

Hebb, D. O. (1949). *The organization of behavior.* New York: Wiley.

Heilbronner, R. L. (2004). A status report on the practice of forensic neuropsychology. *Clinical Neuropsychologist, 18*(2), 312–326.

Hom, J. (2003). Forensic neuropsychology: Are we there yet? *Archives of Clinical Neuropsychology, 18*, 827–845.

Hom, J., & Nici, J. (2004). Forensic neuropsychology. In G. Goldstein & S. R. Beers (Eds.), *Comprehensive handbook of psychological assessment, Volume 1: Intellectual and neuropsychological assessment.* Hoboken, NJ: John Wiley.

Horton, A. M., Jr., & Hartlage, L. C. (2003). *Handbook of forensic neuropsychology.* New York: Springer Publishing Company.

Horton, A. M., Jr., & Wedding, D. (1984). *Clinical and behavioral neuropsychology.* New York: Praeger.

Indianapolis Union Railway v. Walker, Court of Appeals of Indiana, First District, 578–590 (1974).

Kelley, A. E., & Stinus, L. (1984). Neuroanatomical and neurochemical substrates of affective behavior. In N. A. Fox & R. J. Davidson (Eds.), *The psychobiology of affective development.* New York: Lawrence Erlbaum.

Kolb, B., & Whishaw, I. (1990). *Fundamentals of human neuropsychology.* New York: W. H. Freeman.

Lansdell, H. C. (1970). Relation of extent of temporal removals to closure and visuomotor factors. *Perceptual and Motor Skills, 31*, 491–498.

Luria, A. R. (1965). Neuropsychology in the local diagnosis of brain damage. *Cortex, 1*, 2–18.

Luria, A. R. (1966). *Higher cortical functions.* New York: Basic Books.

Milner, B. (1962). Laterality effects in audition. In V. B. Mountcastle (Ed.), *Interhemispheric relations and cerebral dominance.* Baltimore, MD: Johns Hopkins University Press.

Morgan, C. T. (1943). *Physiological psychology.* New York: McGraw-Hill.

Ochs, S. (1965). *Elements of neurophysiology.* New York: Wiley.

Penfield, W. (1958). *The excitable cortex in conscious man.* Liverpool: Liverpool University Press.

Penfield, W., & Boldrey, E. (1937). Somatic motor and sensory representation in the cerebral cortex as studied by electrical stimulation. *Brain, 60*, 389–443.

Penfield, W., & Roberts, L. (1959). *Speech and brain mechanisms.* Princeton, NJ: Princeton University Press.

Phelps, E. A. (2004). Human emotion and memory: Interactions of the amygdala and hippocampal complex. *Current Opinion in Neurobiology, 14*, 198–202.

Puente, A. E. (1997). Forensic clinical neuropsychology as a paradigm for clinical neuropsychological assessment: Basic and emerging issues. In R. J. McCaffrey, A. D. Williams, J. M. Fisher, & L. C. Laing (Eds.), *The practice of forensic neuropsychology: Meeting challenges in the court room.* New York: Plenum Press.

Purish, A. D., & Sbordone, R. J. (1997). Forensic neuropsychology: Forensic issues and practice. In A. M. Horton, Jr., D. Wedding, & J. S. Webster (Eds.), *The neuropsychology handbook* (2nd ed.). New York: Springer Publishing Company.

Reitan, R. M. (1964). *Manual for administering and scoring the Reitan-Indiana Neuropsychological Battery for Children* (aged five through eight). Indianapolis: University of Indiana Medical Center.

Rosenblum, W. I., Greenberg, R. P., Seelig, J. M., & Becker, D. P. (1981). Midbrain lesions: Frequent and significant prognostic features in closed head injury. *Neurosurgery, 9*, 613–620.

Shankweiler, D. (1966). Effects of temporal lobe damage on perception of dichotically presented melodies. *Journal of Comparative and Physiological Psychology, 62,* 115.

Teuber, H. L. (1972). Unity and diversity of frontal lobe functions. *Acta Neurobiologiae Experimentalis, 32,* 615–656.

Valenstein, E. S. (1973). *Brain control.* New York: Wiley.

Zillmer, E. A., & Spiers, M. V. (2001). *Principles of neuropsychology.* Belmont, CA: Wadsworth/Thomson Learning.

Historical Influences in Forensic Neuropsychology

3

Lawrence C. Hartlage
Bruce H. Stern

Although clinical neuropsychology has a robust scientific basis traceable to the 19th century, it was not until the dramatic evolutionary developments of the mid-20th century that the potential application of clinical neuropsychological science to the forensic arena was recognized. Following the formal identification of the relationship between psychology and the law, reflected in the founding of the American Psychology Law Society in 1968 (Fox, 1999), it did not take the legal profession long to recognize the potential of clinical neuropsychology for assisting in clarifying forensic issues.

By the early 1980s, the utility of clinical neuropsychology in describing to the courts the impact of acquired brain injury was well recognized (Blau, 1984; Wright, Bahn, & Rieber, 1980), and more recently forensic neuropsychology has been recognized as a subspecialty of clinical neuropsychology (Bigler, 1986).

Early recognition of the value of clinical neuropsychology's potential contributions to forensic issues did not include formal identification of "forensic neuropsychology" as a professional specialty area. Primarily involving clinical neuropsychologists affiliated with hospital-based programs treating patients with catastrophic and very severe residual brain injury that were clearly identified as to cause and severity, contributions from clinical neuropsychology were sought concerning residual functional limitations in the patient (Reitan & Wolfson, 1997). Testimony from clinical neuropsychologists was initially requested mainly for its contributions in determining levels of support and life care needs related to the ability of the patient to deal with such matters as judgment, planning, and self care.

Early involvement of clinical neuropsychology in quasi-forensic activity grew out of the progressive interest in central nervous system processing dysfunctions as being etiologic in a wide variety of children's learning problems (Chalfant & Scheffelin, 1969; Hartlage & Green, 1971) and the "Great Society" focus on identification of childhood learning problems (Hartlage & Long, 1998). Under the provisions of Public Laws 94–142, children were afforded the opportunity for an administrative hearing if they requested (and were denied) special educational considerations, and with clinical neuropsychology's achievement of recognition as a scientific field with potential for contributing to educational planning for exceptional children, clinical neuropsychologists became involved in providing expert testimony in those hearings (Hartlage, 1975, 1981).

The issues of causality and the etiology of the injury were not initially addressed by clinical neuropsychologists in forensic settings. Burgeoning accumulated research on clinical neuropsychological sensitivity to brain injury, and on the adverse effects of brain injury on a patient's ability to perform in an educational, vocational, or adaptive context, made clinical neuropsychology attractive as a specialty area to help educate the courts concerning how a given brain injury might affect a patient. Whereas neurological and neurosurgical specialists could attest to the fact that a brain injury had occurred in an individual, clinical neuropsychology could provide much more definitive information concerning whether the individual had defects, and of their nature and severity, in cognitive or behavioral domains. This produced a push for clinical neuropsychological testimony to relate findings of neuropsychological impairment/brain injury to a specific event, that is, to produce conclusions about causality (Reitan & Wolfson, 1997). Specifically, did the accident or trauma at issue *cause* the deficits documented on neuropsychological examination. This became an equivocal question, which in turn became a source of considerable litigation.

As early as 1975, in the case of *Simmons v. Mullins*, the issue of whether a clinical neuropsychologist was competent to testify as an expert on organic brain malfunctions resulting from a motor vehicle accident was addressed. There, a minor plaintiff, while running across the street, sustained organic brain injuries when struck down by an automobile. In support of the damage claim, the plaintiff presented the depositions of two expert witnesses, one a medical doctor and the other a clinical neuropsychologist. The defendant's lawyer objected to the testimony of the clinical neuropsychologist, arguing that the clinical neuropsychologist was not competent to testify as an expert on organic brain malfunction, since he was not a medical doctor. Both the Trial Court and the Appellate Court disagreed, ruling that the clinical neuropsychologist was competent to testify as an expert on organic brain malfunction. The Appellate Court held that:

To adopt appellant's view that psychologists are not competent witnesses to testify on physical matters would be to ignore present medical and psychological practice.

Similarly, in *Valiulis v. Scheffeos*, the Illinois Court noted:

Indeed, it would be somewhat anomalous to conclude that [the clinical psychologist and neuropsychologist] would not be qualified to testify about [the cause of plaintiff's injury] when the neurologist and psychiatrist who sought out his expertise and assistance in diagnosing the disease would likely be qualified to do so.

The case of *Huntoon v. T.C.I. Cablevision of Colorado, Inc.* demonstrates the majority view on neuropsychologists providing expert testimony regarding medical opinions. Reversing a Colorado Court of Appeals decision, which "could be read as holding that neuropsychologists lack the qualifications to opine on the physical cause of organic brain injury as a matter of law," the Colorado Supreme Court ruled that "the propriety of such testimony is determined by using the same CRE 702 analysis applicable to all other experts." Acknowledging the "idea that neuropsychologists, as a group, lack the competence necessary to testify on the causation of organic brain injury" as a minority viewpoint, the Colorado Supreme Court adopted the majority viewpoint that found that "neuropsychologists may, with the proper foundation, opine on the physical cause of organic brain injury." The Court wrote:

In our view, this approach is persuasive. We could find no compelling reason for the law to single out a particular class of professionals and categorically bar them from expressing opinions on matters that may well be within their expertise. We therefore join the majority of states that have resisted the creation of artificial barriers to the admission of expert testimony by drawing lines between the various professions, and we continue to require such witnesses to be measured under the well-established perimeters of CRE 702.

Initially, with strong opposition from medical specialists and insurance companies, clinical neuropsychologists were widely precluded from testifying about the etiology of their findings of brain injury, since *causation* was considered to be solely within the purview of medical specialists. In many cases, physicians without neurological specialization and who had not conducted a comprehensive neurological examination had their testimony supersede that of clinical neuropsychologists on the issue of causality. Clinical neuropsychology recognized the crucial significance of this issue, and issued challenges to those courts that denied clinical neuropsychologists permission to testify about causality. In one of the more widely promulgated cases (*Horne v. Goodson, Majestic,* 1986), after the deputy commissioner of the North Carolina Industrial Commission ruled on March 6, 1985, that testimony of a clinical neuropsychologist, Antonio Puente, PhD, ABN, was "neither...competent nor credible, concerning brain injury" (see Docket Number I-1608; IC Number 809927), the American Psychological Association (APA) represented by Bersoff, O'Keefe, and Welch, and the North Carolina Psychological Association (NCPA), represented by Majestic (1986), filed an amici curiae brief asserting, among other issues, that "professional psychologists are qualified to perform forensic psychological evaluations and to testify as experts in...judicial proceedings" and that "neuropsychologists can offer unique perspectives on the presence of brain injury" (Majestic, 1986). The North Carolina Court of Appeals, in its ruling (pp. 43–44), essentially agreed with the arguments presented in the amici curiae, thus providing a milestone in judicial recognition of the role and scope of forensic neuropsychology in testimony concerning multiple aspects of brain injury.

Other courts handled the question of clinical neuropsychological testimony concerning cause of brain injury on a more limited basis. John S. Currie, PhD, an Atlanta, Georgia, area clinical neuropsychologist, had his diagnosis of brain injury due to neurotoxic chemical exposure overturned by the Georgia Court of Appeals on the basis that a clinical neuropsychologist is not qualified to diagnose brain injury, using as a rationale that the Georgia Psychology Licensing Law was a title law, that is, being licensed in Georgia entitled one to call oneself a psychologist (see *Chandler Exterminators, Inc. v. Morris*, 1992). Since no other functions were spelled out in the Georgia licensing law, the Court concluded that licensed psychologists could only do what they were licensed to do, that is, call themselves psychologists. Amended "practice" legislation, specifically listing the diagnosis of brain injury as a function of psychology practice, was introduced and passed in the next session of the Georgia legislature, thus establishing by legislative rather than judicial fiat the competence of clinical neuropsychologists to testify concerning causation of brain injury.

The natural evolution of clinical neuropsychology into a science with strong impact on the law involved clinical neuropsychologists' testimony about their patients with a focus on how a brain injury had affected a patient's cognitive and neurobehavioral status. These preliminary forays in two different forensic arenas were not, or often not, intentionally forensic in focus, but naturally progressed out of clinical neuropsychologists' willingness to help their patients by providing information about the patients' neuropsychological status. In this context, early involvement in forensic practice did not produce a significant impact on clinical neuropsychology practice, insofar as early forensic neuropsychology involved little more than instructing the courts on brain injury and clinical neuropsychology's potential for identifying it and describing its impact on given patients.

Changes in clinical neuropsychology practice due to early forensic involvement tended to be salutary, as clinical neuropsychologists who had been "nailed" on cross-examination for errors in scoring, use of abbreviated versus complete tests, or insufficient data to support conclusions, modified their practice to eliminate such appropriately assailable shortcomings. Those clinical neuropsychologists who anticipated possible future forensic involvement began to give greater consideration to self-education and training issues involving conversations with colleagues involved in forensic activities and pursued continuing education in relevant forensic issues and board certification in neuropsychology. It is probably safe to assert that clinical neuropsychology's early involvement in forensic matters produced a generally positive outcome, with salutary effects on general levels of practice and professionalism, in that practitioners became aware that their activities might become the focus of scrutiny and critical questioning, and thus were reminded to always ensure that meticulous accuracy and careful documentation became a regular part of their practice.

Neuropsychological Evaluation in Criminal Jurisprudence

Mental competence is an area that was addressed as early as 1980 by Wright, Bahn, and Reiber. In addition, there has been a long-standing focus on the determination of whether a given patient is competent to conform his or her behavior to the law (Bigler, 1986). With the progressive recognition of the role of brain function as a determinant of behavior, the forensic arena has seen concurrent progressive recognition of the potential role of neuropsychologists in addressing issues of impaired competence putatively resulting from impaired brain function.

One of the first court decisions to address the admissibility of expert testimony by a clinical psychologist or clinical neuropsychologist as to the existence of a brain injury or mental defect was *Jenkins v. United States*, 1962. In that criminal case, the defense attempted to introduce the testimony of three clinical psychologists who opined that the defendant had a mental disease when he committed the crimes charged. The Court, at the conclusion of the trial, instructed the jury to disregard the testimony of the clinical psychologists, ruling that clinical psychologists were not competent to give a medical opinion as to mental disease or defect because they lacked medical training.

On appeal, the Appellate Court reversed, acknowledging:

> *The general rule is that anyone who is shown to have special knowledge and skill in diagnosing and treating human ailments is qualified to testify as an expert, if his learning and training show that he is qualified to give an opinion on the particular question at issue. It is not essential that the witness be a medical practitioner.*

The kinds of witnesses whose opinions courts have received, even though they lacked medical training and would not be permitted by law to treat the conditions they describe, are legion.

The Court instructed that in determining whether a psychologist had the requisite special knowledge and skill to testify as an expert witness depended upon a review of that psychologist's training and experience, not upon his or her degree or title. The Court opined that "the critical factor in respect to admissibility is the actual experience of the witness and the probable probative value of his opinion."

Seven years later in *United States v. Riggleman*, the Fourth Circuit Court of Appeals similarly was confronted with the issue of whether a psychologist could provide expert testimony that the defendant was not "legally sane" at the time the crime was committed. On appeal, the defendant asserted that only a psychiatrist is permitted to testify as an expert. The Fourth Circuit Court of Appeals disagreed, finding:

> *However, we think the better rule is that the determination of a psychologist's competence to render an expert opinion based on his findings as to the presence or absence of mental disease or defect must depend upon the nature and extent of his knowledge. It does not depend upon his claim to the title of psychologist or psychiatrist.*

By the early 1980s, brain dysfunction had been related to juvenile delinquency and violent crimes (Shanok & Lewis, 1981; Yeudall, Fromm-Auch, & Davies, 1982). In general, clinical neuropsychological data confirming brain impairment have played two principal roles in clinical neuropsychology: determination of guilt versus innocence on the basis of mental competence, and (once convicted) as a factor (mitigating circumstances) in sentencing considerations. In terms of mental competence, determining issues have included the ability to determine right from wrong, the ability to control one's actions, and the ability to participate in one's own defense. The use of the intelligence level as a sentencing consideration in capital punishment has become fairly accepted, whereby in many jurisdictions intelligence below a certain level precludes imposition of the death penalty. Although in earlier years the determination of disordered behavior had been the forensic purview of clinical psychology and psychiatry, neurophysiological substrates of disordered behavior became progressively recognized and clinical neuropsychology's role in such forensic issues evolved (Denney, 2008). While there is general recognition that among criminal offenders there is increased likelihood of neuropsychological impairment, there has as yet not been an equally compelling body of research into possible forensic interrelationships of brain dysfunction and such issues as drug abuse, violence, and other aspects of clinical behavior, but studies are ongoing.

Although not directly related, a clinical neuropsychological and methodological approach to assessing mental competence closely paralleling its approach in criminal matters has been applied to civil competence determinations. In 1991, Freedman, Stuss, and Gordon proposed a set of guidelines for assessing competency and decision making for patients with cognitive deficits due to neurological disorders. Guilmette and Krupp (1999) reviewed some twelve studies relating these sorts of guidelines to mental status measures in civil competency determinations, and Kennedy (1990, 1993) applied this frame of reference to assessing competency to consent to sexual activity in a cognitively impaired population. These research and practice foci were included in the inaugural volume of the *Journal of Forensic Neuropsychology*, whose advent and development serves as yet another milestone in the growth of the field.

Although clinical neuropsychologists have debated for over three decades or more the validity of neuropsychological testing in general and fixed batteries versus flexible testing specifically, these issues for the most part have not been a major subject of debate in United States jurisprudence.

During the past two decades, a revolution has been ongoing with regard to the introduction and admissibility of scientific evidence in general. While the competency of clinical neuropsychologists to provide expert testimony on "medical issues" is now well established, it is not surprising that the validity of neuropsychological testing and the methodology employed by clinical neuropsychological experts would eventually become the subject of court battles.

In 1993, the United States Supreme Court, in the landmark decision of *Daubert v. Merrill Dow Chemical* (1993), held that before scientific testimony would be admitted into the federal courts, the trial court must first serve as a gatekeeper to determine whether or not the methodology and opinions rendered were scientifically valid. In the Daubert case, the Supreme Court held that the Federal Rules of Evidence impose a special obligation upon a trial judge to insure that scientific testimony is not only relevant, but also reliable. The Supreme Court introduced a four-factor test, which included testing, peer review, error rates, and acceptability in the relevant scientific community, that would prove helpful in determining the reliability of a particular scientific theory or technique.

Four years later in *General Electric v. Joiner* (1997), the United States Supreme Court again ruled:

> *Conclusions and methodology are not entirely distinct from one another. Trained experts commonly extrapolate from existing data. But nothing in either Daubert or the Federal Rules of Evidence requires a district court to admit opinion evidence, which is connected to existing data only by the ipse dixit of the expert. A court may conclude that there is simply too great an analytical gap between the data and the opinion offered.*

Therefore, evidence is not admissible simply because the expert says it is reliable.

Following the Supreme Court's decisions in *Daubert* and *Joiner*, a debate arose among the federal circuits as to whether or not *Daubert* should be narrowly applied only to scientific expert testimony, or broadly extended to all expert witness testimony, based upon scientific, technical or other specialized knowledge.

That debate was resolved by the United States Supreme Court decision in *Kumho Tire Co. v. Carmichael* (1999). In that case, the United States Supreme Court held that the *Daubert* factors might apply to testimony by all experts. The Court held that a trial judge, determining the admissibility of expert testimony, might consider one or more of the specific *Daubert* factors. The emphasis on the word "may" reflects *Daubert*'s description of R. 702 inquiry as "a flexible one."

The *Daubert* factors were held not to constitute a definitive checklist or test. Rather, the Court held that the factors that may or may not be pertinent in assessing reliability, depend on the nature of the specific issue, including an expert's particular expertise and the subject matter of his testimony. The Court concluded:

> *The conclusion, in our view, is that we can neither rule out, nor rule in, for all cases and for all times the applicability of the factors mentioned in Daubert, nor can we now do so for subsets of cases categorized by category of expert or by kind of evidence. Too much depends upon the particular circumstances of the particular case at issue.*

To date, this revolution has not yet fully permeated down to the state trial court levels in many states. While some states have embraced it, others have paid it lip service or rejected it in totality. While many states, through either Appellate or Supreme Court decisions, have cited with approval the *Daubert* standard, state trial judges have not used the gatekeeper role to the extent presently seen in our federal courts. It is not unusual, in reading federal court cases, to see expert testimony excluded that certainly, in some state courts, would be admissible.

Forensic Neuropsychology to the Defense

Shortly following the recognition that clinical neuropsychology could be of value for demonstrating (to courts) the relationship between a patient's brain injuries and subsequent impairment in a number of abilities important for vocational, social, and general adjustment functions, legal practices focusing on defense against such claims generally adopted one of two foci.

The first focus, calling into question the scientific validity of clinical neuropsychology and its recognition as a professional specialty, resulted in a number of court challenges. Since 1923, United States courts operated under the *Frye* standard (Greiffenstein, 2008) for admissibility of scientific evidence, requiring that scientific evidence be of the type generally accepted within the relevant scientific community. This precipitated such challenges as to whether the complete Halstead-Reitan Neuropsychology Battery needed to be administered in order to be valid, in evoking research by Hartlage (1983), Hartlage and DeFilippis (1983), and Dean (1995) concerning professional practice in the United States (Reed, 1996). Then, in 1993, the Supreme Court superseded the *Frye* standard with the *Daubert* standard, reflecting a more conservative view of the Federal Rules of Evidence (Fisher, 1994; Larvie, 1994). Although this new standard was apparently more receptive toward neuropsychological evidence (in relying more on proven science and less on general acceptance), it has not been applied to all courts and, in turn, has produced different types of challenges to clinical neuropsychology.

To date, there have been very few court decisions assessing the admissibility of clinical neuropsychological testing under the *Daubert* standard. One of the very few cases to discuss the admissibility of clinical neuropsychological testing under *Daubert* was *Chapple v. Ganger* (1994). There, as a result of a motor vehicle collision, Peggy A. Chapple was killed. Additionally, her 10-year-old son Christopher was severely injured. A wrongful death and survival action, as well as a claim for Christopher, was brought in state court and later removed to federal court. The parties consented to proceed before a United States magistrate and stipulated to an abbreviated bench trial. It was agreed by the parties that a determination of damages would be based upon a review of deposition testimony, submitted by the parties, of their expert witnesses, as well as expert reports, briefing, and argument of counsel.

In support of their claim, the plaintiff produced the deposition transcript of a treating psychologist, Paul J. Domitor, PhD, who utilized the Halstead-Reitan Neuropsychological Battery (HRNB). Dr. Domitor found that Christopher had sustained a traumatic brain injury as a result of the motor vehicle collision, now had mild cognitive problems, moderate behavioral problems involving social appropriateness and his ability to inhibit emotions, and trouble controlling his behavior and understanding social demands, and was experiencing some depression from the loss of his mother. Dr. Domitor opined that these problems would increase as Christopher grew older. Dr. Domitor, however, could not make a prognosis, indicating that it would depend on developments over the next four to five years.

Katherine Mateer, PhD, a clinical neuropsychologist, director of neuropsychology services at the Good Samaritan Hospital, and a research associate professor at the University of Washington, also evaluated Christopher. Dr. Mateer concluded:

> *Christopher is an eleven-year-old male who suffered a moderate to severe traumatic brain injury secondary to a motor vehicle accident....Secondary to his injury, changes have been noted in Christopher's physical, cognitive, and emotional functioning. Christopher now frequently suffers from headaches and has difficulty attending and*

concentrating. He is also noted to be more easily frustrated and has suffered a decline in grades since the accident.

Neuropsychological evaluation revealed a youngster with average-range intellectual skills and solid abilities in the areas of language and visuospatial functioning. Areas of weakness of cognitive deficit were seen on measures assessing attention and concentration and measures of new learning and memory. Though Christopher did score within the normal range on some of these tasks, he appears to have more difficulty with tasks requiring vigilance or a higher level of mental control. Additionally, there is considerable variability within his new learning and his ability to retain information over time. Deficits of attention/concentration and new learning/memory abilities are common sequelae secondary to traumatic brain injury...As such, deficits noted are felt to be directly related to the head injury he sustained in the motor vehicle accident.

During her assessment, Dr. Mateer administered a flexible test battery, testifying that no single test confirms or disconfirms brain impairment. Basically, a neuropsychologist must look at the patterns and profiles and compare them to pre-injury levels of functioning. Dr. Mateer testified that clear functional impairments cannot be demonstrated with all brain injuries. She considered Christopher's injury to be in the moderate to severe range, disagreeing with Dr. Domitor who characterized it as mild. She concluded that the bulk of Christopher's recovery had been made and that he was likely left with permanent residual problems of attention, memory, and executive functions.

The defendant argued that Christopher did not have a permanent brain injury, but that the problems that were now manifesting could have been predicted based upon Christopher's social history before the accident, particularly his declining academic performance and increasing problems with behavior premorbidly. The defendant retained Ralph M. Reitan, PhD, an internationally known clinical neuropsychologist and the co-originator of the Halstead-Reitan Neuropsychological Test Batteries for Adults, Older and Younger Children. Dr. Reitan evaluated Christopher and administered most of the Halstead-Reitan Neuropsychological Test Battery for Older Children. He noted that most of the test scores fell in the normal range, concluding, however, that there were certain mild deviations that could be of significance regarding minor brain dysfunction. Dr. Reitan noted:

Some scores are very good; some scores are below normal; most scores are in the average range. This is exactly what happens with normal "non-brain-damaged" children. In terms of the objective test results, Christopher appears to be essentially normal. Nevertheless, from a clinical point of view, I would postulate that there might be some very mild left cerebral deficits and that Christopher might be having more trouble in school as a result. If brain impairment of a very mild nature is present, it would be compatible with head trauma.

Dr. Reitan criticized the findings of Dr. Domitor, concluding that he (Dr. Domitor) relied on results from adult literature and incorrectly applied these results to children. He also rejected Dr. Mateer's assessment, describing it not as a clinical neuropsychological examination, but instead, "The kind of ability and cognitive testing that might be used to assess a normal child." He argued that Dr. Mateer's test results were never compared with those of brain-damaged children. He concluded that Dr. Mateer's testing and testimony was scientifically invalid and unreliable.

The Trial Court awarded Christopher $29,013 for past medical expenses, $124,000 for future medical expenses, $125,000 in temporary disability, $30,000 for fear, and $325,000 in pain and suffering. However, the Court specifically dismissed any claim for permanent organic brain damage. The Court concluded:

> *Based on the evidence, specifically the lack of medical evidence as to long-term prognosis, the Court is unable to conclude that Christopher has permanent organic brain damage. This conclusion is supported by the rapid recovery of his physical symptoms, Dr. Domitor's assessment that Christopher did not need treatment during the first year after the accident, his fifth-grade performance, his unremarkable visits to New York, and some indication prior to the accident that his academic performance and behavior patterns were on the decline. In substantial part, the Court finds the causation of Christopher's problems during the sixth grade was due to his father's marriage following the death of Christopher's mother, the adjustment of living with a stepmother and stepbrother, as well as the reaction by the other siblings to the remarriage. The Court accepts the test results as they indicate normal scores in most areas. As to those areas which show below normal scores, there is not sufficient scientific evidence to support the conclusion that those scores are indicative of permanent organic brain damage in children.*

Following the *Chapple* decision, in an article entitled "Fixed vs. Flexible Neuropsychological Test Batteries Under the *Daubert* Standard for the Admissibility of Scientific Evidence," Reed wrote:

> *In* Chapple v. Ganger (1994), the Daubert *standard was applied for the very first time to the use of fixed (standardized) versus flexible (non-standardized) neuropsychological test batteries in the federal court. In this personal injury case, the Chapple Court gave far greater weight to the results obtained from a fixed battery than to the results obtained from two flexible neuropsychological test batteries. Significantly, under the* Daubert *standard, the district judge noted the lack of medical and scientific evidence to support the conclusions made by the plaintiff's two expert witnesses, a psychologist and a neuropsychologist, even though each had administered a comprehensive and flexible neuropsychological test battery and had based their conclusions on the test results. However, the judge accepted as scientific evidence the objective test results obtained from the fixed Halstead-Reitan Neuropsychological Test Battery for Older Children administered by the defendant's expert witness, Dr. Ralph Reitan, and also accepted his scientific expert medical testimony, which was closely derived from these data. (Reed, 1996)*

In a presentation before the American Trial Lawyers Association, Dr. Reitan asserted that the Halstead-Reitan Neuropsychological Test Battery had been found scientifically valid and admissible under a *Daubert* analysis, citing Reed. Similarly, in a book review, Bennett wrote:

> *While not reviewed in this volume, the case of* Chapple v. Ganger *(1994) is relevant to both* Daubert *and the use of a fixed vs. a flexible battery approach in forensic*

neuropsychology. In Chapple v. Ganger, *a federal district court ruled that the fixed Halstead-Reitan Neuropsychological Test Battery met the* Daubert *standard for the admissibility of scientific evidence while data obtained using a flexible assessment did not. For a review of this case, see Reed. (Bennett, 1996)*

A reading of *Chapple* does not support this assertion. On reading this decision, one finds that while the Court did discuss the *Daubert* decision, it was not the defendants who raised the *Daubert* issue, but the plaintiffs, who contended that two of the defendants' expert witnesses' testimony did not meet the *Daubert* evidentiary requirements. At no time did the defense or the Court raise any *Daubert* issue with regard to the validity and admissibility of the use of a fixed or a flexible test battery. While the Court ultimately did reject the plaintiff's contention that Christopher had permanent, organic brain damage, the Court's decision was based on non-accident-related factors. Further, in a battle of experts, the Court accepted the testimony of Dr. Reitan over that of Drs. Domitor and Mateer.

Reed, in his article, acknowledged this as well:

In reaching its decision the Chapple *Court specifically emphasized that the lack of medical evidence to support a long-term prognosis rendered the Court unable to conclude that the child had permanent, organic brain injury. It is important to note, however, that the plaintiffs' failure was partly a result of Dr. Reitan's adverse expert witness testimony, which was admitted as medical scientific evidence indicating normal brain functioning.*

Interestingly, important issues were raised in Court regarding the standardized or "fixed" battery assessment method versus the unstandardized or "flexible" neuropsychological battery assessment method. However, after consideration of all of this proffered expert witness testimony, the Chapple *Court limited its holding primarily to scientific and medical evidence (e.g., scientific and medical evidence was weighted very heavily by the Court given that the point at issue was the presence of brain injury caused by the 1992 auto accident). Thus, by acknowledging the body of medical and scientific evidence offered by the defense and the lack of medical and scientific evidence offered by the plaintiffs, the district judge did not discuss the clinical validity or clinical relevance of the two types of neuropsychological battery in her decision.*

Greiffenstein (2008), in an article discussing "various myths surrounding forensic neuropsychology," noted that one of those myths is that "only the fixed battery is admissible under *Daubert*." Greiffenstein attributes this myth to the article cited above by Reed. Greiffenstein wrote:

The assertion of the Halstead-Reitan battery's superior admissibility is a myth for two reasons. It is easily disproved by showing that Reed materially mischaracterized the Chapple *ruling…Second, fifteen years of* Daubert *jurisprudence have not been accompanied by any increase in Halstead-Reitan use or decline in flexible approaches.*

What is clear is the assertion that *Chapple* upheld the use of the fixed test battery and found that the flexible battery did not satisfy the *Daubert* standard simply is incorrect.

The State of New Hampshire proved to be the unlikely battleground for the first major battle between the fixed battery approach and the flexible test approach. There, in the case of *Baxter v. Temple* (2008), the plaintiff's expert was Dr. Barbara Bruno-Golden, who used the Boston process approach in testing the plaintiff. Defendant retained Dr. David Faust, who asserted that for Dr. Bruno-Golden's testimony to be admissible, the comprehensive neuropsychological batteries that she used in evaluating the plaintiff as a whole must have been tested, have been subject to peer review, and have a known or potential error rate. Dr. Faust also asserted that the Boston process approach was not generally accepted in the forensic assessment community.

In a pretrial hearing, the plaintiff called as a rebuttal expert witness Sandra Shaheen, PhD, a member of the Department of Psychiatry of the Harvard Medical School. Dr. Shaheen testified that while the Boston process approach had gained widespread acceptance in the literature, the specific methodology or test used by Dr. Bruno-Golden had not. The Trial Court ruled in favor of the defendants, barring Dr. Bruno-Golden's testimony, and finding that although the plaintiff had shown that Dr. Bruno-Golden's methodology was generally accepted in the appropriate scientific literature in the making of a clinical assessment, the plaintiff had not shown that Dr. Bruno-Golden's methodology was generally accepted in the appropriate scientific literature in the making of a forensic assessment.

This decision by the Trial Court was difficult to comprehend. While it relied upon the *Daubert* standard in making its decision, it ignored the U.S. Supreme Court's mandate in *Kumho Tire v. Carmichael* (1999) that clearly held:

> *The objective of that requirement is to ensure the reliability and relevancy of expert testimony. It is to make certain that an expert, whether basing testimony upon professional studies or personal experience, employs in the courtroom the same level of intellectual rigor that characterizes the practice of an expert in the relevant field.*

In *Kumho Tire*, the U.S. Supreme Court specifically ruled that the test to be applied is whether or not the expert witness's methodology that was used in the litigated case was the same methodology that he or she would use in clinical practice. Thus, the Trial Court's finding that the Boston process approach had gained widespread acceptance in a particular clinical community should have been sufficient for its admission into evidence. Thus, the Trial Court found that the plaintiff had not shown that the methodology was generally accepted in the appropriate scientific literature as reliable in a legal proceeding. In reaching its conclusion, the Trial Court focused on the plaintiff's failure to demonstrate that the specific battery—the entire series of tests viewed as a whole—employed by plaintiff's clinical neuropsychologist was or could be tested, subjected to peer review and publication, or have a known or potential rate of error.

Plaintiff appealed directly to the New Hampshire Supreme Court. The American Academy of Clinical Neuropsychology (AACN) filed an amicus brief, supporting the use of the flexible approach. The purpose of the amicus brief filed on their behalf was to address the issue of the scientific merits and acceptability of the flexible battery approach in clinical neuropsychology, and the contention that the threshold for clinical judgments of clinical neuropsychologists is less than for forensic judgments, that is, data-based clinical judgments do not meet legal admissibility standards.

The AACN asserted that "reliance on a flexible battery approach to neuropsychological testing is empirically proven as a mainstream practice in that the logic of the flexible battery approach is the same as in clinical medicine, namely, selection of different test groupings because of the many forms that brain damage can take."

Rejecting the argument that flexible testing must be validated as a battery, the AACN wrote: "Test validity lies in individual tests, not test batteries as a whole." The AACN pointed out that in four AACN surveys conducted in 1989, 1994, 1999, and 2005, the vast majority of neuropsychologists used a flexible battery. The 2005 survey found that 76% used a flexible battery (variable but routine groups of tests for different types of patients such as head injury, alcoholism, elderly, etc.), 18% used a totally flexible approach (based on the needs of an individual case, not uniform across patients), whereas only 7% used a standardized battery (routine group of tests uniform across patients such as the Halstead-Reitan, Luria-Nebraska, Benton, or other standardized clinical neuropsychology battery).

The New Hampshire Supreme Court, using the standards set forth by the United States Supreme Court in *Daubert*, rejected the Trial Court's determination. The Court held that there does not exist a different standard for testing in the forensic setting as opposed to the clinical setting. The Court noted that the Boston Process Approach (BPA) is a variation of the flexible battery approach that adds "a qualitative element to evaluating brain function." The Court opinion, 22 pages in length, discusses in great detail why the flexible battery approach is admissible under the *Daubert* standard. The Court, soundly rejecting the defendant's contention (defendant's expert was Dr. David Faust) that in order for a "battery" to be admissible in a forensic setting, all of the tests needed to be evaluated as an entire battery in order to determine known error rates, reasoned thus:

> *To conclude otherwise would require the field of neuropsychology to test, peer review, and calculate error rates for an infinite number of test combinations for the interpretations to be reliable. Each time a new validated and reliable test or battery of tests such as the NPSY is developed or even updated, a clinical examiner could not use it as part of a comprehensive battery, since it would be unknown how it interacted with the other tests within that battery. Since the flexible battery approach is the generally accepted approach to conducting neuropsychological assessments, the APA standards could not logically mandate that a neuropsychologist always use a comprehensive test battery that is validated as a whole.*

The New Hampshire Supreme Court also found that the evidence in the record indicated that the BPA as a flexible battery approach could be tested. It stated that while the BPA itself does not have a known or potential error rate, this was not critical to its admissibility. In its opinion, the Supreme Court concluded:

> *Accordingly, we find that, when the BPA is administered in a manner consistent with the flexible battery approach, as described above, it is generally a reliable approach to neuropsychological assessment and is thus a reliable methodology for determining a person's cognitive status.*

For those forensic neuropsychologists from the fixed battery school who have consistently attacked the admissibility of the flexible battery approach, this decision stands as a defeat. Furthermore the Court soundly rejected defense "forensic" neuropsychologists who maintain that there is a distinction between the practice of clinical and forensic neuropsychology.

Although the *Chapple* and *Baxter* decisions are the only published decisions to date discussing the admissibility of neuropsychological testing under *Daubert* or *Kumho*, two state court decisions regarding the admissibility of psychological testimony may prove helpful to understand the direction that these decisions will take.

In *State of Louisiana v. Foret* (1993) the Supreme Court of Louisiana was cause to discuss whether it was error to admit a child psychologist to testify concerning child sexual abuse accommodation syndrome (CSAAS). In that case a jury found the defendant, who was charged with molestation of a juvenile when the offender had controlled supervision over the juvenile, guilty of attempted molestation of a juvenile. Chief among the defendant's claim for a new trial was that the Trial Court erred in allowing, over objection, a psychologist who would examine the victim to testify. The state offered two expert witnesses to support its case. The first was a physician qualified in the field of family medicine who testified that although an examination of the victim after the abuse was reported yielded no positive physical evidence of abuse, that this lack of positive physical evidence was not unusual in this type of case. The second witness was a child psychologist, Dr. William Janzen, who qualified as an expert in the field of psychology with expertise in child sexual abuse. Based largely on the testimony of the victim and bolstered by Dr. Janzen, the defendant was convicted of attempted molestation. In making his diagnosis of child abuse, Dr. Janzen used CSAAS, a psychological phenomenon prevalent among victims of child sexual abuse. This syndrome was first developed by Dr. Roland C. Summit in the late 1970s and early 1980s who listed factors that were "both most characteristic of child sexual abuse and most provocative of rejection in the prevailing adult methodology about legitimate victims." Despite its stated purpose, the "syndrome" came to be used by many as a tool for determining whether or not abuse had occurred, as opposed to the intended use of the "syndrome" as a treatment device.

The Louisiana Supreme Court, rejecting the testimony and reversing the Trial Court decision, found:

> In the instant case, Dr. Janzen used the "dynamics" of the syndrome not as a "common language" to facilitate treatment of the disorder as Dr. Summit and other therapists in the field intended, but as a tool for diagnosing whether or not abuse had occurred.

This use of CSAAS is seen as having highly dubious value by many members of the psychological treatment community because, "Generally speaking, the psychological evaluation of a child suspected of being sexually abused is, at best, an inexact science."

Progressively, the court rulings clarified the legitimate scientific basis and utility of clinical neuropsychology for providing courts with valid and helpful information, although there were along the way a number of rulings concluding that clinical neuropsychologists were not competent to provide scientific testimony about brain injury. These rulings generally were based on medical exclusionary reasoning, that is, the brain and its function is the domain of medical specialties such as neurology, neurosurgery, and psychiatry, and thus valid information about the brain and its functions (or dysfunctions) rested within the purview of these medical specialties. As accumulated court rulings in case law recognized clinical neuropsychology as relevant to the forensic issues involving brain damage, legal challenges became more narrow, addressing such issues as admissibility under *Daubert* criteria and specific neurological practices such as fixed versus flexible neuropsychological batteries (*Chapple v. Ganger*, 1994; Reed, 1996). Indirect support for clinical neuropsychology's scientific recognition came in the American Academy of Neurology's Therapeutic and Technology Assessment Committees (1996), which, although lacking in comprehensiveness, clarified the research-based content of neuropsychological assessment (Hartlage, 2001).

The other defensive focus—one that has had significant impact on both forensic neuropsychology and clinical neuropsychology in general—involves attempting to discredit positive clinical neuropsychological findings under the theory of contaminated or invalid results of testing due to malingering or suboptimal efforts. Interestingly, no such proliferations have affected the neurology literature, where diagnostic impressions based on examination findings are generally unchallenged. Whereas clinical neuropsychologists' measure of grip strength, for example, based on standardized measurement with a grip dynamometer may be challenged as possibly contaminated by suboptimal effort, neurologists' impressions based on having patients squeeze the neurologists' hands are much more likely to go unchallenged. Based largely on psychiatric literature involving inability of practitioners to differentiate real symptoms from malingering, and in the much cited *Diagnostic and Statistical Manual of Mental Disorders* criterion (American Psychiatric Association, 1994) for malingering that includes the possibility of secondary gain, a proliferation of tests of malingering has contributed a significant portion of the papers presented at annual professional meetings at the National Academy of Neuropsychology (NAN), as well as a noticeable number of published articles.

Neuropsychological approaches to tests aimed at detection of malingering have tended to be based on one or two models: symptom validity models or actuarial (e.g., forced choice) models. Methods of symptom validity assessment have been reviewed by Reynolds (1998), Slick, Sherman, and Iverson (1999), and Sweet (1999), and more recently by Biachini, Mathias, and Grove (2001), and Larrabee (2003). A National Academy of Neuropsychology Position Paper (Bush et al., 2005) clarified relevant practice issues and the necessity of being aware of possible contaminants of test data. Such symptom validity procedures typically involved symptoms not commonly reported by brain injury patients, with endorsement of uncommon symptoms supposedly confirmatory of malingering. Unfortunately, the actual identification of malingering versus not malingering patients is almost never known, so that the validation of these tests is almost solely based on either response by individuals (college students told to malinger, by individuals identified as "malingerers" on the basis of performance in the "malingering" range on another test or tests similarly validated). As more and more forensic neuropsychologists create malingering tests to assist their clients, one can expect more *Daubert* and *Frye* challenges regarding their validity.

As Gouvier and his associates have noted (Gouvier, Hayes, & Smiroldo, 1998; Gouvier, Uddo-Crane, & Brown, 1988), although often overlooked, base rates are directly applicable to validity testing. They specifically establish the validity of any assessment procedure and involve examining sensitivity specificity, and the false-positive and false-negative error rates for the procedure (Bar-Hillel, 1980; Duncan & Snow, 1987; Willis, 1984). Unfortunately, it is nearly impossible to determine with precision exactly how much an individual's performance on a given neuropsychological test on a given date may be influenced by such interacting and possibly overlapping factors as litigation status (McKinley, Brooks, & Bond, 1983; Rogers, 1988), task instruction (Martin, Bolter, Todd, Gouvier, & Nicholls, 1993), knowledge of head injury symptoms and motivation (Martin, Gouvier, Todd, Bolter, & Nicholls, 1992), malingering (Trueblood, 1994), performance anxiety, fatigue, or pain (Purisch & Sbordone, 1997), and actual neuropsychological sequelae of impaired brain function. With malingering estimates ranging from 2 to 7% (Schretlen, 1988) to 64% (Heaton, Smith, Lehman & Vogt, 1978), for example, and with malingerers, neither readily identifiable by some distinguishing mark or characteristic, nor likely to self-identify for purposes of helping neuropsychological science clarify matters (Hartlage, 1995), it is very difficult to calculate the base rate of malingering (i.e., *number of cases with condition* divided by *number of cases in population*) (Gouvier, Hayes, & Smiroldo, 1998; Grouvier, Uddo-Crane, & Brown, 1988). Rather it is likely that various populations of patients (litigation vs. non-litigation, coached by attorneys vs. not coached by attorneys, civil vs. criminal) may vary widely. Without even a gross consensus about the number of cases of malingerers within the population, not all clinical neuropsychologists agree that a "test of malingering" can be validated within acceptable criteria for scientific, classificatory accuracy. Because different etiologies of brain injury have been known for many years to produce quite different neurobehavioral outcomes (Della, Sala, Gray, Spinner, & Trivelli, 1998; Hartlage & Williams, 1991; Malloy, Bihrle, & Duffy, 1983), comparing individuals with a brain injury versus "normal individuals" may be too simplistic to produce valid symptom clusters. Furthermore, damage to different brain areas can produce quite different neurobehavioral sequelae (Damasio, Damasio, & VanHoegen, 1982; Golden & Van den Broeck, 1998; Hecaen, 1962; Milner, 1954; Kixmiller, Briggs, Hartlage, & Dean, 1993; Patch & Hartlage, 2001), and sequelae of brain injury may be influenced by the premorbid ability structure of the patient as well as both severity of brain injury and time since brain injury (Hartlage, Wilson, & Patch, 2001; Patch & Hartlage, 2003) among other factors.

Another possible reason for which clinical neuropsychology, much more so than neurology, is challenged in terms of failure to detect possible malingering may relate to the increasing use of technicians in neuropsychological assessment (DeLuca, 1987; Guilmette, Faust, Hart, & Arkes, 1990; Hartlage & Telzrow, 1980; Seretny, Dean, Gray, & Hartlage, 1986). Use of technicians for conducting most of the examination, while serving a number of practical purposes, sharply reduces opportunities for the clinical neuropsychologist to make observations of behaviors throughout extended examination, and to use, as indicated, a number of clinical tests on a continuing basis throughout the examination to assess patient behaviors in terms of their congruence with neurologic substrates of behavior subserving given tests (Hartlage, 1998).

Thus, forensic neuropsychology with a focus on defense issues has significantly altered the research landscape of clinical neuropsychology. Perhaps most illustrative of this conundrum is the literature involving the Fake-Bad Scale scores on the MMPI-2 as being indicative of malingering (Lees-Haley, English, & Glenn, 1991). Butcher and his associates (Arbisi & Butcher, 2004; Butcher, Arbisi, Atlis, & McNulty, 2003) have seriously criticized the Lees-Haley Fake-Bad Scale (FBS). Although the Butcher and colleagues' (2003) criticisms of the FBS scale largely focus on empirical validity and sensitivity issues, they also note that the FBS includes items that occur with general medical conditions. For example, FBS criteria for malingering include positive endorsement of such items as headaches (item 40); sleep disturbances (item 39); finding it hard to keep my mind on a task or job (item 31); having more trouble concentrating than other seems to have (item 325); feeling tired a good deal of the time (item 464); dizzy spells (item 164); headaches (item 176); pain (item 224); tinnitus (item 255); and not having enough energy to do my work (item 561). In light of the fact that research literature concerning complaints reported following brain injury, especially traumatic brain injury, very frequently if not typically reveal many of these problems, raising the possibility that the FBS scale dramatically overdiagnoses malingering (Arbisi & Butcher, 2004; Butcher, Arbisi, Atlis, & McNulty, 2003).

In *Williams v. CSX Transportation, Inc.* (Greiffenstein, 2008), an unreported Florida Trial Court decision, the plaintiff's counsel moved to bar the use and acceptance of the Fake-Bad Scale as a scientific means of assessing effort and malingering. The State of Florida, which has not adopted the *Daubert* standard, but still relies on the older *Frye* standard, conducted a hearing to determine the scientific validity of the FBS. The plaintiff's expert was Dr. James M. Butcher, the lead investigator for the restandardization of MMPI-2 and the author of an article extremely critical of the FBS entitled "The construct validity of the Lees-Haley Fake-Bad Scale: Does this scale measure somatic malingering and feigned emotional distress?" Defendant's expert was Yossef Ben-Porath, PhD, an eminent MMPI-2 researcher.

After a *Frye* hearing, the Court barred the use of the FBS, finding that it lacked objectivity. In support of its decision, the Court noted that the FBS had no scoring or administration manual, interpretation recommendations, or appropriate cautions published by the University of Minnesota (which holds the MMPI-2 copyright), that the FBS was subjective and dependent on the interpretation of the person using the FBS, that the FBS lacked definitive scoring, that cutout scores continually changed, and an acknowledgment by all that it was biased against women and those with serious injuries. The Court found that:

> Unlike every other scale in the MMPI-2, there is no scoring or administration manual for the FBS, and the above recommendations and cautions published by the University of Minnesota press for its use indicate to the Court that FBS is not an objective measurement of effort, malingering, or over-reporting of symptoms. The Court concludes that the FBS is very subjective and dependent on the interpretation of the person using or interpreting it. There is no definitive scoring because the scoring has to be adjusted up and down based on the circumstances, and there is a high degree of probability for false-positives.

As more and more forensic neuropsychologists create malingering tests to assist their clients, one can expect more *Daubert* and *Frye* challenges to their validity.

The reasons for which clinical neuropsychologists (but not neurologists) have historically been challenged in forensic settings concerning the possibility of malingering may be traced to several sources. Perhaps the most likely source relates to clinical neuropsychology's evolution from clinical psychology, which is, of course, subject to the diagnostic ambiguity and overlap involved in psychological test data so thoroughly critiqued by Faust and his colleagues (Faust, Ziskin, & Hiers, 1991). It is highly likely that the active growth of challenges to clinical neuropsychology's participation in forensic issues has accelerated with the omnipresent adversarial focus involved in most forensic efforts. Indeed, Bigler (2007) addresses the issue of challenges of neuropsychological testimony by other neuropsychologists as an issue of critical significance for neuropsychology practice.

Today, in most jurisdictions that have permitted the expert testimony of a clinical neuropsychologist, the courts have focused on the qualifications of the proposed expert clinical neuropsychologist, examining education, training, and work experience to determine whether or not the clinical neuropsychologist is qualified to testify. See *Madrid v. University of California* (1997), *Kinsey v. King* (1982), *Shilling v. Mobile Analytical Services, Inc.* (1992), *Sanchez v. Derby* (1989), *Dutaquier v. Barbera* (1986), *Sabianke v. Weaver* (1988), *Hutchison v. American Family Mutual Insurance Co.* (1994), and *Adamson v. Chiovaro* (1988).

Nevertheless, in a minority of jurisdictions, clinical neuropsychologists have been and still are prohibited from providing expert testimony on the issue of causation or even prognosis. In *Executive Car and Truck Leasing, Inc. v. DeSerio (1985)*, the Florida Court of Appeals held that the Trial Court did not abuse its discretion in allowing a clinical psychologist who was not a medical doctor to testify as to the existence of organic brain injury. The Court indicated that the issue of lack of a medical degree should be raised during cross-examination and closing arguments. The Court held, after acknowledging authorities to the contrary, that the psychologist was not competent, however, to give expert testimony on the issue of causation of the brain injury.

Shortly following the *Executive Car* decision, the Florida Appellate Division addressed the issue again in *GIW Southern Valve Co. v. Smith* (1985). There, the Court, agreeing with the *Executive Car* decision, opined:

> *We believe that the underlying rationale for excluding that type of opinion testimony requires the exclusion of the type of testimony in issue here [prognosis]. That rationale involves the lack of qualifications of a nonmedical witness on a medical subject. We have no doubt that the matter of providing a prognosis as to future physiological effects upon the plaintiff's brain of a particular accident is a medical subject no less than is the subject of causation in the first instance, i.e., whether an accident caused existing brain damage. Just as, relative to causation, a witness who is a psychologist and not a medical doctor lacks qualifications to trace retrospectively what would occur to the brain from a given trauma...so also does the witness lack established qualifications to trace prospectively what would occur to the brain in the future.*

Following the Court's decision in *Executive Car*, the Florida Legislature amended its statute defining the practice of psychology, following which some Florida courts ruled that clinical neuropsychologists were not precluded from testifying as to the cause of brain injury (*Broward County School Board v. Cruz*, 2000). However, in 2003, the Supreme Court of Florida was called upon again to decide what limitations, if any, should be placed upon the testimony of a clinical neuropsychologist in *Grenitz v. Tomlian* (2003). This case involved parents who brought a medical malpractice action on behalf of their son, who was born with cerebral palsy. The plaintiffs called as an expert witness a clinical neuropsychologist who testified that the son sustained significant brain damage, which was caused by oxygen deprivation at birth, but the witness was not permitted to give his opinion as to why the injury had not occurred weeks prior to the birth as contended by the defendants. The Trial Court sustained an objection made by the defendants that a psychologist, who was not a medical doctor, was not qualified to render an opinion as to causation. The District Court reversed the jury verdict for the defendants and remanded the case for a new trial.

On appeal to the Florida Supreme Court, the Court ruled that a "properly trained and qualified neuropsychologist can never testify as to the cause of brain damage, though is permitted to give an opinion as to diagnosis."

In *John v. Im* (2002) the Virginia Supreme Court ruled that a neuropsychologist was not qualified to give expert testimony on the issue of diagnosis or causation. The Court ruled that "An opinion concerning causation of a particular physical human injury is a component of a diagnosis, which is part of the practice of medicine ...." Because Dr. Nash (the clinical neuropsychologist) was not a medical doctor, he was not qualified to state an expert medical opinion regarding the cause of the plaintiff's injury.

In 2005, a Virginia Circuit Court was called upon to apply the earlier decision in a case where a plaintiff asserted that he had sustained a mild traumatic brain injury as the result of a motor vehicle crash (*McCarthy v. Atwood*, 2005). In that case the defendant, pursuant to Court Order, had the plaintiff undergo a neuropsychological evaluation by Scott W. Sautter, PhD, ABN, a nationally known clinical neuropsychologist. Dr. Sautter stated in his report that his overall impression of the plaintiff's neuropsychological and emotional functioning were consistent with generally intact cognitive functions, and that given the history it was probable that the plaintiff did sustain a concussion in the collision. However, he continued, whatever cognitive deficits were present would have been expected to resolve within a few weeks to a few months, according to large, controlled studies of brain injuries. Dr. Sautter asserted that any lingering deficits were due to other factors unrelated to the motor vehicle collision.

At trial, the plaintiff, relying upon *John v. Im*, moved to exclude any opinion by the defense neuropsychologist concerning the cause or extent of the plaintiff's brain injury and resulting cognitive dysfunction and memory loss.

The District Court re-examined the *John v. Im* decision, as well as those cases decided subsequently. The Court also reviewed an article entitled "*John v. Im*: Time for Clarification and Revisiting the Decision by the Supreme Court of Virginia." The District Court concluded that:

> *Dr. Sautter can render medical opinions within his neuropsychological expertise as to plaintiff's mental ailments, conditions, and diseases, as well as the relationship between his conduct and such mental ailments, conditions, and diseases, assuming defendant shows the relevance of such opinions....However, consistent with the Virginia Supreme Court's ruling in* Im, *Dr. Sautter cannot render an opinion that plaintiff did or did not sustain a 'mild traumatic brain injury' as a result of his automobile accident, since such an opinion is an opinion concerning the causation of a physical human injury that could only be rendered by a medical doctor."*

The Court, however, instructed that an appropriate method to introduce such testimony, consistent with *Im*, would be the presentation of testimony of a clinical neuropsychologist for the actual content of the test results and findings, followed by testimony from a medical doctor on the issue of causation relying upon the neuropsychologist's test results and findings.

On the whole, there no longer remains in the vast majority of states any question that clinical neuropsychologists are competent to give expert medical testimony on the issues of diagnosis, causation, and prognosis.

Conclusion

The history of forensic neuropsychology reflects general developments in the fields of clinical neuropsychology and brain sciences, and has, in turn, exhibited a significant and continuing force of both practice parameters and research issues that can be expected to influence the future of clinical neuropsychology and forensic neuropsychology. As the literature reflects in fairly obvious fashion, clinical neuropsychology has had a significant impact on forensic science by providing both scientifically accepted means of confirming the presence or absence of brain injury (Reitan & Wolfson, 1997) and, if present, by providing realistic means of predicting how the brain injury effects may be expected to affect the patient's future. This is obviously of considerable importance for helping calculate damages related to brain injury and for developing appropriate life care planning needs of the brain-injured patient. Less obvious in the literature is the reciprocal effect forensic science has exerted on clinical neuropsychology. From such simple and obviously salutary effects as eliminating shortcuts in test administration and encouraging meticulous accuracy in scoring, to less obvious influences such as increasing the burden on the patient to prove absence of malingering or suboptimal effort by increasing research foci on such issues, involvement with forensic applications has influenced clinical neuropsychology practice, research, and theory.

References

Adamson v. Chiovaro, 308 N.J. Super. 70 (1998).

American Academy of Neurology. (1996). Assessment: Neuropsychological test and adults. Considerations for neurologists. *Neurology, 47,* 592–599.

American Psychiatric Association. (1994). *Diagnostic and statistical manual of mental disorders* (4th ed.). Washington, DC: American Psychiatric Press.

Arbisi, P. A., & Butcher, J. N. (2004). Failure of the FBS to predict what is going of somatic symptoms: Response to critics by Greve and Bianchini and Lees Haley and Fox. *Archives of Clinical Neuropsychology, 19,* 341–345.

Bar-Hillel, M. (1980). The base rate fallacy in probability judgments. *Acta Psychologicia, 44,* 211–233.

Baxter v. Temple, 949 A.2d 167 (NH 2008).

Bersoff, D. N., O'Keefe, A., & Welch, B. (1986). Amici Curia, North Carolina. Court of Appeals Horne V. Goodson.

Bianchini, K. J., Mathis, C., & Grove, K. (2001). Symptom validity testing: A critical review. *Clinical Neuropsychologist, 15*(1), 19–45.

Bigler, E. D. (1986), Forensic issues in neuropsychology. In D. Wedding, A. M. Horton, Jr., & J. Webster (Eds.), *The neuropsychology handbook* (pp. 526–547). New York: Springer Publishing Company.

Bigler, E. D. (2007). A motion to exclude and the " fixed" versus "flexible" battery in forensic neuropsychology: Challenge to the practice of clinical neuropsychology. *Archives of Clinical Neuropsychology, 22,* 45–51.

Blau, J. T. (1984). *The psychologist as expert witness.* New York: Wiley.

Broward County School Board v. Cruz, 761 So.2d 388 (Fla. App. 4 Dist. 2000).

Bush, S. S., Ruff, R. M., Troster, A. T., Barth, J. T., Koffler, S. P., Pliskin, N. H., et al. (2005). Symptom validity assessment: Practice issues and medical necessity in policy planning conferences. *Archives of Clinical Neuropsychology, 20,* 419–427.

Butcher, J. N., Arbisi, P., Atlis, M. M., & McNulty, J. I. (2003). The construct validity of the Lees-Haley Fake-Bad Scale: Does the scale measure somatic malingering and feigned emotional disorders? *Archives of Clinical Neuropsychology, 18,* 473–481.

Chalfant, J. C., & Scheffelin, M. A. (1969). *Central processing dysfunction in children: A review of research.* Bethesda, MD: U.S. Department of Health, Education, and Welfare.

Chandler Exterminators, Inc. v. Morris, 262 Ga. 257, 416 S.E.2d 277 (Ga. 1992).

Chapple v. Ganger, 851 F. Supp. 1481 (E.D. Wash. 1994).

Damasio, A. R., Damasio H., & Van Hoegen, G. W. (1982) Prosopagnosia: Anatomic bases and behavioral mechanisms. *Neurology, 32,* 331–334.

Daubert v. Merrill Dow Chemical, 509 U.S. 579 (1993).

Dean, R. S. (1995). Review of the Halsted-Reitan Neuropsychological Test Battery. In J. V. Mitchell (Ed.), *The ninth mental measurements yearbook.* Lincoln, NE: University of Nebraska Press.

Della Sala, S., Gray, C., Spinner, H.. & Trivelli, A. (1998). Frontal lobe functioning in man: The riddle revisited. *Archives of Clinical Neuropsychology, 13,* 663–682.

DeLuca, J. W. (1987). Neuropsychology technicians in clinical practice. *Clinical Neuropsychologist, 1,* 3–21.

Denney, R. L. (2008). *Foundations of neuropsychological assessment for the criminal courts.* National Academy of Neuropsychology, the 28th annual conference program (p. 34).

Duncan, D., & Snow, W. (1987). Base rates in neuropsychology. *Professional Psychology: Research and Practice, 18*(4), 368–370.

Dutaquier v. Barbera, 490 S. 2d 341 (La. App. 1 Cir. 1986).

Faust, D., Ziskin, J., & Hiers, J. B. (1991). *Brain damage claims: Coping with neuropsychological evidence.* Los Angeles: Law and Psychology Press.

Executive Car and Truck Leasing, Inc. v. DeSerio, 468 S.2d 1027 (Fla. App. 4 Dist. 1985).

Fisher, D. (1994). Daubert v. Merrell Dow Pharmaceuticals: The Supreme Court gives federal judges the keys to admissibility of expert scientific testimony. *San Diego Law Review, 141,* 395.

Fox, D. R. (1999). Psychological scholarship contribution to false consciousness about injustice. *Law and Human Behavior, 23,* 9–30.

Freeman, M., Stuss, D. T., & Gordon, M. (1991) Assessment of competency: The role of neurobehavioral deficits. *Annals of Internal Medicine, 115,* 203–208.

GIW Southern Valve Co. v. Smith, 471 So. 2d 81 (Fla. App. 2 Dist. 1985).

General Electric v. Joiner, 522 U.S. 136 (1997).

Golden, C. J., & Van den Broeck, A. (1998) Potential impact at age of education, scores on H.RNB. score patterns in patients with focal brain injury. *Archives of Clinical Neuropsychology, 13,* 63–694.

Gouvier, W. D., Hayes, J. S., & Smiroldo, B. B. (1998). The significance of base rates test sensitivity, test specificity, and subjects' knowledge of symptoms in assessing TBI sequelae and malingering. In C. Reynolds (Ed.), *Detection of malingering during head injury litigation* (pp. 56–79). New York: Plenum.

Gouvier, W. D., Uddo-Crane, M., & Brown, L. (1998). Base rates of postconcussional symptoms. *Archives of Clinical Neuropsychology, 3,* 273–278.

Greiffenstein, M. F. (2008). Clinical myths of forensic neuropsychology. *Clinical Neuropsychologist, 22*(1), 1–11.

Greiffenstein, M. F., Baker, W. J., Gola, T., Danders, J., & Miller, J. (2002). The fake bad scale in atypical and severe closed head injury litigants. *Journal of Clinical Psychology, 58,* 1591–1600.

Grenitz v. Tomlian, 858 So.2d 999 (Fla. 2003).

Guillmette, J. J., Faust, D., Hart, K., & Arkes, A. R. (1990). A national survey of psychologists will offer neuropsychological services. *Archives of Clinical Neuropsychology, 5,* 373–392.

Hartlage, L. C. (1975). Neuropsychological approaches to predicting outcome of remedial educational strategies for learning disabled children. *Pediatric Psychology, 3*(3), 23.

Hartlage, L. C. (1981). Clinical application of neuropsychological data. *School Psychology Review, 10*(3), 362–366.

Hartlage, L. C. (1983). The evolution of professional neuropsychology. *Bulletin of the National Academy of Neuropsychologists, 3,* 3–4.

Hartlage, L. C. (1995). Neuropsychological complaint base rates in personal injury, revisited. *Archives of Clinical Neuropsychology, 10,* 279–280.

Hartlage, L. C. (1998). Clinical detection of malingering. In C. R. Reynolds (Ed.), *Detection of malingering during head injury litigation* (pp. 239-261). New York: Plenum.

Hartlage, L. C. (2001). Neuropsychological testing of adults: Further considerations for neurologists. *Archives of Clinical Neuropsychology, 16,* 201–213.

Hartlage, L. C., & DeFilippis, N. (1983). History of neuropsychological assessment. In C. J. Golden & P. T. Vicente (Eds.), *Foundations of clinical neuropsychology* (pp. 1–23). New York: Plenum.

Hartlage, L. C., & Green, J. B. (1971). EEG differences in children's reading, spelling and arithmetic ability. *Perceptual and Motor Skills, 32,* 133–134.

Hartlage, L. C., & Long, C. J. (1998). Development of neuropsychology and a professional psychological specialty: History and credentialing. In C. R. Reynolds & E. Fletcher-Jansen (Eds.), *Handbook of clinical child psychology* (2nd ed., pp. 3–16). New York: Plenum.

Hartlage, L. C., & Telzrow, C. F. (1980). The practice of neuropsychology in the US. *Clinical Neuropsychology, 2,* 200–202.

Hartlage, L. C., & Williams B. L. (1991). Assessment of behavioral sequelae of traumatic and CNS insult. *Archives of Clinical Neuropsychology, 6,* 279–286.

Hartlage, L. C., Wilson, D. D., & Patch, P. C. (2001). Persistent neurobehavioral problems following mild traumatic brain injury. *Archives of Clinical Neuropsychology, 16,* 561–570.

Heaton, R., Smith, H., Lehman, R., & Vogt, A. (1978). Prospects for faking behavioral deficits on neuropsychological testing. *Journal of Consulting and Clinical Psychology, 46,* 892–900.

Hecaen, H. (1962). Clinical symptomatology in right and left hemiplegic lesions. In U. B. Mountcastle (Ed.), *Interhemisperic relations and cerebral dominance.* Baltimore: Johns Hopkins Press.

Josephs, K., Whitwell, J. L., Vemuri, P., Senjem, M. L., Boeve, B. F., Knopman, D. S., et al. (2008). The anatomical correlate in semantic dementia. *Neurology, 71,* 1628–1633.

Huntoon v. T.C.I. Cablevision of Colorado, Inc., 969 P.2d 681, 687 (Colo. 1998).

Hutchison v. American Family Mutual Ins. Co., 514 N.W.2d 882 (Iowa 1994).

Jenkins v. United States, 307 F.2d 637 (D.C. Cir. 1962).

John v. Im, 559 S.E.2d 694 (Va. 2002).

Kennedy, C. H. (1993). *Sexual consent and education assessment.* Philadelphia: Drexel University.

Kennedy, C. H. (1999). Assessing competence to consent to sexual activity in the cognitively impaired population. *Journal of Forensic Neuropsychology, 1,* 17–37.

Kinsey v. King, 103 Ill. App. 3d 933, 431 N.E.2d 1316 (Ill. App. 1st Dist. 1982).

Kixmiller, J. S., Briggs, J. R., Hartlage, L. C., & Dean, R. S. (1993). Factor structure of emotional and cognitive behaviors for normals and neurological impaired patients. *Journal of Clinical Psychology, 49*(2), 233–241.

Kumho Tire Co. v. Carmichael, 526 U.S. 137 (1999).

Larrabee, G. J. (2003). Exaggerated MMPI-2 symptom report in personal injury litigants with malingered neurocognitive deficit. *Archives of Clinical Neuropsychology, 18,* 673–686.

Larvie, V. (1994). Evidence: Admissibility of scientific evidence in federal courts. Daubert v. Pharmaceuticals, 1135. Ct. 2786. *Lane & Wafer Law Review, 29,* 275.

Lees-Haley, P. R., English, L. T., & Glenn, W. J. (1991). A fake bad scale on the MMPI-2 for personal injury claimants. *Psychological Reports, 68,* 203–210.

Madrid v. University of California, 105 N.M. 715, 737 P2d 74 (N.M. 1987).

Majestic, A. L. (1986). Amici Curia, North Carolina Psychological Association. N. Carolina Court of Appeals, Horne v. Goodson.

Malloy, P., Bihrle, A., & Duffy, J. (1983) The orbitomedial frontal indexes. *Archives of Clinical Neuropsychology, 8,* 185–201.

Martin, R., Bolter, J., Todd, M., Gouvier, W., & Nicholls, R. (1993). Effects of sophistication and motivation on the detection of malingered memory performance using a computerized forced choice test. *Journal of Clinical and Experimental Neuropsychology, 15,* 867–888.

Martin, R., Gouvier, W., Todd, M., Bolter, J., & Nicholls, R. (1992). Effects of test instructions on malingered memory performance. *Forensic Reports, 5,* 390–397.

McCarthy v. Atwood, 67 Va. Cir. 237, 2005 WL 937271 (Va. Cir. Ct. 2005).

McKinley, W., Brooks, D., & Bond, M. (1983). Post-concessional symptoms, financial compensation and outcomes of severe blunt trauma injury. *Journal of Neurology, Neurosurgery and Psychiatry, 46,* 1084–1091.

Milner, B. (1954). Intellectual function of the temporal lobes. *Psychological Bulletin, 51,* 42–62.

Patch, P. C., & Hartlage, L. C. (2001). Neurological and emotional sequelae of exposure to ethylene oxide. *International Journal of Neuroscience, 106,* 101–107.

Patch, P. C., & Hartlage, L. C. (2003). Behavioral outcomes of mild traumatic brain injury. In A. M. Horton, Jr., & L. Hartlage (Eds.), *Handbook of forensic neuropsychology* (pp. 215–236). New York: Springer Publishing Company.

Purish, A. D., & Sbordone, R. J. (1997). Forensic neuropsychology: Clinical issues and practices. In A. M. Horton, Jr., D. Wedding, & J. Webster (Eds.), The *neuropsychology handbook* (Vol. 2, pp. 215–236). New York: Springer Publishing Company.

Reed, J. E. (1996) . Fixed versus flexible neuropsychological test batteries under the Daubert standard for the admissibility of scientific evidence. *Behavioral Sciences and the Law, 14*, 315–322.

Reitan, R. M., & Wolfson, D. (1997). *The use of the Halstead-Reitan Battery to diagnose brain damage* (pp. 1–3). Presented at the American Trial Lawyers Association Meeting, San Diego, CA.

Reynolds, C. R. (1998). *Detection of malingering during head injury litigation.* New York: Plenum.

Rogers, R. (1988). *Clinical assessment of malingering and deception.* New York: Guilford Press.

Sabianke v. Weaver, 527 S. 2d 1253 (Ala. 1988).

Sanchez v. Derby, 230 Neb. 782, 433 N.W. 2d 523 (Neb. 1989).

Schretlen, D. (1988). The use of psychological tests to identify malingered symptoms of mental disorders. *Clinical Psychology Review, 8*, 451–476.

Seretny, M. L., Dean, R. S., Gray, J. W., & Hartlage, L. C. (1986). The practice of clinical neuropsychology in the United States. *Archives of Clinical Neuropsychology, 1*, 5–12.

Shanok, S. S., & Lewis, D. O. (1981). Medical histories of female delinquents. *Archives of General Psychiatry, 38*, 211–213.

Shilling v. Mobile Analytical Services, Inc., 602 N.E. 2d 1154 (Oh. 1992).

Simmons v. Mullins, 231 PA. Super. 199, 331 A2d 892 (PA Super. 1975).

Slick, D. J., Sherman, E. M. S., & Iverson, G. L. (1999). Diagnostic criteria for malingering cognitive dysfunction: Proposed standards for clinical practice and research. *Clinical Neuropsychologist, 13*, 545–561.

State of Louisiana v. Foret, 628 So. 2d 1116 (LA. 1993).

Sweet, J. J. (1999). Malingering differential diagnosis. In J. J. Sweet (Ed.), *Forensic neuropsychology: Fundamentals and practice* (pp. 255-285). Lisse, The Netherlands: Swets and Zeitlinger.

Trueblood, W. (1994). Qualitative and quantitative characteristics of malingered and other invalid WAIS-R and clinical memory data. *Journal of Clinical and Experimental Neuropsychology, 16*, 597–607.

United States v. Riggleman, 411 F.2d 1190 (4th Cir. 1969).

Willis, W. (1984). Re-analysis of an actuarial approach to neuropsychological diagnosis and consideration of base rates. *Journal of Consulting and Clinical Psychology, 52*(4), 567–569.

Valiulis v. Scheffeos, 191 Ill. App. 3d. 775, 547 N.E. 2d 1289 (Ill. App. 1989).

Wright, F., Bahn, C., & Rieber, R. W. (1980). *Forensic psychology and psychiatry* (Vol. 347). New York: New York Academy of Sciences.

Yeudall, L. T., Fromm-Auch, D., & Davies, S. D. (1982). Neuropsychological impairment of persistent delinquency. *Journal of Nervous and Mental Disease, 170*, 257–265.

Neuropsychology of Intelligence: Forensic Implications

4

Cecil R. Reynolds
Christine L. Castillo
Arthur MacNeill Horton, Jr.

Intellectual functions are largely a product of the overall physiological efficiency of the central nervous system, especially the brain itself. Because neuropsychology is the study of brain-behavior relationships, neuropsychologists have a strong interest in intelligence from both theoretical and clinical perspectives. An individual's level of intelligence is important to establish in clinical exams, as is a baseline of overall cognitive function against which more specific cognitive skills may be compared. This chapter will review the concept of intelligence from a forensic clinical neuropsychological perspective as an aid to understanding implications of normal as well as abnormal intellectual functioning in forensic practice through the discussion of bio-behavioral paradigms related to intelligence. Intelligence as an abstract clinical bio-behavioral concept was first used by Alfred Binet, when the public school officials of Paris, France, requested that Binet develop a proce-

This chapter is based in part on a prior work by the first two authors: Reynolds, C. R., & French, C. (2003). The neuropsychological basis of intelligence. In A. Horton & L. Hartlage (Eds.), *Handbook of forensic neuropsychology*. New York: Springer Publishing Company.

dure to determine which children should be in special education (Binet & Simon, 1905, 1908). Binet, of course, devised the first standardized intelligence test specifically designed for this task. Later, David Wechsler, in New York, developed an intelligence test for adults as a standardized mental status examination to aid in clinical assessment (Wechsler, 1939). Interestingly, Wechsler's older brother was a neurologist and Wechsler saw that the need for a standardized mental status examination for neurological patients was clear. Wechsler had been a research assistant during World War I when 17 million men were assessed with a variety of psychological tests commonly used at that time to determine which men had the intellectual potential to become officers (Wechsler, 1939). Wechsler selected those psychological tests that had been most successful for selecting officers during World War I and then standardized the administration and scoring, and established norms for the intelligence test in large national samples of adults (Wechsler, 1952, 1955). Clinical neuropsychology as a field has had a long-term interest in evaluating intelligence (Horton & Wedding, 1984) and in elaborating in even greater detail specific aspects of cognitive function. Initial clinical neuropsychological assessments were seen as a way of addressing limitations of intelligence testing for the comprehensive assessment of clinical patients, supplementing such batteries as the Wechsler Scales to obtain a more through assessment of intellectual functions.

The Role of "*g*" in Neuropsychological Models of Intelligence

The ancient Greek philosopher Aristotle, tutor of Alexander the Great, first suggested that assessment of intellect may be based on a single mental ability variable, "*g*" (*g*) (Detterman, 1982). The abstract psychometric concept of *g* is a single measure used to describe higher-level human mental abilities. The notion of *g* can be conceptualized as the average of an individual's higher-level mental abilities as assessed by multiple diverse cognitive tasks. Although *g* is an important measure of higher-level mental abilities relative to specific tasks, an individual's scope of cognitive abilities may be best described by assessing task-specific skills (Kaufman, 1994).

Researchers have found *g* to be an extremely important and useful means of conceptualizing overall intellectual ability (Aluja-Fabregat, Colom, Abad, & Juan-Espinosa, 2000; Kane, 2000). Jensen (1998) reviewed the empirical research basis for the presence of a general cognitive ability factor in intelligence. Jensen observed that when a sufficiently large number of tests have been used to assess a sufficiently wide spectrum of mental abilities a *g* factor is always indentified. Jensen also postulated that failures to identify a *g* factor in previous research were based on a failure to utilize a large enough number of tests with a sufficiently large number of diverse item types. Reynolds and French (2003) subsequently averred that the study of *g* and the study of cognitive processing styles should be undertaken as complementary areas of clinical neuropsychology and intelligence research investigation.

Research that noted evidence for simultaneous and successive information processes in the human brain can be viewed as complementary to the concept of a *g* factor. For example, the verbal and performance factors identified in multiple research studies of intelligence testing are examples of separate but related factors in many diverse populations (Reynolds, 1981). The concept of g is also supported by individual differences in the level or efficiency of information processing (Das, Kirby, & Jarman, 1979; Detterman, 1982). Indeed, Travers (1977), Luborsky, Auerbach, Chandler, Cohen, and Bachrach (1971), and Lezak (1995) found in studies of psychotherapy-outcome research that the best predictor of success was the general intellectual level (i.e., g) of the individual receiving psychotherapy. Similarly, the best predictor of rehabilitative success of patients with a number of neurological diseases and disorders is the premorbid level of general intellectual functioning (Golden, 1978). Similar to Halstead's notion of biological intelligence, the concept of g is considered to be limited by the biological integrity and physiological efficiency of the human brain (Brand, 1996; Vernon, 1998). Harmony (1997) and Languis and Miller (1992) reported that research studies using EEG measures, auditory evoked responses, visual evoked responses, and event-related potentials have suggested that physiological measures could be utilized to assess aspects of cognitive ability. Similarly, Jensen's research (1978, 1998) on reaction times and the study of evoked potentials suggests that g is the general physiological efficiency of the central nervous system. Future conceptualizations of intelligence will require elucidation of the method and components of information processing in the brain, as well as the mental ability to use the various information-processing strategies to their fullest potential, conceptualized as the g factor. At the same time, elucidation of brain-behavior models may contribute to understanding the biological basis of intelligence.

Luria's Brain-Behavior Model

Alexander R. Luria, MD, PhD, the noted Russian neuropsychologist, made major contributions to the scientific discipline of neuropsychology. Luria contributed to clinical neuropsychology the concept of the complex functional system (i.e., multiple diverse brain areas subserving particular behavioral abilities) as well as a model of the brain's functioning. Luria used a variety of neuropsychological research tasks based on a cultural-historical theory of higher cognitive functioning to obtain a qualitative evaluation of an individual's neurological status (Horton, 1987). Luria (1970) described sensory and motor functions of the brain as having highly specific functional localizations, while higher-level mental processes required coordination of multiple areas of the brain. Higher-level cognitive functions require multiple areas of the brain to subserve specific complex behaviors, but simple sensory motor functions may be localized in a specific area of the brain (Reynolds, 1981). Specialization for higher-level cognitive tasks is very process specific, and complex processing of information requires coordination of several anatomical sections of the cortex (Ashman & Das, 1980). Luria postulated a paradigm of the brain's higher-level mental processing, which is organized into three major brain components (Luria, 1970). Luria's first component consists of the brain stem, including the reticular formation, midbrain, pons, and medulla. Luria's second component consists of the parietal, occipital, and temporal lobes. Luria's third component of the brain consists of the cerebral cortex anterior to the central sulcus, and the sensory-motor strip. These three brain components were postulated by Luria to function in a dynamic interaction between and among the three brain areas to produce higher-level mental processes (Reynolds, 1981).

Luria owes an intellectual debt to Hughlings Jackson, an English physician who lived in the nineteenth century (Horton, 1987), for the notion of the brain as a dynamic functional system. Luria (1964) noted that successful higher mental processes were based on multiple diverse brain areas communicating and working together. Luria (1961, 1964) also observed that higher-level mental functions may be disrupted by the destruction of a communication channel of the functional system. In addition, Luria (1964) found that disturbances of the higher-level mental functions are mediated in different ways based on the specific localization of the brain damage. Put another way, the functional system may need to use a completely different structure to perform behavioral tasks, if there is specific brain damage (Luria, 1964). Luria qualitatively analyzed the difficulty experienced in performing a neuropsychological task, using his three-component model of brain functioning, to determine the localizing significance of the behavioral disturbance (Luria, 1964). Each component of Luria's brain functioning model is described below, in an overly simplistic fashion, as blocks (Horton, 1987; Reynolds, 1981).

Block One

The first component of the brain includes the brain stem and involves maintaining consistent arousal, attention, and concentration abilities over time. Only if the energy level and tone of the entire cortex provides a stable basis, is it possible to organize the various other functions and processes of the brain. The first brain block includes the reticular formation, the posterior hypothalamic and brain stem portions of the brain. When the first block of the brain has been impaired, there is a lowering of the level of consciousness in the cortex, giving rise to disorganized behavior.

Block Two

The second component of the brain is the area posterior to the central sulcus (i.e., the parietal, occipital, and temporal lobes) and involves receiving sensory input, and integrating and storing information. Block two subserves analysis and synthesis of sensory stimuli (e.g., auditory in the temporal lobes, visual in the occipital lobes, and tactile in the parietal lobes), and each lobe is organized into three hierarchical zones. The *primary zone* sorts and records incoming sensory stimuli. The *secondary zone* receives sensory information from the *primary zone* and organizes the sensory information. The *tertiary zone* merges sensory information from multiple *secondary zones* and organizes complex human behavior. This second block of the brain is primarily receptive in nature.

Block Three

The third component of the brain consists of the frontal lobes and involves the initiation, development, and monitoring of plans for behavior. The third block is postulated to have an executive/managerial role and receives and evaluates organized sensory input from the first and second blocks of the brain (Obrzut & Obrzut, 1982). For example, the frontal lobes are directly connected to the reticular formation in the first block of the brain, and this reciprocal communication mediates the activation of the remainder of the cortex. The frontal lobes thereby regulate arousal, and monitor and direct attention and concentration processes in the brain. Similarly, there are direct connections between the first and second areas of the brain that allow reciprocal communication that facilitates decision making based on sensory input. In the first component of the brain, of course, inputs from both the second and third components are integrated to facilitate the initiation, development, and monitoring of behavioral plans and their timely, efficient, and effective evaluation. The third block of the brain is primarily expressive and generative, and has important regulatory function over higher mental processes. Therefore, human higher-level mental functioning is the result of the dynamic interplay of the three blocks of the brain (Luria, 1964). Because Luria was primarily focused on researching and validating the cultural-historical theory of higher-level mental abilities for the majority of his career, and not on providing clinical services to brain-injured patients (except for his neurological service during World War II in a rehabilitation hospital in the Ural mountains), he did not devote time and effort toward the development of standardized assessment procedures based on his theoretical brain model (Horton, 1987). Rather, in response to clinical interest in Luria's neuropsychological assessment procedures, a standardized version of those procedures was later developed (after Luria's death) in the United States for adults (Golden, Purisch, & Hammeke, 1979) and children (Golden, 1987).

Simultaneous and Successive Cognitive Processes

Complementary to Luria's (1964) theoretical brain model's second block, simultaneous and successive (or sequential) cognitive processes are types of information-processing strategies (Naglieri, 1997). Types of sensory stimuli may be processed more efficiently through either simultaneous or successive means but cognitive processing of stimuli is possible through either simultaneous or successive processing means (Kaufman, 1979). Simultaneous and successive processes are essentially independent of any specific sensory modality (i.e., auditory, visual, tactile, etc.) or type of stimulus (verbal, nonverbal) (Ashman & Das, 1980). The choice of either simultaneous or successive cognitive processing used for a task can depend on the task demands, attention demands required by the task, and preferred means for completing the task (Hall, Gregory, Billinger, & Fisher, 1988; Watters & English, 1995; Willis, 1985). For example, verbal communications can be processed efficiency through linear successive methods such as writing a letter. Alternatively, drawing a visual picture may be processed more efficiently through simultaneous processing strategies.

Simultaneous Processing

Das, Kirby, and Jarman (1979) describe simultaneous processing as the synthesis of separate elements into spatially related groups in which any separate element can be accessed directly. Right occipital and parietal lobes of the brain, in Luria's second block of the brain, are postulated to subserve simultaneous information processing (Naglieri, Kamphaus, & Kaufman, 1983; Willis, 1985). Spatial ability tests, as is well known, are often used as measures of simultaneous processing (Kirby & Das, 1977).

Successive Processing

Das, Kirby, and Jarman (1979) describe successive (sequential) processing as the linear accessing of information in a serial fashion. The left temporal lobe of the brain, in Luria's second block of the brain, is postulated to subserve successive (sequential) processing (Naglieri, Kamphaus, & Kaufman, 1983; Willis, 1985). Maintenance of a temporal order of input of information is crucial to successful successive processing. For example, learning to read, as is well known, is based on a phonetic approach that requires rapid identification of each letter of a word in succession and conceptualizing the word based on the sounds each letter makes and is best accomplished by means of successive processing (Gunnison, Kaufman, & Kaufman, 1982).

Hemispheric Specialization and Simultaneous and Successive Cognitive Processes

As may be seen from the above material, different cerebral hemispheres appear to be somewhat more efficient in either simultaneous or successive processing. This information processing distinction is extremely oversimplified here, but it appears that the left cerebral hemisphere may be more efficient in performing linguistic, serial, and analytical tasks. Similarly, the right hemisphere it appears may be more efficient in performing visual-spatial and holistic tasks (Bever, 1975; Bogen, 1969; Dean & Reynolds, 1997; Gazzaniga, 1970; Harnad, Doty, Goldstein, Jaynes, & Krauthamer, 1977; Kinsbourne, 1978a, 1997; Naglieri, Kamphaus, & Kaufman, 1983; Schwartz, Davidson, & Maer, 1975; Segalowitz & Gruber, 1977; Willis, 1985). Table 4.1 describes modes of information processing related to hypothesized differences in cerebral hemispheric processing. Use of specific cognitive processing modes may optimize the efficiency of these hemispheric brain functions.

As previously noted, cerebral hemispheric asymmetries of functioning are preferences for *process-specific* strategies rather than *stimulus-specific* strategies. Simply put, the mode of cognitive processing for the task performance selected is determined by multiple factors that include, but are not limited to, specific task demands, level of attention required for the task, individual mental abilities, genetics, and cultural traditions (Cumming & Rodda, 1985; Hall, Gregory, Billinger, & Fisher, 1988; McCallum & Merritt, 1983; Watters & English, 1995; Willis, 1985). In addition, the need for specific types of manipulation of stimuli may be the source of hemispheric differences (see, for example, Grimshaw, 1998; Mateer, Rapport, & Kettrick, 1984; Obrzut, Obrzut, Bryden, & Bartels, 1985; Ornstein, Johnstone, Herron, & Swencionis, 1980; Piccirilli, D'Alessandro, Mazzi, Sciarma, & Testa, 1991; Tous, Fusté, & Vidal, 1995). Preferences for either simultaneous or successive processing may have significant implications for successful adaptive human functioning (Reynolds, 1981).

4.1 Functions of the Right and Left Hemispheres*

Right Hemisphere		Left Hemisphere	
Processing Modes	**Representative Reference**	**Processing Modes**	**Representative Reference**
Simultaneous	Hall, Gregory, Billinger, & Fisher, 1988	Sequential	Bell, 1990; Bloom, 2000
Holistic Visual/ Nonverbal	Dimond & Beaumont, 1974 Sperry, 1974	Temporal Analytic	Mills, 1977 Morgan, McDonald, & McDonald, 1971
Imagery Spatial Reasoning	Seamon & Gazzaniga, 1973 Sperry, 1974		
Nonverbal Functions	**Representative Reference**	**Verbal Functions**	**Representative Reference**
Depth Perception	Carmon & Bechtoldt, 1969	Speech	Wada, 1949 Reitan, 1955
Melodic Perception	Shankweiler, 1966	General Language/Verbal Abilities	Mateer, Rapport, & Kettrick, 1984
Tactile Perception (Integration)	Boll, 1974	Calculation/Arithmetic	Mitsuda, 1991
Haptic Perception	Wittelson, 1974	Abstract Verbal Thought	Watters & English, 1995 Reynolds & Horton, 2006
Nonverbal Sound Recognition	Wright & Ashman, 1991	Writing (Composition)	Hecaen & Marcie, 1974
Motor Integration	Gorynia & Egenter, 2000 Reynolds, 2000	Complex Motor Functions	Dimond & Beaumont, 1974 Reynolds, 2003
Visual Constructive Performance	Capruso, Hamsher, & Benton, 1995	Body Orientation	Gerstmann, 1957
Pattern Recognition	Capruso, Hamsher, & Benton, 1995	Vigilance	Dimond & Beaumont, 1974

*Adapted from Dean (1984) and Kamphaus and Reynolds (1987).

Hemisphericity and Cognitive Processing

Hemisphericity (Reynolds, 1981) has been conceptualized as preference for a particular cognitive information-processing style but is unrelated to an individual's personal cerebral dominance. A frequently used definition is that hemisphericity is the tendency of an individual to rely primarily upon the information-processing style of one hemisphere (Reynolds, 1981). Luria's theoretical brain model appears to be essentially consistent with hemispheric specialization, because the extant empirical neuropsychological research on hemisphericity supports Luria's model (Dean & Reynolds, 1997). In recent years, the emerging conceptualization of preferred higher-level cognitive style (hemisphericity) has subsumed and elaborated upon the earlier notion of cerebral dominance as a major theoretical contribution in understanding human brain-behavior relationships. The dominant information-processing modality of an individual may or may not be optimal for adaptive functioning in specific situations. Optimal adaptive functioning is conceptualized as requiring the utilization of both modes of information processing, either separately or in conjunction with one another, and also being able to shift the cognitive information processing mode in response to multiple factors (Gazzaniga, 1974, 1975). On the other hand, dysfunctional hemisphericity is conceptualized to possibly impede adaptive functioning (Newell & Rugel, 1981; Roubinek, Bell, & Cates, 1987). As earlier mentioned, the original concept of cerebral dominance (which traditionally referred simply to the hemisphere of the brain responsible for language, but which has since lost this meaning and has become a vague term used in many nonspecific ways in the literature as well as in popular media) has evolved into the more sophisticated theoretical notion of hemispheric specialization (Reynolds, 1981). Recent research has demonstrated that identifying a student's preferred mode of cognitive information processing (hemisphericity) may be advantageous in terms of remediating children's academic learning problems (Faust, Kravetz, & Babkoff, 1993; Gunnison, Kaufman, & Kaufman, 1982; Paquette, Tosoni, Lassonde, & Peretz, 1996; Roubinek, Bell, & Cates, 1987; Sonnier, 1992; Sonnier & Goldsmith, 1985).

Thus far, the research on intelligence and clinical neuropsychology has focused on intelligence as a single factor (g), a brain-based behavior model, and two different modes of cognitive information processing. The next section will focus on further elaboration of higher level mental abilities directly related to landmark research that formed the empirical basis for many of the most frequently used measures in contemporary clinical neuropsychology.

Halstead's Theory of Biological Intelligence

Halstead (1947) established a very influential experimental brain-behavior research program at the University of Chicago Medical School around the time of World War II. As a result of Halstead's experimental research program many experimental psychometric measures were first identified and initially validated as neuropsychological tests, sensitive to the biological integrity of the human brain (Horton & Wedding, 1984). Halstead was essentially interested in the mental abilities subserved by the intact human frontal lobes in a theoretical sense. This theoretical interest clearly overlapped with the concept of intelligence (Halstead, 1947). Halstead theorized that there were two types of human intelligence: biological intelligence and psychometric intelligence. Psychometric intelligence was postulated by Halstead to be what was measured by the intelligence tests of that time, such as the Stanford-Binet of the day, or the contemporary Wechsler intelligence tests (Halstead, 1947). Biological intelligence as distinct from psychometric intelligence was postulated by Halstead as human adaptive abilities subserved by an intact uninjured brain. He developed the concept of biological intelligence because he saw that the measures of psychometric intelligence in his day were extremely limited in terms of comprehensively assessing patients who had been previously brain injured (Halstead, 1947). Halstead observed that many brain injured patients were able to score well on measures of psychometric intelligence despite very significant and well documented brain damage. Halstead postulated that the intelligence tests, available for use before, during, and after World War II were extremely limited in their ability to comprehensively assess human adaptive abilities. Therefore, he theorized that there must be some other abstract theoretical construct that was sensitive to human adaptive abilities. Halstead later developed a research program to determine the nature of the hypothesized missing abstract theoretical construct. He termed his postulated abstract theoretical construct, of course, "biological intelligence." Halstead's (1947) experimental research program had a number of exceptional features. First, he performed naturalistic observations (including involvement in social situations such as parties) of well documented, formerly brain injured patients to determine in which everyday work and social situations brain damaged patients had adaptive problems. Second, he assessed the brain damaged former patients on a wide variety of the experimental psychology tasks of that time to determine on which measures brain damaged individuals had deficits in their day-to-day application of cognitive skills to life functions. Third, he then selected ten measures that were most sensitive to deficits, from the much larger number of experimental psychology tests, for further study in his research program on biological intelligence (Halstead, 1947). Halstead then assessed large numbers of well documented brain damaged individuals with these highly specific measures of cognitive skills. He postulated that his selected set of sensitive measures represented the abstract concept of biological intelligence and were distinct from psychometric intelligence.

Halstead (1947) then factor analyzed the intercorrelation matrix of the more specific tests. Four basic factors of biological intelligence were extracted. Halstead described the four adaptive behavior factors as follows:

C—The Integrative Field Factor

This factor is the ability to adapt to new situations and to integrate new experiences and information (Reitan, 1994). Factor C had loadings on the Halstead Category Test, the Henmon-Nelson Tests of Mental Ability, the Speech-Sounds Perception Test, the Halstead Finger Oscillation Test, and the Halstead Time-Sense Test (Halstead, 1947).

A—The Abstraction Factor

This factor is the ability to draw meaning from a series of events or to hold in mind abstract nonverbal ideas without the use of past experience. Factor A had loadings from the Carlo Hollow-Square Performance Test for Intelligence, the Halstead Category Test, the Halstead Tactual Performance Test (memory component), and Halstead Tactual Performance Test (localization component) (Halstead, 1947).

P—The Power

This factor is the reserve power available to an amplifier not already functioning at peak ability. Factor P had loadings on the Halstead Flicker-Fusion Test, the Halstead Tactual Performance Test (recall component), the Halstead Dynamic Visual Field Test (central form), and the Halstead Dynamic Visual Field Test (central color) (Halstead, 1947).

D—The Directional Factor

This factor is an attentional component. Factor D had loadings on the Halstead Tactual Performance Test (speed component) and the Halstead Dynamic Visual Field Test (peripheral component) (Halstead, 1947). The first three factors, C, A, and P, were postulated as process factors of biological intelligence, and D is the factor through which expression of these processes was directed.

It was postulated that individuals with known brain damage have suffered impairment in their ability to perform tasks represented by the factors. Halstead's tests measuring the four factors differentiated between individuals with documented head injury and individuals with no documented history of head injury, and an average of the measures performed better than any single measure in differentiating these individuals (Halstead, 1947). Halstead combined the ten best discriminating test scores with equal weighting and averaged the ten test scores to create an index of impairment, which was named the Halstead Impairment Index (HII) (Reitan, 1994). While Halstead (1947) had thought that the HII was related to the integrity of the frontal lobes, subsequent experimental research studies couldn't cross-validate a relationship between the frontal lobes and HII (Reitan, 1975).

Halstead's first doctoral student, Ralph Reitan (1994) recognized the need for a comprehensive clinical battery of neuropsychological tests in order to make behavioral diagnoses of brain damaged patients. Reitan (1975) felt that Halstead's original battery of tests could serve as the core of a comprehensive clinical battery of neuropsychological tests. Interestingly, prior to meeting Halstead, Reitan, the son of a Lutheran minister, had planned to study counseling psychology with Carl Rogers at Ohio State University, but while working at a Veterans Hospital to earn money for graduate school, Reitan encountered a physician who had had a stroke but scored above the 85th percentile on all of the psychological tests available to Reitan at that time (immediately after World War II). Despite the excellent psychological test scores, the physician who had had a stroke still complained of significant difficulties practicing medicine. Reitan visited Halstead because he had learned of Halstead's research program on the frontal lobes and biological intelligence, and the behavioral effects of brain damage in humans. After meeting Reitan and learning that Reitan intended to go to graduate school, Halstead invited Reitan to join him at the University of Chicago as a doctoral student. After graduating, Halstead later developed a clinical brain-behavior research program at the University of Indiana Medical School (Reitan, 1994). A unique feature of Reitan's research program was that neuropsychological testing of neurology and neurosurgical clinical patients with documented brain damage was assessed "blindly." The blind assessment research procedure was similar in intent to blind review of research manuscripts submitted to a peer-reviewed scientific journal or double-blind research study designs that prevent nonspecific factors from influencing scientific judgments or research results. Reitan had all brain-damaged patients assessed by neuropsychological technicians and saw only the test results, not the patients. This procedure was instituted in order to validate that his diagnostic judgments were based solely on the neuropsychological test results and not on clinical impressions from observing the brain-damaged patients. Put another way, Reitan needed to prove to neurologists and neurosurgeons that his neuropsychological tests were of value for diagnosing brain-damaged patients in the context of a neurology or neurosurgery ward. Based on diagnostic errors in interpreting neuropsychological test results on brain-damaged patients with well documented lesion over many years, Reitan (1994) modified and augmented the neuropsychological test battery based on Halstead's tests as a core to improve diagnostic accuracy (Hevern, 1980; Reed, 1985; Swiercinsky, 1979). It is noteworthy that formal intelligence testing (the age-appropriate Wechsler Intelligence Scale of the day) has always been included as an integral portion of Reitan's comprehensive clinical neuropsychological test battery, in addition to Halstead's core tests and a number of additional test procedures that were added to assess brain areas not identified by the aforementioned measures.

Reitan's work (Reitan, 1955, 1964a, 1966, 1975; Reitan & Davison, 1974; Wheeler & Reitan, 1962) has been well supported by empirical research. Over many years, Reitan developed and validated, as sensitive to the effects of brain damage in human beings, the Halstead-Reitan Neuropsychological Test Battery (HRNTB). The HRNTB is the most extensively researched, comprehensive neuropsychological assessment battery (Reitan & Wolfson, 1996), and versions of the HRNTB are widely used throughout the United States and internationally. There is a misconception that the HRNTB is a "fixed neuropsychological battery" that cannot be augmented or adapted to the clinical needs of patients. Rather, the recommended approach is to include additional neuropsychological tests when indicated by clinical and educational needs while still maintaining a standard battery that is given to all patients capable of completing the test.

Although Halstead and Reitan's work (Horton & Wedding, 1984) identified a number of brain-behavior sensitive measures, their factor structure in some ways is very similar to the factor structure found for the age-appropriate Wechsler scales (Kamphaus, 2001; Kaufman, 1994).

Subsequent factor analysis studies with various age groups found comparable results. For example research with adult neuropsychiatric patients (Fowler, Zillmer, & Newman, 1988) found five factors (verbal comprehension, perceptual organization, sensory-attention, primary-motor and tactual-spatial abilities). A study of older children ages 9–14 (Brooks, Dean, & Gray, 1989) found four factors (simple motor, tactile kinesthesis, memory/attention and nonverbal visual-spatial memory). A study with children ages 9 to 12 (Francis, Fletcher, Rourke, & York, 1992) found a five-factor model (simple motor skill, complex visual-spatial relations, simple spatial motor operations, motor steadiness, and speeded motor sequencing). In addition, a study with children age 5 to 7 (Foxcroft, 1989) found six factors (analytic-synthetic visual motor ability, perceptual organization, cross-modality motoric efficiency, directed motor speed patterned critical discrimination and strength). In sum, the multiple-factor analysis studies are relatively similar to research results found from the age-appropriate Wechsler scales (Kamphaus, 2001; Kaufman, 1994). Thus, conceptualizations of intelligence have progressed far beyond the single measure "g," two cognitive information processing modes, and the multiple neuropsychological factors identified by Halstead (1947). In the next section, a new conceptualization of clinical neuropsychology and intelligence will be briefly described.

Carroll's Theory of Intelligence

Carroll's (1993) seminal and often cited three-stratum theory of intelligence has demonstrated that the latent traits tapped by intelligence tests were test-battery independent. Carroll demonstrated that numerous tests measured the same crystallized, visual-perceptual, and memory abilities. Stratum three is composed of one construct only, g. Multiple studies of intelligence have demonstrated that psychometric g accounts for the major portion of variance assessed by intelligence test batteries. In addition, the consistent finding that the correlations of intelligence tests with important social outcomes, such as academic achievement and occupational attainment, are directly related to the amount of g measured by the intelligence test. Put another way, tests that include large amounts of g are better predictors of important outcomes than are tests with low amounts of g. While the essential nature of g is not yet fully understood, tests with large amounts of g have important purposes in society, especially in terms of prediction of mental abilities and success in school and the workplace. The psychometric concept of g remains useful even though the actual mechanisms of action are not yet completely understood by scientists.

Carroll's second-stratum theoretical hierarchy consists of traits that are assessed by combinations of first-stratum measures. First-stratum measures are typically single subtests that measure a trait of interest. Combinations of first-stratum measures can become second-stratum measures and can result in enhanced measurement of complex traits such as verbal and nonverbal intelligence. Second-stratum measures can be combined into a composite measure that will allow for the measurement of a complex third-stratum trait, such as intelligence.

Second-stratum traits include concepts such as fluid intelligence, crystallized intelligence, general memory and learning, broad visual perception, and broad auditory perception and processing speed. It is important to appreciate that multiple scientific studies have found that second-stratum traits can be ranked in terms of their ability to assess g (Kamphaus, 2001). For example, those subtests that involve reasoning abilities are superb measures of g. Higher-order abstraction abilities include general sequential reasoning, induction, deduction, syllogisms, series tasks, matrix reasoning, analogies, and quantitative reasoning among others (Carroll, 1993).Therefore those second-stratum factors that are the best measures of g are the best measures to include in an intelligence test that seeks to accurately and effectively assess important social outcomes. The recently published Reynolds Intellectual Assessment Scale (RIAS) (Reynolds & Kamphaus, 2003) follows the more contemporary Carroll (1993) theoretical model of intelligence and has demonstrated impressive evidence for exemplary validity and reliability, as well as being very user friendly for administration and scoring. Another very noteworthy feature of the RIAS is the fact the test has been demonstrated not to have disparate impact when used to assess members of minority groups. The RIAS has been demonstrated to be a significant advance in the assessment of intelligence.

Discussion: Neuropsychology of Intelligence

The concept of intelligence is related to the biological integrity of the brain. Clearly, this chapter has demonstrated that the concept of intelligence can be assessed as a single measure, two cognitive information processing modes, as well as a handful of different cognitive factors derived from factor-analysis research studies. As conceptualized by Carroll's (1993) three-stratum theory of intelligence, the latent mental traits are test-battery independent. Carroll also demonstrated that numerous tests measured the same latent mental traits tapped by intelligence tests. Carroll's third-stratum is composed of one construct only, g. As mentioned earlier, multiple research studies have demonstrated that psychometric g accounts for the major portion of variance assessed by intelligence test batteries. Also, Carroll's second stratum consists of traits that are assessed by combinations of first-stratum measures. In turn, first-stratum measures are typically single subtests that measure a trait of interest. Combinations of first-stratum measures can form second-stratum measures and measure higher-level cognitive mental abilities such as fluid intelligence, crystallized intelligence, general memory and learning, broad visual perception, broad auditory perception, and processing speed. Moreover, second-stratum measures can be also be combined into a complex third-stratum trait, such as general intelligence conceptualized as g.

Therefore, intelligence can be conceptualized on multiple theoretical levels. Intelligence can be seen as represented by a single score that has impressive predictive abilities, two different cognitive processing modes that have implications for mental functioning, and multiple other higher-level mental ability factors that represent important cognitive skills. Carroll's 1993 theoretical model seems to include aspects of the various conceptualizations of intelligence. Further elucidations of the concept of intelligence are likely to require a better understanding of how biology and human experience relate to human brain functioning.

Various hemispheric brain-mechanism developments are assisted by a wealth of cultural experiences, as suggested by Luria (1966, 1973). Intelligence appears to be both genetically based and dependent on the nurturance of the environment pre- and postnatally. Intelligence has been conceptualized as largely influenced by the person's environmental history (for a discussion of Luria's cultural-historical theory, see Horton, 1987, and Reynolds, 1981), but also with a genetic influence mediating the functional development of the various anatomical structures of the brain. Intelligence appears to be facilitated by both the physiological efficiency of the brain and the hemispheric information processing strategies through which intelligence is externalized. Put another way, intelligence is related to an individual's level of mental function as well as an individual's ability to adapt to various life circumstances (Pallier, Roberts, & Stankov, 2000).

This chapter has focused primarily on previously developed theories of intelligence and related neuropsychological studies that support the biology of intelligence. The further developments of the theoretical foundations of intelligence appear likely to continue to elucidate how the human brain carries out higher-order thinking (Reynolds & Horton, 2006). Nonetheless, the important concept of g would appear very likely to remain central to any future theory of human intelligence. Also, the most interesting contemporary conceptualization of intelligence appears to be Carroll's (1993) theoretical model. In addition, it is likely that new knowledge regarding the different modes of cognitive processing in the human, as noted by Das, Kirby, and Jarman (1979), will be important for further elaboration of the mental mechanisms and biological substrates of higher-order thinking. Although a number of new measures of intelligence have been developed in the past two decades (see, for example, Kaufman & Kaufman, 1983; Naglieri & Das, 1996; Reynolds & Kamphaus, 2003), much additional research concerning the elaboration of mental factors related to the neuropsychology of intelligence is urgently needed. In the future, the pace of new knowledge is expected to increase, and new, more differentiated and complex understandings of human intelligence are expected (Reynolds & Horton, 2006). The hope and expectation is that the material included in this chapter may be of some value in facilitating this area of research and contribute to the amelioration of human suffering and the promotion of the development of increasingly more effective neuropsychological services for children, adolescents, adults, and the elderly.

References

Aluja-Fabregat, A., Colom, R., Abad, F., & Juan-Espinosa, M. (2000). Sex differences in general intelligence defined as g among young adolescents. *Personality and Individual Differences, 28,* 813–820.

Ashman, A. F., & Das, J. P. (1980). Relation between planning and simultaneous-successive processing. *Perceptual and Motor Skills, 51,* 371–382.

Bever, T. G. (1975). Cerebral asymmetries in humans are due to the differentiation of two incompatible processes: Holistic and analytic. In D. Aaronson & R. Reiber (Eds.), *Developmental psycholinguistics and communication disorders.* New York: New York Academy of Sciences.

Binet, A., & Simon, T. (1905). New methods for the diagnosis of the intellectual level of subnormals. *L'annee Psychologique, 11,* 191–244.

Binet, A., & Simon, T. (1908). The development of intelligence in the child. *L'annee Psychologique, 14,* 1–90.

Bogen, J. E. (1969). The other side of the brain: Parts I, II, and III. *Bulletin of the Los Angeles Neurological Society, 34,* 73–105, 135–162, 191–203.

Brand, C. (1996). Doing something about g. *Intelligence, 22,* 311–326.

Brooks, D. A., Dean, R. S., & Gray, J. W. (1989). HRNB factors with simultaneous-successive marker variables. *International Journal of Neuroscience, 46*(3–4), 157–160.

Carroll, J. B. (1993). *Human cognitive abilities: A survey of factor analytic studies.* New York: Cambridge University Press.

Cumming, C. E., & Rodda, M. (1985). The effects of auditory deprivation on successive processing. *Canadian Journal of Behavioural Science, 17,* 232–245.

Das, J. P., Kirby, J. R., & Jarman, R. F. (1979). *Simultaneous and successive cognitive processes.* New York: Academic Press.

Dean, R. S., & Reynolds, C. R. (1997). Cognitive processing and self-report of lateral preference. *Neuropsychology Review, 7,* 127–142.

Detterman, D. K. (1982). Does "g" exist? *Intelligence, 6,* 99–108.

Faust, M., Kravetz, S., & Babkoff, H. (1993). Hemisphericity and top-down processing of language. *Brain and Language, 44,* 1–18.

Fowler, P. C., Zillmer, E., & Newman, A. C. (1988). A multifactor model of the Halstead-Reitan Neuropsychological Test Battery and its relationship to cognitive status and psychiatric diagnosis. *Journal of Clinical Psychology, 44*(6), 898–906.

Foxcroft, C. D. (1989). Factor analysis of the Reitan-Indiana Neuropsychological Test Battery. *Perceptual and Motor Skills, 69*(3, Pt. 2), 1303–1313.

Francis, D. J., Fletcher, J. M., Rourke, B. P., & York, M. J. (1992). A five-factor model for the motor, psychomotor and visual-spatial tests used in the neuropsychological assessment of children. *Journal of Clinical and Experimental Neuropsychology, 14*(4), 625–637.

Gazzaniga, M. S. (1970). *The bisected brain*. New York: Appleton.

Gazzaniga, M. S. (1974). Cerebral dominance viewed as a decision system. In S. Dimond & J. Beaumont (Eds.), *Hemisphere functions in the human brain*. London: Halstead Press.

Gazzaniga, M. S. (1975, May). Recent research on hemispheric lateralization of the human brain: Review of the split-brain. *UCLA Educator*, pp. 9–12.

Golden, C. J. (1978). *Diagnosis and rehabilitation in clinical neuropsychology*. Springfield, IL: Charles C. Thomas.

Golden, C. J. (1987). *Luria-Nebraska Neuropsychological Battery Children's Revision*. Los Angeles: Western Psychological Services.

Golden, C. J., Purisch, A. D., & Hammeke, T. A. (1979). *The Luria-Nebraska Neuropsychological Test Battery: A manual for clinical and experimental uses*. Lincoln, NE: The University of Nebraska Press.

Grimshaw, G. M. (1998). Integration and interference in the cerebral hemispheres: Relations with hemispheric specialization. *Brain and Cognition, 36*, 108–127.

Gunnison, J., Kaufman, N. L., & Kaufman, A. S. (1982). Reading remediation based on sequential and simultaneous processing. *Academic Therapy, 17*, 297–306.

Hall, C. W., Gregory, G., Billinger, E., & Fisher, T. (1988). Field independence and simultaneous processing in preschool children. *Perceptual and Motor Skills, 66*, 891–897.

Halstead, W. C. (1947). *Brain and intelligence*. Chicago: University of Chicago Press.

Harmony, T. (1997). Psychophysiological evaluation of neuropsychological disorders in children. In C. R. Reynolds & E. Fletcher-Janzen (Eds.), *Handbook of clinical child neuropsychology* (2nd ed., pp. 356–370). New York: Plenum Press.

Harnad, S., Doty, R. W., Goldstein, L., Jaynes, J., & Krauthamer, G. (Eds.). (1977). *Lateralization in the nervous system*. New York: Academic Press.

Hevern, V. W. (1980). Recent validity studies of the Halstead-Reitan approach to clinical neuropsychological assessment: A critical review. *Clinical Neuropsychology, 2*, 49–61.

Horton, A. M., Jr. (1987). Luria's contributions to clinical and behavioral neuropsychology. *Neuropsychology, 1*(2), 39–44.

Horton, A. M., Jr., & Wedding, D. (1984) *Clinical and behavioral neuropsychology*. New York: Praeger.

Jensen, A. R. (1978, September). *"g": Outmoded concept or unconquered frontier?* Address at the annual meeting of the American Psychological Association, New York.

Jensen, A. R. (1998). *The g factor: The science of mental ability*. Westport, CT: Praeger.

Kamphaus, R. W. (2001). *Clinical assessment of child and adolescent intelligence* (2nd ed.). Boston: Allyn and Bacon.

Kane, H. D. (2000). A secular decline in Spearman's g: Evidence from the WAIS, WAIS-R and WAIS-III. *Personality and Individual Differences, 29*, 561–566.

Kaufman, A. S. (1979). Cerebral specialization and intelligence testing. *Journal of Research and Development in Education, 12*, 96–107.

Kaufman, A. S. (1994). *Intelligence testing with the WISC-III*. New York: John Wiley.

Kaufman, A. S., & Kaufman, N. L. (1983). *Administration and scoring manual for the Kaufman Assessment Battery for Children*. Circle Pines, MN: American Guidance Service.

Kinsbourne, M. (1978). Biological determinants of functional bisymmetry and asymmetry. In M. Kinsbourne (Ed.), *Asymmetrical function of the brain*. Cambridge: Cambridge University Press.

Kinsbourne, M. (1997). Mechanisms and development of cerebral lateralization in children. In C. R. Reynolds & E. Fletcher-Janzen (Eds.), *Handbook of clinical child neuropsychology* (2nd ed., pp. 102–119). New York: Plenum Press.

Kirby, J. R., & Das, J. P. (1977). Reading achievement, IQ, and simultaneous-successive processing. *Journal of Educational Psychology, 69*, 564–570.

Languis, M. L., & Miller, D. C. (1992). Luria's theory of brain functioning: A model for research in cognitive psychophysiology. *Educational Psychologist, 27*, 493–511.

Lezak, M. D. (1995). *Neuropsychological assessment* (3rd ed.). New York: Oxford University Press.

Luborsky, L., Auerbach, A. H., Chandler, M., Cohen, J., & Bachrach, H. M. (1971). Factors influencing the outcome of psychotherapy: A review of quantitative research. *Psychological Bulletin, 75*, 145–185.

Luria, A. R. (1961). *The role of speech in the regulation of normal and abnormal behavior*. Oxford: Pergamon Press.

Luria, A. R. (1964). Neuropsychology in the local diagnosis of brain damage. *Cortex, 1*, 3–18.

Luria, A. R. (1966). *Higher cortical functions in man*. New York: Basic Books.

Luria, A. R. (1970). The functional organization of the brain. *Scientific American, 222*, 66–78.

Luria, A. R. (1973). *The working brain*. London: Penguin.

Mateer, C. A., Rapport, R. L., & Kettrick, C. (1984). Cerebral organization of oral and signed language responses: Case study evidence from amytal and cortical stimulation studies. *Brain and Language, 21*, 123–135.

McCallum, R. S., & Merritt, F. M. (1983). Simultaneous-successive processing among college students. *Journal of Psychoeducational Assessment, 1*, 85–93.

Naglieri, J. A. (1997). Planning, attention, simultaneous, and successive theory and the Cognitive Assessment System: A new theory-based measure of intelligence. In D. P. Flanagan, J. L. Genshaft, & P. L. Harrison (Eds.), *Contemporary intellectual assessment: Theories, tests, and issues* (pp. 247–267). New York: Guilford Press.

Naglieri, J. A., & Das, J. P. (1996). *Das-Naglieri cognitive assessment system.* Chicago: Riverside.

Naglieri, J. A., Kamphaus, R. W., & Kaufman, A. S. (1983). The Luria-Das simultaneous-successive model applied to the WISC-R. *Journal of Psychoeducational Assessment, 1*, 25-34.

Newell, D., & Rugel, R. P. (1981). Hemispheric specialization in normal and disabled readers. *Journal of Learning Disabilities, 14*, 296–298.

Obrzut, J. E., & Obrzut, A. (1982). Neuropsychological perspectives in pupil services: Practical application of Luria's model. *Journal of Research and Development in Education, 15*, 38–47.

Obrzut, J. E., Obrzut, A., Bryden, M. P., & Bartels, S. G. (1985). Information processing and speech lateralization in learning-disabled children. *Brain and Language, 25*, 87–101.

Ornstein, R., Johnstone, J., Herron, J., & Swencionis, C. (1980). Differential right hemisphere engagement in visuospatial tasks. *Neuropsychologia, 18*, 49–64.

Pallier, G., Roberts, R. D., & Stankov, L. (2000). Biological versus psychometric intelligence: Halstead's (1947) distinction revisted. *Archives of Clinical Neuropsychology, 15*, 205–226.

Paquette, C., Tosoni, C., Lassonde, M., & Peretz, I. (1996). Atypical hemispheric specialization in intellectual deficiency. *Brain and Language, 52*, 474–483.

Piccirilli, M., D'Alessandro, P., Mazzi, P., Sciarma, T., & Testa, A. (1991). Cerebral organization for language in Down's Syndrome patients. *Cortex, 27*, 41–47.

Reed, J. (1985). The contributions of Ward Halstead, Ralph Reitan and their associates. *International Journal of Neuroscience, 25*, 289–293.

Reitan, R. M. (1955). Certain differential effects of left and right cerebral lesions in human adults. *Journal of Comparative and Physiological Psychology, 48*, 474–477.

Reitan, R. M. (1964a). Psychological deficits resulting from cerebral lesions in man. In J. M. Warren & K. Akert (Eds.), *The frontal granular cortex and behavior.* New York: McGraw-Hill.

Reitan, R. M. (1964b). Relationships between neurological and psychological variables and their implications for reading instruction. In K. A. Robinson (Ed.), *Meeting individual differences in reading.* Chicago: University of Chicago Press.

Reitan, R. M. (1966). A research program on the psychological effects of brain lesions in human beings. *International Review of Research in Mental Retardation, 1*, 153–218.

Reitan, R. M. (1975). Assessment of brain-behavior relationships. In P. McReynolds (Ed.), *Advances in psychological assessment: Vol. III.* San Francisco: Jossey-Bass.

Reitan, R. M. (1994). Ward Halstead's contributions to neuropsychology and the Halstead-Reitan Neuropsychological Test Battery. *Journal of Clinical Psychology, 50*, 47–69.

Reitan, R. M., & Davison, L. A. (1974). *Clinical neuropsychology: Current status and applications.* Washington, DC: V. H. Winston.

Reitan, R. M., & Wolfson, D. (1996). Theoretical, methodological, and validational bases of the Halstead-Reitan Neuropsychological Test Battery. In I. Grant & K. M. Adams (Eds.), *Neuropsychological assessment of neuropsychiatric disorders* (2nd ed., pp. 3–42). New York: Oxford University Press.

Reynolds, C. R. (1981). The neuropsychological basis of intelligence. In G. Hynd & J. Obrzut (Eds.), *Neuropsychological assessment and the school-aged child.* New York: Grune & Stratton.

Reynolds, C. R., & French, C. (2003). Neuropsychological basis of intelligence: Revisited. In A. M. Horton, Jr., & L. C. Hartlage (Eds.), *Handbook of forensic neuropsychology.* New York: Springer Publishing Company.

Reynolds, C. R., & Horton, A. M., Jr. (2006). *Test of verbal conceptualization and fluency: Examiner's manual.* Austin TX: PRO-ED.

Reynolds, C. R., & Kamphaus, R. W. (2003). *Reynolds intellectual assessment scales.* Odessa, FL: PAR.

Roubinek, D. L., Bell, M. L., & Cates, L. A. (1987). Brain hemispheric preference of intellectually gifted children. *Roeper Review, 10*, 120–122.

Schwartz, G. E., Davidson, R. J., & Maer, F. (1975). Right hemisphere lateralization for emotion in the human brain: Interactions with cognition. *Science, 190*, 286–288.

Segalowitz, S. J., & Gruber, F. A. (Eds.). (1977). *Language development and neurological theory*. New York: Academic Press.

Sonnier, I. L. (1992). Hemisphericity as a key to understanding individual differences. In I. L. Sonnier (Ed.), *Hemisphericity as a key to understanding individual differences* (pp. 6–8). Springfield, IL: Charles C Thomas.

Sonnier, I. L., & Goldsmith, J. (1985). The nature of human brain hemispheres: The basis for some individual differences. In I. L. Sonnier (Ed.), *Methods and techniques of holistic education* (pp. 17–25). Springfield, IL: Charles C Thomas.

Swiercinsky, D. P. (1979). Factorial pattern description and comparison of functional abilities in neuropsychological assessment. *Perceptual and Motor Skills, 48*, 231–241.

Tous, J. M., Fusté, A., & Vidal, J. (1995). Hemispheric specialization and individual differences in cognitive processing. *Personality and Individual Differences, 19*, 463–470.

Travers, R. M. W. (1977). *Essentials of learning* (4th ed.). New York: MacMillan.

Vernon, P. A. (1998). From the cognitive to the biological: A sketch of Arthur Jensen's contributions to the study of *g*. *Intelligence, 26*, 267–271.

Watters, J. J., & English, L. D. (1995). Children's application of simultaneous and successive processing in inductive and deductive reasoning problems: Implications for developing scientific reasoning skills. *Journal of Research in Science Teaching, 32*, 699–714.

Wechsler, D. (1939). *The measurement of adult intelligence*. Baltimore, MD: Williams & Wilkins.

Wechsler, D. (1952). *The range of human capacities*. Baltimore, MD: Williams & Wilkins.

Wechsler, D. (1955). *The manual for the Wechsler adult intelligence scale*. New York: Psychological Corporation.

Wheeler, L., & Reitan, R. M. (1962). The presence and laterality of brain damage predicted from responses to a short aphasia screening test. *Perceptual and Motor Skills, 15*, 783–799.

Willis, W. G. (1985). Successive and simultaneous processing: A note on interpretation. *Journal of Psychoeducational Assessment, 4*, 343–346.

Normative Data and Scaling Issues in Neuropsychology

5

Charles J. Golden
Lindsay Hines

Normative Data and Scaling Issues

Neuropsychology has recognized across all of its theoretical orientations the need to compare performances across tests in order to identify relationships between performances on different tests that allow for the isolation of specific deficits. For example, it is well recognized that a test like Block Design (Wechsler, 1997) can be failed because of a wide variety of deficits, which include motor speed, visual skills, spatial skills, planning, and organization. By comparing performance on the Block Design test to tests of spatial skills without a motor component, as well as to tests of motor skills without a spatial component, the neuropsychologist can begin to identify which specific factor is impaired.

Although the comparison of neuropsychological tests is recognized as our most effective method of evaluating functional aspects of brain injury, significant errors may result from a lack of understanding of the psychometrics underlying normative data and scaling. These issues will be discussed along with the integrative procedures that are recognized as being the most useful in interpreting a battery of tests. Each of these concerns should be considered when interpreting any kind of extensive test battery.

Normative Populations

One of the most substantial pitfalls in the comparison of tests is the use of measures normed on different populations. The underlying samples for the scores on different tests vary considerably in terms of many important variables. The most substantial of these variables are age, education, gender, culture, language, when the norms were collected, where they were collected, and size of the sample. Each of these may have a significant impact on how scores are interpreted, both independently as well as in comparisons across a battery of tests.

Age and Education

Comparing a test corrected for age and education to one that is not corrected is potentially very harmful. For example, if Test A is normed on a 50-year-old group with a 10th grade education, a score by a 30-year-old with 14 years of education and a moderate brain injury may appear to be normal. However, if Test B is normed on a group with an average age of 24 with 18 years of education (graduate students), the score is likely to be abnormal. This may lead to the conclusion that the client is more impaired on Test B when in fact the difference is solely due to the differences in the underlying norm groups. The examiner must be aware of such differences for any tests he or she adopts.

This is primarily an issue with those tests that do not provide age or education norms or corrections. However, even when those norms are presented, they are often only age corrected or education corrected. In such a case, some tests may have age groups that do not have comparable educational levels, or other tests may present norms based on education groups containing different ages. None of this represents insurmountable problems, but such deviations must be considered before the results of two tests can be compared.

For example, an elderly man with 6 years of education would often receive significantly better scores on a test with age and education corrections. When that result was compared with the same test based on an uncorrected score, one would conclude that the uncorrected test showed a "deficit" that was solely due to the lack of correction for age and education. While this would be obvious if one was using the same test twice, it is less obvious when different tests are employed. Thus, if we compare the age-, education-, and gender-corrected norms of the Halstead Category Test with uncorrected norms on the Rey Figure, we may again get differences resulting from the scoring procedures, rather than from real neuropsychological findings. This is also a common problem when the age-corrected Wechsler Intelligence Tests are compared with tests that are both age and education corrected, or not corrected al all.

This may become a critical issue when properly normed tests are compared with modified procedures or qualitative procedures used without proper normative data. In such cases, the interpretation of the severity of the score is based upon the clinician's judgment that is biased by that individual's own background and experience, which will differ considerably among neuropsychologists.

Gender

Gender corrections are also an issue, although the impact of this issue on most neuropsychological tests is much smaller than those for age, education, when the results were collected, or cultural group. They must be attended to on those tests where there is a documented influence and it must always be kept in mind when they have not been properly analyzed (many normative samples, for example, come from Veterans Administration samples, which are predominantly male).

Geography

Where the data is collected may also have a substantial impact. If we pick equivalent populations, which we match for age, education, gender, and race in a high school in Des Moines, Iowa, and one in Bradenton, Florida, we are likely to get different results on a variety of tests in the normal population. Thus, the normative data chosen in scaling will have an impact in a battery of tests, and may add variation to scores considered normal and those considered abnormal. In neuropsychology, the site of data gathering may vary widely by geography (e.g., urban, rural, different states, different countries), setting (e.g., academic, medical, community), and inclusion and exclusion criteria.

Stratified normative data is also available for some major tests, such as the WAIS-III and WMS-III. In such cases, the data should represent the general population, and is often modeled after U.S. Census data. Thus, a group may include the same percentage of males and females as the general population, drawn in proportion from each region of the country, from urban and rural environments, and include each ethnic or cultural group in the percentages that they represent in the general population. Despite the fact that tests are routinely exchanged among the English-speaking countries, it is at best unclear whether norms gathered in the U.S. are appropriate in Great Britain or Australia and vice versa.

Culture and Language

Cross-cultural and cross-ethnic group problems are also substantial. Data collected from different cultural and ethnic groups cannot be generalized to other groups whether the tests are verbal or nonverbal. While differences are often clearer on verbal tests (whether translated into another language or not), there are also differences on nonverbal tests, which may reflect differences in style, differences in the meaning of age and education corrections, differences in cultural experiences, and other factors. Although some specific problems from focal brain injuries (such as severe construction dyspraxia, dysfluency, loss of receptive skills, paralysis) are indeed cross cultural, performances on more complex standardized tests do not hold up as well without renorming and reanalysis.

In general, neuropsychology (and psychology as a whole) has done a poor job of demonstrating the cross-cultural effectiveness of normative, validity, and reliability information. Applications to these populations must be cautious at best, and the impact on adequate evaluation of the pattern of test results should be considered. It cannot be assumed that all tests are equally affected by culture, because this is unlikely and certainly unproven. Test data that have been clearly analyzed for these issues are rare.

Consideration of the variance within members of an ethnic or cultural group is important as well. Golden (1973), for example, studied Japanese university students in Hawaii who were assigned to groups based on whether they were first-, second-, or third-generation Hawaiians. All participants were proficient in English. Golden found that individuals whose families had been in Hawaii the longest performed differently from the other groups on both verbal and nonverbal tests and were most similar to a Caucasian control group. Similarly, it may be inferred that minority individuals from different socio-economic levels will also show differences from one another.

Finally, simply including minority groups and different cultures within a standardization group does not make the norms for that test "culture free." For example, the standardization for the Wechsler Adult and Intelligence Scale-III (WAIS-III) made a major effort to include members of different ethnic and cultural groups based on their percentages in the population. Such an effort likely created norms that are as representative of the normal population in the U.S. as any other test currently available. Thus, we can compare the performance of anyone who is motivated and cooperative with the test procedure with the U.S. population as a whole.

This, however, does not tell us the standing of those individuals within their own community, or their cultural or ethnic group. Such information is capable of yielding results that are often more appropriate for use in neuropsychological analysis. If the individual is unimpaired compared with his or her own reference group (rather than with the U.S. population as a whole), there is much less likelihood of neuropsychological dysfunction. Conversely, evidence of deficits in comparison with one's own reference group is likely to be an accurate representation of neuropsychological dysfunction. In any case, norms that are stratified for such constructs may result in decreased sensitivity to, or failure to identify, neuropsychological abnormalities.

The impact of culture and ethnicity is further complicated by the impact of language. It is not uncommon for variations in Standard English to be evident across ethnic groups, such as verb conjugation and grammatical structure. Such differences may change scores on language-based tests in ways that will mislead pattern analysis when scores are based on the general population.

Time Frame

Another related issue is when the norms were generated. In general, research has found that norms collected in the 1950s and 1960s are not comparable to those gathered more recently. Increases in performance are estimated to range from 3 to 9 points per decade, dependent on the test (Flynn, 2000). This appears to have a greater impact on the more complex cognitive tests rather than on tests of simple motor performance or simple recognition. When older norms are used, they may substantially overrepresent how "good" a given performance may actually be. This effect can be seen clearly in the Wechsler Intelligence Tests where the normative data of the four versions of the test show increasing normal performance across nearly all areas even when the items remain essentially unchanged. It has been suggested that normative data is reliable for 15 to 20 years as long as the test items themselves do not become outdated (Tulsky, Saklofske, & Zhu, 2003).

An additional concern with regard to time frame is the possible impact of recent research on neuropsychologists' interpretation of a test. This is of particular importance in forensic neuropsychology, because our understanding of the brain-behavior relationship continues to evolve and become more accurate. Failing to stay abreast of recent research about commonly used measures can be potentially harmful in litigation.

Size of Data Set

A common practice among neuropsychologists is to demographically adjust all scores in a battery using normative data collected from various studies and compiled into one common resource. It is important to consider the positive and negative implications of such adjustments when interpreting scores. Although many data sets comprise a large N, they yield small cell sizes when demographically divided into subgroups. As a result, each score is corrected based on normative data for very few individuals, rather than a large, comprehensive population (Strauss, Sherman, & Spreen, 2006).

Statistical analyses are also commonly used to increase the size of each subgroup, such as case weighting. Though this method results in a partially estimated score, it is relatively common in widely used tests such as the Wechsler scales.

Unrelated Diagnoses

A related issue is the impact of non-neuropsychological diagnoses. In many cases, normative samples only look at normal people, excluding individuals with psychiatric diagnoses, histories of learning problems, or substantial medical problems, as well as individuals who are hospitalized or involved in litigation. However, many people tested for the impact of a neuropsychological insult will be in hospitals, have pain or other problems relating to accidents or aging, be on major medications, be suing someone, or have a psychiatric diagnosis such as major depression or schizophrenia. All of these conditions may have an impact on the outcome of neuropsychological testing.

As a result, it is beneficial to consider normative data that represent the demographic characteristics of the individual being assessed in addition to stratified samples more closely representing the general population. This may aid in reducing the possible confusion of comparing "normal" normative samples, because they may show deficits that are not neurologically based, but rather are related to these exclusionary conditions. Mitrushina, Boone, Ranzani, and D'Elia's (2005) text on normative data is based on this theory, according to which the patient's performance is compared with a data set that most closely represents his or her demographic characteristics, purportedly resulting in an interpretation appropriate to each individual. For many tests, such data do not exist, compromising the accuracy of the interpretive strategies employed.

In all cases, there should be an attempt to use norms that are properly corrected for age, education, and gender, when these factors influence test performance. In the absence of such norms, the possible impact of these variables must be clinically considered before any clinical conclusions are reached.

Classification of Scores

Once a normative group is finalized, the question arises as to how a test is actually scored: using deviation scores, cutoffs, or a combination of both. Although neuropsychological evaluation was founded on tests using cutoff scores such as the Luria Nebraska and the Halstead-Reitan, more recent work has shown increased use of deviation scores (Heaton, Miller, Taylor, & Grant, 2004; Mitrushina, Boone, Ranzani, & D'Elia, 2005). Cutoff scores typically dichotomize test performance as normal or impaired in an attempt to identify scores that represent brain injury rather than just a deviation from the population average. This, in turn, is often based on underlying assumptions that certain performances are characteristic of brain injury. Cutoffs fail to tell us the severity of a problem and often fail to tell us the likelihood of a misclassification of the deficit. While cutoffs can be useful, they can also limit the clinicians' ability to accurately compare performance across tests.

Defining the Brain Injury Group

To define a cutoff, it is usually necessary to define a brain injury group with which the normative group can be compared. This process is fraught with potential problems, since all of the issues that apply to the choice of a normal group apply here, along with the additional issues of defining a general brain injury group. These additional problems include consideration of the cause of the brain injury, the severity, the location, the chronicity, and the degree of treatment. Despite recent gains in understanding traumatic brain injury, significant variations remain evident in the classification of mild, moderate, and severe trauma (McCrea, 2008; Moser et al., 2007). Variations in each of these factors can impact how the brain injured group performs, and in turn, how the cutoff is determined.

Cause of the Brain Injury

Brain injury may, of course, arise from multiple causes. The common causes include strokes, head injuries, tumors, dementia, demyelinating diseases, Parkinson's disease, anoxia, poisoning, and metabolic disorders. Many of these groups can be broken down even further. For example, strokes differ considerably (hemorrhagic, occlusive, etc.), their size, and their location. Each type typically produces (when considered with the other factors listed above) a modal pattern of deficits and strengths. Brain injured groups used in norming will differ considerably depending on which population the group came from.

Evaluation of different tests will show that the causes of brain injury in the normative group differ widely from test to test, some being all head injury, some being all stroke, some being all dementia, and some reflecting an idiosyncratic combination, usually based on where the study was done (samples of convenience rather than planned samples, which are very rare). This has a major impact on the pattern of test results and, in turn, will affect the cutoff points when they are calculated.

Depending on the makeup and the severity of the group, the cutoff points that are established between groups will vary, ranging typically from one to two standard deviations above the normal mean. This will result in widely different error rates in misclassifying normal and brain injured clients. This method of establishing cutoffs normally is based on a procedure that optimizes correct classification of clients.

The difficulty with such procedures lies in three major areas. First, the cutoff is dependent on the exact sample used. For example, if one test's cutoff is determined between a matched sample of above average controls and brain injured clients, that will not be the same optimal cutoff as when a sample of matched, below average normal and brain injured clients has been used. The efficacy of the cutoff when applied to a specific brain injured client will vary greatly depending on how appropriate it is for the client being considered. For example, if a study establishes an optimal cutoff for a test when comparing severe head injured clients with normal clients, it is likely that a client with a mild head injury will be misclassified as normal.

Another major, but related, problem is that cutoffs are often not adequately cross-validated across different populations, again leaving their efficacy in question. Often a cutoff set up in a single study within a single population is applied across the board to new replication samples to see if such a cutoff is stable even in similar populations. Since population characteristics can potentially affect cutoff points, such replication studies are important to support the generalization of the cutoff across clinical populations.

A second problem is that cutoffs will differ in how many brain injured clients are misclassified as normal, and how many normal clients are misclassified as brain injured. Test A may reach an optimal cutoff by classifying 100% of brain injured correctly, but only 60% of normal clients (for an 80% hit rate), while Test B may classify 100% of normal clients correctly, but only 60% of brain injured clients (for an 80% hit rate.) When used in practice, Test A is much more likely to call someone brain injured while Test B is more likely to call someone normal. In such cases, finding a pattern of brain injured performance on Test A and normal performance on Test B may not reflect differential performance of the client, but rather the ways in which the cutoffs were selected.

A third problem is that cutoffs are usually based on samples of "very normal" normal clients screened for psychiatric problems, history of neurological problems, history of learning problems, and so on, and very clearly brain injured clients with well documented injuries. Unfortunately, such samples represent the easiest form of distribution and do not address real-life clinical questions (e.g., Did the person with severe depression, who wasn't paying attention while driving, get hurt in the automobile accident?). While such studies meet rigorous, traditional research standards, such information may not translate into real life. Studies that use controls of individuals with other illnesses (such as orthopedic illnesses or psychiatric disorders) will offer more conservative but perhaps more relevant cutoff points.

Discriminant Analysis

This is similar to the optimization level except that it is decided by a statistical procedure. This procedure is heavily influenced by sample characteristics and can vary widely with changes in the sample and sample size (especially in situations where sample sizes are uneven). When multiple groups are involved (normal, depressed, and brain injured, for example), the weightings of each group can heavily influence the outcome. Seemingly small changes in options in running discriminant computer programs can also lead to substantial changes in the results. Such programs are unconcerned with the type of error made, leading to cutoffs that may yield highly skewed results. Formulas generated to make discriminations based on groups of tests may be overly influenced by chance and not be easily replicable across populations. While again this can be a useful technique, the use of such cutoffs must be regarded with caution. In general, all of the issues related to optimization also must be considered when discriminant functions are used.

Cutoffs From Normal Distributions

Increasing numbers of tests use cutoffs based on the normal distribution. Such studies may identify the mean and standard deviation of normal individuals, and then select a point on the normal curve that is said to indicate brain injury. This may be two standard deviations from the mean—a very rigorous criterion—but most often only one standard deviation or slightly more. Such studies may present a single cutoff, or ideally may offer cutoffs on scores adjusted for age, education, and gender.

These cutoffs also have disadvantages. First, cutoffs based on normal clients do not tell us how well the test will identify brain injured clients (which will also be influenced by the point on the normal curve that defines the cutoff). In some cases, a one standard deviation cutoff may identify 60% of brain injured clients, or 80% or 30%. This depends on the distribution of the score in brain injured clients, which in turn is also influenced by how skewed or how flat both the normal and brain injured sample curves are, as well as their relative position to one another. Such issues are important in analyzing neuropsychological data because distributions are often skewed and may indeed not even be truly normal, due to floor and ceiling effects, as well as the basic nature of many of the measures employed. In such situations, cutoffs that appear to be equal in sensitivity actually vary greatly.

One attempt to deal with the issue of normality is to force the scores into a normal distribution using statistical techniques. This was done with the various Wechsler scales, where scores are forced into a normal distribution with a mean of 10 and a standard deviation of 3. This was also done by Heaton, Grant, and Matthews (1991) when norming their extended version of the Halstead-Reitan. In general, such procedures force scores into a range from 1 to 19, so that all raw scores are shrunk to fit a distribution up to 3 standard deviations from the mean.

Although this procedure can correct for the distribution problems discussed above, it also introduces several problems, especially with neuropsychological data. In neuropsychological populations, scores can be 10 or even 20 standard deviations from the average of normal individuals. Thus, a wide range of scores are forced together at the bottom of the distribution. As a result, scores that differ in large degree when compared as raw scores, end up all being represented by a single-scale score at the bottom of the distribution. This is not a problem when the possible scores in the distribution fall into a limited range that does not extend outside the 3 standard deviation limit, but is an issue with scores like the time to complete the Trail Making Test, when scores 10 standard deviations from the mean are not unusual.

The question which then arises is whether these raw score differences are meaningful in terms of an understanding of the degree of the client's dysfunction and, by extension, the nature and prognosis of the client's problem. This may be of specific concern in cases in which serial assessment is warranted, such as developmental or degenerative disorders. In such instances, test scores may indicate basal-level performance, and may fail to identify evident changes in functioning over time. Research pertaining to extremely low performance and specific diagnostic groups has remained limited and fragmented for this reason.

Second, such cutoffs may be affected by minor changes in scores that end up being overinterpreted. Thus the difference between a "normal" T score of 40.01 and an "abnormal" T score of 39.99 may indeed be minuscule and not worthy of the sudden interpretive emphasis given to the lower score. Cutoffs will clearly vary if we choose one, two, or some other number of standard deviations to indicate the cutoff point. Even using the same cutoff point (one standard deviation, for example) across tests will result in differing levels of sensitivity and specificity, influencing overall accuracy. This problem, however, exists with all cutoff points that attempt to dichotomize performance as "normal" or "abnormal."

Third, different tests may use cutoffs at 1, 2, 1.5, or some other number of standard deviations, again leading to misleading classifications of test results. As with other cutoffs, sample characteristics may substantially influence results and lead to questionable generalizability.

Age and Education Corrections

The importance of considering age and education issues in adult samples is obvious. However, they may lead to several pitfalls, some of which are obvious and others that are more subtle. First, different test norms and cutoffs may address age, education, a combination of both, or neither. This, of course, makes information from the different tests difficult to compare directly, although these scores may be regarded as equivalent by the user. When one test corrects for age and education and is compared with one that corrects for age only, then apparent differences in scores may again be illusory. In general, tests that correct for all of these factors are seen as more conservative in diagnosing brain injury in populations with higher ages and lower education, but more liberal in populations with higher educations and lower ages.

A second problem arises from how the corrections are made. Vastly different results may emerge from samples that correct for "over 45" and "under 45" versus those that correct by year using regression formulas. Similarly, bunching of education in groups of "9–11 years" or "16+ years" may cause similar problems. In samples that use "bunching" techniques, sample characteristics among normative groups for each education level may cause variations in norms that are unrelated to brain injury. However, regression formulas that assume linearity of relationships between test performance and demographic variables also may err if the underlying relationship is not linear. In all of these cases the actual magnitude of the effect of age, education, or other demographic factors influences the importance of these issues.

In some cases, however, age and education corrections can lead to serious problems when the corrections correct for brain injury itself. In many samples of older normal clients, we may see decline because of unidentified neurological factors or as a result of systemic disorders (e.g., diabetes, peripheral joint disorders, etc.) that act to bias norms towards the impaired side, masking real problems. Similarly, a group of individuals with only a sixth-grade education may have received the sixth-grade education because they were unable to go any further because of a neurological disorder, while others may have dropped out for economic or other reasons. The effect, however, is to make the test less sensitive to actual (although pre-existing) disorders.

Cultural and Ethnic Diversity Issues

This is a less researched (unfortunately) but extremely important area. The administration of tests to ethnic minorities and to groups whose primary and original language is other than the language the test was normed in is questionable, even in the case of so-called nonverbal tests. Our own work (e.g., Demsky, Mittenberg, Quintar, Katell, & Golden, 1998) suggests that even nonverbal tests yield different results in normal populations, let alone in brain injured samples. Unless a test is appropriately standardized for a group, the use of the norms and cutoffs must be done very cautiously and with strong attention to these factors.

A recent trend in psychological and neuropsychological assessment has been to use nonverbal tests designed specifically for culturally and linguistically diverse groups. Although these measures are proposed to eliminate language barriers and produce greater accuracy than traditional methods, research other than that provided by the test authors is not yet available.

It is our belief that simply including a group in a more general normative sample does not make the norms culturally fair or accurate. While we may represent ethnic group X in the normative sample in the same 3% ratio it represents in the U.S. population, this does not make the resultant norms fairer or more accurate. (It does make the norms more representative of the true mean, if we tested everyone in the U.S., but this is irrelevant to the question of neuropsychological dysfunction.) Only if the norms are appropriately evaluated within that group with an adequate sample can we determine if the norms are fair.

The issues involved in such norms are complex. For example, when working in Hawaii our senior author found that norms for second-generation Japanese residents were not equivalent to those for third-generation Japanese residents. Norms for Spanish speakers from Cuba may not be the same as for Spanish speakers from Mexico. Norms for a client who is truly bilingual may not be the same for someone who still thinks predominantly in his or her native language. These issues are unfortunately endless, but must be considered when reaching conclusions.

When analyzing the results of "translated tests," differences of up to 2/3 of a standard deviation (10 standard score points) may be seen in "nonverbal" tests, while differences twice as large (4/3 of a standard deviation, or up to 20 points) may be due solely to issues of translation and culture. If a test is translated inappropriately or in an idiosyncratic method, the expected changes in norms—even in a normal population—may even be larger.

Interpretive Implications

Interpreting a series of tests with traditional cutoffs for each test can result in many distortions. As was described above, many factors may influence how a cutoff is picked and the degree to which the cutoff generates errors in normal clients (false positives, when we call a normal person brain injured) and in brain-injured clients (false negatives, when we call a brain-injured client normal). If

Test A generates a high rate of false positives, and Test B generates a high rate of false negatives, differences in classification of the tests may not be the result of differences in level of performance but differences in how the cutoffs are set.

This creates the potential for substantive errors, because tests differ widely in their overall sensitivity, as well as the occurrence of false negative and false positive outcomes. Users of such cutoffs must be familiar with the psychometric properties of the specific tests that are employed in order to be able to judge the accuracy of a given classification. Even in such circumstances, however, reliance on cutoff points to classify clients across a set of tests is likely to be misleading due to these factors.

A related interpretive issue is the impact of random chance and premorbid levels when using cutoffs with multiple tests. Probability rules tell us that by chance alone some tests will be performed at levels below the cutoff point, with the likelihood directly related to the degree to which the test is likely to show false positive results. The more frequently tests are given, the higher the likelihood of such chance findings. For example, if a battery includes fifteen tests or subtests each of which has a cutoff score and an average false positive rate of 20%, three of the tests would be expected by chance alone to fall below preset cutoffs (Ingraham & Aiken, 1996). This is made worse by many of the other issues that have already been discussed, such as appropriateness of the normative group initially.

Despite this issue, it is not unusual to see users of such tests interpret the three or four "findings" as having neuropsychological significance and thus indicating the presence of brain injury. This represents a substantial overinterpretation of the data and false findings of the presence of brain injury. Similarly, one can argue that chance fluctuations can cause false negatives as well, so that apparently normal profiles are misinterpreted as indicating the absence of brain dysfunction.

Premorbid levels clearly influence these outcomes as well. If a client's premorbid performance on one or more tests is below the cutoff, the impact of a current condition (such as a head injury) will be overinterpreted. In cases in which a large number of tests are poorly performed premorbidly (e.g., in cases of mental retardation or significant learning disabilities), cutoff scores may be essentially useless. Similarly, high-functioning clients may show a decline in function but still remain above cutoffs, again causing misclassification of the client as uninjured.

It has been argued that the above interpretive problems can be avoided by adjusting cutoffs for such factors as age and education. While such procedures offer better results, they do not eliminate these problems, because such cutoffs are set for the average person at a given age and education. Thus, if we looked at all individuals who are 40 years old with twelve years of education, then half of that population would perform better than the mean while half would perform worse. While we would expect that the overall standard deviation for such a group would be smaller than in a more heterogeneous population, there would still be those who were premorbidly very high and very low compared with that average. This would produce the same problems, but hopefully reduce false positive and false negative rates so as to minimize the impact of these concerns.

Similar concerns would apply to corrections for gender, ethnic group, race, geographical region, language, and so on. The impact of first language on a person whose second language is English would depend on the degree to which the person was fully bilingual and likely the language the person thinks in (with a poorer performance expected if the individual has to continuously translate back and forth between the languages).

Pattern Analysis

Although cutoffs give us rough ideas of the level of performance of a client, the use of pattern analysis across tests that ignore cutoffs but rather focus on internal variations in the client's own results with respect to the client's own baseline of current and previous performance offers a much more powerful tool, especially in more subtle cases or those cases where we wish to understand the true deficits that underlie a brain injury or whether a brain injury has even occurred. Such a technique ideally translates all scores into a standard score system with appropriate demographic corrections.

Translation of the scores into a common system is made difficult by the presence of many scoring systems using demographically corrected and uncorrected scores, T-scores, standard scores, z-scores, raw scores, Wechsler scale scores, and percentiles. These scores must be translated into a common system (most often T-scores or standard scores), which are ideally corrected on the same demographic variables. For example, if we evaluate a client with six years of education and who is 45 years of age, we will get widely different results with or without an education correction. If we corrected only for age, an achievement score equivalent to five years of education would yield a very low score, while correcting for education as well might yield a normal score. If different tests are corrected for different demographic factors, apparent differences in the pattern of scores may only be related to the differences in the scoring corrections.

Though a common practice is to use a comprehensive data set to correct for demographic variables, it should be noted that adjustments are made for raw scores on some tests, and for previously adjusted scores on others. For example, one can use a comprehensive normative data set to find age, education, and gender corrections for the number of errors on the Halstead Category test, as well as for an age-adjusted scaled score from the WAIS-III, which uses case weighting. Although this is the most effective method for making adjustments across an assessment battery, additional variances may result.

Client Profile

Once scores have been converted into a common scoring system, client profiles may be plotted or analyzed, looking for score differences that suggest neuropsychological significance. Such analysis must consider the issue of individual variation. When looking at an overall profile, one can calculate the individual's expected scores across all tests administered. In most cases, the FSIQ (premorbid) will represent this score. In less severe cases, the current FSIQ is often a good estimate, or even the client's average score. In general, research on test batteries seems to suggest that scores for normal clients will vary about one standard deviation from these average scores (fifteen points for standard scores on either side of the average, ten points on either side for T-scores). This works, however, only when such factors as ceiling or floor limits, demographic equations, or skewed distributions do not influence the profile.

There are several other major exceptions to these rules. First, very high-functioning clients (90th percentile and above) may show skewed distribution of scores so that there is a greater variability for scores below their average and lesser variability for scores above their average. For example, a client with an FSIQ of 145 may have few scores above, but the range for scores below may be as high as two standard deviations. Similarly, individuals at the low end of the spectrum may have a tendency to show more high scores than expected (often in motor, sensory, attention, and some memory domains), so the range may be up to two standard deviations above the expected score.

Profiles where scores show less variation than expected are generally considered within the normal range (although that does not prove someone is normal). Profiles with greater variations suggest an unusual degree of variation, which may indicate the presence of cognitive problems or may simply indicate any of the problems with specific tests or scoring procedures that have been discussed already. Overall, in all clients, a range of scores that reflects only two standard deviations is normal; ranges between two and three standard deviations are likely to be borderline; ranges greater than three standard deviations suggest that there is a disability (assuming that the differences are not due to any of the statistical and methodological flaws already discussed).

Variations Between Scores

Below the level of overall profile differences, scores can be compared directly with one another. The degree of difference between scores necessary for neuropsychological significance varies depending on the underlying relationships of the tests as well as variations in the normative samples employed.

The easiest comparisons are between scores representing identical motor or sensory performance on opposite sides of the body. These scores should be very close to one another and are usually normed on the same population with the same scoring methods, therefore minimizing errors from these sources. Thus, differences of one-half of one standard deviation may be significant.

The second class is tests that are moderately correlated with one another (verbal and performance IQ, performance on two similar drawing tests). If both sets of scores have similar normative populations, then differences of one standard deviation between scores are usually neuropsychologically significant. If the tests use very different normative populations or different correction methods (e.g., one corrects for education, one does not), a more conservative difference of one and one-half standard deviations should be used.

The third class consists of tests that are independently normed but represent areas that theoretically overlap, such as achievement and IQ, executive performance and IQ, or spatial reasoning and construction skills. Such tests normally require differences of $1^1/2$ standard deviations before neuropsychological differences can be reliably implied. In limited cases, a more liberal difference of one standard deviation can be applied, but only when there is clear research to back up such an assumption. In most cases, such research is not available, and the more liberal one standard deviation should not be employed.

The final class is made up of tests that are generally unrelated (block design and grammatical skills) and normed on different populations. In such cases, the most conservative criterion of two standard deviations should be employed.

It should be noted, however, that the presence of a significant deficit between tests does not mean there is a brain injury or a disability. Since normal people have scores that are typically one standard deviation above and one standard deviation below their average or base score, the difference between scores at the extremes is often two standard deviations. Only a combination of clear and consistent differences among sets of tests, along with a definite abnormal range of scores, can be clearly interpreted as indicating a disability or brain injury.

Observations

In addition to an analysis of scores, much information can be gained from the qualitative analysis of how a client achieved a score. While it can be argued that an extensive test battery could be organized so that many or even most qualitative variations would be reflected in the quantitative scores, the state of testing at the present time does not have a research base that allows us to demonstrate this argument. Differences between tests as discussed above, as well as simple error variance, obscure fine differences in client performance. Such problems have less effect on simple classification of performance as "impaired," but have many more implications as we attempt to make finer discriminations as to specific problems or specific etiologies.

Under these circumstances, qualitative observations become an important source of collateral information that should be integrated with the actual data. It is important to recognize that neither quantitative nor qualitative data is either better or more perfect, but that both offer insights that, when combined, create a more accurate and detailed description of the client. Thus, such observations should be routinely made, along with testing the limits of procedures when they can further elucidate the reasons for a client's behavior. All individuals who administer tests, whether they are doctoral psychologists or technicians, should be trained in making and reporting such observations.

Premorbid Baseline

Although the level of performance measures compares a client's performance with population norms, and pattern analysis looks at current intra-individual variations, there has always been a desire to compare the client's current functioning with the client's own premorbid level of functioning. This has traditionally been attempted in two ways: using formulas to estimate premorbid levels, and using performance on current "hold" tests to estimate premorbid levels.

The use of formulas has generally focused on the prediction of full-scale IQ as a measure of g, with which all other test scores can be compared. These systems have many problems because they tend to lump clients into heterogeneous groups that are not descriptive of the individual. Most of the success of such formulas lies in classifying those in the middle of the normal distribution as being in the middle, but adding little by simply assuming that everyone is normal. When these scores are used, errors of up to 15 standard score points from baseline must be assumed, with scores needing to deviate an additional 15 points before one can reach the conclusion that a score has changed.

The second method involves estimation from "hold" tests, typically a test of reading recognition (such as the WRAT-III or WTAR), or vocabulary tests (such as the PPVT-R or vocabulary from the WAIS-III). These tests offer decent correlations with "g" and are easy to give. In the absence of aphasia or severe visual problems they offer reasonable estimates of the premorbid level, especially when combined with historical information on a person's actual accomplishments. However, even in the best of circumstances, these scores are accurate only within 5–7 standard score points at the 68% confidence level, and 10–12 points at the 95% confidence level. This range of error must be considered in any comparisons.

A final caution is in order concerning the appropriateness of these baselines. While they may offer some useful information for premorbid general IQ, they do not predict performance on tests of motor performance, drawing, attention, and other important skills. Thus, care should be taken before generalizing such baselines to such tests where the accuracy rate may drop to as low as 20–30 standard score points. There is a paucity of research on the relation of these areas to premorbid scores, and any generalization must be made very cautiously and take into account the other issues discussed in this chapter.

Summary

Although there are many issues to consider when analyzing a comprehensive test battery, such an approach remains by far the most accurate and useful method of neuropsychological evaluation. When quantitative and qualitative information are properly integrated with consideration of the issues described above, valid and useful descriptions of client deficits may be identified.

References

Demsky, Y., Mittenberg, W., Quintar, B., Katell, A. D., & Golden, C. J. (1998). Bias in the use of standard American norms with Spanish translations of the Wechsler Memory Scale-Revised. *Assessment, 5*, 115–121.

Flynn, J. R. (2000). IQ gains and fluid *g. American Psychologist, 55*(5), 543-543.

Golden, C. J. (1973). *Cognitive differences among different generations of immigrants to Hawaii.* Unpublished masters thesis, University of Hawaii, Honolulu, HI.

Heaton, R., Grant, I., & Matthews, C. (1991). *Comprehensive norms for an expanded Halstead-Reitan battery: Demographic corrections, research findings, and clinical applications.* Odessa, FL: Psychological Assessment Resources.

Heaton, R. K., Miller, W. S., Taylor, M. J., & Grant, I. (2004). *Revised comprehensive norms for an expanded Halstead-Reitan battery: Demographically adjusted neuropsychological norms for African American and Caucasian adults (HRB).* Tampa, FL: Psychological Assessment Resources.

Ingraham, L. J., & Aiken, C. B. (1996). An empirical approach to determining criteria for abnormality in test batteries with multiple measures. *Neuropsychology, 10*, 120–124.

McCrea, M. A. (2008). *Mild traumatic brain injury and post concussion syndrome: The new evidence base for diagnosis and treatment.* New York: Oxford.

Mitrushina, M., Boone, K. B., Ranzani, J., & D'Elia, L. F. (2005). *Handbook of normative data for neuropsychological assessment* (2nd ed.). New York: Oxford.

Moser, R. S., Iverson, G. L., Echemendia, R. J., Lovell, M. R., Schatz, P., Webbe, F. M., Ruff, R. M., & Barth, J. T. (2007). Neuropsychological evaluation in the diagnosis and management of sports-related concussion. *Archives of Clinical Neuropsychology, 22*, 909–916.

Strauss, E., Sherman, E., & Spreen, O. (2006). *A compendium of neuropsychological tests: Administration, norms, and commentary* (3rd ed.). New York: Oxford.

Tulsky, D. S., Saklofske, D. H., & Zhu, J. (2003). Revising a standard: An evaluation of the origin and development of the WAIS-III. In D. S. Tulsky, D. H. Saklofske, G. J. Chelune, R. K. Heaton, R. Ivnik, R. Bornstein, A. Prifitera, & M. F. Ledbetter (Eds.), *Clinical interpretation of the WAIS-III and WMS-III* (pp. 43–92). New York: Academic Press.

Wechsler, D. (1997). *WAIS-III: Administration and scoring manual.* San Antonio: Psychological Corporation.

Detecting Exaggeration, Poor Effort, and Malingering in Neuropsychology

6

Grant L. Iverson

Introduction

Effort testing is standard practice in forensic neuropsychology (Bush et al., 2005; Heilbronner, Sweet, Morgan, Larrabee, & Millis, in press). Effort testing should be done in every forensic evaluation. This is because (a) poor effort during testing is common (Larrabee, 2003b; Mittenberg, Patton, Canyock, & Condit, 2002), (b) poor effort has a very large adverse effect on neuropsychological test results (Vickery, Berry, Inman, Harris, & Orey, 2001), (c) there are well-validated tests for detecting poor effort that have low false positive rates, and (d) in forensic cases, practitioners pay special attention to issues relating to causation and try to rule out factors that might lead to incorrect inferences or interpretation.

The context of the evaluation is critically important. Gervais and colleagues (2001) examined 96 patients with fibromyalgia (FM) with two effort tests. Approximately half of the patients were seen in the context of a disability-related evaluation

This chapter was adapted, revised, and updated from two previous works by Grant L. Iverson (2003, 2008).

($N = 46$). For the 50 patients who were not involved in a disability-related evaluation, 4% failed one effort test, and none of them failed the other effort test. In contrast, effort-test failure ranged from 24–30% of patients seeking disability benefits. In a follow-up large-scale study, Gervais and colleagues (2004) reported that failure rates on different effort tests in a sample of 326 patients being evaluated within a compensation context (e.g., worker's compensation or personal injury) ranged from 17–43%. None of these patients were being evaluated for lingering effects of a brain injury or toxic exposure. They were all being evaluated for chronic pain, psychological problems, or both.

Iverson and colleagues (2007) recruited 54 community-dwelling adults with FM to participate in a study (these were not clinical referrals and no reports were generated). These subjects reported high levels of depression, chronic pain, and disability on questionnaires. However, not a single research subject failed effort testing. Etherton and colleagues induced moderate pain in healthy young adults, using the cold-presser technique, and demonstrated that this acute pain did not have an adverse effect on effort-test results (Etherton, Bianchini, Ciota, & Greve, 2005; Etherton, Bianchini, Greve, & Ciota, 2005). This series of studies clearly illustrate that acute and chronic pain, in isolation, does not lead to effort-test failure. However, effort-test failure is common in patients with chronic pain who are involved in a compensation-related evaluation.

Whitney and colleagues (2009) conducted a retrospective chart review study of Operation Iraqi Freedom/Operation Enduring Freedom patients at a Polytrauma Network Site who were referred for a neuropsychological evaluation. Of the 23 military personnel and veterans evaluated, four (17%) failed effort testing. The patients who failed effort testing had experienced, at most, mild traumatic brain injuries characterized by brief or no loss of consciousness and post-traumatic amnesia lasting less than 10 minutes.

As part of an early intervention program for mild traumatic brain injury, we conduct cognitive screening evaluations that include effort testing. These patients are referred to the early intervention program by their Worker's Compensation case managers because they are slow to recover. The patients were evaluated, on average, 2.1 months ($SD = 1.3$; Range $= 1–6$) postinjury. Nearly all endorsed symptoms severe enough to warrant an *ICD-10 (International Statistical Classification of Diseases*, World Health Organization, 1992) diagnosis of postconcussion syndrome, none were working, and all were receiving benefits. Cognitive test results, based on the Neuropsychological Assessment Battery Screening Module (NAB) (Stern & White, 2003), stratified by effort-test results, are presented in Figure 6.1. Based on the first 40 evaluations that we conducted, 25% failed effort testing. As seen in Figure 6.1, effort-test failure had a dramatic effect on neuropsychological test results. On average, patients who passed effort testing had broadly normal cognitive functioning, and those who failed had "mildly impaired" cognitive functioning.

Clinicians should not assume, however, that poor effort occurs only in a forensic context. Poor effort can occur in a research context and thus contaminate the findings. This was illustrated, unexpectedly and persuasively, by Stulemeijer and colleagues (2007). These researchers sent a letter and questionnaire to 618 consecutive patients who attended the emergency department, as part of a longitudinal prospective cohort study on outcome after mild traumaic brain injury (MTBI). The information was sent at six months post injury. Of the 299 patients

6.1

Effects of poor effort on cognitive test results in Worker's Compensation patients with *ICD-10* postconcussion syndrome.

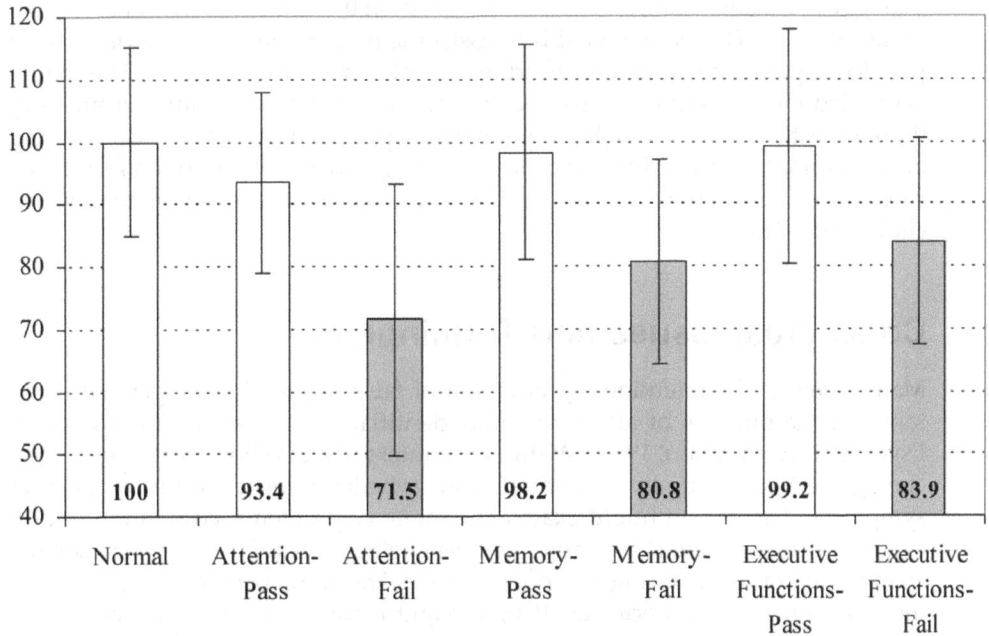

Note: Scores are for the Attention, Memory, and Executive Functions Indexes from the NAB Screening Module. The sample size is 40, 10 of whom failed the Test of Memory Malingering.

that returned the questionnaire, 113 patients were also willing to undergo a neuropsychological evaluation. The final sample consisted of 110 patients. In this sample of research participants with a history of MTBI, 27% failed effort testing. Poor effort was associated with significantly worse performance on neuropsychological testing. Poor effort was also associated with increased reporting of symptoms of psychological distress.

There is no question that effort testing is critically important. Clinicians are encouraged to conceptualize poor effort, exaggeration, and malingering, not in simple dichotomous terms, but in continuous terms, through probabilistic considerations. Practitioners need to identify and explain test scores that simply do not make biological or psychometric sense. If the examinee demonstrates clear evidence of poor effort on any test within the evaluation, the entire set of test results is questionable. The results might not be "invalid," but one should have less confidence in their reliability and validity. In that situation, one cannot assume that even broadly normal test scores represent the person's true ability. Some broadly normal scores might also be diminished due to variable effort. Accordingly, the more conservative conclusion would be that the obtained scores represent the examinee's minimum overall performance at the time of the evaluation.

Practitioners should avoid trying to use clinical judgment (i.e., making "educated" guesses) to determine which test performances are valid, questionable, or biased. In general, psychologists should avoid overstating effort-test results in either direction ("excellent" effort or "poor" effort). Rather, psychologists should use phraseology that is clear, objective, reasoned, and unambiguous.

The purpose of this chapter is to provide a critical review and discussion of poor effort, exaggeration, and malingering within the context of neuropsychological assessment. The explicit goal is to assist the practitioner in developing a best-practice approach for assessing effort in clinical and forensic contexts. The chapter is divided into the following six sections: (a) conceptual issues and terminology, (b) diagnostic criteria for malingering in neuropsychology, (c) assessing for exaggerated symptom reporting, (d) conceptualizing and assessing poor effort in neuropsychology, (e) ethical issues, and (f) conclusions and recommendations for clinical practice.

Conceptual Issues and Terminology

Malingering is the intentional production of false or greatly exaggerated symptoms for the purpose of attaining some identifiable external reward (American Psychiatric Association, 1994). Within the context of a psychological or neuropsychological evaluation, an individual who is malingering typically exaggerates symptoms. The person might exaggerate memory problems, concentration difficulty, depression, anxiety, pain, dizziness, sleep disturbance, or personality change, for example. During neuropsychological testing, a person who is malingering deliberately underperforms. People might malinger to (a) influence the outcome of a personal injury lawsuit, (b) receive worker's compensation or disability benefits, (c) obtain prescription medications, (d) avoid prosecution for criminal activities (by means of a determination of incompetence to stand trial), or (e) avoid criminal responsibility (i.e., not guilty by reason of insanity).

Resnick (1997) described three types of malingering, labeled *pure malingering, partial malingering,* and *false imputation.* Pure malingering is characterized by a complete fabrication of symptoms. Partial malingering is defined by exaggerating actual symptoms or by reporting past symptoms as if they have been ongoing. False imputation refers to the deliberate misattribution of actual symptoms to the compensable event. That is, a person reports legitimate symptoms and problems, reasonably accurately, but deliberately attributes them to a false cause (such as a motor vehicle accident). False imputation, without question, occurs in forensic evaluations. It can be difficult, even impossible at times, to determine if a person is deliberately attributing symptoms or problems falsely to a compensable cause (i.e., false imputation to a personal injury tort). In general, attribution of cause, by a patient, claimant, or plaintiff, falls on a continuum of accuracy, as illustrated in Figure 6.2. These false attributions can be intentional or unintentional.

Appreciating different types of malingering is important because mental health and legal professionals might have a simplistic view of malingering (i.e., only pure malingering is considered malingering). Many lawyers and health care professionals adopt a rather extreme and simplistic position regarding malingering. They assume that malingering represents total fabrication (i.e., fraud). An extreme example would be the person who pretends to not be able to walk caught

6.2

Continuum of accuracy of causal attributions.

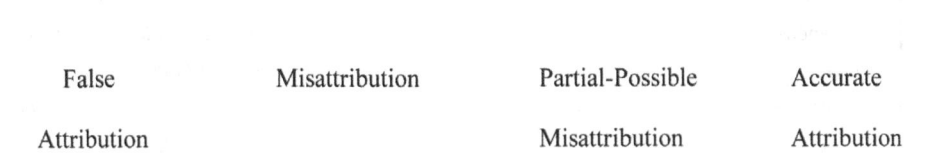

False	Misattribution	Partial-Possible	Accurate
Attribution		Misattribution	Attribution

on videotape walking. Less blatant malingering is conceptualized differently, such as deliberate exaggeration. Exaggeration is seen as common in personal injury litigation, and part of the function of the adversarial system is to illustrate to the trier of fact that exaggeration is present. Some professionals are tempted to believe that if a person has a well-documented psychiatric condition or visible brain damage on magnetic resonance imaging (MRI), the person could not be malingering or exaggerating. However, it is naïve to assume that a person with a psychiatric problem or the lingering effects of a traumatic brain injury could not malinger. That would be tantamount to concluding that people with these conditions are not capable of engaging in goal-directed behavior (e.g., exaggeration of symptoms to influence their litigation).

Exaggeration is a core feature of malingering, but exaggeration is not synonymous with malingering. The pervasive negativism and cognitive distortions seen in some patients with major depressive disorder can result in self-reported symptoms and problems that appear to be, and frequently are, exaggerated. Some patients with chronic pain conditions and somatoform disorders behaviorally and interpersonally evolve to the point of describing their symptoms and problems in an exaggerated manner. That is, their interpersonal style changes over time, through environmental factors and social reinforcement, to include verbal and nonverbal behaviors that appear, and likely are, exaggerated. Some patients fear their problems will be dismissed or minimized by their physician. In response, they might exaggerate the frequency, intensity, severity, or duration of these problems, or some combination thereof. Some patients might exaggerate their problems to influence the dynamics of the physician-patient relationship. From the patient perspective, the exaggeration might bring them more attention and make them a more interesting patient in the eyes of their physician. Of course, some patients have a deep-seated psychological need to be in the sick role. These

6.1   Factors and Incentives Relating to Exaggeration and Malingering

Psychosocial Factors	Incentives/Motivational Factors
Entitlement	Avoiding Responsibilities
Justification	Attention from Spouse
Neediness	Special Medical Attention
Anger	Obtain Medications
Frustration	Avoid Criminal Prosecution
Greed	Influence Sentencing
Somatization	Disability Benefits
Reinforced Behavior Pattern (e.g., in chronic pain)	Personal Injury Settlement
Depressive Negativistic Thinking	
Personality Characteristics & Disorders	
Nocebo Effect	
Misattribution	
"Good-Old-Days" Bias	
External Gain (e.g., financial or legal)	

This table was adapted from information presented in Iverson (2007).

patients deliberately exaggerate their symptoms and problems in order to maintain themselves in this sick role, and they would therefore meet diagnostic criteria for a factitious disorder. In forensic evaluations, clinicians are often expected to make an inference regarding the underlying motivation or reasons for presumed exaggeration or fabrication of symptoms. Factors related to, and incentives that can be derived from, exaggeration and malingering are summarized in Table 6.1. These factors can occur singly or in combination.

There are numerous factors, such as feelings of entitlement, anger, frustration, and somatization, and certain personality characteristics that can influence the decision to exaggerate symptoms and problems. Certain factors, such as reinforced behavior patterns and secondary gain are bidirectional in their influence. Social-psychological factors can influence how a person perceives and reports his or her symptoms. Examples include (a) the nocebo effect—negative expectations about sickness or symptoms are causally linked to the sickness or symptoms, that is, one's mindset or belief system can affect the outcome of his or her health, independent of other risk factors; (b) misattribution—normal, everyday symptoms, or symptoms that are due to another cause, are incorrectly attributed to a specific injury, illness, or condition, and (c) a "good-old-days" bias—a response bias in which patients retrospectively recall themselves as being healthier in the past and experiencing fewer pre-injury or pre-illness symptoms than the base rates of those symptoms in the healthy population, thus overestimating the degree of change.

Without question, it can be very difficult to conceptualize the underlying cause, or causes, of exaggeration. First, the "cry for help" euphemism implies that the person has serious psychological or psychiatric problems and is desperately seeking recognition of, and attention for, these problems. There is a long history of conceptualizing exaggeration as a cry for help in psychology and neuropsychology, whereas in psychiatry and general medicine clinicians are inclined to attribute exaggeration to "psychological factors," "psychiatric problems," "nonorganic factors," or "secondary gains." Some physicians even use vague and obfuscating terms like "supratentorial" to communicate that the patient's problems are "in his head" (technically, the location of the problems would be above the tentorium cerebri). Clinicians are cautioned not to use the "cry for help" explanation for exaggeration unless there is converging evidence that this seems plausible. An elevated validity scale on a psychological test, for example, is not evidence that a "cry for help" underlies symptom overendorsement. Some psychologists seem to uncritically accept that because a computerized interpretive printout lists a "cry for help" as a possible cause, it is therefore the cause.

Second, neuropsychologists experienced with conducting civil forensic evaluations know that claimants and plaintiffs often feel angry about being injured and by their perceived mistreatment from an insurance company or the worker's compensation system. Some people feel strong justification for aggressively pursuing their litigation and feel entitled to generous compensation. Some people become preoccupied, consumed, and overwhelmed with their disability case or litigation. Through a series of independent evaluations they might feel the need to exaggerate their symptoms or problems for fear of not being taken seriously, or to communicate how bad off they were in the past. Moreover, there might be a number of reinforcing benefits relating to exaggerating one's problems, such as attention from family and friends, or avoidance of unpleasant activities.

Third, it is important to appreciate that some people with depression have an extremely negative view of themselves, the world, and their future. This negative thinking can manifest in exaggeration of symptoms and problems. When this happens, it is usually obvious. The person appears frankly and obviously depressed during the interview—and the pervasive negativism is easily noted.

Fourth, some people have a personality style that is prone to dramatizing and exaggerating their problems.

Fifth, a person might deliberately exaggerate because he has a deep-seated psychological need to be perceived as sick and disabled. The motivation is not the litigation per se, but to be seen and treated as a sick and disabled person. Under these circumstances, the person would meet the diagnostic criteria for factitious disorder.

Finally, a person might deliberately exaggerate because he is trying to influence the outcome of his evaluations in order to influence the outcome of his litigation (or disability evaluation). This latter behavior is what we consider malingering. In every evaluation, clinical or forensic, the reporting of symptoms and problems falls on a continuum, from under-reporting, to accurate reporting, to exaggeration, as illustrated in Figure 6.3. A person's reporting of symptoms and problems can move along this continuum during an evaluation, and over time from evaluation to evaluation.

Over the past 20 years, many terms have been used to describe reduced effort during neuropsychological testing, including but not limited to nonoptimal effort, suboptimal effort, incomplete effort, poor effort, biased responding, negative response bias, and noncredible test performance. Faking, feigning, simulating,

6.3

Continuum of symptom reporting.

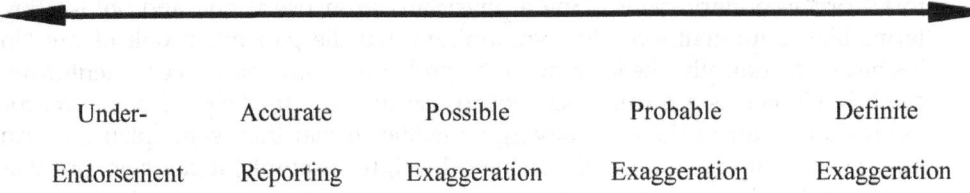

| Under- | Accurate | Possible | Probable | Definite |
| Endorsement | Reporting | Exaggeration | Exaggeration | Exaggeration |

dissimulating, magnifying, amplifying, over-reporting, and exaggerating are some of the terms used to describe interview behaviors, responses on psychological tests, and performance on neuropsychological tests. Those familiar with the literature will appreciate that nearly all of the above terms have been used to describe both test performance and symptom endorsement.

It is important conceptually to separate test performance and symptom endorsement. My preferred terms are poor effort for describing underperforming on neuropsychological tests and exaggeration for describing self-reported symptoms and problems during interviews or on psychological tests such as the MMPI-2. When there is clear and converging evidence, I will use these terms in a report without a hint of equivocation. Sometimes the terms poor effort or exaggeration seem too strong for the clinical situation where there is somewhat equivocal evidence for their presence. There are also occasions when I might describe a person's effort on testing as suboptimal or variable. I try to use the word *variable* on rare occasions. I occasionally use the expressions over-reporting or magnifying in relation to symptom reporting.

In general, the terms poor effort and exaggeration are simple, descriptive, and communicative. Many researchers and clinicians have adopted the expression *symptom validity assessment*, used in the NAN position paper (Bush et al., 2005), to refer to all methods and procedures upon which the practitioner can draw to make inferences regarding poor effort during testing and exaggeration of symptoms or problems during interviews or on psychological tests. There is nothing wrong with this terminology provided that the conceptual issues conveyed by the terminology are clearly understood. I think there has been longstanding conceptual confusion among clinicians and researchers regarding the similarities and differences between exaggeration and poor effort. Exaggeration and poor effort are related, but not synonymous, behavioral constructs. Unfortunately, the distinction between them is often blurred. For example, clinicians frequently refer to poor performance on an effort test as exaggeration, such as symptom exaggeration or cognitive exaggeration. The term "exaggeration" is less ambiguous conceptually if it is used to describe symptom reporting during interviewing, symptom over-endorsement on psychological tests, or behavioral observations (e.g., facial expressions or pain behaviors). Poor effort, on the other hand, refers to clearly suboptimal effort during testing. This simply means the person underperformed during testing. The clinician might wish to infer that this underperformance constitutes exaggeration of problems, such as memory problems, but it is important to appreciate that this is a secondary clinical inference. Rather, the primary clinical inference is poor effort, underperformance, or submaximal effort.

Diagnostic Criteria for Malingering in Neuropsychology

Slick, Sherman, and Iverson (1999) proposed diagnostic criteria for definite, probable, and possible malingering (see Table 6.2 for a partial reproduction of the criteria). These criteria have been used in numerous studies (e.g., Ardolf, Denney, & Houston, 2007; Bianchini, Greve, & Love, 2003; Bianchini et al., 2003; Bianchini, Love, Greve, & Adams, 2005; Curtis, Greve, Bianchini, & Brennan, 2006; Etherton, Bianchini, Greve, & Heinly, 2005; Greve et al., 2006; Greve, Bianchini, & Doane, 2006; Greve et al., 2009; Greve, Bianchini, Love, Brennan, & Heinly, 2006; Greve, Bianchini, Mathias, Houston, & Crouch, 2002, 2003; Greve et al., 2007; Heinly, Greve, Bianchini, Love, & Brennan, 2005; Larrabee, 2003c; Mathias, Greve, Bianchini, Houston, & Crouch, 2002). For a diagnosis of definite malingering, there must be clear and compelling evidence of poor effort on testing (i.e., below chance performance). To be considered malingering, the person's behavior should be conceptualized as volitional and rational. In addition, there must not be plausible alternative explanations for this behavior (e.g., factitious disorder or somatoform disorder). Moreover, it should be determined that the exaggeration or fabrication of impairment is not the result of diminished capacity to appreciate laws or mores against malingering or an inability to conform behavior to such standards, as may be the case in persons with certain psychiatric (e.g., a schizophrenia spectrum disorder), developmental (e.g., mental retardation), or neurological disorders (e.g., dementia).

The foundation of an opinion regarding malingered cognitive impairment is deliberately poor performance on testing. Evidence of poor effort on neuropsychological testing can be demonstrated by one of the following: (a) below-chance performance ($p < .05$) on one or more forced-choice measures of cognitive function; (b) poor effort on one or more well-validated tests or embedded indices designed to measure this behavior; (c) compelling inconsistency between test results and known patterns of brain functioning (e.g., biological severity indexing); (d) compelling inconsistency between test results and observed behavior; (e) compelling inconsistency between test results and reliable collateral reports; and (f) compelling inconsistency between test results and documented background history.

According to Slick and colleagues (1999), evidence from the patient's self-report can be used to support a diagnosis of malingering. The following factors

6.2 Criteria for Definite, Probable, and Possible Malingering of Cognitive Impairment

Definite Malingering is indicated by the presence of clear and compelling evidence of volitional exaggeration or fabrication of cognitive impairment, and the absence of plausible alternative explanations. The specific diagnostic criteria necessary for Definite Malingering are listed below.

1. Presence of a substantial external incentive [Criterion A]
2. Definite poor effort on testing characterized by below-chance performance [Criterion B1]
3. Behaviors meeting necessary criteria from group B are not fully accounted for by Psychiatric, Neurological, or Developmental factors [Criterion D]

Probable Malingering is indicated by the presence of evidence strongly suggesting volitional exaggeration or fabrication of cognitive impairment, and the absence of plausible alternative explanations. The specific diagnostic criteria necessary for Probable Malingering are listed below.

1. Presence of a substantial external incentive [Criterion A]
2. Two or more types of evidence from neuropsychological testing, excluding definite (i.e., below-chance) poor effort [two or more of Criteria B2–B6]
OR
One type of evidence from neuropsychological testing, excluding definite poor effort, and one or more types of evidence from Self-Report [one of Criteria B2–B6 and one or more of Criteria C1–C5]
3. Behaviors meeting necessary criteria from groups B or C are not fully accounted for by Psychiatric, Neurological, or Developmental Factors [Criterion D]

Possible Malingering is indicated by the presence of evidence suggesting volitional exaggeration or fabrication of cognitive impairment, and the absence of plausible alternative explanations. Alternatively, Possible Malingering is indicated by the presence of criteria necessary for Definite or Probable Malingering, except that other possible causes cannot reasonably be ruled out. The specific diagnostic criteria for Possible Malingering are listed below.

1. Presence of a substantial external incentive [Criterion A]
2. Evidence from Self-Report [one or more of Criteria C1–C5]
3. Behaviors meeting necessary criteria from groups B or C are not fully accounted for by Psychiatric, Neurological, or Developmental factors [Criterion D]
OR
Criteria for Definite or Probable Malingering are met except for Criterion D (i.e., primary psychiatric, neurological, or developmental etiologies cannot reasonably be ruled out). In such cases, the alternate etiologies that cannot be ruled out should be specified.

Adapted with minor terminology modifications from Slick, Sherman, & Iverson (1999). Reprinted with permission.

may be considered suspect, and should be examined carefully: (a) self-reported history that is inconsistent with documented history; (b) self-reported symptoms that are inconsistent with known patterns of brain functioning; (c) self-reported symptoms that are inconsistent with behavioral observations; (d) self-reported symptoms that are inconsistent with information obtained from reliable collateral informants; or (e) evidence of exaggerated or fabricated self-reported problems on psychological tests (e.g., the MMPI-2). A checklist for using the diagnostic criteria is provided in Table 6.3.

6.3	Malingering Criteria Checklist
A.	Clear and substantial external incentive
B1.	Definite poor effort (below chance)
B2.	Probable poor effort
B3.	Discrepancy between known patterns of brain function/dysfunction and test data
B4.	Discrepancy between observed behavior and test data
B5.	Discrepancy between reliable collateral reports and test data
B6.	Discrepancy between history and test data
C1.	Self-reported history is discrepant with documented history
C2.	Self-reported symptoms are discrepant with known patterns of brain functioning
C3.	Self-reported symptoms are discrepant with behavioral observations
C4.	Self-reported symptoms are discrepant with information obtained from collateral informants
C5.	Evidence of exaggerated or fabricated psychological dysfunction on standardized measures
D.	Behaviors satisfying Criteria B and/or C were volitional and directed at least in part towards acquiring or achieving external incentives as defined in Criteria A
E.	The patient adequately understood the purpose of the examination and the possible negative consequences of exaggerating or fabricating cognitive impairments
F.	Test results contributing to Criteria B are sufficiently reliable and valid (see Slick, Sherman, & Iverson, 1999)

Checklist from Iverson (2003), with slight modifications.

Limitations and Suggested Refinements to the Malingering Criteria

Larrabee, Greiffenstein, Greve, and Bianchini (2007) provided a review of the strengths and limitations of the 1999 malingering criteria. Their review and critique was informed by an extraordinary amount of research done between 1999 and 2007, and their combined and extensive clinical experience with the criteria. They noted the five limitations listed below.

1. The focus on cognitive malingering tends to minimize important evidence of malingering in other behavioral domains (e.g., emotional and physical).
2. Certain combinations of variables may predict malingering with a very high degree of specificity, but because they all represent the same B criterion (usually either B2 or B6), they are not sufficient for a probable malingering diagnosis.
3. There is an over-reliance on cognitive test findings (particularly B1, B2, and B6 findings). Other findings (e.g., C5), although potentially strongly indicative of malingering, are weighted less.

4. The C criteria are largely clinician dependent. The reliability and accuracy of clinical judgments of atypical self-reports or implausible-sounding symptom development depends heavily on the depth and breadth of fundamental neurological knowledge of the neuropsychologist.
5. The criteria might be too conservative (e.g., requiring two B6 hits for a positive B6).

Larrabee and colleagues (2007) offered the following recommendations for improving the criteria: (a) allow multiple psychometric findings to define probable malingering, (b) require only one B6 hit to meet the B6 criterion, (c) require multiple qualitative, subjective criteria, and (d) give C criteria equal weight. In contrast, Boone (2007a) encourages clinicians to move away from diagnosing malingering, arguing that it is extremely difficult, and perhaps unnecessary, to form an opinion regarding conscious intent. She recommended that the terminology in the criteria be changed from malingering to *noncredible neurocognitive function*. Further, she recommended that the criteria for definite noncredible neurocognitive performance be determined by (a) failure on at least three validated effort measures with minimal shared variance and with cutoffs set to ≥ 90% specificity, and (b) behavioral evidence of noncredible symptoms.

Assessing for Exaggerated Symptom Reporting

Several multiscale psychological tests have validity scales. These validity scales have varying degrees of accuracy for detecting exaggeration. Examples of tests with validity scales include the *Minnesota Multiphasic Personality Inventory—Second Edition* (MMPI-2) (Butcher et al., 2001), Personality Assessment Inventory (PAI) (Morey, 1991), Ruff Neurobehavioral Inventory (Ruff & Hibbard, 2003), and the Behavior Rating Inventory of Executive Function–Adult Version (BRIEF-A) (Roth, Isquith, & Gioia, 2005).

Minnesota Multiphasic Personality Inventory– Second Edition

There is an enormous literature relating to detecting exaggeration on the *Minnesota Multiphasic Personality Inventory–Second Edition (MMPI-2)* (Butcher et al., 2001) (see, for example, reviews by Greene, 2000; Guriel & Fremouw, 2003; Iverson & Lange, 2005; Lees-Haley, Iverson, Lange, Fox, & Allen, 2002; Meyers, Millis, & Volkert, 2002; Nelson, Sweet, & Demakis, 2006; and Rogers, Sewell, Martin, & Vitacco, 2003). Researchers frequently have reported that the traditional and supplemental infrequency validity scales, such as F, F$_B$, and F (p) are effective for identifying exaggeration. There is no doubt that some personal injury litigants will substantially elevate these scales. When this occurs, it often represents frank and somewhat unsophisticated exaggeration. It is important to note, however, that these scales are more useful for identifying exaggeration of severe mental illness, such as in criminal forensic evaluations involving competency to stand trial.

Validity scales and indices that might be more useful for identifying exaggeration in civil forensic evaluations include the Fake Bad Scale, the Henry-Heilbronner Index, and the Malingered Mood Disorder Scale, among others. Iverson and Lange (2005) provided numerous tables summarizing the literature on a variety of older-generation validity scales. A meta-analysis is essential reading for practitioners using the *MMPI-2* validity scales (Nelson et al., 2006). Nelson and colleagues concluded that the Fake Bad Scale performed as well or better than the other *MMPI-2* validity scales for identifying exaggeration. Based on a large literature (see, for example, Bagby, Nicholson, Buis, & Bacchiochi, 2000; Dean et al., 2008; Dearth et al., 2005; Greiffenstein, Baker, Axelrod, Peck, & Gervais, 2004; Greiffenstein, Baker, Gola, Donders, & Miller, 2002; Guez, Brannstrom, Nyberg, Toolanen, & Hildingsson, 2005; Henry, Heilbronner, Mittenberg, Enders, & Stanczak, 2008; Larrabee, 1997, 1998, 2003a, 2003c; Lees-Haley, 1992; Lees-Haley, English, & Glenn, 1991; Nelson et al., 2006; Ross, Millis, Krukowski, Putnam, & Adams, 2004; Tsushima & Tsushima, 2001; and Wygant et al., 2007), this scale seems particularly useful in civil forensic neuropsychological evaluations.

Meyers and colleagues developed the MMPI-2 Validity Index (Meyers et al., 2002). The Validity Index combines seven validity scales from the *MMPI-2* (i.e., F-K, F, FBS, F (p), Ds-r, Es, and O-S). Each validity index is assigned a weight of 1 or 2 points based on an arbitrarily defined score range on each validity scale. Scores on the Validity Index can range from 0 to 14. A cutoff score of 5 or higher was recommended as a preliminary criterion for exaggeration based on the Validity Index scores of 100 nonlitigant chronic pain patients, 100 litigating chronic pain patients, and 30 sophisticated simulators instructed to feign the emotional and cognitive difficulties demonstrated by chronic pain patients. Using a cutoff score of 5 or above, 100% of nonlitigant chronic pain patients were successfully classified as honest responders, and 86% of the simulators were correctly identified as exaggerating symptomatology. In the litigating chronic-pain patient sample, 33% scored 5 points or higher on this index. These authors conclude that the MMPI-2 Validity Index appears to be superior to any single validity scale, although replication of these findings was recommended.

Aguerrevere and colleagues reanalyzed large data sets using an abbreviated version of the Meyers Validity Index (Aguerrevere, Greve, Bianchini, & Meyers, 2008). This was done because two of the seven validity scales (Obvious minus Subtle and Dissimulation-revised) are not reported by the commercially available Pearson computerized scoring system. The authors concluded that the abbreviated Meyers Index can be used as a substitute of the original Meyers Index without decrements in classification accuracy.

Greve and colleagues published a sophisticated, elaborate, and clinically useful study on interpreting the *MMPI-2* validity scales in brain injury litigation (Greve et al., 2006). They examined the *MMPI-2* validity scales in 259 patients with traumatic brain injuries in comparison with 133 patients not involved in litigation who were referred for neuropsychological evaluations for a variety of neurological, medical, or psychiatric reasons. Fb, DS-r, and Ego Strength appeared to be the most effective scales. The Fake Bad Scale and Myers Validity Index also were useful. The authors provided sensitivity, specificity, and predictive value statistics for various cutoffs on the validity scales. This article is essential reading for anyone using the *MMPI-2* in civil forensic neuropsychological evaluations.

The Response Bias Scale (RBS) (Gervais, Ben-Porath, Wygant, & Green, 2007) is a 28-item *MMPI-2* scale that was developed to predict failure on effort tests. Multiple regression analyses were used to select items that independently predicted failure on one or more effort tests, and the resulting items formed the RBS scale. Not surprisingly, given the methodology for scale construction, the initial validation of the RBS found that the scale outperformed the MMPI-2 F, F_P, and FBS in predicting failure on effort tests such as the Computerized Assessment of Response Bias (CARB), Word Memory Test (WMT), and the Medical Symptom Validity Test (MSVT). A cutoff score of 17 had very high positive predictive power and specificity, indicating that (a) scoring in this range is highly associated with effort-test failure, and (b) the false positive rate is low. However, the RBS had relatively low sensitivity (i.e., 25–30% of people who failed effort testing were accurately identified). Whitney and colleagues reported that the RBS was associated with effort-test failure in an outpatient veteran's sample (Whitney, Davis, Shepard, & Herman, 2008). Additional research, however, is needed on this scale.

The Henry-Heilbronner Index (HHI) (Henry, Heilbronner, Mittenberg, & Enders, 2006; Henry et al., 2008) is a 15-item, empirically derived scale designed to identify exaggeration and malingering in personal injury litigants and disability claimants. In the original validation study, the HHI was reportedly superior to the FBS for identifying symptom exaggeration in litigating patients versus nonlitigating head-injury control subjects. A cutoff score of ≥ 8 was associated with 80% sensitivity and 89% specificity. Additional research is needed on this scale.

Henry and colleagues (2008) developed the Malingered Mood Disorder Scale (MMDS). This scale, consisting of 15 items, was empirically derived from the original 32-item Malingered Depression Scale (MDS) (Steffan, Clopton, & Morgan, 2003). The authors reported that the MMDS was superior to the original MDS for identifying symptom exaggeration in personal-injury litigants and disability claimants compared with nonlitigating head-injured control subjects. A score of ≥ 8 was associated with 100% positive predictive power (no false positive errors). This study suggests that the MMDS may be useful in identifying personal-injury litigants who exaggerate psychological problems on the *MMPI-2*. Additional research on this scale is needed.

The *MMPI-2* is the most thoroughly researched and well-validated psychological test for identifying exaggerated symptom reporting. Over decades, the research has evolved from identifying fake-bad to malingered insanity to exaggerated physical and psychological problems in forensic psychological and neuropsychological evaluations.

Personality Assessment Inventory

The Personality Assessment Inventory (PAI) (Morey, 1991) is an objective personality inventory designed to measure psychological functioning across multiple domains. Unlike the *MMPI-2*, there is no item overlap on the scales. In addition, items are answered on a 4-point Likert scale as opposed to a true/false format. In addition to the clinical scales, the PAI has four validity scales. The Inconsistency scale comprises 10 highly correlated items. The Infrequency scale contains 8 items that are rarely endorsed by healthy adults, and these items are believed to be minimally related to psychopathology. The Positive Impression Management scale is designed to evaluate a response style involving denial or minimization of shortcomings, and the Negative Impression Management scale (NIM) contains nine items that are rarely endorsed by persons in the general population and are considered to reflect exaggerated psychological problems. Morey (1996) described eight score patterns that comprise a Malingering Index on the PAI. If the patient demonstrates three or more of these score patterns, malingering is suspected; five or more score patterns represent likely malingering. A raw score of 2 on the Malingering Index corresponds to a T score of 71, a score of 3 corresponds to a T score of 84, and a score of 4 corresponds to a T score of 98. The vast majority of mental health patients in the PAI clinical sample obtained a score of 2 or less on the Malingering Index. Rogers and colleagues conducted a large-scale study of the PAI validity scales using undergraduates and psychology graduate students as simulators. A discriminant function analysis provided better classification accuracy than the single validity scales (Rogers, Sewell, Morey, & Ustad, 1996). This discriminant function is included in the computerized scoring program for the PAI.

In general, the Personality Assessment Inventory is a well-designed and validated measure for identifying psychological, behavioral, and personality problems. There is a growing body of research directed toward identifying exaggeration and malingering on the PAI, and most has been related to identifying severe psychopathology (Bagby, Nicholson, Bacchiochi, Ryder, & Bury, 2002; Baity, Siefert, Chambers, & Blais, 2007; Boccaccini, Murrie, & Duncan, 2006; Calhoun, Earnst, Tucker, Kirby, & Beckham, 2000; Edens, Poythress, & Watkins-Clay, 2007; Hawes & Boccaccini, 2009; Hopwood, Morey, Rogers, & Sewell, 2007; Hopwood, Talbert, Morey, & Rogers, 2008; King & Sullivan, 2009; Kucharski, Duncan, Egan, & Falkenbach, 2006; Kucharski, Toomey, Fila, & Duncan, 2007; Liljequist, Kinder, & Schinka, 1998; Morey & Lanier, 1998; Rogers, Ornduff, & Sewell, 1993; Rogers, Sewell, Cruise, Wang, & Ustad, 1998; Rogers et al., 1996; Sumanti, Boone, Savodnik, & Gorsuch, 2006; Veazey, Wagner, Hays, & Miller, 2005; Wang et al., 1997; Whiteside, Dunbar-Mayer, & Waters, 2009). Hawes and Boccaccini (2009) conducted a meta-analysis of the literature. They concluded that scores of ≥ 81 on the Negative Impression Management scale and ≥ 3 on the Malingering Index resulted in the highest overall classification rates for identifying exaggeration.

Psychologists should be cautious about over-relying on the Negative Impression Management scale or the Malingering Index. These measures are more likely to detect extreme and bizarre symptom reporting, such as that seen in a criminal forensic evaluation of someone who is faking insanity. These measures might be less sensitive to exaggeration in civil forensic evaluations. Nonetheless, when patients involved in compensation-related evaluations elevate these validity scales, they also have pronounced elevations on the clinical scales. Sumanti and colleagues presented PAI data from a large sample of patients ($N = 233$) who were undergoing psychological evaluations in connection with a worker's compensation claim (Sumanti et al., 2006). They defined exaggeration using the following cutoff scores: NIM, ≥ 84T, Malingering Index raw score, ≥ 3, or Roger's Discriminant Function, ≥ 60T. The prevalence of exaggeration in their sample, based on these cutoff scores, was 9% on NIM, 16% on the Malingering Index, and 29% on Roger's Discriminant Function. Interestingly and unexpectedly, there were few differences on the PAI clinical scales in those who were believed to be exaggerating versus not exaggerating on the Roger's Discriminant Function. In contrast, claim-

6.4

Comparing worker's compensation claimants with elevated Malingering Index scores on other PAI scales.

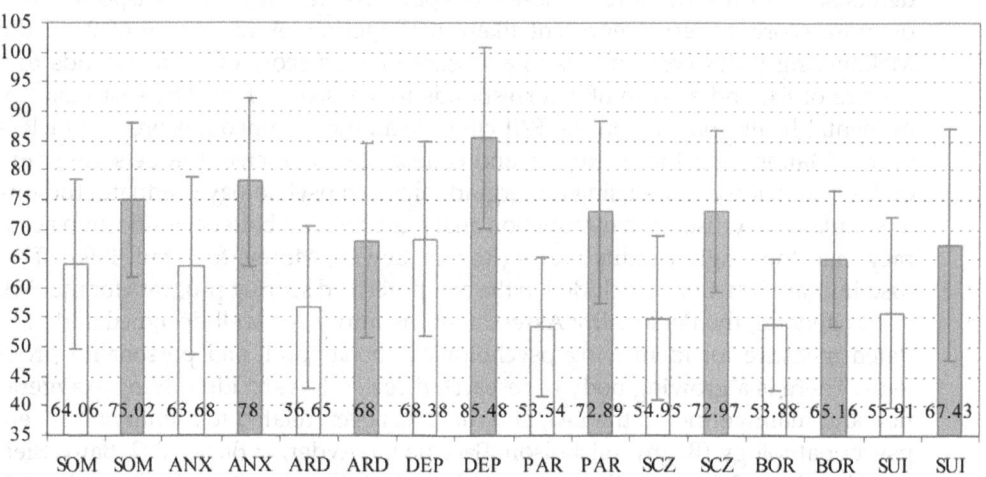

Note: Worker's compensation claimants (N = 233) undergoing psychological evaluations; 16% had elevated Malingering Index scores. Mean scores for the exaggeration group are illustrated with gray bars. The error lines represent 1 SD. SOM = Somatic Complaints, ANX = Anxiety, ARD = Anxiety-Related Disorders, DEP = Depression, PAR = Paranoia, SCZ = Schizophrenia, BOR = Borderline Features, and SUI = Suicidal Ideation.

ants with elevated NIM or Malingering Index scores also had more elevated scores on numerous clinical scales.

The PAI clinical scales that differed between worker's compensation claimants who had elevated Malingering Index scores versus those who did not are illustrated in Figure 6.4. Scores between 40 and 60 are broadly normal for healthy, community-dwelling adults, and scores above 70 are highly elevated for healthy adults. Notice that the average score for the exaggerating group exceeds a T score of 70 for the Somatic Complaints, Anxiety, Depression, Paranoia, and Schizophrenia scales.

From a clinical perspective, another method for screening for exaggeration is to determine whether the person's symptom reporting seems extreme relative to the clinical sample. If so, do the assessment results converge to suggest that this extreme symptom reporting is reflective of the person's true condition? That is, when considering interview findings, behavioral observation, medical records, and other collateral information, does it make sense that the person could be experiencing the extreme symptoms and problems reported on this test (such as depression and anxiety in excess of 90% of the clinical sample)?

Selected clinical scales and subscales are presented in Table 6.4. The PAI scoring program plots a line indicating where 2 standard deviations above the mean for the PAI clinical sample falls. To supplement this information, I calculated the raw score that corresponds to 1 standard deviation above the mean, and the

	Selected PAI Clinical Scales and Subscales: Census-Matched Normative T Scores Corresponding to Unusual and Highly Unusual Symptom Reporting in the Clinical Sample			
6.4				
Clinical Scales & Subscales	**1 SD Raw**	**>1 SD Normative T**	**90th % Raw**	**> 90th % Normative T**
Somatic Complaints (SOM)	33.7	72	38.2	78
Conversion (SOM-C)	10.7	75	12.4	81
Somatization (SOM-S)	12.3	73	13.8	75
Hypochondriasis (SOM-H)	12.4	71	14.2	76
Anxiety (ANX)	44.0	77	48.8	81
Anxiety-Cognitive (ANX-C)	16.7	75	18.6	80
Anxiety-Affective (ANX-A)	15.9	75	17.6	81
Anxiety-Physiological (ANX-P)	12.7	75	14.2	81
Anxiety-Related Disorders (ARD)	40.7	75	44.5	80
Traumatic Stress (ARD-T)	16.4	82	18.5	87
Depression (DEP)	42.5	80	47.2	86
Depression-Cognitive (DEP-C)	13.7	78	15.4	84
Depression-Affective (DEP-A)	15.2	83	17.1	88
Depression-Physiological (DEP-P)	15.2	72	16.9	77
Irritability (MAN-I)	14.9	67	16.4	71
Thought Disorder (SCZ-T)	12.9	75	14.5	81
Affective Instability (BOR-A)	12.8	75	14.2	81

Note: The raw scores are for the Clinical Sample presented in the PAI manual (N = 1,246). The T scores are for the Census-Matched Standardization Sample (N = 1,000). The T scores for healthy adults represent raw scores that are greater than 1 SD above the mean, and greater than the 90th percentile for the Clinical Sample. Scores above 1 SD are uncommon, and scores above the 90th percentile are very uncommon in the PAI Clinical Sample.

90th percentile for the clinical sample. I then looked up the corresponding T scores from the normative sample. Thus, if evaluating a patient who obtains an Anxiety Scale score of ≥ 81 and a Depression Scale T score of ≥ 86, these scores are greater than 90% of the PAI clinical sample, they should be considered very uncommon. There should be clear and obvious converging evidence to suggest that the patient is suffering from a high degree of depression and anxiety. Otherwise, scores in this range could easily reflect exaggeration.

Ruff Neurobehavioral Inventory

The Ruff Neurobehavioral Inventory (RNBI) (Ruff & Hibbard, 2003) is a 243-item, self-report questionnaire that assesses a person's perception of the important dimensions of his or her daily life activities following a traumatic brain injury.

The RNBI uses two different types of questions to assess both pre-injury and post-injury functioning. The test yields four validity scales, four composite scores (i.e., Cognitive, Emotional, Physical, and Quality of Life), and 18 basic scales (e.g., Learning & Memory, Executive Functions, Anger & Aggression, Depression, Pain, Activities of Daily Living, and Vocation & Finance). Premorbid and postmorbid normative scores are derived for nearly every scale.

The Inconsistency Scale contains 12 pairs of items with similar content that are scattered throughout the test. Respondents are expected to answer the items consistently. The Infrequency Scale contains items that were endorsed in an extreme manner by the normative sample and the clinical validation sample. Six items from the premorbid scales and six items from the postmorbid scales were selected based on low levels of endorsement. There are two Negative Impression scales. These scales contain six items from the premorbid scales and six from the postmorbid scales. These scales are designed to identify frank exaggeration. The items describe unusually negative and exaggerated problems. Most of the items are emotional or psychological in content. There are two Positive Impression scales that contain six items each, premorbid and postmorbid. These scales are designed to measure a person's denial of flaws or difficulties.

By design, the validity scales seem promising for identifying random or highly inconsistent responding; fairly extreme exaggeration, primarily in the psychological/emotional domain; and positive response bias, such as denying common faults and presenting oneself in an overly favorable light. To my knowledge, however, there has been no published research as of early 2009 relating to detecting exaggeration or malingering using the RNBI validity scales.

The self-report of symptoms and problems, especially in cases involving personal injury litigation or disability-related evaluations, has obvious inherent limitations. Getting the person's perspective, nonetheless, is critical. The RNBI is an excellent instrument for gathering comprehensive and diverse information on the patient's perspective. We use the RNBI on a regular basis because of its large normative sample, unique design, and obvious clinical relevance. To date, we have rarely seen any elevated validity scales in patients seen for forensic evaluations. On several occasions I have evaluated patients with extreme symptom reporting and frank effort-test failures who have not elevated the validity scales. I anticipate that a new RNBI validity scale will need to be developed and validated to more reliably identify exaggeration in civil forensic neuropsychological evaluations. After that development, we can have increased confidence in the reliability and accuracy of the symptom reporting on this inventory.

Behavior Rating Inventory of Executive Function–Adult Version

The Behavior Rating Inventory of Executive Function–Adult Version (BRIEF-A) (Roth et al., 2005) contains 75 items that yield nine nonoverlapping theoretically and clinically derived scales that measure different aspects of executive functioning. The clinical scales are combined to form two broad index scores, the Behavioral Regulation Index and the Metacognition Index, and an overall composite score, the Global Executive Composite. The clinical scales comprising the Behavioral Regulation Index are labeled Inhibit, Shift, Emotional Control, and Self-Monitor.

The clinical scales comprising the Metacognition Index are labeled Initiate, Working Memory, Plan/Organize, Task Monitor, and Organization of Materials. The BRIEF-A can be completed rapidly (approximately 15 minutes), it has broad coverage of executive functioning, and it is normed based on self-report and informant-report. Norming the test for use with a collateral informant (e.g., a spouse or family member) makes it inherently useful in mainstream clinical practice.

The BRIEF-A contains three validity scales labeled Negativity, Infrequency, and Inconsistency. Each validity scale is on the self-report and informant-report versions of the test. The Negativity scale contains 10 items. They are scored only if the respondent rates them in the most extreme direction (i.e., to get a point they must be rated as Often, versus Never or Sometimes). Thus, there is a maximum score of 10 points for the scale. Obtaining a raw score of 6 or greater on this scale occurs in less than 1% of the normative sample and the clinical sample. The Infrequency scale is designed to measure the extent to which individuals respond to the test in an atypical manner. The scale contains 5 items that people would customarily respond to in a single direction. These items, if responded to in the extreme directions might represent an overly favorable or overly negative point of view. Elevations on this scale might also reflect a haphazard approach to completing the test. A cutoff score is provided, above which 1% or fewer of the normative sample or clinical sample scored. The Inconsistency scale contains 10 pairs of items with similar content. Thus, barring an insufficient reading level, it is expected that a person who carefully and thoughtfully responds to the items will rate these pairs similarly. Extreme cutoff scores for the Inconsistency scale are provided (i.e., a person must score above 99.7% of the combined normative and clinical samples to be considered to have responded inconsistently). To my knowledge, as of early 2009, there has been no published research evaluating the BRIEF-A validity scales. Similar to the RNBI, it might be necessary, over time, for clinical researchers to develop modified or alternative validity scales and indices that can reliably and accurately identify exaggeration. In the meantime, of course, research is needed on the current validity scales.

Conceptualizing and Assessing Poor Effort in Neuropsychology

Neuropsychological testing is exquisitely dependent upon effort. Effort is a state, not a trait. Effort is variable, not constant. Effort is behavior that falls on a continuum. On occasion, in clinical practice, we assess people who are *extremely* motivated to perform well. Most of the time, however, our patients' effort is likely to be only *good* or *adequate* for the purposes of the evaluation. It is likely that the normative data upon which we compare our patients' test results comprise subjects who gave *adequate, good,* or *excellent* effort (with the possibility of a subset of subjects who gave relatively *poor* effort due to lack of interest or other reasons). Most subjects in normative studies likely gave *good* or *adequate* effort, although this assumption is ultimately unknowable.

A continuum for conceptualizing effort is illustrated in Figure 6.5. This figure reminds us to approach effort as a spectrum of behavior, not simply a dichotomous construct. It would be a mistake to conclude, for example, that a person provided

6.5

Continuum of effort.

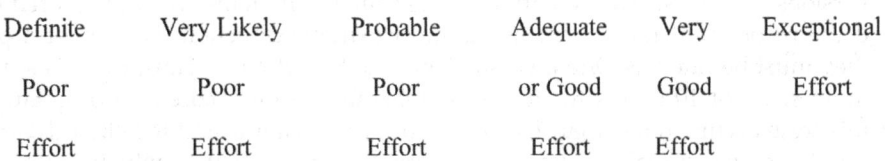

Definite	Very Likely	Probable	Adequate	Very	Exceptional
Poor	Poor	Poor	or Good	Good	Effort
Effort	Effort	Effort	Effort	Effort	

Note: Some people provide exceptional effort. They are extremely motivated to perform well on tests. Most people provide adequate effort during testing. A person's effort can vary along this continuum within a single evaluation.

exceptional effort, or even *good* effort, on the basis of performing normally on a single effort test. *Conclusions about level of effort should be based on several sources of converging evidence, not on a single test score.* As a general rule, passing one or more effort tests suggests *adequate* effort, or possibly *good* effort, provided that there are no other indicators in the battery or in the behavioral observations of possible *poor* effort.

There are two types of tests that are used to identify poor effort in neuropsychology: traditional and specialized. Traditional tests are simply tests that have been developed to measure a specific skill or ability, and that have been used by researchers to identify poor effort. Examples of traditional tests that have been used to identify poor effort are provided in Table 6.5. This list is not exhaustive. Many tests have been similarly used in this manner. Traditional tests have embedded measures (e.g., reliable digit span; errors on Subtests I or II of the Category Test; Logical Memory Rarely Missed Index), or cut-off scores or score patterns that are associated with poor effort. Specialized tests, in contrast, have been designed and validated specifically for the detection of poor effort. Examples of specialized tests are provided in Table 6.6.

Clinicians know that poor effort can result in a global suppression of neuropsychological test performance or scattered low scores across a battery of tests. Researchers have reported that poor effort results in suppressed test scores on a variety of neuropsychological tests (e.g., Backhaus, Fichtenberg, & Hanks, 2004; Constantinou, Bauer, Ashendorf, Fisher, & McCaffrey, 2005; Henry, 2005).

6.5 Examples of Traditional Tests, With Embedded Markers, That Have Been Used to Identify Poor Effort

California Verbal Learning Test
Ashendorf, O'Bryant, & McCaffrey (2003); Demakis (1999); Moore & Donders (2004); Baker, Donder, & Thompson (2000); Coleman, Rapport, Millis, Ricker, & Farchione (1998); Trueblood (1994); Trueblood & Schmidt (1993); Millis, Putnam, Adams, & Ricker (1995); Slick, Iverson, & Green (2000); Sweet et al. (2000); Demakis (2004); Bauer, Yantz, Ryan, Warden, & McCaffrey (2005); Greve, Curtis, Bianchini, & Ord (2008); Donders & Boonstra (2007); Root, Robbins, Chang, & Van Gorp (2006); Curtis, Greve, Bianchini, & Brennan (2006).

Category Test
DiCarlo, Gfeller, & Oliveri (2000); Forrest, Allen, & Goldstein (2004); Sweet & King (2002); Tenhula & Sweet (1996); Williamson, Green, Allen, & Rohling (2003); Greve, Bianchini, & Robertson (2007).

Digit Span, Reliable Digit Span, & Vocabulary-Digit Span Difference Scores
DiCarlo, Gfeller, & Oliveri (2000); Forrest, Allen, & Goldstein (2004); Sweet & King (2002); Tenhula & Sweet (1996); Binder & Willis (1991); Greiffenstein, Baker, & Gola (1994); Meyers & Volbrecht (1998); Iverson & Franzen (1994, 1996); Iverson & Tulsky (2003); Meyers & Volbrecht (1998); Suhr, Tranel, Wefel, & Barrash (1997); Trueblood & Schmidt (1993); Merten, Green, Henry, Blaskewitz, & Brockhaus (2005); Heinly et al. (2005); Etherton, Bianchini, Greve, & Heinly (2005); Etherton, Bianchini, et al. (2005); Fisher & Rose (2005); Axelrod & Rawlings (1999); Iverson & Tulsky (2003); Mittenberg, Theroux-Fichera, Zielinski, & Heilbronner (1995); Millis, Ross, & Ricker (1998); Miller, Ryan, Carruthers, & Cluff (2004); Vagnini et al. (2006); Babikian, Boone, Lu, & Arnold (2006); Shum, O'Gorman, & Alpar (2004); Larrabee (2003a); Nelson et al. (2003); Greve et al. (2003); Mittenberg, Aguila-Puentes, Patton, Canyock, & Heilbronner (2002); Larrabee, Millis, & Meyers (2009); Dean, Victor, Boone, Philpott, & Hess (2008); Greiffenstein & Baker (2008); Ruocco et al. (2008); Greve et al. (2007); Schwarz, Gfeller & Oliveri (2006); Axelrod, Fichtenberg, Millis, & Wertheimer (2006).

Rey Auditory Verbal Learning Test
Barrash, Suhr, & Manzel (2004); Suhr, Gunstad, Greub, & Barrash (2004); Powell, Gfeller, Hendricks, & Sharland (2004); Sherman, Boone, Lu, & Razani (2002); Bernard, Houston, & Natoli (1993); Silverberg & Barrash (2005); Boone, Lu, & Wen (2005); Russeler, Brett, Klaue, Sailer, & Munte (2008); Dean et al. (2008).

Recognition Memory Test
Iverson & Franzen (1994, 1998); Iverson & Binder (2000); Millis (1992, 1994); Millis & Dijkers (1993); Barrash et al. (2004); Silverberg & Barrash (2005); Nelson et al. (2003); Ross, Putnam, & Adams (2006); Tardif, Barry, Fox, & Johnstone (2000); Millis (2002); Dean, Victor, Boone, Philpott, & Hess (2008); Dean, Victor, Boone, & Arnold (2008).

Wechsler Memory Scale–Third Edition (WMS-III)
Killgore & DellaPietra (2000a, 2000b); Langeluddecke & Lucas (2003); Glassmire et al. (2003); Hilsabeck et al. (2003); Miller et al. (2004); Lange, Sullivan, & Anderson (2005); Mittenberg et al. (2002); Langeluddecke & Lucas (2004); Ord, Greve, & Bianchini (2008); Swihart, Harris, & Hatcher (2007); Lange, Iverson, Sullivan, & Anderson (2006); Langeluddecke & Lucas (2005).

6.6 Examples of Specialized Tests That Have Been Used to Identify Poor Effort

Amsterdam Short-Term Memory Test

Merten et al. (2005); van Hout, Schmand, Wekking, Hageman, & Deelman (2003); Bolan, Foster, Schmand, & Bolan (2002); van der Werf, Prins, Jongen, van der Meer, & Bleijenberg (2000); Schmand et al. (1998); Schagen, Schmand, de Sterke, & Lindeboom (1997); Jelicic, Merckelbach, Candel, & Geraerts (2006); Merten, Bossink, & Schmand (2007); Stulemeijer, Andriessen, Brauer, Vos, & Van Der Werf (2007).

b Test

Vilar-Lopez, Gomez-Rio, Caracuel-Romero, Llamas-Elvira, & Perez-Garcia (2008); Dean et al. (2008); Vilar-Lopez et al. (2007); Nelson et al. (2003); Boone et al. (2000); Boone & Lu (2007).

Computerized Assessment of Response Bias

Allen, Conder, Green, & Cox (1997); Green & Iverson (2001a, 2001b); Allen, Iverson, & Green (2002); Lynch (2004); Gervais et al. (2004); Dunn, Shear, Howe, & Ris (2003); Iverson (2001); Slick, Iverson, & Green (2000).

Dot Counting Test

Erdal (2004); Nelson et al. (2003); Strauss et al. (2002); Vickery, Berry, Inman, Harris, & Orey (2001); Lee et al. (2000); Rose, Hall, Szalda-Petree, & Bach (1998); Hayes, Hale, & Gouvier (1998); Arnett & Franzen (1997); Binks, Gouvier, & Waters (1997); Boone et al. (1995); Beetar & Williams (1995); Frederick (2002a); Brennan & Gouvier (2006); Erdal (2009); Vilar-Lopez, Gomez-Rio, Santiago-Ramajo, et al. (2008b); Dean et al. (2008); Marshall & Happe (2007); Hunt, Ferrara, Miller, & Macciocchi (2007); Sumanti, Boone, Savodnik, & Gorsuch (2006); Boone & Lu (2007).

Medical Symptom Validity Test

Green (2004); Merten et al. (2005); Richman et al. (2006); Carone (2008); Blaskewitz, Merten, & Kathmann (2008); Stevens, Friedel, Mehren, & Merten (2008); Chafetz (2008); Howe, Anderson, Kaufman, Sachs, & Loring (2007).

Portland Digit Recognition Test

Binder (1993); Binder & Kelly (1996); Binder & Willis (1991); Ju & Varney (2000); Rose et al. (1998); Doane, Greve, & Bianchini (2005); Temple, McBride, David Horner, & Taylor (2003); Larrabee (2003b); Bianchini, Mathias, Greve, Houston, & Crouch (2001); Gunstad & Suhr (2001); Binder, Salinsky, & Smith (1994); Vickery et al. (2001); Binder, Kelly, Villanueva, & Winslow (2003); Rosen & Powel (2003); Binder (2002); Gunstad & Suhr (2004); Greve, Bianchini, Etherton, Ord, & Curtis (2009); Greve, Binder, & Bianchini (2009); Greve, Ord, Curtis, Bianchini, & Brennan (2008); Greve et al. (2008); Greve & Bianchini (2006a).

Rey 15-Item Test

Arnett, Hammeke, & Schwartz (1995); Bernard & Fowler (1990); Goldberg & Miller (1986); Greiffenstein, Baker, & Gola (1996); Guilmette, Hart, Giuliano, & Leininger (1994); Hays, Emmons, & Stallings (2000); Lee, Loring, & Martin (1992); Millis & Kler (1995); Iverson & Binder (2000); Kelly, Baker, van den Broek, Jackson, & Humphries (2005); Reznek (2005); Fisher & Rose (2005); McCaffrey, O'Bryant, Ashendorf, & Fisher (2003); Frederick (2002a); Brennan & Gouvier (2006); Russeler et al. (2008); Blaskewitz et al. (2008); Whitney, Hook, Steiner, Shepard, & Callaway (2008); Vilar-Lopez et al. (2008a); McGuire (2006); Boone & Lu (2007).

(continued)

Table 6.6 *(continued)*

Test of Memory Malingering
Tombaugh (1996, 1997); Rees, Tombaugh, Gansler, & Moczynski (1998); Ashendorf, Constantinou, & McCaffrey (2004); Constantinou & McCaffrey (2003); Hill, Ryan, Kennedy, & Malamut (2003); Rees, Tombaugh, & Boulay (2001); Teichner & Wagner (2004); Weinborn, Orr, Woods, Conover, & Feix (2003); Powell et al. (2004); Yanez, Fremouw, Tennant, Strunk, & Coker (2006); Greve & Bianchini (2006b); Donders (2005); Duncan (2005); Gierok, Dickson, & Cole (2005); Etherton, Bianchini, Greve, Ciota, et al. (2005); Gavett, O'Bryant, Fisher, & McCaffrey (2005); Moore & Donders (2004); van Hout et al. (2003); Vagnini et al. (2006); Horner, Bedwell, & Duong (2006); O'Bryant & Lucas (2006); Haber & Fichtenberg (2006); Greve, Bianchini, Black, et al. (2006); Vallabhajosula & van Gorp (2001); McCaffrey et al. (2003); Tombaugh (2002); Bolan et al. (2002); Brennan & Gouvier (2006); Greve et al. (2009); Whiteside, Dunbar-Mayer, & Waters (2009); Whitney, Hooks, et al. (2008); Greiffenstein, Greve, Bianchini, & Baker (2008); Batt, Shores, & Chekaluk (2008); Walters, Berry, Rogers, Payne, & Granacher (2008); Greve et al. (2008); Vilar-Lopez et al. (2008); Blaskewitz et al. (2008); Chafetz (2008); Ruocco et al. (2008); Vagnini, Berry, Clark, & Jiang (2008); O'Bryant et al. (2008); Locke, Smigielski, Powell, & Stevens (2008); DenBoer & Hall (2007); Bauer, O'Bryant, Lynch, McCaffrey, & Fisher (2007); Iverson et al. (2007).

21-Item Test
Arnett & Franzen (1997); Gontkovsky & Souheaver (2000); Iverson, Franzen, & McCracken (1991, 1994); Iverson (1998); Rose et al. (1998); Vickery et al. (2001).

Validity Indicator Profile
Frederick (1997, 2000); Frederick & Crosby (2000); Frederick, Crosby, & Wynkoop (2000); Frederick & Foster (1991); Frederick, Sarfaty, Johnston, & Powel (1994); Rose et al. (1998); Vallabhajosula & van Gorp (2001); Frederick (2002b); Frederick & Bowden (2009); Frazier, Frazier, Busch, Kerwood, & Demaree (2008).

Victoria Symptom Validity Test
Doss, Chelune, & Naugle (1999); Grote et al. (2000); Slick, Hopp, Strauss, Hunter, & Pinch (1994); Slick, Hopp, Strauss, & Spellacy (1996); Slick, Hopp, Strauss, & Thompson (1997); Loring, Lee, & Meador (2005); Macciocchi, Seel, Alderson, & Godsall (2006); Vagnini et al. (2006); Thompson (2002); Walters et al. (2008); Vilar-Lopez et al. (2008); Frazier et al. (2008); Haggerty, Frazier, Busch, & Naugle (2007); Loring, Larrabee, Lee, & Meador (2007); Vilar-Lopez et al. (2007); Frazier, Youngstrom, Naugle, Haggerty, & Busch (2007).

Word Memory Test
Green, Allen, & Astner (1996); Green, Iverson, & Allen (1999); Iverson, Green, & Gervais (1999); Dunn et al. (2003); Gervais et al. (2004); Gervais et al. (2001); Gorissen et al. (2005); Green & Flaro (2003); Green, Lees-Haley, & Allen (2002); Green, Rohling, Iverson, & Gervais (2003); Green, Rohling, Lees-Haley, & Allen (2001); Rohling, Allen, & Green (2002); Rohling, Green, Allen, & Iverson (2002); Tan, Slick, Strauss, & Hultsch (2002); Green & Iverson (2001a); Williamson et al. (2003); O'Bryant & Lucas (2006); Frederick & Bowden (2009); Greve et al. (2009); Batt et al. (2008); Greiffenstein et al. (2008); Greve et al. (2008); Gervais, Ben-Porath, Wygant, & Green (2008); Suhr, Hammers, Dobbins-Buckland, Zimak, & Hughes (2008); Allen, Bigler, Larsen, Goodrich-Hunsaker, & Hopkins (2007); Stevens et al. (2008); Morel (2008); Sullivan, May, & Galbally (2007); Bauer et al. (2007); Flaro, Green, & Robertson (2007); Merten et al. (2007); Donders & Boonstra (2007); Green (2007); Bowden, Shores, & Mathias (2006); Osmon, Plambeck, Klein, & Mano (2006).

Bayesian Methods/Diagnostic Accuracy Statistics/ Odds Ratios

How do we draw accurate inferences regarding possible, probable, very likely, or definite poor effort? For several years, researchers have been encouraging the use of Bayesian methods (e.g., Mossman, 2000, 2003) for effort testing (see Barrash, Suhr, & Manzel, 2004; Bianchini, Matthias, Greve, & Houston, 2001; Etherton, Bianchini, Greve, & Heinly, 2005; Glassmire et al., 2003; Greve et al., 2003; Lange, Sullivan, & Anderson, 2005; Millis & Volinsky, 2001; Slick, Hopp, Strauss, & Thompson, 1997). This encouragement is similar to other areas of professional neuropsychological research and practice (see Barr & McCrea, 2001; Benedict et al., 2004; Benedict et al., 2003; Iverson, Mendrek, & Adams, 2004; Ivnik et al., 2001; Labarge, McCaffrey, & Brown, 2003; Rasquin, Lodder, Visser, Lousberg, & Verhey, 2005; Sawrie et al., 1998; Shapiro, Benedict, Schretlen, & Brandt, 1999; Tierney, Szalai, Dunn, Geslani, & McDowell, 2000; Woods, Weinborn, & Lovejoy, 2003). Unfortunately, Bayesian methods and other interesting statistical methodologies (see Crawford, Garthwaite, Howell, & Venneri, 2003; Godber, Anderson, & Bell, 2000), including odds and likelihood ratios (see Bieliauskas, Fastenau, Lacy, & Roper, 1997; Dori & Chelune, 2004; Ivnik et al., 2001; Ivnik et al., 2000), are rarely used in mainstream clinical practice.

O'Bryant and Lucas (2006) calculated predictive value statistics for the Test of Memory and Malingering (TOMM) based on data published by Gervais and colleagues (2004). The sample was 519 non-head-injured disability evaluation cases. The predictive value statistics for the TOMM were based on two assumptions: (a) claimants failing the Word Memory Test provided poor effort (i.e., the WMT was the gold standard), and (b) the base rate of poor effort in disability claimants was 30%. With these assumptions, predictive value statistics for the TOMM were computed. The positive predictive value was .98 and the negative predictive value was .78. This means that the clinician can be 98% sure that a person who fails the TOMM is providing poor effort. Moreover, a clinician can be 78% sure that a person who passes the TOMM is not providing obviously poor effort. Note that the TOMM is much more specific than sensitive, meaning it will fail to identify poor effort in a subset of cases. Thus, using predictive value statistics, a clinician can have much more confidence conceptualizing a patient's poor effort along the continuum presented in Figure 6.5.

Two-group contingency analyses also can be used to provide meaningful information regarding effort-test scores. Two-group analyses can be conducted by collecting or combining large groups of subjects with similar characteristics. Using the TOMM as an example, Iverson (2008) summarized performances from highly specific groups reported in the literature and combined them to create specific two-group comparisons. Odds ratios were calculated to represent the likelihood of belonging to one group versus another based on poor effort on Trial 2 of the TOMM. The results of these two-group comparisons are listed below.

1. People who score below the cut-off on Trial 2 of the TOMM are 1,069 times more likely to be in the laboratory malingering group than the traumatic brain injury group (95% confidence interval = 165.4 to 6,600.5).
2. People who score below the cut-off on Trial 2 of the TOMM are 1,144 times more likely to be in the laboratory malingering group than in the combined group of adults with depression, severe mental illness, or chronic pain (95% confidence interval = 266.4 to 4,767.6).
3. People who score below the cut-off on Trial 2 of the TOMM are 1,828 times more likely to be in the laboratory malingering group than in the combined

group of children and elderly subjects (95% confidence interval = 426.7 to 7,602.9).

4. People who score below the cut-off on Trial 2 of the TOMM are 1,115 times more likely to be in the laboratory malingering group than in a group of children with psychiatric or neurological problems (95% confidence interval = 172.6 to 6,882.3).

Based on a large literature to date, when a person fails the TOMM, clinicians can be confident that this performance reflects probable poor effort. However, clinicians should be very cautious about overinterpreting the results of patients who pass the TOMM. The TOMM is highly specific to poor effort, but its sensitivity might be lower than other related tests. Gervais and colleagues have suggested that the TOMM is less sensitive to poor effort than the Word Memory Test (Gervais et al., 2004). Tan and colleagues also reported that the TOMM is less sensitive than the Word Memory Test (Tan, Slick, Strauss, & Hultsch, 2002), and the TOMM appears to be less sensitive to poor effort than the Amsterdam Short-Term Memory Test (van Hout, Schmand, Wekking, Hageman, & Deelman, 2003).

The two-group contingency analysis reported above for the TOMM can also be applied to the Medical Symptom Validity Test (MSVT) (Green, 2004). This Windows-based program is patterned after the Word Memory Test, but it is a briefer and easier task. The examiner reads aloud the instructions while the patient sits at the computer. The patient is asked to watch the screen while a list of 10 word pairs is presented twice at a rate of 6 seconds per pair. Then, the computer successively presents one word from each pair that was shown previously (i.e., the target) and one that was not shown (i.e., a foil), and the person is required to select the word shown previously in the original list. This produces a total of 20 test items on the immediate recognition trial (IR). After a 10-minute filled delay (for example, with nonverbal testing), the same recognition testing is performed again using different foil words in the delayed recognition trial (DR). A consistency score (CNS) between the two trials is calculated with a computer. After the DR trial, testing proceeds to the paired associates trial (PA), in which the person is asked to sit where the computer screen cannot be seen. The examiner reads the first word of each pair from the screen and the person is asked to say the word that went with it in the original list. Finally, the person is asked to recall as many words as possible from the original list in the free recall trial (FR). The examiner records the person's responses using the computer.

In the MSVT manual, data from 228 Brazilians (tested in Portuguese) between the ages of 6 and 68, who were instructed to try their best can be compared with data from 70 additional subjects instructed to simulate memory impairment. Of those instructed to try their best, 96% scored above the cutoffs on Immediate Recognition, Delayed Recognition, and Consistency. In contrast, 97% of those instructed to simulate memory impairment scored below the cutoff on at least one of these measures. Therefore, a person who scores below the cutoff on any one of the three scales is 827 times more likely to be in the group simulating memory impairment than in the normal effort group (95% confidence interval = 188.4 to 3,515.3).

To further illustrate the ease of the MSVT effort scales, healthy children were compared with adults seen for civil forensic evaluations who were very likely to be providing poor effort. The children were in Grades 2 through 5 ($N = 75$)[1].

---

[1]Data provided by Lloyd Flaro, PhD.

The adults were seen for disability-related evaluations involving chronic pain, psychological problems, or both (N = 37[2]). All of these adults failed the TOMM relatively early in the evaluation process. The children performed nearly perfectly on the MSVT's Immediate Recognition (M = 98.9, SD = 3.6), Delayed Recognition (M = 98.6, SD = 3.9), and Consistency scales (M = 98.1, SD = 5.5). Only one child scored below 85 on any of these scales. In contrast, adults known to be providing poor effort performed very poorly on the Immediate Recognition (M = 74.3, SD = 21.9), Delayed Recognition (Mean = 68.0, SD = 24.8), and Consistency (Mean = 69.6, SD = 20.6) scales, and 70% frankly failed the MSVT. Based on these data, a person who failed the MSVT is 174.9 times more likely to fall in the poor-effort adult group than in the healthy-child group (95% confidence interval = 26.6 to 1,096.3).

Without question, there is a significant gap between research and practice regarding the use of innovative statistical and psychometric approaches to identifying exaggerated symptoms and poor effort. As a profession, we are close to being able to provide clinical inferences regarding where a person falls on the continuum of symptom reporting (Figure 6.3) and effort (Figure 6.5) using predictive accuracy statistics with known confidence intervals. Clinicians should be encouraged to conceptualize poor effort, exaggeration, and malingering not in simple dichotomous terms, but through probabilistic estimations. The use of Bayesian methods can provide strong statistical evidence to underpin a clinical inference regarding where a person falls along the spectrum of symptom reporting accuracy (Figure 6.3) and effort (Figure 6.5).

Ethical Issues

The central issues regarding effort and validity testing, from an ethical perspective, relate to competence, objectivity, clarity in communication, and the proper use of tests. Common sense dictates that effort testing is essential. It is, however, by its very nature, controversial. Ten ethical concerns, issues, and considerations are summarized below. These ethical concerns and issues are discussed in detail elsewhere (Iverson, 2006).

1. Failing to use well-researched effort tests.
2. Using effort tests only for defence cases.
3. Using more or fewer effort tests, systematically, depending on whether you were retained by the defendant or the plaintiff.
4. Using different effort tests or using effort tests differently, depending on which side retains you, for example, using the Rey 15 Item Test for plaintiff cases and the Word Memory Test for defence cases. The former test has lower sensitivity (see Arnett, Hammeke, & Schwartz, 1995; Guilmette, Hart, Guiliano, & Leininger, 1994; Iverson & Binder, 2000; and Millis & Kler, 1995). Therefore, the clinician would be systematically, with forethought, reducing the likelihood of detecting poor effort. An obvious example of using the same test differently would be to give simple effort tests at the end of the evaluation, or after much more difficult

---

[2]Data provided by Roger Gervais, PhD.

tests, such as a battery of memory tests. Researchers have cautioned that from a common-sense perspective, this practice might reduce the sensitivity of the effort test (see Bernard, 1990 and Iverson, 2003), and there is some empirical support for this concern (see Guilmette, Whelihan, Hart, Sparadeo, & Buongiorno, 1996).

5. Warning or prompting patients immediately before taking an effort test.

6. Systematically interpreting effort test results differently, depending on which side retains you. The most extreme examples would be to systematically interpret effort-test failure as a cry for help or distraction due to psychological factors or pain for plaintiff cases and due to malingering for defence cases. Of course, these examples are extreme. The point is to be careful and self-reflective of one's clinical approach to interpreting effort-test results. It might be useful for clinicians to write out, for personal reflection, their decision rules or clinical criteria for inferring a patient's probable underlying motivation for exaggeration or poor effort.

7. Assuming that someone who passes a single effort test gave his full, complete, or best effort during the entire evaluation. Passing an effort test simply means the person passed the effort test. It cannot be used, especially in isolation, to infer that the client gave his best effort throughout the evaluation. It can be one piece of converging evidence to suggest adequate or good effort throughout the evaluation. It is important to understand that most effort tests are quite simple and easily passed by children or adults with significant brain damage. Thus, they don't measure the continuum of effort (see Figure 6.5).

8. Interpreting effort test failure or exaggerated symptoms, in isolation, as malingering. The research literature is replete with inappropriate use of the term malingering. In many studies, the term is used synonymously with poor effort. Clinicians should be careful not to assume, automatically, that the probable poor effort is diagnostic of malingering. Concluding that someone is malingering requires multiple sources of converging evidence, and the systematic ruling out of probable alternative explanations (Bush et al., 2005; Heilbronner, Sweet, Morgan, Larrabee, & Millis, in press; Slick et al., 1999).

9. Inappropriately interpreting exaggeration or poor effort as a cry for help. A clinician should provide the foundations for an opinion of a cry for help as the probable underlying cause of exaggeration or poor effort, or both, just as a clinician needs to provide the foundations for an opinion regarding malingering. Unfortunately, most clinicians who rely regularly on the euphemistic cry for help do not provide the foundations for this clinical inference.

10. Competent, responsible, informed use of tests. Practitioners cannot simply rely on test manuals. The literature on specific tests is constantly evolving. Thus, clinicians should actively keep up with the literature for the specific tests used. The citations in Tables 6.5 and 6.6 are provided to assist the clinician with this exercise.

Clinicians can avoid most ethical problems by following four recommendations. First, neuropsychologists should routinely assess for poor effort and exaggerated symptoms and problems. Second, neuropsychologists should explain to examinees that it is important to provide their best effort and to report their symptoms and problems accurately. Third, neuropsychologists should be familiar with the literature on poor effort, exaggeration, and malingering, and keep up to date with the literature regarding the specific tests and measures used. Finally,

6.6

Assessment of malingering.

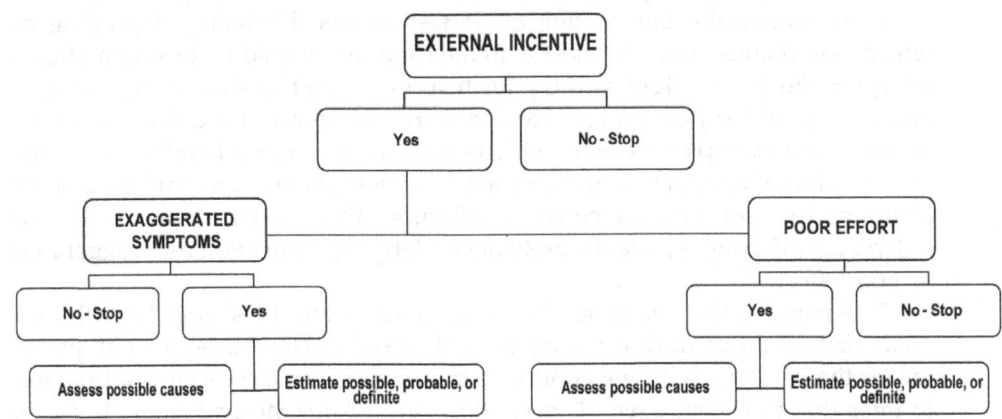

Note: A person might exaggerate symptoms and/or perform poorly on effort testing yet not be malingering. There is always the possibility of a false positive diagnosis (except if the person admits to malingering, of course). See Slick, Sherman, and Iverson for a complete discussion of criteria for possible, probable, and definite malingering. The practitioner must consider carefully the possible underlying cause, or causes, for exaggeration and/or poor effort. If exaggeration and/or poor effort are present, practitioners should be just as cautious ruling out possible malingering as they are concluding probable or definite malingering.

neuropsychologists should state carefully, explicitly, and clearly their conclusions about poor effort, exaggeration, and malingering.

Conclusions and Recommendations for Clinical Practice

Neuropsychological test performance is exquisitely dependent upon effort. Effort is variable, not constant, and when conceptualized globally it falls on a continuum. This has not been articulated well in the literature over the past twenty years. Passing one or more effort tests does not mean that the patient provided excellent, good, or adequate effort throughout the entire evaluation. Passing one or more effort tests does not ensure that the patient was not exaggerating symptoms and problems. Failing one or more effort tests does not necessarily mean that the patient is malingering. Failing one or more effort tests does not necessarily mean that the patient was exaggerating his symptoms or problems. A flowchart for the assessment of malingering is presented in Figure 6.6.

Hundreds of studies and reviews relating to the detection of exaggerated symptoms, poor effort during neuropsychological testing, and malingering have been published in the past twenty years. It is virtually impossible for practitioners to keep up with all the research in this area. Fortunately, there are many good books and reviews of this literature (see, for example, Bianchini, Mathias, & Greve,

2001; Boone, 2007b; Hayes, Hilsabeck, & Gouvier, 1999; Hom & Denney, 2003; Iverson, 2003; Iverson, 2008; Iverson & Binder, 2000; Larrabee, 2005, 2007; Millis & Volinsky, 2001; Reynolds, 1998; Rogers, 1997; Sweet, 1999; and Vickery et al., 2001). Specific guidelines and recommendations for identifying malingering in a neuropsychological evaluation have been available for several years (Slick et al., 1999), and have recently been published for pain-related disability evaluations (Bianchini, Greve, & Glynn, 2005). The key for practitioners is to (a) have a solid plan for how to conduct and interpret this aspect of the evaluation, and (b) stay abreast of the literature relating to the specific tests used.

In 2005 the National Academy of Neuropsychology (NAN) published a position paper on symptom validity assessment (Bush et al., 2005). In that paper, symptom validity assessment refers to all methods and procedures upon which the practitioner can draw to make inferences regarding poor effort during testing, and exaggeration of symptoms or problems during interviews or on psychological tests. The NAN position paper clearly states that symptom validity assessment is not optional. This position paper solidifies the recommendation for routine effort and validity testing made by clinical researchers for many years. In 2008 a consensus conference on the topic was held at the annual meeting of the American Academy of Clinical Neuropsychology. A consensus statement is soon forthcoming (Bush et al., 2005; Heilbronner et al., in press).

In forensic practice, clinicians who fail to properly administer and interpret effort testing are not conducting a thorough or competent independent neuropsychological evaluation. This is because (a) poor effort during testing is, unfortunately, common (Larrabee, 2003a; Mittenberg et al., 2002), (b) the effect of poor effort on neuropsychological test results is major (Vickery et al., 2001), and, in fact, dwarfs the effect of mild traumatic brain injuries or other conditions that have modest effects on cognitive functioning, (c) there are well-validated tests for detecting poor effort that have low false positive rates, (d) in forensic practice special effort must be made to address causation and to rule out factors that might lead to incorrect inferences or interpretations, and (e) it is considered standard practice in forensic psychology and neuropsychology to do so. Effort testing should not, however, be limited to forensic practice. Screening for poor effort should also be part of routine clinical assessments.

Clinicians should be encouraged to conceptualize poor effort, exaggeration, and malingering, not in simple dichotomous terms, but through probabilistic considerations. Without doubt, we are faced with clinical, statistical, and ethical challenges, issues, and considerations associated with the assessment of poor effort. Commercially available tests, well-written manuals, and dozens of research studies facilitate, but do not ensure, proper and responsible test use. Individual practitioners, clinical researchers, professional organizations, and regulatory bodies are all stakeholders in responsible test use, but the ultimate responsibility lies with the practitioner. I recommend that the clinician keep abreast of the literature and follow the multistep procedure listed below.

1. Approach the evaluation proactively, not reactively. Plan for the evaluation of poor effort and exaggerated symptoms just as you would plan to evaluate any specific area of functioning.
2. Don't wait for obvious evidence of poor effort or exaggeration before giving specialized tests. Evaluate for poor effort or exaggerated symptoms with the

same or greater diligence as you would employ to evaluate other things like concentration, memory, or depression.

3. Use a combination of approaches, including specialized tests, and examination of performance patterns and embedded markers on traditional tests.

4. Use well-validated, specialized tests (e.g., Word Memory Test, Medical Symptom Validity Test, Victoria Symptom Validity Test, CARB, or TOMM). Give simple specialized tests (e.g., TOMM, Rey 15 Item Test, or 21 Item Test) at the beginning of the evaluation, not the middle or end.

5. Intersperse effort and validity indicators throughout the evaluation.

It is the responsibility of the neuropsychologist to identify and explain test scores that do not make biological or psychometric sense. If the patient demonstrates clear evidence of poor effort on any test within the evaluation, the entire set of test results is questionable. Practitioners should avoid trying to use clinical judgment (i.e., making an educated guess) to determine which test performances are valid, questionable, or biased. When poor effort is suspected, the evaluation results are best conceptualized as underestimating the person's true ability.

Some patients who give poor effort might have demonstrable evidence of structural brain damage documented on neuroimaging (Bianchini, Greve, et al., 2003a; Boone & Lu, 2003; Iverson, 2003). Obviously, it would be inappropriate to conclude that they have no neuropsychological decrements or subjective symptoms. Rather, the clinician is encouraged to conclude that because the patient did not put forth his or her best performance, it is not possible to determine relative strengths or weaknesses in the neuropsychological profile.

Some neuropsychologists are very reluctant to infer the underlying motivation for exaggerated symptoms or deliberately poor test performance. Without inferring the underlying motivation (i.e., the antecedents), it is impossible to differentiate malingering from a factitious disorder, somatoform disorder, or uncooperativeness. Those psychologists who refuse to infer motivation with regard to exaggerated symptoms should be equally cautious with regard to inferring motives for less contentious behaviors. The neuropsychologist might simply wish to state: "There is considerable evidence that the patient exaggerated his level of disability and gave poor effort during neuropsychological testing. I am not comfortable, based on the evidence available to me, providing an opinion as to whether this behavior was motivated by general uncooperativeness, a desire for monetary gain (i.e., malingering), or a psychological need to assume the sick or disabled role (i.e., factitious disorder)."

A comprehensive forensic neuropsychological assessment should in most cases comprise (a) review of records (e.g., medical and educational), (b) interviews with the plaintiff and other informants such as spouse or employer, if possible, (c) behavioral observations, (d) neuropsychological measures covering all major domains of cognitive function, (e) measures of psychological adjustment and psychiatric symptoms, and (f) measures for detecting poor effort (Slick & Iverson, 2003). An evaluation that does not include the elements listed above might lead to incorrect conclusions about the nature and cause of any observed deficits, and may thus be considered to have been conducted incompetently. A thorough assessment provides the best, and in many cases, the only, acceptable basis for an expert opinion.

References

Aguerrevere, L. E., Greve, K. W., Bianchini, K. J., & Meyers, J. E. (2008). Detecting malingering in traumatic brain injury and chronic pain with an abbreviated version of the Meyers Index for the MMPI-2. *Archives of Clinical Neuropsychology, 23*(7-8), 831–838.

Aizenstein, H. J., Butters, M. A., Wu, M., Mazurkewicz, L. M., Stenger, V. A., Gianaros, P. J., et al. (2009). Altered functioning of the executive control circuit in late-life depression: Episodic and persistent phenomena. *American Journal of Geriatric Psychiatry, 17*(1), 30–42.

Allen, L. M., Conder, R. L., Green, P., & Cox, D. R. (1997). *CARB 97 manual for the computerized assessment of response bias.* Durham, NC: CogniSyst.

Allen, L. M., Iverson, G. L., & Green, P. (2002). Computerized Assessment of Response Bias in forensic neuropsychology. *Journal of Forensic Neuropsychology, 3*, 205–225.

Allen, M. D., Bigler, E. D., Larsen, J., Goodrich-Hunsaker, N. J., & Hopkins, R. O. (2007). Functional neuroimaging evidence for high cognitive effort on the Word Memory Test in the absence of external incentives. *Brain Injury, 21*(13–14), 1425–1428.

American Psychiatric Association. (1994). *Diagnostic and statistical manual of mental disorders* (4th ed.) Washington, DC: American Psychiatric Press.

Ardolf, B. R., Denney, R. L., & Houston, C. M. (2007). Base rates of negative response bias and malingered neurocognitive dysfunction among criminal defendants referred for neuropsychological evaluation. *The Clinical Neuropsychologist, 21*(6), 899–916.

Arnett, P. A., & Franzen, M. D. (1997). Performance of substance abusers with memory deficits on measures of malingering. *Archives of Clinical Neuropsychology, 12*(5), 513–518.

Arnett, P. A., Hammeke, T. A., & Schwartz, L. (1995). Quantitative and qualitative performance on Rey's 15-Item Test in neurological patients and dissimulators. *Clinical Neuropsychologist, 9*(1), 17–26.

Ashendorf, L., Constantinou, M., & McCaffrey, R. J. (2004). The effect of depression and anxiety on the TOMM in community-dwelling older adults. *Archives of Clinical Neuropsychology, 19*(1), 125–130.

Ashendorf, L., O'Bryant, S. E., & McCaffrey, R. J. (2003). Specificity of malingering detection strategies in older adults using the CVLT and WCST. *Clinical Neuropsychologist, 17*(2), 255–262.

Axelrod, B. N., Fichtenberg, N. L., Millis, S. R., & Wertheimer, J. C. (2006). Detecting incomplete effort with Digit Span from the Wechsler Adult Intelligence Scale-Third edition. *Clinical Neuropsychologist, 20*(3), 513–523.

Axelrod, B. N., & Rawlings, D. B. (1999). Clinical utility of incomplete effort WAIS-R formulas: A longitudinal examination of individuals with traumatic brain injuries. *Journal of Forensic Neuropsychology, 1*, 15–27.

Babikian, T., Boone, K. B., Lu, P., & Arnold, G. (2006). Sensitivity and specificity of various digit span scores in the detection of suspect effort. *Clinical Neuropsychologist, 20*(1), 145–159.

Backhaus, S. L., Fichtenberg, N. L., & Hanks, R. A. (2004). Detection of sub-optimal performance using a floor effect strategy in patients with traumatic brain injury. *Clinical Neuropsychologist, 18*(4), 591–603.

Bagby, R. M., Nicholson, R. A., Bacchiochi, J. R., Ryder, A. G., & Bury, A. S. (2002). The predictive capacity of the MMPI-2 and PAI validity scales and indexes to detect coached and uncoached feigning. *Journal of Personality Assessment, 78*(1), 69–86.

Bagby, R. M., Nicholson, R. A., Buis, T., & Bacchiochi, J. R. (2000). Can the MMPI-2 validity scales detect depression feigned by experts? *Assessment, 7*(1), 55–62.

Baity, M. R., Siefert, C. J., Chambers, A., & Blais, M. A. (2007). Deceptiveness on the PAI: A study of naive faking with psychiatric inpatients. *Journal of Personality Assessment, 88*(1), 16–24.

Baker, R., Donders, J., & Thompson, E. (2000). Assessment of incomplete effort with the California Verbal Learning Test. *Applied Neuropsychology, 7*(2), 111–114.

Barr, W. B., & McCrea, M. (2001). Sensitivity and specificity of standardized neurocognitive testing immediately following sports concussion. *Journal of the International Neuropsychological Society, 7*(6), 693–702.

Barrash, J., Suhr, J., & Manzel, K. (2004). Detecting poor effort and malingering with an expanded version of the Auditory Verbal Learning Test (AVLTX): Validation with clinical samples. *Journal of Clinical and Experimental Neuropsychology, 26*(1), 125–140.

Batt, K., Shores, E. A., & Chekaluk, E. (2008). The effect of distraction on the Word Memory Test and Test of Memory Malingering performance in patients with a severe brain injury. *Journal of the International Neuropsychological Society, 14*(6), 1074-1080.

Bauer, L., O'Bryant, S. E., Lynch, J. K., McCaffrey, R. J., & Fisher, J. M. (2007). Examining the Test of Memory Malingering Trial 1 and Word Memory Test Immediate Recognition as screening tools for insufficient effort. *Assessment, 14*(3), 215–222.

Bauer, L., Yantz, C. L., Ryan, L. M., Warden, D. L., & McCaffrey, R. J. (2005). An examination of the California Verbal Learning Test II to detect incomplete effort in a traumatic brain-injury sample. *Applied Neuropsychology, 12*(4), 202–207.

Beetar, J. T., & Williams, J. M. (1995). Malingering response styles on the memory assessment scales and symptom validity tests. *Archives of Clinical Neuropsychology, 10*(1), 57–72.

Benedict, R. H., Cox, D., Thompson, L. L., Foley, F., Weinstock-Guttman, B., & Munschauer, F. (2004). Reliable screening for neuropsychological impairment in multiple sclerosis. *Multiple Sclerosis, 10*(6), 675–678.

Benedict, R. H., Munschauer, F., Linn, R., Miller, C., Murphy, E., Foley, F., et al. (2003). Screening for multiple sclerosis cognitive impairment using a self-administered 15-item questionnaire. *Multiple Sclerosis, 9*(1), 95–101.

Bernard, L. C. (1990). Prospects for faking believable memory deficits on neuropsychological tests and the use of incentives in simulation research. *Journal of Clinical and Experimental Neuropsychology, 12*(5), 715–728.

Bernard, L. C., & Fowler, W. (1990). Assessing the validity of memory complaints: Performance of brain-damaged and normal individuals on Rey's task to detect malingering. *Journal of Clinical Psychology, 46*(4), 432–436.

Bernard, L. C., Houston, W., & Natoli, L. (1993). Malingering on neuropsychological memory tests: Potential objective indicators. *Journal of Clinical Psychology, 49*(1), 45–53.

Bianchini, K. J., Greve, K. W., & Glynn, G. (2005). On the diagnosis of malingered pain-related disability: Lessons from cognitive malingering research. *Spine Journal, 5*(4), 404–417.

Bianchini, K. J., Greve, K. W., & Love, J. M. (2003). Definite malingered neurocognitive dysfunction in moderate/severe traumatic brain injury. *Clinical Neuropsychologist, 17*(4), 574–580.

Bianchini, K. J., Houston, R. J., Greve, K. W., Irvin, T. R., Black, F. W., Swift, D. A., et al. (2003). Malingered neurocognitive dysfunction in neurotoxic exposure: An application of the Slick criteria. *Journal of Occupational and Environmental Medicine, 45*(10), 1087–1099.

Bianchini, K. J., Love, J. M., Greve, K. W., & Adams, D. (2005). Detection and diagnosis of malingering in electrical injury. *Archives of Clinical Neuropsychology, 20*(3), 365–373.

Bianchini, K. J., Mathias, C. W., & Greve, K. W. (2001). Symptom validity testing: A critical review. *The Clinical Neuropsychologist, 15*(1), 19–45.

Bianchini, K. J., Mathias, C. W., Greve, K. W., Houston, R. J., & Crouch, J. A. (2001). Classification accuracy of the Portland Digit Recognition Test in traumatic brain injury. *Clinical Neuropsychologist, 15*(4), 461–470.

Bieliauskas, L. A., Fastenau, P. S., Lacy, M. A., & Roper, B. L. (1997). Use of the odds ratio to translate neuropsychological test scores into real-world outcomes: From statistical significance to clinical significance. *Journal of Clinical and Experimental Neuropsychology, 19*(6), 889–896.

Binder, L. M. (1993). An abbreviated form of the Portland Digit Recognition Test. *Clinical Neuropsychologist, 7,* 104–107.

Binder, L. M. (2002). The Portland Digit Recognition Test: A review of validation data and clinical use. *Journal of Forensic Neuropsychology, 2*(3/4), 27–42.

Binder, L. M., & Kelly, M. P. (1996). Portland Digit Recognition Test performance by brain dysfunction patients without financial incentives. *Assessment, 3,* 403–409.

Binder, L. M., Kelly, M. P., Villanueva, M. R., & Winslow, M. M. (2003). Motivation and neuropsychological test performance following mild head injury. *Journal of Clinical and Experimental Neuropsychology, 25*(3), 420–430.

Binder, L. M., Salinsky, M. C., & Smith, S. P. (1994). Psychological correlates of psychogenic seizures. *Journal of Clinical and Experimental Neuropsychology, 16*(4), 524–530.

Binder, L. M., & Willis, S. C. (1991). Assessment of motivation after financially compensable minor head trauma. *Psychological Assessment, 3,* 175–181.

Binks, P. G., Gouvier, W. D., & Waters, W. F. (1997). Malingering detection with the dot counting test. *Archives of Clinical Neuropsychology, 12*(1), 41–46.

Blaskewitz, N., Merten, T., & Kathmann, N. (2008). Performance of children on symptom validity tests: TOMM, MSVT, and FIT. *Archives of Clinical Neuropsychology, 23*(4), 379–391.

Boccaccini, M. T., Murrie, D. C., & Duncan, S. A. (2006). Screening for malingering in a criminal-forensic sample with the personality assessment inventory. *Psychological Assessment, 18*(4), 415–423.

Bolan, B., Foster, J. K., Schmand, B., & Bolan, S. (2002). A comparison of three tests to detect feigned amnesia: The effects of feedback and the measurement of response latency. *Journal of Clinical and Experimental Neuropsychology, 24*(2), 154–167.

Boone, K. B. (2007a). A reconsideration of the Slick et al. (1999) criteria for malingered neurocognitive dysfunction. In K. B. Boone (Ed.), *Assessment of feigned cognitive impairment: A neuropsychological perspective* (pp. 29–49). New York: Guilford Press.

Boone, K. B. (Ed.). (2007b). *Assessment of feigned cognitive impairment: A neuropsychological perspective.* New York: Guilford Press.

Boone, K. B., & Lu, P. (2003). Noncredible cognitive performance in the context of severe brain injury. *Clinical Neuropsychologist, 17*(2), 244–254.

Boone, K. B., Lu, P., Sherman, D., Palmer, B., Back, C., Shamieh, E., et al. (2000). Validation of a new technique to detect malingering of cognitive symptoms: The b Test. *Archives of Clinical Neuropsychology, 15*(3), 227–241.

Boone, K. B., Lu, P., & Wen, J. (2005). Comparison of various RAVLT scores in the detection of noncredible memory performance. *Archives of Clinical Neuropsychology, 20*(3), 301–319.

Boone, K. B., & Lu, P. H. (2007). Non-Forced-Choice Effort Measures. In G. J. Larrabee (Ed.), *Assessment of malingered nuropsychological deficits* (pp. 27–43). New York: Oxford University Press.

Boone, K. B., Savodnik, I., Ghaffarian, S., Lee, A., Freeman, D., & Berman, N. G. (1995). Rey 15-item memorization and Dot counting scores in a "stress" claim worker's compensation population: Relationship to personality (MCMI) scores. *Journal of Clinical Psychology, 51*(3), 457–463.

Bowden, S. C., Shores, E. A., & Mathias, J. L. (2006). Does effort suppress cognition after traumatic brain injury? A re-examination of the evidence for the Word Memory Test. *Clinical Neuropsychologist, 20*(4), 858–872.

Brennan, A. M., & Gouvier, W. D. (2006). Are we honestly studying malingering? A profile and comparison of simulated and suspected malingerers. *Applied Neuropsychology, 13*(1), 1–11.

Bush, S. S., Ruff, R. M., Troster, A. I., Barth, J. T., Koffler, S. P., Pliskin, N. H., et al. (2005). Symptom validity assessment: Practice issues and medical necessity NAN policy & planning committee. *Archives of Clinical Neuropsychology, 20*(4), 419–426.

Butcher, J. N., Graham, J. R., Ben-Poranh, Y. S., Tellegen, A., Dahlstrom, W. G. & Kaemmer, B. (2001). *MMPI-2 Manual for administration scoring and interpretation* (rev. ed.) Minneapolis, MN: University of Minnesota Press.

Calhoun, P. S., Earnst, K. S., Tucker, D. D., Kirby, A. C., & Beckham, J. C. (2000). Feigning combat-related posttraumatic stress disorder on the personality assessment inventory. *Journal of Personality Assessment, 75*(2), 338–350.

Carone, D. A. (2008). Children with moderate/severe brain damage/dysfunction outperform adults with mild-to-no brain damage on the Medical Symptom Validity Test. *Brain Injury, 22*(12), 960–971.

Chafetz, M. D. (2008). Malingering on the social security disability consultative exam: Predictors and base rates. *Clinical Neuropsychologist, 22*(3), 529–546.

Coleman, R. D., Rapport, L. J., Millis, S. R., Ricker, J. H., & Farchione, T. J. (1998). Effects of coaching on detection of malingering on the California Verbal Learning Test. *Journal of Clinical and Experimental Neuropsychology, 20*(2), 201–210.

Constantinou, M., Bauer, L., Ashendorf, L., Fisher, J. M., & McCaffrey, R. J. (2005). Is poor performance on recognition memory effort measures indicative of generalized poor performance on neuropsychological tests? *Archives of Clinical Neuropsychology, 20*(2), 191–198.

Constantinou, M., & McCaffrey, R. J. (2003). Using the TOMM for evaluating children's effort to perform optimally on neuropsychological measures. *Neuropsychology, Development, and Cognition. Section C, Child Neuropsychology, 9*(2), 81–90.

Crawford, J. R., Garthwaite, P. H., Howell, D. C., & Venneri, A. (2003). Intra-individual measures of association in neuropsychology: Inferential methods for comparing a single case with a control or normative sample. *Journal of the International Neuropsychological Society, 9*(7), 989–1000.

Curtis, K. L., Greve, K. W., Bianchini, K. J., & Brennan, A. (2006). California verbal learning test indicators of Malingered Neurocognitive Dysfunction: Sensitivity and specificity in traumatic brain injury. *Assessment, 13*(1), 46–61.

Dean, A. C., Boone, K. B., Kim, M. S., Curiel, A. R., Martin, D. J., Victor, T. L., et al. (2008). Examination of the impact of ethnicity on the Minnesota Multiphasic Personality Inventory-2 (MMPI-2) Fake Bad Scale. *Clinical Neuropsychologist, 22*(6), 1054–1060.

Dean, A. C., Victor, T. L., Boone, K. B., & Arnold, G. (2008). The relationship of IQ to effort test performance. *Clinical Neuropsychologist, 22*(4), 705–722.

Dean, A. C., Victor, T. L., Boone, K. B., Philpott, L. M., & Hess, R. A. (2008). Dementia and effort test performance. *Clinical Neuropsychologist, 22,* 1–20.

Dearth, C. S., Berry, D. T., Vickery, C. D., Vagnini, V. L., Baser, R. E., Orey, S. A., et al. (2005). Detection of feigned head injury symptoms on the MMPI-2 in head injured patients and community controls. *Archives of Clinical Neuropsychology, 20*(1), 95–110.

Demakis, G. J. (1999). Serial malingering on verbal and nonverbal fluency and memory measures: An analog investigation. *Archives of Clinical Neuropsychology, 14*(4), 401–410.

Demakis, G. J. (2004). Application of clinically-derived malingering cut-offs on the California Verbal Learning Test and the Wechsler Adult Intelligence Test-Revised to an analog malingering study. *Applied Neuropsychology, 11*(4), 222–228.

DenBoer, J. W., & Hall, S. (2007). Neuropsychological test performance of successful brain injury simulators. *Clinical Neuropsychologist, 21*(6), 943–955.

DiCarlo, M. A., Gfeller, J. D., & Oliveri, M. V. (2000). Effects of coaching on detecting feigned cognitive impairment with the Category test. *Archives of Clinical Neuropsychology, 15*(5), 399–413.

Doane, B. M., Greve, K. W., & Bianchini, K. J. (2005). Agreement between the abbreviated and standard Portland Digit Recognition Test. *Clinical Neuropsychologist, 19*(1), 99–104.

Donders, J. (2005). Performance on the test of memory malingering in a mixed pediatric sample. *Neuropsychology, Development, and Cognition. Section C, Child Neuropsychology, 11*(2), 221–227.

Donders, J., & Boonstra, T. (2007). Correlates of invalid neuropsychological test performance after traumatic brain injury. *Brain Injury, 21*(3), 319–326.

Dori, G. A., & Chelune, G. J. (2004). Education-stratified base-rate information on discrepancy scores within and between the Wechsler Adult Intelligence Scale–Third edition and the Wechsler Memory Scale–Third edition. *Psychological Assessment, 16*(2), 146–154.

Doss, R. C., Chelune, G. J., & Naugle, R. I. (1999). Victoria Symptom Validity Test: Compensation-seeking vs. non-compensation-seeking patients in a general clinical setting. *Journal of Forensic Neuropsychology, 1*(4), 5–20.

Duncan, A. (2005). The impact of cognitive and psychiatric impairment of psychotic disorders on the test of memory malingering (TOMM). *Assessment, 12*(2), 123–129.

Dunn, T. M., Shear, P. K., Howe, S., & Ris, M. D. (2003). Detecting neuropsychological malingering: Effects of coaching and information. *Archives of Clinical Neuropsychology, 18*(2), 121–134.

Edens, J. F., Poythress, N. G., & Watkins-Clay, M. M. (2007). Detection of malingering in psychiatric unit and general population prison inmates: A comparison of the PAI, SIMS, and SIRS. *Journal of Personality Assessment, 88*(1), 33–42.

Erdal, K. (2004). The effects of motivation, coaching, and knowledge of neuropsychology on the simulated malingering of head injury. *Archives of Clinical Neuropsychology, 19*(1), 73–88.

Erdal, K. (2009). Why one fakes a head injury affects how one fakes a head injury. *Applied Neuropsychology, 16*(1), 42–48.

Etherton, J. L., Bianchini, K. J., Ciota, M. A., & Greve, K. W. (2005). Reliable digit span is unaffected by laboratory-induced pain: Implications for clinical use. *Assessment, 12*(1), 101–106.

Etherton, J. L., Bianchini, K. J., Greve, K. W., & Ciota, M. A. (2005). Test of Memory Malingering Performance is unaffected by laboratory-induced pain: Implications for clinical use. *Archives of Clinical Neuropsychology, 20*(3), 375–384.

Etherton, J. L., Bianchini, K. J., Greve, K. W., & Heinly, M. T. (2005). Sensitivity and specificity of reliable digit span in malingered pain-related disability. *Assessment, 12*(2), 130–136.

Fisher, H. L., & Rose, D. (2005). Comparison of the effectiveness of two versions of the Rey memory test in discriminating between actual and simulated memory impairment, with and without the addition of a standard memory test. *Journal of Clinical and Experimental Neuropsychology, 27*(7), 840–858.

Flaro, L., Green, P., & Robertson, E. (2007). Word Memory Test failure 23 times higher in mild brain injury than in parents seeking custody: The power of external incentives. *Brain Injury, 21*(4), 373–383.

Forrest, T. J., Allen, D. N., & Goldstein, G. (2004). Malingering indexes for the Halstead Category Test. *Clinical Neuropsychologist, 18*(2), 334–347.

Frazier, T. W., Frazier, A. R., Busch, R. M., Kerwood, M. A., & Demaree, H. A. (2008). Detection of simulated ADHD and reading disorder using symptom validity measures. *Archives of Clinical Neuropsychology, 23*(5), 501–509.

Frazier, T. W., Youngstrom, E. A., Naugle, R. I., Haggerty, K. A., & Busch, R. M. (2007). The latent structure of cognitive symptom exaggeration on the Victoria Symptom Validity Test. *Archives of Clinical Neuropsychology, 22*(2), 197–211.

Frederick, R. I. (1997). *Validity indicator profile manual*. Minnetonka, MN: NCS Assessments.

Frederick, R. I. (2000). A personal floor effect strategy to evaluate the validity of performance on memory tests. *Journal of Clinical and Experimental Neuropsychology, 22*(6), 720–730.

Frederick, R. I. (2002a). A review of Rey's strategies for detecting malingered neuropsychological impairment. *Journal of Forensic Neuropsychology, 2*(3/4), 1–26.

Frederick, R. I. (2002b). Review of the Validity Indicator Profile. *Journal of Forensic Neuropsychology, 2*(3/4), 125–146.

Frederick, R. I., & Bowden, S. C. (2009). Evaluating constructs represented by symptom validity tests in forensic neuropsychological assessment of traumatic brain injury. *Journal of Head Trauma Rehabilitation, 24*(2), 105–122.

Frederick, R. I., & Crosby, R. D. (2000). Development and validation of the Validity Indicator Profile. *Law and Human Behavior, 24*(1), 59–82.

Frederick, R. I., Crosby, R. D., & Wynkoop, T. F. (2000). Performance curve classification of invalid responding on the Validity Indicator Profile. *Archives of Clinical Neuropsychology, 15*(4), 281–300.

Frederick, R. I., & Foster, H. G. (1991). Multiple measures of malingering on a forced-choice test of cognitive ability. *Psychological Assessment, 3*(4), 596–602.

Frederick, R. I., Sarfaty, S. D., Johnston, J. D., & Powel, J. (1994). Validation of a detector of responses bias on a forced-choice test of nonverbal ability. *Neuropsychology, 8*, 118–125.

Gavett, B. E., O'Bryant, S. E., Fisher, J. M., & McCaffrey, R. J. (2005). Hit rates of adequate performance based on the test of memory malingering (TOMM) Trial 1. *Applied Neuropsychology, 12*(1), 1–4.

Gervais, R. O., Ben-Porath, Y. S., Wygant, D. B., & Green, P. (2007). Development and validation of a Response Bias Scale (RBS) for the MMPI-2. *Assessment, 14*(2), 196–208.

Gervais, R. O., Ben-Porath, Y. S., Wygant, D. B., & Green, P. (2008). Differential sensitivity of the Response Bias Scale (RBS) and MMPI-2 validity scales to memory complaints. *Clinical Neuropsychologist, 22*(6), 1061–1079.

Gervais, R. O., Rohling, M. L., Green, P., & Ford, W. (2004). A comparison of WMT, CARB, and TOMM failure rates in non-head injury disability claimants. *Archives of Clinical Neuropsychology, 19*(4), 475–487.

Gervais, R. O., Russell, A. S., Green, P., Allen, L. M., 3rd, Ferrari, R., & Pieschl, S. D. (2001). Effort testing in patients with fibromyalgia and disability incentives. *Journal of Rheumatology, 28*(8), 1892–1899.

Gierok, S. D., Dickson, A. L., & Cole, J. A. (2005). Performance of forensic and non-forensic adult psychiatric inpatients on the Test of Memory Malingering. *Archives of Clinical Neuropsychology, 20*(6), 755–760.

Glassmire, D. M., Bierley, R. A., Wisniewski, A. M., Greene, R. L., Kennedy, J. E., & Date, E. (2003). Using the WMS-III faces subtest to detect malingered memory impairment. *Journal of Clinical and Experimental Neuropsychology, 25*(4), 465–481.

Godber, T., Anderson, V., & Bell, R. (2000). The measurement and diagnostic utility of intrasubtest scatter in pediatric neuropsychology. *Journal of Clinical Psychology, 56*(1), 101–112.

Goldberg, J. O., & Miller, H. R. (1986). Performance of psychiatric inpatients and intellectually deficient individuals on a test that assesses the validity of memory complaints. *Journal of Clinical Psychology, 42*, 792–795.

Gontkovsky, S. T., & Souheaver, G. T. (2000). Are brain-damaged patients inappropriately labelled as malingering using the 21-item Test and the WMS-R Logical Memory Forced Choice Recognition Test. *Psychological Reports, 87*(2), 512–514.

Gorissen, M., Sanz, J. C., & Schmand, B. (2005). Effort and cognition in schizophrenia patients. *Schizophrenia Research, 78*(2–3), 199–208.

Green, P. (2004). *Green's Medical Symptom Validity Test for Windows user's manual*. Edmonton, AB: Green's Publishing.

Green, P. (2007). The pervasive influence of effort on neuropsychological tests. *Physical Medicine and Rehabilitation Clinics of North America, 18*(1), 43–68, vi.

Green, P., Allen, L. M., & Astner, K. (1996). *The Word Memory Test: A user's guide to the oral and computer-administered forms, US Version 1.1*. Durham, NC: CogniSyst.

Green, P., & Flaro, L. (2003). Word memory test performance in children. *Neuropsychology, Development, and Cognition. Section C, Child Neuropsychology, 9*(3), 189–207.

Green, P., & Iverson, G. L. (2001a). Effects of injury severity and cognitive exaggeration on olfactory deficits in head injury compensation claims. *NeuroRehabilitation, 16*(4), 237–243.

Green, P., & Iverson, G. L. (2001b). Validation of the Computerized Assessment of Response Bias in litigating patients with head injuries. *Clinical Neuropsychologist, 15*, 492–497.

Green, P., Iverson, G. L., & Allen, L. (1999). Detecting malingering in head injury litigation with the Word Memory Test. *Brain Injury, 13*(10), 813–819.

Green, P., Lees-Haley, P. R., & Allen, L. M. (2002). The Word Memory Test and the validity of neuropsychological test scores. *Journal of Forensic Neuropsychology, 2*(3/4), 97–124.

Green, P., Rohling, M. L., Iverson, G. L., & Gervais, R. O. (2003). Relationships between olfactory discrimination and head injury severity. *Brain Injury, 17*(6), 479–496.

Green, P., Rohling, M. L., Lees-Haley, P. R., & Allen, L. M., 3rd. (2001). Effort has a greater effect on test scores than severe brain injury in compensation claimants. *Brain Injury, 15*(12), 1045–1060.

Greene, R. L. (2000). *The MMPI-2: An interpretive manual, second edition.* Boston: Allyn and Bacon.

Greiffenstein, M. F., & Baker, W. J. (2008). Validity testing in dually diagnosed post-traumatic stress disorder and mild closed head injury. *Clinical Neuropsychologist, 22*(3), 565–582.

Greiffenstein, M. F., Baker, W. J., Axelrod, B., Peck, E. A., & Gervais, R. (2004). The Fake Bad Scale and MMPI-2 F-family in detection of implausible psychological trauma claims. *Clinical Neuropsychologist, 18*(4), 573–590.

Greiffenstein, M. F., Baker, W. J., & Gola, T. (1994). Validation of malingered amnesia measures with a large clinical sample. *Psychological Assessment, 6*, 218–224.

Greiffenstein, M. F., Baker, W. J., & Gola, T. (1996). Comparison of multiple scoring methods for Rey's malingered amnesia measures. *Archives of Clinical Neuropsychology, 11*, 283–293.

Greiffenstein, M. F., Baker, W. J., Gola, T., Donders, J., & Miller, L. (2002). The Fake Bad Scale in atypical and severe closed head injury litigants. *Journal of Clinical Psychology, 58*(12), 1591–1600.

Greiffenstein, M. F., Greve, K. W., Bianchini, K. J., & Baker, W. J. (2008). Test of Memory Malingering and Word Memory Test: A new comparison of failure concordance rates. *Archives of Clinical Neuropsychology, 23*(7–8), 801–802.

Greve, K. W., & Bianchini, K. J. (2006a). Classification accuracy of the Portland Digit Recognition Test in traumatic brain injury: Results of a known-groups analysis. *Clinical Neuropsychologist, 20*(4), 816–830.

Greve, K. W., & Bianchini, K. J. (2006b). Should the Retention trial of the Test of Memory Malingering be optional? *Archives of Clinical Neuropsychology, 21*(1), 117–119.

Greve, K. W., Bianchini, K. J., Black, F. W., Heinly, M. T., Love, J. M., Swift, D. A., et al. (2006). Classification accuracy of the Test of Memory Malingering in persons reporting exposure to environmental and industrial toxins: Results of a known-groups analysis. *Archives of Clinical Neuropsychology, 21*(5), 439–448.

Greve, K. W., Bianchini, K. J., & Doane, B. M. (2006). Classification accuracy of the test of memory malingering in traumatic brain injury: Results of a known-groups analysis. *Journal of Clinical and Experimental Neuropsychology, 28*(7), 1176–1190.

Greve, K. W., Bianchini, K. J., Etherton, J. L., Ord, J. S., & Curtis, K. L. (2009). Detecting malingered pain-related disability: Classification accuracy of the Portland Digit Recognition Test. *Clinical Neuropsychologist, 23*(3), 1–20.

Greve, K. W., Bianchini, K. J., Heinly, M. T., Love, J. M., Swift, D. A., & Ciota, M. (2008). Classification accuracy of the Portland Digit Recognition Test in persons claiming exposure to environmental and industrial toxins. *Archives of Clinical Neuropsychology, 23*(3), 341–350.

Greve, K. W., Bianchini, K. J., Love, J. M., Brennan, A., & Heinly, M. T. (2006). Sensitivity and specificity of MMPI-2 validity scales and indicators to malingered neurocognitive dysfunction in traumatic brain injury. *Clinical Neuropsychologist, 20*(3), 491–512.

Greve, K. W., Bianchini, K. J., Mathias, C. W., Houston, R. J., & Crouch, J. A. (2002). Detecting malingered performance with the Wisconsin card sorting test: A preliminary investigation in traumatic brain injury. *Clinical Neuropsychologist, 16*(2), 179–191.

Greve, K. W., Bianchini, K. J., Mathias, C. W., Houston, R. J., & Crouch, J. A. (2003). Detecting malingered performance on the Wechsler Adult Intelligence Scale. Validation of Mittenberg's approach in traumatic brain injury. *Archives of Clinical Neuropsychology, 18*(3), 245–260.

Greve, K. W., Bianchini, K. J., & Roberson, T. (2007). The Booklet Category Test and malingering in traumatic brain injury: Classification accuracy in known groups. *Clinical Neuropsychologist, 21*(2), 318–337.

Greve, K. W., Binder, L. M., & Bianchini, K. J. (2009). Rates of below-chance performance in forced-choice symptom validity tests. *Clinical Neuropsychologist, 23*(3), 534–544.

Greve, K. W., Curtis, K. L., Bianchini, K. J., & Ord, J. S. (2008). Are the original and second edition of the California Verbal Learning Test equally accurate in detecting malingering? *Assessment, 14*, 12–21.

Greve, K. W., Ord, J., Curtis, K. L., Bianchini, K. J., & Brennan, A. (2008). Detecting malingering in traumatic brain injury and chronic pain: A comparison of three forced-choice symptom validity tests. *Clinical Neuropsychologist, 22*(5), 896–918.

Greve, K. W., Springer, S., Bianchini, K. J., Black, F. W., Heinly, M. T., Love, J. M., et al. (2007). Malingering in toxic exposure: Classification accuracy of reliable digit span and WAIS-III Digit Span scaled scores. *Assessment, 14*(1), 12–21.

Grote, C. L., Kooker, E. K., Garron, D. C., Nyenhuis, D. L., Smith, C. A., & Mattingly, M. L. (2000). Performance of compensation seeking and non-compensation seeking samples on the Victoria symptom validity test: Cross-validation and extension of a standardization study. *Journal of Clinical and Experimental Neuropsychology, 22*(6), 709–719.

Guez, M., Brannstrom, R., Nyberg, L., Toolanen, G., & Hildingsson, C. (2005). Neuropsychological functioning and MMPI-2 profiles in chronic neck pain: A comparison of whiplash and non-traumatic groups. *Journal of Clinical and Experimental Neuropsychology, 27*(2), 151–163.

Guilmette, T. J., Hart, K. J., Guiliano, A. J., & Leininger, B. E. (1994). Detecting simulated memory impairment: Comparison of the Rey Fifteen-Item Test and the Hiscock forced-choice procedure. *Clinical Neuropsychologist, 8*, 283–294.

Guilmette, T. J., Whelihan, W. M., Hart, K. J., Sparadeo, F. R., & Buongiorno, G. (1996). Order effects in the administration of a forced-choice procedure for detection of malingering in disability claimants' evaluations. *Perceptual and Motor Skills, 83*(3, Pt. 1), 1007–1016.

Gunstad, J., & Suhr, J. A. (2001). Efficacy of the full and abbreviated forms of the Portland Digit Recognition Test: Vulnerability to coaching. *Clinical Neuropsychologist, 15*(3), 397–404.

Gunstad, J., & Suhr, J. A. (2004). Use of the Abbreviated Portland Digit Recognition Test in simulated malingering and neurological groups. *Journal of Forensic Neuropsychology, 4*(1), 33–48.

Guriel, J., & Fremouw, W. (2003). Assessing malingered posttraumatic stress disorder: A critical review. *Clinical Psychology Review, 23*(7), 881–904.

Haber, A. H., & Fichtenberg, N. L. (2006). Replication of the Test of Memory Malingering (TOMM) in a traumatic brain injury and head trauma sample. *Clinical Neuropsychologist, 20*(3), 524–532.

Haggerty, K. A., Frazier, T. W., Busch, R. M., & Naugle, R. I. (2007). Relationships among Victoria Symptom Validity Test indices and personality assessment inventory validity scales in a large clinical sample. *Clinical Neuropsychologist, 21*(6), 917–928.

Hawes, S. W., & Boccaccini, M. T. (2009). Detection of overreporting of psychopathology on the Personality Assessment Inventory: A meta-analytic review. *Psychological Assessment, 21*(1), 112–124.

Hayes, J. S., Hale, D. B., & Gouvier, W. D. (1998). Malingering detection in a mentally retarded forensic population. *Applied Neuropsychology, 5*(1), 33–36.

Hayes, J. S., Hilsabeck, R. C., & Gouvier, W. D. (1999). Malingering in traumatic brain injury: Current issues and caveats in assessment and classification. In N. R. Varney & R. J. Roberts (Eds.), *The evaluation and treatment of mild traumatic brain injury* (pp. 249–290). Mahwah, NJ: Lawrence Erlbaum.

Hays, J. R., Emmons, J., & Stallings, G. (2000). Dementia and mental retardation markers on the Rey 15-item Visual Memory Test. *Psychological Reports, 86*(1), 179–182.

Heilbronner, R. L., Sweet, J. J., Morgan, J. E., Larrabee, G. J., & Millis, S. (in press). American Academy of Clinical Neuropsychology Consensus Conference Statement on the neuropsychological assessment of effort, response bias, and malingering. *Clinical Neuropsychologist*.

Heinly, M. T., Greve, K. W., Bianchini, K. J., Love, J. M., & Brennan, A. (2005). WAIS digit span-based indicators of malingered neurocognitive dysfunction: Classification accuracy in traumatic brain injury. *Assessment, 12*(4), 429-444.

Henry, G. K. (2005). Probable malingering and performance on the test of variables of attention. *Clinical Neuropsychologist, 19*(1), 121–129.

Henry, G. K., Heilbronner, R. L., Mittenberg, W., & Enders, C. (2006). The Henry-Heilbronner Index: A 15-item empirically derived MMPI-2 subscale for identifying probable malingering in personal injury litigants and disability claimants. *Clinical Neuropsychologist, 20*(4), 786–797.

Henry, G. K., Heilbronner, R. L., Mittenberg, W., Enders, C., & Roberts, D. M. (2008). Empirical derivation of a new MMPI-2 scale for identifying probable malingering in personal injury litigants and disability claimants: The 15-item Malingered Mood Disorder Scale (MMDS). *Clinical Neuropsychologist, 22*(1), 158–168.

Henry, G. K., Heilbronner, R. L., Mittenberg, W., Enders, C., & Stanczak, S. R. (2008). Comparison of the Lees-Haley Fake Bad Scale, Henry-Heilbronner Index, and restructured clinical scale 1 in identifying noncredible symptom reporting. *Clinical Neuropsychologist, 22*(5), 919–929.

Hill, S. K., Ryan, L. M., Kennedy, C. H., & Malamut, B. L. (2003). The relationship between measures of declarative memory and the Test of Memory Malingering in patients with and without temporal lobe dysfunction. *Journal of Forensic Neuropsychology, 3*(3), 1–18.

Hilsabeck, R. C., Thompson, M. D., Irby, J. W., Adams, R. L., Scott, J. G., & Gouvier, W. D. (2003). Partial cross-validation of the Wechsler Memory Scale-Revised (WMS-R) General Memory-Attention/Concentration Malingering Index in a nonlitigating sample. *Archives of Clinical Neuropsychology, 18*(1), 71–79.

Hom, J., & Denney, R. L. (2003). *Detection of response bias in forensic neuropsychology*. New York: Haworth Medical Press.

Hopwood, C. J., Morey, L. C., Rogers, R., & Sewell, K. (2007). Malingering on the Personality Assessment Inventory: Identification of specific feigned disorders. *Journal of Personality Assessment, 88*(1), 43–48.

Hopwood, C. J., Talbert, C. A., Morey, L. C., & Rogers, R. (2008). Testing the incremental utility of the negative impression-positive impression differential in detecting simulated personality assessment inventory profiles. *Journal of Clinical Psychology, 64*(3), 338–343.

Horner, M. D., Bedwell, J. S., & Duong, A. (2006). Abbreviated form of the test of memory malingering. *International Journal of Neuroscience, 116*(10), 1181–1186.

Howe, L. L., Anderson, A. M., Kaufman, D. A., Sachs, B. C., & Loring, D. W. (2007). Characterization of the Medical Symptom Validity Test in evaluation of clinically referred memory disorders clinic patients. *Archives of Clinical Neuropsychology, 22*(6), 753–761.

Hunt, T. N., Ferrara, M. S., Miller, L. S., & Macciocchi, S. (2007). The effect of effort on baseline neuropsychological test scores in high school football athletes. *Archives of Clinical Neuropsychology, 22*(5), 615–621.

Iverson, G. L. (1998). *21 Item Test research manual*. Unpublished manuscript.

Iverson, G. L. (2001). Can malingering be identified with the judgment of the line orientation test? *Applied Neuropsychology, 8*(3), 167–173.

Iverson, G. L. (2003). Detecting malingering in civil forensic evaluations. In A. M. Horton & L. C. Hartlage (Eds.), *Handbook of forensic neuropsychology*. New York: Springer Publishing Company.

Iverson, G. L. (2006). Ethical issues associated with the assessment of exaggeration, poor effort, and malingering. *Applied Neuropsychology, 13*(2), 77–90.

Iverson, G. L. (2007). Identifying exaggeration and malingering. *Pain Practice, 7*(2), 94–102.

Iverson, G. L. (2008). Assessing for exaggeration, poor effort, and malingering in neuropsychological assessment. In A. M. Horton, Jr., & D. Wedding (Eds.), *Neuropsychology handbook* (3rd ed., pp. 125–182). New York: Springer Publishing Company.

Iverson, G. L., & Binder, L. M. (2000). Detecting exaggeration and malingering in neuropsychological assessment. *Journal of Head Trauma Rehabilitation, 15*(2), 829–858.

Iverson, G. L., & Franzen, M. D. (1994). The Recognition Memory Test, Digit Span, and Knox Cube Test as markers of malingered memory impairment. *Assessment, 1*, 323–334.

Iverson, G. L., & Franzen, M. D. (1996). Using multiple objective memory procedures to detect simulated malingering. *Journal of Clinical and Experimental Neuropsychology, 18*(1), 38–51.

Iverson, G. L., & Franzen, M. D. (1998). Detecting malingered memory deficits with the Recognition Memory Test. *Brain Injury, 12*(4), 275–282.

Iverson, G. L., Franzen, M. D., & McCracken, L. M. (1991). Evaluation of a standardized instrument for the detection of malingered memory deficits. *Law and Human Behavior, 15*, 667–676.

Iverson, G. L., Franzen, M. D., & McCracken, L. M. (1994). Application of a forced-choice memory procedure designed to detect experimental malingering. *Archives of Clinical Neuropsychology, 9*(5), 437–450.

Iverson, G. L., Green, P., & Gervais, R. (1999). Using the Word Memory Test to detect biased responding in head injury litigation. *Journal of Cognitive Rehabilitation, 2*, 4–8.

Iverson, G. L., & Lange, R. T. (2005). Detecting exaggeration and malingering in psychological injury claims. In W. J. Koch, K. S. Douglas, T. L. Nicholls, & M. O'Neill (Eds.), *Psychological injuries: Forensic assessment, treatment and law* (pp. 76–112). New York: Oxford University Press.

Iverson, G. L., LePage, J., Koehler, B. E., Shojania, K., & Badii, M. (2007). TOMM scores are not affected by chronic pain or depression in patients with fibromyalgia. *Clinical Neuropsychologist, 21*(3), 532–546.

Iverson, G. L., Mendrek, A., & Adams, R. L. (2004). The persistent belief that VIQ-PIQ splits suggest lateralized brain damage. *Applied Neuropsychology, 11*(2), 85–90.

Iverson, G. L., & Tulsky, D. S. (2003). Detecting malingering on the WAIS-III. Unusual Digit Span performance patterns in the normal population and in clinical groups. *Archives of Clinical Neuropsychology, 18*(1), 1–9.

Ivnik, R. J., Smith, G. E., Cerhan, J. H., Boeve, B. F., Tangalos, E. G., & Petersen, R. C. (2001). Understanding the diagnostic capabilities of cognitive tests. *Clinical Neuropsychologist, 15*(1), 114–124.

Ivnik, R. J., Smith, G. E., Petersen, R. C., Boeve, B. F., Kokmen, E., & Tangalos, E. G. (2000). Diagnostic accuracy of four approaches to interpreting neuropsychological test data. *Neuropsychology, 14*(2), 163–177.

Ju, D., & Varney, N. R. (2000). Can head injury patients simulate malingering? *Applied Neuropsychology, 7*(4), 201–207.

Kelly, P. J., Baker, G. A., van den Broek, M. D., Jackson, H., & Humphries, G. (2005). The detection of malingering in memory performance: The sensitivity and specificity of four measures in a UK population. *British Journal of Clinical Psychology, 44*(Pt. 3), 333–341.

Killgore, W. D., & DellaPietra, L. (2000a). Item response biases on the logical memory delayed recognition subtest of the Wechsler Memory Scale-III. *Psychological Reports, 86*(3, Pt. 1), 851–857.

Killgore, W. D., & DellaPietra, L. (2000b). Using the WMS-III to detect malingering: Empirical validation of the rarely missed index (RMI). *Journal of Clinical and Experimental Neuropsychology, 22*(6), 761–771.

King, J., & Sullivan, K. A. (2009). Deterring malingered psychopathology: The effect of warning simulating malingerers. *Behavioral Sciences and the Law, 27*(1), 35–49.

Kucharski, L. T., Duncan, S., Egan, S. S., & Falkenbach, D. M. (2006). Psychopathy and malingering of psychiatric disorder in criminal defendants. *Behavioral Sciences and the Law, 24*, 311–322.

Kucharski, L. T., Toomey, J. P., Fila, K., & Duncan, S. (2007). Detection of malingering of psychiatric disorder with the personality assessment inventory: An investigation of criminal defendants. *Journal of Personality Assessment, 88*(1), 25–32.

Labarge, A. S., McCaffrey, R. J., & Brown, T. A. (2003). Neuropsychologists' abilities to determine the predictive value of diagnostic tests. *Archives of Clinical Neuropsychology, 18*(2), 165–175.

Lange, R. T., & Chelune, G. J. (2006). Application of new WAIS-III/WMS-III discrepancy scores for evaluating memory functioning: Relationship between intellectual and memory abilities. *Journal of Clinical and Experimental Neuropsychology, 28*(4), 592–604.

Lange, R. T., Iverson, G. L., Sullivan, K., & Anderson, D. (2006). Suppressed working memory on the WMS-III as a marker for poor effort. *Journal of Clinical and Experimental Neuropsychology, 28*(3), 294–305.

Lange, R. T., Sullivan, K., & Anderson, D. (2005). Ecological validity of the WMS-III rarely missed index in personal injury litigation. *Journal of Clinical and Experimental Neuropsychology, 27*(4), 412–424.

Langeluddecke, P. M., & Lucas, S. K. (2003). Quantitative measures of memory malingering on the Wechsler Memory Scale–Third edition in mild head injury litigants. *Archives of Clinical Neuropsychology, 18*(2), 181–197.

Langeluddecke, P. M., & Lucas, S. K. (2004). Validation of the Rarely Missed Index (RMI) in detecting memory malingering in mild head injury litigants. *Journal of Forensic Neuropsychology, 4*(1), 49–64.

Langeluddecke, P. M., & Lucas, S. K. (2005). WMS-III findings in litigants following moderate to extremely severe brain trauma. *Journal of Clinical and Experimental Neuropsychology, 27*(5), 576–590.

Larrabee, G. J. (1997). Neuropsychological outcome, post concussion symptoms, and forensic considerations in mild closed head trauma. *Seminars in Clinical Neuropsychiatry, 2*(3), 196–206.

Larrabee, G. J. (1998). Somatic malingering on the MMPI and MMPI-2 in litigating subjects. *Clinical Neuropsychologist, 12*, 179–188.

Larrabee, G. J. (2003a). Detection of malingering using atypical performance patterns on standard neuropsychological tests. *Clinical Neuropsychologist, 17*(3), 410–425.

Larrabee, G. J. (2003b). Detection of symptom exaggeration with the MMPI-2 in litigants with malingered neurocognitive dysfunction. *Clinical Neuropsychologist, 17*(1), 54–68.

Larrabee, G. J. (2003c). Exaggerated MMPI-2 symptom report in personal injury litigants with malingered neurocognitive deficit. *Archives of Clinical Neuropsychology, 18*(6), 673–686.

Larrabee, G. J. (2005). Assessment of malingering. In G. J. Larrabee (Ed.), *Forensic neuropsychology: A scientific approach* (pp. 115–158). New York: Oxford University Press.

Larrabee, G. J. (Ed.). (2007). *Assessment of malingered neuropsychological deficits.* New York: Oxford University Press.

Larrabee, G. J., Greiffenstein, M. F., Greve, K. W., & Bianchini, K. J. (2007). Refining diagnostic criteria for malingering. In G. J. Larrabee (Ed.), *Assessment of malingered neuropsychological deficits* (pp. 27–43). New York: Oxford University Press.

Larrabee, G. J., Millis, S. R., & Meyers, J. E. (2009). 40 plus or minus 10, a new magical number: Reply to Russell. *Clinical Neuropsychologist, 23*(1), 1–9.

Lee, A., Boone, K. B., Lesser, I., Wohl, M., Wilkins, S., & Parks, C. (2000). Performance of older depressed patients on two cognitive malingering tests: False positive rates for the Rey 15-item memorization and dot counting tests. *Clinical Neuropsychologist, 14*(3), 303–308.

Lee, G. P., Loring, D. W., & Martin, R. C. (1992). Rey's 15-Item visual memory test for the detection of malingering: Normative observations on patients with neurological disorders. *Psychological Assessment, 4,* 43–46.

Lees-Haley, P. R. (1992). Efficacy of MMPI-2 validity scales and MCMI-II modifier scales for detecting spurious PTSD claims: F, F-K, Fake Bad Scale, ego strength, subtle-obvious subscales, DIS, and DEB. *Journal of Clinical Psychology, 48*(5), 681–689.

Lees-Haley, P. R., English, L. T., & Glenn, W. J. (1991). A Fake Bad Scale on the MMPI-2 for personal injury claimants. *Psychological Reports, 68*(1), 203–210.

Lees-Haley, P. R., Iverson, G. L., Lange, R. T., Fox, D. D., & Allen, L. M. (2002). Malingering in forensic neuropsychology: *Daubert* and the MMPI-2. *Journal of Forensic Neuropsychology, 3,* 167–203.

Liljequist, L., Kinder, B. N., & Schinka, J. A. (1998). An investigation of malingering posttraumatic stress disorder on the Personality Assessment Inventory. *Journal of Personality Assessment, 71*(3), 322–336.

Locke, D. E., Smigielski, J. S., Powell, M. R., & Stevens, S. R. (2008). Effort issues in post-acute outpatient acquired brain injury rehabilitation seekers. *NeuroRehabilitation, 23*(3), 273–281.

Loring, D. W., Larrabee, G. J., Lee, G. P., & Meador, K. J. (2007). Victoria Symptom Validity Test performance in a heterogenous clinical sample. *Clinical Neuropsychologist, 21*(3), 522–531.

Loring, D. W., Lee, G. P., & Meador, K. J. (2005). Victoria Symptom Validity Test performance in non-litigating epilepsy surgery candidates. *Journal of Clinical and Experimental Neuropsychology, 27*(5), 610–617.

Lynch, W. J. (2004). Determination of effort level, exaggeration, and malingering in neurocognitive assessment. *Journal of Head Trauma Rehabilitation, 19*(3), 277–283.

Macciocchi, S. N., Seel, R. T., Alderson, A., & Godsall, R. (2006). Victoria Symptom Validity Test performance in acute severe traumatic brain injury: Implications for test interpretation. *Archives of Clinical Neuropsychology, 21*(5), 395–401.

Marshall, P., & Happe, M. (2007). The performance of individuals with mental retardation on cognitive tests assessing effort and motivation. *Clinical Neuropsychologist, 21*(5), 826–840.

Mathias, C. W., Greve, K. W., Bianchini, K. J., Houston, R. J., & Crouch, J. A. (2002). Detecting malingered neurocognitive dysfunction using the reliable digit span in traumatic brain injury. *Assessment, 9*(3), 301–308.

McCaffrey, R. J., O'Bryant S, E., Ashendorf, L., & Fisher, J. M. (2003). Correlations among the TOMM, Rey-15, and MMPI-2 validity scales in a sample of TBI litigants. *Journal of Forensic Neuropsychology, 3*(3), 45–54.

McGuire, B. E. (2006). Response mode and performance on the Rey 15-item test: A preliminary study. *Brain Injury, 20*(6), 647–651.

Merten, T., Bossink, L., & Schmand, B. (2007). On the limits of effort testing: Symptom validity tests and severity of neurocognitive symptoms in nonlitigant patients. *Journal of Clinical and Experimental Neuropsychology, 29*(3), 308–318.

Merten, T., Green, P., Henry, M., Blaskewitz, N., & Brockhaus, R. (2005). Analog validation of German-language symptom validity tests and the influence of coaching. *Archives of Clinical Neuropsychology, 20*(6), 719–726.

Meyers, J. E., Millis, S. R., & Volkert, K. (2002). A validity index for the MMPI-2. *Archives of Clinical Neuropsychology, 17*(2), 157–169.

Meyers, J. E., & Volbrecht, M. (1998). Validation of reliable digits for detection of malingering. *Assessment, 5*(3), 303–307.

Miller, L. J., Ryan, J. J., Carruthers, C. A., & Cluff, R. B. (2004). Brief screening indexes for malingering: A confirmation of vocabulary minus digit span from the WAIS-III and the Rarely Missed Index from the WMS-III. *e Clinical Neuropsychologist, 18*(2), 327–333.

Millis, S. R. (1992). The Recognition Memory Test in the detection of malingered and exaggerated memory deficits. *Clinical Neuropsychologist, 6,* 406–414.

Millis, S. R. (1994). Assessment of motivation and memory with the Recognition Memory Test after financially compensable mild head injury. *Journal of Clinical Psychology, 50*(4), 601–605.

Millis, S. R. (2002). Warrington's Recognition Memory Test in the detection of response bias. *Journal of Forensic Neuropsychology, 2,* 147–166.

Millis, S. R., & Dijkers, M. (1993). Use of the Recognition Memory Test in traumatic brain injury: Preliminary findings. *Brain Injury, 7*(1), 53–58.

Millis, S. R., & Kler, S. (1995). Limitations of the Rey Fifteen-Item Test in the detection of malingering. *Clinical Neuropsychologist, 9*(3), 241–244.

Millis, S. R., Putnam, S. H., Adams, K. H., & Ricker, J. H. (1995). The California Verbal Learning Test in the detection of incomplete effort in neuropsychological testing. *Psychological Assessment, 7,* 463–471.

Millis, S. R., Ross, S. R., & Ricker, J. H. (1998). Detection of incomplete effort on the Wechsler Adult Intelligence Scale-Revised: A cross-validation. *Journal of Clinical and Experimental Neuropsychology, 20*(2), 167–173.

Millis, S. R., & Volinsky, C. T. (2001). Assessment of response bias in mild head injury: Beyond malingering tests. *Journal of Clinical and Experimental Neuropsychology, 23*(6), 809–828.

Mittenberg, W., Aguila-Puentes, G., Patton, C., Canyock, E. M., & Heilbronner, R. L. (2002). Neuropsychological profiling of symptom exaggeration and malingering. *Journal of Forensic Neuropsychology, 3*(1/2), 227–240.

Mittenberg, W., Patton, C., Canyock, E. M., & Condit, D. C. (2002). Base rates of malingering and symptom exaggeration. *Journal of Clinical and Experimental Neuropsychology, 24*(8), 1094–1102.

Mittenberg, W., Theroux-Fichera, S. T., Zielinski, R. E., & Heilbronner, R. L. (1995). Identification of malingered head injury on the Wechsler Adult Intelligence Scale–Revised. *Professional Psychology: Research and Practice, 26*, 491–498.

Moore, B. A., & Donders, J. (2004). Predictors of invalid neuropsychological test performance after traumatic brain injury. *Brain Injury, 18*(10), 975–984.

Morel, K. R. (2008). Comparison of the Morel Emotional Numbing Test for Posttraumatic Stress Disorder to the Word Memory Test in neuropsychological evaluations. *Clinical Neuropsychologist, 22*(2), 350–362.

Morey, L. C. (1991). *Personality Assessment Inventory professional manual.* Odessa, FL: Psychological Assessment Resources.

Morey, L. C. (1996). *An interpretive guide to the Personality Assessment Inventory (PAI).* Odessa, FL: Psychological Assessment Resources.

Morey, L. C., & Lanier, V. W. (1998). Operating characteristics of six response distortion indicators for the personality assessment inventory. *Assessment, 5*(3), 203–214.

Mossman, D. (2000). The meaning of malingering data: Further applications of Bayes' theorem. *Behavioral Sciences and the Law, 18*(6), 761–779.

Mossman, D. (2003). Daubert, cognitive malingering, and test accuracy. *Law and Human Behavior, 27*(3), 229–249.

Nelson, N. W., Boone, K., Dueck, A., Wagener, L., Lu, P., & Grills, C. (2003). Relationships between eight measures of suspect effort. *Clinical Neuropsychologist, 17*(2), 263–272.

Nelson, N. W., Sweet, J. J., & Demakis, G. J. (2006). Meta-analysis of the MMPI-2 fake bad scale: Utility in forensic practice. *Clinical Neuropsychologist, 20*(1), 39–58.

O'Bryant, S. E., Gavett, B. E., McCaffrey, R. J., O'Jile, J. R., Huerkamp, J. K., Smitherman, T. A., et al. (2008). Clinical utility of Trial 1 of the Test of Memory Malingering (TOMM). *Applied Neuropsychology, 15*(2), 113–116.

O'Bryant, S. E., & Lucas, J. A. (2006). Estimating the predictive value of the Test of Memory Malingering: An illustrative example for clinicians. *e Clinical Neuropsychologist, 20*(3), 533–540.

Ord, J. S., Greve, K. W., & Bianchini, K. J. (2008). Using the Wechsler Memory Scale-III to detect malingering in mild traumatic brain injury. *Clinical Neuropsychologist, 22*(4), 689–704.

Osmon, D. C., Plambeck, E., Klein, L., & Mano, Q. (2006). The word reading test of effort in adult learning disability: A simulation study. *Clinical Neuropsychologist, 20*(2), 315–324.

Powell, M. R., Gfeller, J. D., Hendricks, B. L., & Sharland, M. (2004). Detecting symptom- and test-coached simulators with the test of memory malingering. *Archives of Clinical Neuropsychology, 19*(5), 693–702.

Rasquin, S. M., Lodder, J., Visser, P. J., Lousberg, R., & Verhey, F. R. (2005). Predictive accuracy of MCI subtypes for Alzheimer's disease and vascular dementia in subjects with mild cognitive impairment: A 2-year follow-up study. *Dementia and Geriatric Cognitive Disorders, 19*(2-3), 113–119.

Rees, L. M., Tombaugh, T. N., & Boulay, L. (2001). Depression and the Test of Memory Malingering. *Archives of Clinical Neuropsychology, 16*(5), 501–506.

Rees, L. M., Tombaugh, T. N., Gansler, D. A., & Moczynski, N. P. (1998). Five validation experiments of the Test of Memory Malingering (TOMM). *Psychological Assessment, 10*, 10–20.

Resnick, P. J. (1997). Malingering of posttraumatic disorders. In R. Rogers (Ed.), *Clinical assessment of malingering and deception* (2nd ed., pp. 130–152). New York: Guilford Press.

Reynolds, C. R. (Ed.). (1998). *Detection of malingering during head injury litigation.* New York: Plenum Press.

Reznek, L. (2005). The Rey 15-item memory test for malingering: A meta-analysis. *Brain Injury, 19*(7), 539–543.

Richman, J., Green, P., Gervais, R., Flaro, L., Merten, T., Brockhaus, R., et al. (2006). Objective tests of symptom exaggeration in independent medical examinations. *Journal of Occupational and Environmental Medicine, 48*(3), 303–311.

Rogers, R. (1997). *Clinical assessment of malingering and deception* (2nd ed.). New York: Guilford Press.

Rogers, R., Ornduff, S. R., & Sewell, K. W. (1993). Feigning specific disorders: A study of the Personality Assessment Inventory (PAI). *Journal of Personality Assessment, 60*(3), 554–560.

Rogers, R., Sewell, K. W., Cruise, K. R., Wang, E. W., & Ustad, K. L. (1998). The PAI and feigning: A cautionary note on its use in forensic-correctional settings. *Assessment, 5*(4), 399–405.

Rogers, R., Sewell, K. W., Martin, M. A., & Vitacco, M. J. (2003). Detection of feigned mental disorders: A meta-analysis of the MMPI-2 and malingering. *Assessment, 10*(2), 160–177.

Rogers, R., Sewell, K. W., Morey, L. C., & Ustad, K. L. (1996). Detection of feigned mental disorders on the personality assessment inventory: A discriminant analysis. *Journal of Personality Assessment, 67*(3), 629–640.

Rohling, M. L., Allen, L. M., & Green, P. (2002). Who is exaggerating cognitive impairment and who is not? *CNS Spectrums, 7*(5), 387–395.

Rohling, M. L., Green, P., Allen, L. M., & Iverson, G. L. (2002). Depressive symptoms and neurocognitive test scores in patients passing symptom validity tests. *Archives of Clinical Neuropsychology, 17*(3), 205–222.

Root, J. C., Robbins, R. N., Chang, L., & Van Gorp, W. G. (2006). Detection of inadequate effort on the California Verbal Learning Test-Second edition: Forced choice recognition and critical item analysis. *Journal of the International Neuropsychological Society, 12*(5), 688–696.

Rose, F. E., Hall, S., Szalda-Petree, A. D., & Bach, P. J. (1998). A comparison of four tests of malingering and the effects of coaching. *Archives of Clinical Neuropsychology, 13*(4), 349–363.

Rosen, G. M., & Powel, J. E. (2003). Use of a Symptom Validity Test in the forensic assessment of Posttraumatic Stress Disorder. *Journal of Anxiety Disorders, 17*(3), 361–367.

Ross, S. R., Millis, S. R., Krukowski, R. A., Putnam, S. H., & Adams, K. M. (2004). Detecting incomplete effort on the MMPI-2: An examination of the Fake-Bad Scale in mild head injury. *Journal of Clinical and Experimental Neuropsychology, 26*(1), 115–124.

Ross, S. R., Putnam, S. H., & Adams, K. M. (2006). Psychological disturbance, incomplete effort, and compensation-seeking status as predictors of neuropsychological test performance in head injury. *Journal of Clinical and Experimental Neuropsychology, 28*(1), 111–125.

Roth, R. S., Isquith, P. K., & Gioia, G. A. (2005). *BRIEF-A: Behavior Rating Inventory of Executive Function—Adult version.* Lutz, FL: Psychological Assessment Resources.

Ruff, R. M., & Hibbard, K. M. (2003). *Ruff neurobehavioral inventory.* Lutz, FL: Psychological Assessment Resources.

Ruocco, A. C., Swirsky-Sacchetti, T., Chute, D. L., Mandel, S., Platek, S. M., & Zillmer, E. A. (2008). Distinguishing between neuropsychological malingering and exaggerated psychiatric symptoms in a neuropsychological setting. *Clinical Neuropsychologist, 22*(3), 547–564.

Russeler, J., Brett, A., Klaue, U., Sailer, M., & Munte, T. F. (2008). The effect of coaching on the simulated malingering of memory impairment. *BMC Neurology, 8,* 37.

Sawrie, S. M., Martin, R. C., Gilliam, F. G., Roth, D. L., Faught, E., & Kuzniecky, R. (1998). Contribution of neuropsychological data to the prediction of temporal lobe epilepsy surgery outcome. *Epilepsia, 39*(3), 319–325.

Schagen, S., Schmand, B., de Sterke, S., & Lindeboom, J. (1997). Amsterdam Short-Term Memory test: A new procedure for the detection of feigned memory deficits. *Journal of Clinical and Experimental Neuropsychology, 19*(1), 43–51.

Schmand, B., Lindeboom, J., Schagen, S., Heijt, R., Koene, T., & Hamburger, H. L. (1998). Cognitive complaints in patients after whiplash injury: The impact of malingering. *Journal of Neurology, Neurosurgery and Psychiatry, 64*(3), 339–343.

Schwarz, L. R., Gfeller, J. D., & Oliveri, M. V. (2006). Detecting feigned impairment with the digit span and vocabulary subtests of the Wechsler Adult Intelligence Scale-third edition. *Clinical Neuropsychologist, 20*(4), 741–753.

Shapiro, A. M., Benedict, R. H., Schretlen, D., & Brandt, J. (1999). Construct and concurrent validity of the Hopkins Verbal Learning Test-revised. *Clinical Neuropsychologist, 13*(3), 348–358.

Sherman, D. S., Boone, K. B., Lu, P., & Razani, J. (2002). Re-examination of a Rey auditory verbal learning test/Rey complex figure discriminant function to detect suspect effort. *Clinical Neuropsychologist, 16*(3), 242–250.

Shum, D. H., O'Gorman, J. G., & Alpar, A. (2004). Effects of incentive and preparation time on performance and classification accuracy of standard and malingering-specific memory tests. *Archives of Clinical Neuropsychology, 19*(6), 817–823.

Silverberg, N., & Barrash, J. (2005). Further validation of the expanded auditory verbal learning test for detecting poor effort and response bias: Data from temporal lobectomy candidates. *Journal of Clinical and Experimental Neuropsychology, 27*(7), 907–914.

Slick, D., Hopp, G., Strauss, E., Hunter, M., & Pinch, D. (1994). Detecting dissimulation: Profiles of simulated malingerers, traumatic brain-injury patients, and normal controls on a revised version of Hiscock and Hiscock's Forced-Choice Memory Test. *Journal of Clinical and Experimental Neuropsychology, 16*(3), 472–481.

Slick, D., Hopp, G., Strauss, E., & Spellacy, F. J. (1996). Victoria Symptom Validity Test: Efficiency for detecting feigned memory impairment and relationship to neuropsychological tests and MMPI-2 validity scales. *Journal of Clinical and Experimental Neuropsychology, 18*(6), 911–922.

Slick, D., Hopp, G., Strauss, E., & Thompson, G. (1997). *The Victoria Symptom Validity Test*. Odessa, FL: PAR.

Slick, D., & Iverson, G. L. (2003). Ethical issues arising in forensic neuropsychological assessment. In I. Z. Schultz & D. O. Brady (Eds.), *Handbook of psychological injuries* (pp. 2014–2034). Chicago: American Bar Association.

Slick, D., Iverson, G. L., & Green, P. (2000). California Verbal Learning Test indicators of suboptimal performance in a sample of head-injury litigants. *Journal of Clinical and Experimental Neuropsychology, 22*(5), 569–579.

Slick, D., Sherman, E. M., & Iverson, G. L. (1999). Diagnostic criteria for malingered neurocognitive dysfunction: Proposed standards for clinical practice and research. *Clinical Neuropsychologist, 13*(4), 545–561.

Steffan, J. S., Clopton, J. R., & Morgan, R. D. (2003). An MMPI-2 scale to detect malingered depression (Md scale). *Assessment, 10*(4), 382–392.

Stern, R. A., & White, T. (2003). *Neuropsychological Assessment Battery*. Lutz, FL: Psychological Assessment Resources.

Stevens, A., Friedel, E., Mehren, G., & Merten, T. (2008). Malingering and uncooperativeness in psychiatric and psychological assessment: Prevalence and effects in a German sample of claimants. *Psychiatry Research, 157*(1–3), 191–200.

Strauss, E., Slick, D. J., Levy-Bencheton, J., Hunter, M., MacDonald, S. W., & Hultsch, D. F. (2002). Intraindividual variability as an indicator of malingering in head injury. *Archives of Clinical Neuropsychology, 17*(5), 423–444.

Stulemeijer, M., Andriessen, T. M., Brauer, J. M., Vos, P. E., & Van Der Werf, S. (2007). Cognitive performance after mild traumatic brain injury: The impact of poor effort on test results and its relation to distress, personality and litigation. *Brain Injury, 21*(3), 309–318.

Suhr, J., Gunstad, J., Greub, B., & Barrash, J. (2004). Exaggeration index for an expanded version of the auditory verbal learning test: Robustness to coaching. *Journal of Clinical and Experimental Neuropsychology, 26*(3), 416–427.

Suhr, J., Hammers, D., Dobbins-Buckland, K., Zimak, E., & Hughes, C. (2008). The relationship of malingering test failure to self-reported symptoms and neuropsychological findings in adults referred for ADHD evaluation. *Archives of Clinical Neuropsychology, 23*(5), 521–530.

Suhr, J., Tranel, D., Wefel, J., & Barrash, J. (1997). Memory performance after head injury: Contributions of malingering, litigation status, psychological factors, and medication use. *Journal of Clinical and Experimental Neuropsychology, 19*(4), 500–514.

Sullivan, B. K., May, K., & Galbally, L. (2007). Symptom exaggeration by college adults in attention-deficit hyperactivity disorder and learning disorder assessments. *Applied Neuropsychology, 14*(3), 189–207.

Sumanti, M., Boone, K. B., Savodnik, I., & Gorsuch, R. (2006). Noncredible psychiatric and cognitive symptoms in a workers' compensation "stress" claim sample. *Clinical Neuropsychologist, 20*(4), 754–765.

Sweet, J. J. (1999). Malingering: Differential diagnosis. In J. J. Sweet (Ed.), *Forensic neuropsychology: Fundamentals and practice*. Lisse: Swets & Zeitlinger.

Sweet, J. J., & King, J. H. (2002). Category Test validity indicators: Overview and practice recommendations. *Journal of Forensic Neuropsychology, 3*(1/2), 241–274.

Sweet, J. J., Wolfe, P., Sattlberger, E., Numan, B., Rosenfeld, J. P., Clingerman, S., et al. (2000). Further investigation of traumatic brain injury versus insufficient effort with the California Verbal Learning Test. *Archives of Clinical Neuropsychology, 15*(2), 105–113.

Swihart, A. A., Harris, K. M., & Hatcher, L. L. (2007). Inability of the Rarely Missed Index to identify simulated malingering under more realistic assessment conditions. *Journal of Clinical and Experimental Neuropsychology, 1-7.*

Tan, J. E., Slick, D. J., Strauss, E., & Hultsch, D. F. (2002). How'd they do it? Malingering strategies on symptom validity tests. *Clinical Neuropsychologist, 16*(4), 495–505.

Tardif, H. P., Barry, R. J., Fox, A. M., & Johnstone, S. J. (2000). Detection of feigned recognition memory impairment using the old/new effect of the event-related potential. *International Journal of Psychophysiology, 36*(1), 1–9.

Teichner, G., & Wagner, M. T. (2004). The Test of Memory Malingering (TOMM): normative data from cognitively intact, cognitively impaired, and elderly patients with dementia. *Archives of Clinical Neuropsychology, 19*(3), 455–464.

Temple, R. O., McBride, A. M., David Horner, M. D., & Taylor, R. M. (2003). Personality characteristics of patients showing suboptimal cognitive effort. *Clinical Neuropsychologist, 17*(3), 402–409.

Tenhula, W. N., & Sweet, J. J. (1996). Double cross-validation of the booklet category test in detecting malingered traumatic brain injury. *Clinical Neuropsychologist, 10*, 104-116.

Thompson, G. B. (2002). The Victoria Symptom Validity Test: An enhanced test of symptom validity. *Journal of Forensic Neuropsychology, 2*(3/4), 43–68.

Tierney, M. C., Szalai, J. P., Dunn, E., Geslani, D., & McDowell, I. (2000). Prediction of probable Alzheimer disease in patients with symptoms suggestive of memory impairment. Value of the Mini-Mental State Examination. *Archives of Family Medicine, 9*(6), 527–532.

Tombaugh, T. N. (1996). *Test of Memory Malingering*. North Tonawanda, NY: Multi-Health Systems.

Tombaugh, T. N. (1997). The Test of Memory Malingering (TOMM): Normative data from cognitively intact and cognitively impaired individuals. *Psychological Assessment, 9*(3), 260–268.

Tombaugh, T. N. (2002). The Test of Memory Malingering (TOMM) in forensic psychology. *Journal of Forensic Neuropsychology, 2*(3/4), 69–96.

Trueblood, W. (1994). Qualitative and quantitative characteristics of malingered and other invalid WAIS-R and clinical memory data. *Journal of Clinical and Experimental Neuropsychology, 16*(4), 597-607.

Trueblood, W., & Schmidt, M. (1993). Malingering and other validity considerations in the neuropsychological evaluation of mild head injury. *Journal of Clinical and Experimental Neuropsychology, 15*(4), 578–590.

Tsushima, W. T., & Tsushima, V. G. (2001). Comparison of the Fake Bad Scale and other MMPI-2 validity scales with personal injury litigants. *Assessment, 8*(2), 205-212.

Vagnini, V. L., Berry, D. T., Clark, J. A., & Jiang, Y. (2008). New measures to detect malingered neurocognitive deficit: Applying reaction time and event-related potentials. *Journal of Clinical and Experimental Neuropsychology*, 1–11.

Vagnini, V. L., Sollman, M. J., Berry, D. T., Granacher, R. P., Clark, J. A., Burton, R., et al. (2006). Known-groups cross-validation of the letter memory test in a compensation-seeking mixed neurologic sample. *Clinical Neuropsychologist, 20*(2), 289–304.

Vallabhajosula, B., & van Gorp, W. G. (2001). Post-Daubert admissibility of scientific evidence on malingering of cognitive deficits. *Journal of the American Academy of Psychiatry and the Law, 29*(2), 207–215.

van der Werf, S. P., Prins, J. B., Jongen, P. J., van der Meer, J. W., & Bleijenberg, G. (2000). Abnormal neuropsychological findings are not necessarily a sign of cerebral impairment: A matched comparison between chronic fatigue syndrome and multiple sclerosis. *Neuropsychiatry, Neuropsychology, and Behavioral Neurology, 13*(3), 199–203.

van Hout, M. S., Schmand, B., Wekking, E. M., Hageman, G., & Deelman, B. G. (2003). Suboptimal performance on neuropsychological tests in patients with suspected chronic toxic encephalopathy. *Neurotoxicology, 24*(4-5), 547–551.

Veazey, C. H., Wagner, A. L., Hays, J. R., & Miller, H. A. (2005). Validity of the Miller forensic assessment of symptoms test in psychiatric inpatients. *Psychological Reports, 96*(3, Pt. 1), 771–774.

Vickery, C. D., Berry, D. T., Inman, T. H., Harris, M. J., & Orey, S. A. (2001). Detection of inadequate effort on neuropsychological testing: A meta-analytic review of selected procedures. *Archives of Clinical Neuropsychology, 16*(1), 45–73.

Vilar-Lopez, R., Gomez-Rio, M., Caracuel-Romero, A., Llamas-Elvira, J., & Perez-Garcia, M. (2008). Use of specific malingering measures in a Spanish sample. *Journal of Clinical and Experimental Neuropsychology, 30*(6), 710–722.

Vilar-Lopez, R., Gomez-Rio, M., Santiago-Ramajo, S., Rodriguez-Fernandez, A., Puente, A. E., & Perez-Garcia, M. (2008). Malingering detection in a Spanish population with a known-groups design. *Archives of Clinical Neuropsychology, 23*(4), 365–377.

Vilar-Lopez, R., Santiago-Ramajo, S., Gomez-Rio, M., Verdejo-Garcia, A., Llamas, J. M., & Perez-Garcia, M. (2007). Detection of malingering in a Spanish population using three specific malingering tests. *Archives of Clinical Neuropsychology, 22*(3), 379–388.

Walters, G. D., Berry, D. T., Rogers, R., Payne, J. W., & Granacher, R. P., Jr. (2008). Feigned neurocognitive deficit: Taxon or dimension? *Journal of Clinical and Experimental Neuropsychology*, 1–10.

Wang, E. W., Rogers, R., Giles, C. L., Diamond, P. M., Herrington-Wang, L. E., & Taylor, E. R. (1997). A pilot study of the Personality Assessment Inventory (PAI) in corrections: Assessment of malingering, suicide risk, and aggression in male inmates. *Behavioral Sciences and the Law, 15*(4), 469–482.

Weinborn, M., Orr, T., Woods, S. P., Conover, E., & Feix, J. (2003). A validation of the test of memory malingering in a forensic psychiatric setting. *Journal of Clinical and Experimental Neuropsychology, 25*(7), 979–990.

Whiteside, D. M., Dunbar-Mayer, P., & Waters, D. P. (2009). Relationship between Tomm performance and PAI validity scales in a mixed clinical sample. *Clinical Neuropsychologist, 23*(3), 523–533.

Whitney, K. A., Davis, J. J., Shepard, P. H., & Herman, S. M. (2008). Utility of the response bias scale (RBS) and other MMPI-2 validity scales in predicting TOMM performance. *Archives of Clinical Neuropsychology, 23*(7-8), 777–786.

Whitney, K. A., Hook, J. N., Steiner, A. R., Shepard, P. H., & Callaway, S. (2008). Is the Rey 15-Item Memory Test II (Rey II) a valid symptom validity test?: Comparison with the TOMM. *Applied Neuropsychology, 15*(4), 287–292.

Whitney, K. A., Shepard, P. H., Williams, A. L., Davis, J. J., & Adams, K. M. (2009). The Medical Symptom Validity Test in the evaluation of Operation Iraqi Freedom/Operation Enduring Freedom soldiers: A preliminary study. *Archives of Clinical Neuropsychology*, acp020.

Williamson, D. J. G., Green, P., Allen, L., & Rohling, M. L. (2003). Evaluating effort with the Word Memory Test and Category Test—Or not: Inconsistencies in a compensation-seeking sample. *Journal of Forensic Neuropsychology, 3*(3), 19–44.

Woods, S. P., Weinborn, M., & Lovejoy, D. W. (2003). Are classification accuracy statistics underused in neuropsychological research? *Journal of Clinical and Experimental Neuropsychology, 25*(3), 431–439.

World Health Organization. (1992). *International statistical classification of diseases* (10th ed.). Geneva: Author.

Wygant, D. B., Sellbom, M., Ben-Porath, Y. S., Stafford, K. P., Freeman, D. B., & Heilbronner, R. L. (2007). The relation between symptom validity testing and MMPI-2 scores as a function of forensic evaluation context. *Archives of Clinical Neuropsychology, 22*(4), 489–499.

Yanez, Y. T., Fremouw, W., Tennant, J., Strunk, J., & Coker, K. (2006). Effects of severe depression on TOMM performance among disability-seeking outpatients. *Archives of Clinical Neuropsychology, 21*(2), 161–165.

Neuroimaging of Aggression: Empirical Findings and Implications

7

Laura L. Hoskins
Robert M. Roth
Peter R. Giancola

Introduction

Aggressive and violent acts occur in diverse populations of individuals and across a variety of settings. In the United States, homicide is the second most common cause of death among young adults, and the 12th leading cause of death for all age groups (Saver, 2002). There are an estimated six million violent crimes against U.S. residents age 12 or older annually (Rand & Catalano, 2007), not to mention the many such crimes committed against children under 12 years of age. Nearly 4% of individuals commit at least one violent act each year, and the lifetime prevalence of aggressive acts is estimated to be 24% according to a population-based survey (Swanson, Holzer, Ganju, & Jono, 1990). Other studies indicate that 11% of wives and 11–17% of husbands have struck (assaulted) their spouse (Saver, 2002). Upwards of 40% of psychiatric inpatients committed a physically aggressive act just prior to admission, and 37% assaulted staff or other patients during hospitalization (Saver, 2002). Approximately 70% of individuals who have sustained a traumatic brain injury exhibit irritability and aggression (McKinlay,

Brooks, Bond, Martinage, & Marshall, 1981). Understanding the etiology of human aggression and violence has therefore become an increasingly important goal for the mental health community and policy makers.

The study of the etiology of human aggression and violence has intrigued theorists from a myriad of backgrounds since the early 1900s (Sestir & Bartholow, 2007). Unfortunately, some of the early efforts aimed at understanding the biological underpinnings of criminal behavior, both in the United States and abroad, were tainted by racist overtones, and research was used to support eugenics and related public policies (Miczek et al., 2007; Scarpa & Raine, 2007). More recently, technological advances in the medical sciences have facilitated the examination of potential biological factors underlying aggression, such as genetic and neurobiological influences (Cairns & Stoff, 1996). For example, in just the past few years, research has identified the biochemical, and specifically neurochemical, abnormalities (de Almeida, Ferrari, Parmigiani, & Miczek, 2005; Eriksson & Lidberg, 1997), low HDL cholesterol levels (Buydens-Branchey, Branchey, Hudson, & Fergeson, 2000), and various genetic polymorphisms (Cadoret, Leve, & Devor, 1997; Fresan et al., 2007) associated with aggression.

Although complex human traits and behaviors such as aggression and violence result from a multifaceted interplay of disparate influences, it is now widely accepted that any conceptually sound theory of aggression must include an appreciation of brain-behavior relationships (Filley et al., 2001). Exploration of the neurobiology of aggression and violence has also garnered increasing interest over recent years with the wider availability of structural and functional neuroimaging techniques, along with greater attention to related legal, ethical, and sociological implications.

The current chapter provides a review of neuroimaging studies of adult humans who demonstrate aggression and violence, and findings are considered in the context of methodological limitations and their implications for forensic neuropsychology, including court admissibility. For the purposes of this review, "aggression" is defined by Baron and Richardson (1994) as *"any form of behavior directed toward the goal of harming or injuring another living being who is motivated to avoid such treatment"* (p. 7). Similar definitions have also been advanced by other leading aggression theorists (Anderson & Bushman, 2002; Berkowitz, 1993; Geen, 2001).

The Aggression Construct

Human aggressive behavior is the result of a complex interplay of biological, psychological, and social influences and may be broadly divided into at least two partly overlapping phenomenological forms: a defensive impulsive-affective subtype, and an offensive controlled-instrumental predatory subtype (Das, Barkataki, Kumari, & Sharma, 2002; Saver, 2002; van Elst, Woermann, Lemieux, Thompson, & Trimble, 2000). Affective aggression is considered defensive in nature; as such, it is not premeditated and is characterized by elevated levels of emotional arousal and associated vocalizations of fear and distress. In contrast, predatory aggression is characterized by goal-directed behaviors devoid of emotional arousal. Most forms of human aggression are thought to be affective, that is, reactionary toward a perceived threat (Albert, Walsh, & Jonik, 1993). Human aggression, however, has been found to be heterogeneous even among antisocial individuals (Barratt, Stanford, Kent, & Felthous, 1997).

Aggression is an innate, adaptive impulse found in all mammals; thus, most aggressive behaviors serve as a functional response to an external event, important for fulfilling needs and for survival (Blake & Grafman, 2004; Fishbein, 1992; Saver, 2002). However, this fundamental trait is uniquely mediated in human beings by higher cognitive abilities (King, Blair, Mitchell, Dolan, & Burgess, 2006; Saver, 2002; Sestir & Bartholow, 2007). Neuropsychological research has provided abundant data elucidating cognitive functions that may be implicated in human aggression, with evidence pointing most strongly to impaired executive functioning (Blake & Grafman, 2004; Fishbein, 2000; Giancola, 1995; Giancola, Mezzich, & Tarter, 1998; Giancola, Roth, & Parrott, 2006; Hawkins & Trobst, 2000; Rucco & Platek, 2006; Seguin & Zelazo, 2005). Executive functions are higher-order cognitive abilities that regulate purposeful, independent, goal-directed behavior (Lezak, Howieson, & Loring, 2004), which are thought to be subserved primarily by the frontal lobes and its reciprocal interconnections with other cortical and subcortical regions of the brain, such as the limbic system, basal ganglia, and the reticular activating system (Chow & Cummings, 1999; Roth, Randolph, Koven, & Isquith, 2006; Stuss & Alexander, 2000; Stuss & Levine, 2002). Despite the abundance of converging empirical evidence from animal brain-lesion studies and human neuropsychological, neurological, and neurophysiological studies implicating prefrontal cortex dysfunction in aggressive behavior, the proposed brain-behavior relationship between the prefrontal cortex and the expression of aggressive behavior has yielded considerable debate (Giancola, 1995).

Historical Perspective on the Neuroanatomical Basis

The notion that the underlying mechanisms of human aggression, as well as other emotional and behavioral problems, may be rooted in our neuroanatomical makeup is not particularly novel and predates Phineas Gage's historical 1848 brain injury, in which a 13-pound dynamite tamping rod, 2 inches in diameter, shot through his left cheekbone into the ventromedial region of his prefrontal cortex (PFC), changing his personality into that of a fitful, disinhibited, aggressive, irreverent drifter (Cato, Delis, Abildskov, & Bigler, 2004; Damasio, 1994; Damasio, Grabowski, Frank, Galaburda, & Damasio, 1994; Glicksohn, 2002; Stuss, Gow, & Hetherington, 1992). Gage's now well-known injury has become the archetypal case supporting a theorized relationship between prefrontal cortical damage and subsequent alteration in social behavior. Postmortem analysis of the trajectory of the tamping rod revealed circumscribed orbital and mesial prefrontal damage extending to the anterior-most portion of the anterior cingulate gyrus, but no dorsolateral prefrontal involvement was indicated (Damasio et al., 1994). These findings implicate the role of the basal-orbital prefrontal area in the regulation of emotion and/or behavioral inhibition; such that damage to this region may result in disinhibited behavior and potentially aggression (Giancola, 1995). Consistent with the hypothesis that the orbital prefrontal cortex (OFC) is involved in the modulation of aggressive behavior, a functional decrease in the neural activity of the medial OFC has been observed on PET imaging in healthy individuals when aggressive behavior was evoked through script-driven mental imagery (Pietrini, Guazzelli, Basso, Jaffe, & Grafman, 2000). However, orbitofrontal abnormality contributing to aggression has not been consistently supported in the literature. In animals with orbital frontal lesions, reduced aggressive behaviors and increased withdrawal behaviors in the context of increased emotional blunting have been observed (Butter, Synder, & McDonald, 1970; Miller & Levine, 1977); similar observations have been noted in animals with amygdaloid lesions (Butter & Synder, 1971). Further, both animal and human studies of aggression have provided at least some evidence to indicate that the dorsolateral prefrontal cortex may be involved in the expression of aggression (Giancola & Zeichner, 1994; Grafman et al., 1996; Kamback & Rogal, 1973; Mass & Kling, 1975; Miller, 1976). Despite the profuse amount of empirical support implicating a relationship between the PFC and aggression, the precise nature and manifestation of its functional role with regard to aggressive behaviors unfortunately still remains unclear (Giancola, 1995).

The empirical investigation of brain-behavior relationships underlying aggression began over a half century ago when it was discovered that aggressive behavior could be elicited in cats with the application of electrical stimulation to the hypothalamus (Hess & Akert, 1955). Later studies found that stimulation localized at either the medial or lateral hypothalamus produced seemingly distinct types of aggressive behavior (Vergnes & Karli, 1969, 1972; Wasman & Flynn, 1962), while simultaneous stimulation of the lateral PFC and hypothalamus suppressed aggression elicited via the hypothalamus (Siegel, Edinger, & Dotto, 1975; Siegel, Edinger, & Koo, 1977). Additional animal studies (Butter, Mishkin, & Mirsky, 1968; Kamback, 1973) specifically comparing the effects of dorsolateral and orbital lesions on aggression have found increased aggression in monkeys with bilateral ablations of the dorsolateral prefrontal region, and reduced aggression with bilateral ablations of the orbital region. Based on findings indicating increased aggression following dorsolateral lesions, it has been argued that the dorsolateral prefrontal cortex may serve to provide inhibitory influences on aggressive impulses originating in subcortical areas (Giancola, 1995). The reduction of aggression and the increase of withdrawal behaviors seen in lesions of the OFC implicate this particular prefrontal cortical region in the processing, regulation, and expression of affective information emanating from the amygdala, which is known to play a central role in the production of emotions via its direct connections with the orbital prefrontal cortex (Canli, Desmond, Zhao, Glover, & Gabrieli, 1988; Chow & Cummings, 1999; Filley, 2008; Giancola, 1995; LeDoux, 2000; Lezak et al., 2004; Müller et al., 2003; Schneider et al., 1997; Siever, 2008; Silver, Anderson, & Yudofsky, 2003). Combined, the above-mentioned findings provide some credence for distinct forms of aggression (i.e., offensive/predatory and defensive/affective) controlled by discrete neuroanatomical substrates. Other early efforts to understand the neurobiology of aggression were characterized by approaches focusing on single causative factors, such as specific neurotransmitters or hormones (Balaban, Alper, & Kasamon, 1996; Kavoussi, Armstead, & Coccaro, 1997; Lee & Coccarro, 2001; Young & Balaban, 2003).

Advances in neuroimaging over the last decade have provided an opportunity to examine *in vivo* neuroanatomical structures in relation to aggression. Aggression and associated behaviors have been linked to the presence of focal brain lesions in a variety of regions such as the frontal lobe (Anderson, Bechara, Damasio,

Tranel, & Damasio, 1999; Grafman et al., 1996; Raine, Buchsbaum, & LaCasse, 1997; Raine et al., 1994), the hypothalamus (Anderson & Silver, 1998; Tonkonogy & Geller, 1992), and the paralimbic areas of the temporal lobe (Tonkonogy, 1991; van Elst, Woermann, Lemieux, Thompson, & Trimble, 2000). Functional animal and human brain-imaging studies have also identified neuroanatomical circuits that play critical regulatory roles in the control of aggression (Davidson, Putnam, & Larson, 2000; Ferris et al., 2008; Mattson, 2003; Raine et al., 2002).

Briefly, a complex neural circuit implicated in emotional regulation appears to be involved in aggression and violence (Davidson et al., 2000; Gregg, 2003; King et al., 2006; Miczek et al., 2007; Nelson & Trainor, 2007). This includes several regions of the PFC, amygdala, hippocampus, hypothalamus, anterior cingulate cortex (ACC), insular cortex, ventral striatum, and other interconnected structures. It is posited that aggressive behaviors, specifically impulsive aggression, arise as a consequence of a failure of emotional regulation. Individuals without brain dysfunction are able to volitionally regulate their affect, as well as behavioral manifestation of affect, and benefit from inhibitory environmental cues. Davidson and colleagues (2000) suggested that individuals with aggressive and violent tendencies have an aberration in the central circuitry responsible for such adaptive behavioral strategies.

The core elements of the above-mentioned circuitry model are the orbitofrontal cortex (OFC) and its interconnected structures, which include the ACC and the amygdala. The amygdala, in particular, is essential for modulation of emotion and has been posited to play a role in fear-induced aggression, a subtype of affective aggression (LeDoux, 2000; Trimble & van Elst, 1999; van Elst, Woermann, Lemieux, Thompson, & Trimble, 2000). It is argued that overactivation of the amygdala results in excessive negative affect towards social cues that regulate emotion, while a paucity of activation results in a decreased sensitivity to such cues. Activation of the amygdala may also result in long-term alterations in the physiological makeup of the limbic system that enhance aggressive responses to stimuli (Saver, 2002; Silver, Yudofsky, & Anderson, 2005; Trimble & van Elst, 1999). Indeed, violent behavior resulting from partial damage to the amygdala has been reported in patients with herpes simplex encephalitis (Anderson & Silver, 1998; Tonkonogy, 1991). The OFC, via its connections with other prefrontal cortical areas and with the amygdala, plays a critical inhibitory role by restraining impulsive expression of negative emotional behaviors, and the ACC engages interconnected neural structures, in response to perceived threat or conflict. In neuroanatomically intact individuals, activations that occur in these brain regions during negative emotional arousal serve to restrain impulsive behaviors. Thus, impairments in circuitry responsible for emotional regulation are hypothesized to increase an individual's vulnerability to impulsive aggression (Davidson et al., 2000). Because of the possible association between neuroanatomical circuitry and aggression, various neuroimaging studies have been conducted to examine whether aggressive and violent individuals have structural or functional brain abnormalities that could explain their behavior. Our understanding of the precise relationship between the brain and human aggression to date has ultimately been impeded by the confines of the scientific state of the art in comparison with the convoluted nature of human behavior, the often diffuse nature of brain injury, as well as the ethical limitations on human subject research (Giancola, 1995; Lee & Coccarro, 2001).

Neuroimaging of Aggression

The brain-behavior relationships underlying aggression have remained elusive, given the challenges inherent in traditional neuropsychological methods. Recent advances in neuroimaging, however, are beginning to provide a more detailed picture of these relationships. In the present chapter we provide a brief description of the structural and functional neuroimaging techniques most commonly employed to study human aggression. Readers are referred to several other sources for more detailed explanations of these techniques (Broderick, 2005; Cabeza & Kingstone, 2006; Dougherty, Rauch, & Rosenbaum, 2004; Friston et al., 1995; Grossman & Yousem, 2003; Jezzard, Matthews, & Smith, 2001; Ogawa, Menon, Kim, & Ugurbil, 1998). We then review neuroimaging studies investigating aggressive/violent behavior in selected psychiatric and neurological disorders, as well as studies that do not directly address the issue of aggression, but report on patient populations that are characterized by tendencies towards aggression.

Neuroimaging Basics

The two main structural neuroimaging techniques used by clinicians and neuroscientists are computerized tomography (CT), also known as computerized axial tomography (CAT), and magnetic resonance imaging (MRI). Although these two techniques use fundamentally different physical properties and have correspondingly different strengths and limitations, they both provide information regarding the morphology of brain regions and detect tissue abnormalities.

CT, was one of the first noninvasive imaging techniques for visualization of neuroanatomic structures, and essentially utilizes the same basic technology as X-rays. CT measures tissue interactions with X-rays transmitted through the patient's brain from an external source, and consists of a series of tomograms, or slices, through sections of the brain, rendering measurements primarily reflecting tissue density (Jaqust, 1999; Park & Gonzalez, 2004). Despite the excellent resolution obtained with CT, discrimination between gray and white matter is relatively poor due to weak contrast sensitivity (Jaqust, 1999; Park & Gonzalez, 2004). MRI, which does not involve radiation, exploits the magnetic properties of the atomic components within biological matter to create a visual representation of each tissue type (Goldstein & Price, 2004). MRI provides significantly better neuroanatomical resolution than CT, which is important in identifying smaller or subtle abnormalities. For example, MRI is more sensitive than CT with regards to detection of both lesions and diffuse axonal injuries in patients with mild traumatic brain injury (McAllister, Sparling, Flashman, & Saykin, 2001; Metting, Rodiger, De Keyser, & van der Naalt, 2007).

Structural neuroimaging techniques, while informative, are unable to provide insight into functional neuroanatomical changes that may be associated with aggression. Functional neuroimaging techniques are powerful tools that allow for the identification of brain regions involved in processing and responding to stimuli. The most commonly employed techniques are positron emission tomography (PET) and functional MRI (fMRI), and to a lesser extent, single photon emission computed tomography (SPECT). While still largely research tools, there is burgeoning interest and clinical utility for these methodologies (Dougherty, Rauch, & Fischman, 2004; Price & Friston, 2002; Wishart, Saykin, & McAllister, 2002).

PET enables visualization of brain function via the detection of small amounts of radioactively labeled compounds that are injected (e.g., water or glucose) or inhaled (e.g., oxygen) shortly before or during scans/tasks. Upon decay, the radioactive atoms in the compound release positrons (i.e., small, positively charged particles), which subsequently collide with negatively charged electrons. This collision results in the creation of photons, which are a pair of particles of light that are picked up by detectors in the scanner. Brain regions involved in a given task have the greatest accumulation of the labeled compound, and are identified through computer programs designed to analyze the information and to generate three-dimensional, cross-sectional images. In order to provide more accurate localization of activation, PET is increasingly used in combination with CT and structural MRI. SPECT differs from PET in several important ways, including the radioactive process measured (Dougherty, Rauch, & Fischman, 2004), and while SPECT can only provide an indirect indicator of brain metabolism via cerebral blood-flow measurement, PET can measure both cerebral blood flow and glucose metabolism as indices of neuronal activity (Dougherty, Rauch, & Fischman, 2004; Metting et al., 2007). fMRI takes advantage of the different magnetic properties of oxygenated and deoxygenated hemoglobin, and is based on the observation that hemodynamic activity is closely related to neural activity (Arthurs & Boniface, 2002; Bassarath, 2001; Kwong et al., 1992; Logothetis, 2002; Roth et al., 2006). Greater oxygen utilization is required by brain regions when engaged in a task than when not engaged, resulting in changes in the local magnetic field that are detected by the MRI scanner and used to generate three-dimensional images.

Neuroimaging of Aggression in Selected Populations

A significant association between violent behavior and mental disorders has been found, despite discrepant methodological approaches across studies (Eronen, Angermeyer, & Schulze, 1998; Swanson et al., 1990; Tehrani, Brennan, Hodgins, & Mednick, 1998). Given the concern about violent behaviors and the burgeoning evidence of over-representation of antisocial behaviors among the mentally ill, early interest in the etiology of human violence focused on individuals with chronic and severe mental illnesses. Many investigations of the relationship between aggression and mental illness, unfortunately, do not make a distinction between various diagnostic groups, instead utilizing heterogeneous samples of psychiatric inpatients with a history of violent behavior. Despite this limitation, these early studies provide some insights into the relationship between mental disorder and aggression.

Mixed Psychiatric Samples

In a PET study of four psychiatrically hospitalized males with a history of recurrent violent behaviors resulting in arrest (e.g., attempted homicide, attempted suicide, rape, physical assault, arson), decreased metabolic activity in the frontal and left temporal cortex was demonstrated (Volkow & Tancredi, 1987). In all four patients, there was decreased cerebral blood flow to the left temporal cortex as measured by PET; 50% of the patients also had decreased flow in the frontal lobes. Abnormalities on CT were seen in only two patients, illustrating that functional imaging may help detect abnormalities that are not seen using structural techniques. The authors concluded that the occurrence of aggressive and violent acts was facilitated by cerebral dysfunction related to metabolic abnormalities in the temporal and frontal lobes. Similar results were obtained in another PET study examining regional brain glucose metabolism in eight male psychiatric inpatients (three of whom were diagnosed with a psychotic disorder) with a history of repetitive violent behavior (Volkow et al., 1995). In the latter study, lower metabolic rates were found in the medial temporal cortex and PFC of violent patients than in healthy, nonviolent comparison subjects.

Another study utilized SPECT with 40 adolescents and adults who had demonstrated aggressive behavior within six months of being evaluated (Amen, Stubblefield, Carmichael, & Thisted, 1996). The subject group comprised 30 males and 10 females from both inpatient and outpatient psychiatric populations. The diagnostic composition of the sample was heterogeneous, including attention-deficit/hyperactivity disorder (ADHD), major depression, depressive disorder not otherwise specified (NOS), panic disorder, generalized anxiety disorder, and posttraumatic stress disorder (PTSD). Additionally, the researchers examined a control group consisting of 40 psychiatric patients without a history of aggressive behavior, matched according to age, sex, and diagnosis. Although right-sided pathology was commensurate for both groups, 95% of the aggressive group had findings of increased activity in the left hemisphere, compared with only 25% of the nonaggressive group. Furthermore, 60% of the aggressive group demonstrated decreased PFC activity, compared with only 35% of the nonaggressive group. Significantly increased activity in the anteromedial portions of the frontal lobes was observed in 85% of the aggressive group, compared with only 25% of the nonaggressive group. Also, 72.5% of the aggressive group had increased left temporal lobe activity, as compared with 7.5% in the other group. Other findings included increased activity in the basal ganglia and limbic system in the aggressive group. The authors suggested that violent or aggressive patients may be identified by a brain SPECT profile consisting of decreased perfusion in the PFC, and increased perfusion in any or all of the left temporal lobe, medial frontal lobes, basal ganglia, or limbic system. More generally, they conclude that left hemisphere abnormalities are more prominent in individuals with elevated levels of aggression.

Schizophrenia

Among the severe mental disorders, schizophrenia is among the most frequently implicated in aggression and violence (Angermeyer, 2000; Angermeyer, Cooper, & Link, 1998; Arango, Calcedo Barba, González-Salvador, & Calcedo Ordóñez, 1999; Das et al., 2002; Eronen et al., 1998; Junginger & McGuire, 2004; Link, Stueve, & Phelan, 1998; Narayan et al., 2007; Tardiff, 1998; Volavka, 1999). In most cases, the onset of psychosis precedes the onset of violence (Das et al., 2002). Related disorders, such as schizoaffective disorder, have also been implicated in aggression and violence (Arango et al., 1999). About 8–10% of individuals with schizophrenia experience violent episodes within a 12-month period, compared with 2% of the general population (Swanson et al., 1990).

Diffuse dysfunction across domains in neuropsychological testing, including executive dysfunction and memory impairment, has been observed among individuals with schizophrenia (Heinrichs & Zakzanis, 1998). Deficits in executive functioning have been found to be more pronounced in violent compared with nonviolent individuals with schizophrenia (Barkataki et al., 2005; Foster, Hillbrand, & Silverstein, 1993; Rasmussen, Levander, & Sletvold, 1995; Serper, Beech, Harvey, & Dill, 2008) but not all (Fullam & Dolan, 2008; Lapierre et al., 1995). Additionally, a deficit in facial affect recognition has been reported in relation to violence in this population (Fullam & Dolan, 2006).

Several areas of research have implicated dysfunction of brain regions crucial to integrating cognitive and emotional processes, such as frontal lobe and mesial temporal lobe structures, in schizophrenia (Davidson & Heinrichs, 2003; Flashman et al., 2001; Fornito, Yücel, Dean, Wood, & Pantelis, 2008; Nelson, Saykin, Flashman, & Riordan, 1998; Pantelis et al., 1997; Pantelis et al., 2005; Rose et al., 2006; Roth, Flashman, Saykin, McAllister, & Vidaver, 2004; Seidman et al., 2003). In a detailed review of 17 studies of neurobiological correlates of violent behavior in patients with schizophrenia, Naudts and Hodgins (2006) suggested that inconsistent and, at times, contradictory results due to methodological differences could be clarified and explained by age of illness onset and persistence of violent behavior. Thus, among individuals with schizophrenia, those who have displayed a stable pattern of aggressive, antisocial behavior since childhood, as compared with those who have not demonstrated such a lifelong pattern, show fewer neurological soft signs and perform better on neuropsychological tests measuring dorsolateral and mesial PFC and verbal abilities, but perform worse on measures of orbitofrontal functions, such as measures of impulsivity. They also display larger reductions in volume of the amygdala, more structural abnormalities of white matter in the amygdala-orbitofrontal system, and smaller reductions in volumes of the hippocampus. Given these findings, Naudts and Hodgins theorized that amygdala-orbitofrontal system abnormality might underlie persistent, impulsive antisocial and violent behavior, and that individuals with schizophrenia and a history of violence may exhibit structural abnormalities in the amygdala from early life, resulting in a reduced capacity to experience emotions.

In an MRI study of violent male psychiatric inpatients (six with schizophrenia and four with personality disorders), 6 out of 10 patients were found to have mesial temporal atrophy (Chesterman, Taylor, Cox, Hill, & Lumsden, 1994; Naudts & Hodgins, 2006). In these six patients, unilateral hippocampal atrophy was more commonly lateralized to the left rather than the right hemisphere. The findings of this study, however, are limited by the small size and heterogeneous nature of the sample utilized. An MRI study comparing 15 nonviolent and 13 violent men with schizophrenia [diagnoses included paranoid ($n = 21$), undifferentiated ($n = 5$), disorganized ($n = 1$) and residual ($n = 1$) sub-types] and 15 healthy men without a history of violence, found increased lateral ventricular size in both patient groups, but only the violent group showed increased putamen size and reduced whole brain and hippocampal volumes (Barkataki, Kumari, Das, Taylor, & Sharma, 2006). Although significantly reduced amygdala size was found in the nonviolent patient group, this was accounted for by differences in the severity of psychopathology between the two patient samples.

A [^{18}F]fluorodeoxyglucose (FDG) PET study examined repetitive and nonrepetitive violent offenders with schizophrenia and schizoaffective disorder having no apparent gross neuroanatomical abnormalities. A total of 31 male patients in a maximum-security psychiatric hospital (17 repetitive and 14 nonrepetitive violent offenders) were compared with six healthy-comparison (HC) subjects (Wong, Fenwick, Lumsden, et al., 1997). Results revealed reduced FDG uptake in bilateral anterior-inferior temporal regions in the nonrepetitive offenders, but only in left anterior-inferior temporal regions in repetitive offenders. FDG uptake in right anterior-inferior temporal regions was significantly lower among nonrepetitive than among repetitive violent offenders. These results were interpreted as indicating that abnormality of anterior-inferior temporal regions may be related to frequency of violent offending in inpatients with schizophrenia. Failure to include a nonviolent group with schizophrenia renders it impossible, however, to determine the extent to which the abnormalities are specific to violent individuals with schizophrenia, rather than schizophrenia more generally.

In another study, Wong, Fenwick, Fenton, and colleagues (1997) examined 39 offenders with schizophrenia or schizoaffective disorder from a maximum-security psychiatric hospital (20 repetitive and 19 nonrepetitive violent offenders) and 14 healthy comparison subjects, using both MRI and PET. A higher prevalence of MRI and PET abnormalities was found among violent offenders. In the repetitive violent offending group, 35% of MRI and 10% of PET findings were abnormal, as compared with 25% of MRI and 30% of PET scans in the nonrepetitive group. Asymmetric goral patterns at the temporal-parietal region were particularly common in the repetitive violent offender group, but absent in nonrepetitive violent offenders. These findings support the hypothesis that structural and metabolic changes in the brain may be associated with repetitive violent offending behavior in patients with schizophrenia.

Hoptman and collegues (2005) examined the relationship between OFC volume on MRI and aggression in 49 treatment-refractory patients (6 female, 43 male) diagnosed with schizophrenia or schizoaffective disorder. Of the 49 patients in the study, 25 (51%) had a diagnosis of co-occurring alcohol-use disorder, and 29 (59%) had a co-occurring substance-use disorder; however, patients were hospitalized and thus were presumed to be free of alcohol or other psychoactive substances at the time of the study. Aggression was measured with the Overt Aggression Scale (OAS) and the Positive and Negative Syndrome Scale (PANSS) by trained raters during a 14-week period. Results indicated that larger total OFC volumes, as well as larger left OFC gray-matter volumes and larger bilateral OFC white-matter volumes, were associated with higher levels of aggression. An association between OFC abnormality and aggression is consistent with the role of this brain region in the regulation of socially appropriate behavior and response inhibition (Chow & Cummings, 1999). In a further investigation of these same patients, Hoptman and colleagues (2006) found that a larger left caudate volume was associated with decreased impulse control and greater aggressiveness during the 14-week study period, independent of age or the presence of an alcohol- or substance-use disorder. Patients who had any aggressive incident during the study period had larger caudate volumes, particularly in the left hemisphere, than did those who had no such incidents. The authors posited that the relationship between aggression and caudate volumes may be related to the iatrogenic effects of increased long-term treatment of violent patients with typical antipsychotic agents, or possibly to direct etiological involvement of the caudate. While the implication of larger caudate volumes in patients remains unclear, such an abnormality may interfere with the normal functioning of the frontal-subcortical circuitry, particularly the OFC.

Few studies have examined the brain during task performance in patients with schizophrenia and a history of aggression. A SPECT study assessed the relationship between PFC and aggression in 15 inpatients with schizophrenia (Spalletta et al., 2001). Participants were evaluated both at rest and during performance on the Wisconsin Card Sorting Test (WCST) (Heaton, Chelune, Talley, Kay, & Curtis, 1993), a neuropsychological measure generally considered sensitive to PFC integrity. Evaluation of aggression was based on clinical staff documentation of patient behavior during the first week of hospitalization; three patients were classified as aggressive and 12 were not. No significant differences in PFC regional cerebral blood flow (rCBF) were found between aggressive and nonaggressive patients at rest. In contrast, reduction of rCBF in the right middle and right inferior prefrontal gyri was seen during the WCST in the aggressive group. It was suggested that reduced rCBF in aggressive individuals supports proposed theories arguing that individuals with prefrontal dysfunction are more vulnerable to impulsive aggression due to impaired self-control and difficulties with modifying and inhibiting behavior.

Kumari and colleagues (2006) applied fMRI to investigate brain activation during a working-memory task (n-back) in men with schizophrenia. They studied four groups of men: 10 violent men with antisocial personality disorder (APD), 13 violent inpatients with schizophrenia mandated to detention in either a high- or medium-security hospital due to their dangerous, violent, or criminal propensities (VS), 12 nonviolent outpatients with schizophrenia (NVS), and 13 men without a history of violence or mental illness. Results revealed subtle working-memory deficits in the NVS and APD groups, but severe deficits emerged in the VS group relative to the healthy comparison group. During the working-memory task, the VS group showed decreased bilateral activation in the frontal lobe and precuneus compared with the controls, and in the right inferior parietal region compared with the NVS group. Across all patients with schizophrenia, a more extensive history of violence, established using clinical and forensic records was associated with less bilateral frontal and right inferior parietal, lobe activation. Relative to healthy comparison subjects, patients with APD showed less activation in the left frontal lobe, anterior cingulate gyrus, and precuneus. The findings suggest that reduced functional response in the frontal and inferior parietal regions contributes to violence in schizophrenia, perhaps as a result of impaired executive functioning.

Narayan and colleagues (2007) used MRI data to investigate regional differences in cortical thickness in 14 male inpatients with APD and 12 male inpatients with schizophrenia having a history of violence, 15 men with schizophrenia without a history of violence living in the community, and 15 healthy, nonviolent men. All violent inpatients resided in a high-security hospital. None of the individuals in the APD group met criteria for psychopathy as assessed by the Psychopathy Checklist–Screening version or had a comorbid diagnosis of schizophrenia. Similarly, none of the patients with schizophrenia met diagnostic criteria for APD. All participants had been abstinent from alcohol and psychoactive substances for a minimum of 2 years (confirmed by regular random urine screens in secure hospitals) at the time of scanning for this study. Significant regional effects of violence and schizophrenia were observed for cortical gray-matter thickness. Violence was associated with cortical thinning in the medial inferior frontal and lateral sensory motor cortex, particularly in the right hemisphere, and surrounding association areas. Subjects with APD showed significant bilateral thinning of the medial inferior frontal cortices and right-hemisphere thinning of sensory-motor areas, compared with controls, but only violent subjects with APD exhibited cortical thinning in inferior medial frontal cortices. Violent subjects with schizophrenia showed deficits in sensory-motor areas compared with nonviolent patients with schizophrenia. The neuroanatomical pathways of violent behavior thus appear to differ between APD and schizophrenia, the medial frontal cortex playing an important role in APD, while the sensorimotor cortex appears related to violent behavior in both APD and schizophrenia.

Joyal and colleagues (2007) used an fMRI go/no-go response inhibition task with 24 male homicide offenders with paranoid schizophrenia, half of whom had comorbid diagnoses of APD and substance use disorder (Sz+APD+SUD), as well as with 12 noncriminal men screened for psychiatric diagnoses. Results showed that only the Sz+APD+SUD group failed to show increased activation in the OFC during response inhibition. Between-group comparisons revealed that inferior or orbital activations in the PFC were significantly higher in both the healthy comparison and schizophrenia-only groups than in the Sz+APD+SUD group. In contrast, significantly higher activations in frontal motor, premotor, and anterior cingulate regions were observed in the Sz+APD+SUD group than in the schizophrenia-only group.

Mixed Personality Disorder Samples

Some personality disorders (PD), particularly *DSM* cluster-B disorders such as antisocial personality disorder (APD) and borderline personality disorder (BPD) have been linked to increased rates of aggression, particularly impulsive aggression (Narayan et al., 2007; Tardiff, 1998). However, the relationship between personality disorders and violence is less clear than the relationship between psychosis and violence, partly due to methodological differences employed in measuring personality and antisocial behavior (Barkataki et al., 2005; Fountoulakis, Leucht, & Kaprinis, 2008). Nonetheless, evidence has emerged that impulsive, aggressive individuals with personality disorders have impaired performance on neuropsychological measures of executive functioning (Dolan, Deakin, Roberts, & Anderson, 2002a; Dolan & Park, 2002) as well as in other domains of functioning (Barkataki et al., 2005; Burgess, 1992). Collectively, these studies suggest the presence of frontal-lobe dysfunction in individuals with personality disorders that are associated with impulsive/aggressive behaviors (Johnson, Hurley, Benkelfat, Herpertz, & Taber, 2003; McCloskey, Phan, & Coccaro, 2005; Stein et al., 1993; Völlm, Dolan, et al., 2007).

PET and SPECT in mixed groups of individuals with personality disorders have revealed prefrontal abnormalities in those prone to aggression. Goyer and colleagues (1994) found PFC abnormalities in a heterogeneous group of 17 adult military inpatients (12 males and 5 females) with various personality disorders, compared with 43 healthy comparison civilian subjects using PET to examine cerebral metabolic rate of glucose (CMRG). Diagnoses within the PD group included antisocial ($n = 6$), borderline ($n = 6$), dependent ($n = 2$), and narcissistic ($n = 3$), and 13 of 17 patients also had a comorbid Axis I disorder. Results indicated that greater impulsive aggression, as measured by the Modified Aggression Scale

(MAS), was associated with decrements in metabolism in OFC. Further examination of the data revealed significantly decreased metabolic rate in the inferior, and increased rate in the superior, frontal cortex in the BPD patients with a life history of aggression, while patients with APD and a history of aggression (of whom 4 had a history of alcohol abuse) did not differ from the healthy comparison subjects. Goyer and Semper (1996) supported this finding by extending the Goyer and colleagues' (1994) study to include 14 healthy controls and 10 male combat veterans with post-traumatic stress disorder (PTSD) and a history of substance abuse. An inverse relationship between upper OFC metabolism and life history of aggression scores, as measured by the Civilian Aggression Scale (CAS), was found in both groups. This result provides preliminary support to the purported relationship between a life-long pattern of aggressive behavior and impaired frontal cortex functioning.

In a SPECT study of a mixed sample of 37 patients with BPD or APD (with no comorbid Axis I diagnosis) compared with 34 healthy comparison subjects, reduced cerebral blood flow was observed in the right lateral temporal cortex, the right frontopolar cortex, and the right ventrolateral prefontal cortex (Goethals et al., 2005). This finding supports previous research indicating that DSM cluster-B personality disorders, characterized in part by impulsiveness, are associated with abnormality in the frontal lobe circuitry.

Dolan, Deakin, Roberts, and Anderson (2002b) examined 51 male offenders with personality disorders detained in a maximum-security hospital and 24 healthy comparison subjects recruited from the hospital staff. All subjects underwent an assessment using the Special Hospital Assessment of Personality and Socialization (SHAPS) and neuropsychological testing. Based on the SHAPS, 44 of the patients were rated as psychopathic and highly impulsive and 7 were rated nonpsychopathic with low impulsiveness. The psychopathic inpatient group met criteria for multiple cluster-B *(DSM-III-R)* personality disorders such as APD, while the nonpsychopathic inpatient group predominantly comprised cluster-A and cluster-C personality disorders (e.g., obsessive-compulsive, schizoid). A subset of 24 patients (18 psychopaths, 6 nonpsychopaths) and 19 comparison subjects also had quantitative measurement of frontal and temporal lobe volumes on magnetic resonance imaging (MRI). No volumetric differences were observed between the groups, despite the fact that high impulsive, psychopathic patients showed worse executive functioning than nonpsychopathic, low impulsive patients and the healthy group, even after controlling for between-group differences in IQ.

Völlm and colleagues (2004) investigated the neural substrates of response inhibition using fMRI and a Go/No-Go task in patients with cluster-B personality disorders. Specifically, they were interested in elucidating which neuronal networks are involved in inhibiting behaviors such as aggression, and whether these networks differ in activation from that seen in healthy subjects. Impulsivity was assessed using the Barratt Impulsivity Scale (BIS) and the Impulsiveness-Venturesomeness-Empathy (IVE) inventory in eight male psychiatric inpatients with a *DSM-IV* diagnosis of BPD or APD and eight healthy comparison subjects. The personality disorder group tended to make more impulsive errors during the task, and showed more bilateral, extended activation across the medial, superior, and inferior frontal gyri into the ACC. The finding of more widespread activations in the patient group may reflect recruitment of additional cortical resources in order to successfully inhibit responding.

In another fMRI study, Völlm and colleagues (2007) investigated the effects of positive and negative reinforcement (i.e., monetary reward and loss) on brain activation in two target selection tasks. Eight male psychiatric inpatient participants with impulsivity-related *DSM-IV* cluster-B (APD and BPD) personality disorders were recruited from an inpatient therapeutic community and a private forensic–psychiatric unit and compared with 14 healthy comparison subjects. All patients had a preadmission history of impulsive behavior including offending. Two patients fulfilled diagnostic criteria for both APD and BPD, five for BPD only, and one for APD only. Results demonstrated an absence of PFC activation and reduced activation in the subcortical reward system during positive reinforcement in the personality disorder group. Furthermore, greater impulsivity was associated with less activation of the OFC during both monetary reward and loss in the patient group.

That the OFC should be abnormal in patients with cluster-B personality disorders appears consistent with the impulsive-aggressive features of these disorders (Fossati et al., 2007), and the functional properties of this brain region. The OFC has been found to be one of the critical structures in large-scale neural systems mediating decision making and impulse control, with abnormality increasing the likelihood of poor, risky decisions and impulsive, antisocial behaviors (Bechara, 2004, 2005; Bechara & van der Linden, 2005). Abnormality of the OFC may also contribute to dysfunctional reinforcement processing, which may underpin behavioral dysregulation by making it difficult to utilize previous experience and environmental feedback to guide behavior (Dinn & Harris, 2000).

The anatomical connectivity between the OFC and amygdala, and the role of this circuitry in emotional regulation, has led some investigators to examine whether the circuitry is involved in impulsive aggression. fMRI responses to emotional faces was investigated in 10 healthy adults and 10 adults (half of whom were male) with intermittent explosive disorder and at least one Axis II personality disorder (6 with PD not otherwise specified, 1 with borderline, 1 with narcissistic, 1 with obsessive compulsive [OCPD], 1 with paranoid PD and narcissistic, and 1 with OCPD). Five of the patients had a comorbid Axis I disorder (Coccaro, McCloskey, Fitzgerald, & Phan, 2007). Results demonstrated exaggerated amygdala and decreased OFC reactivity to faces expressing anger in the patient group. Furthermore, a more extensive history of aggressive behavior across subjects was associated with greater amygdala and OFC activation to angry faces. While a significant inverse relationship was noted between the amygdala and OFC in the healthy group, this was not seen in the patient sample. These findings provide additional support for the link between aggression and a dysfunctional cortical-limbic circuitry, emphasizing abnormal neural responding to socially threatening stimuli in personality disordered individuals with a history of impulsive aggressive behavior.

Antisocial Personality Disorder

Along with schizophrenia, antisocial personality disorder (APD) is one of the most frequently implicated psychiatric disorders in aggressive and violent behavior (Barkataki et al., 2005; Barkataki et al., 2006; Narayan et al., 2007; Tardiff, 1998). The most recent data support the relationship between antisocial personality and violence, especially when substance abuse is also present, although the presence of confounding factors in the diagnostic criteria suggests caution in the interpreta-tion of the neuroscience literature (Fountoulakis et al., 2008). Consistent with the literature on aggression in heterogeneous samples of personality disorders, evidence has emerged that impulsive aggressive individuals with APD have impaired performance on neuropsychological measures of executive functioning, particularly those purportedly sensitive to orbitofrontal dysfunction (Brower & Price, 2001; Deckel, Hesselbrock, & Bauer, 1996; Dinn & Harris, 2000; Dolan et al., 2002a; Dolan & Park, 2002). Additionally, impairments in emotional memory have been found and surmised to be related to a variety of emotional and atten-tional processes linked with prefrontal-limbic neural circuitry (Bergvall, Wessely, Forsman, & Hansen, 2001; Dolan & Fullam, 2005).

In an MRI study of 13 violent men with APD and comorbid personality disorders (8 with BPD, 3 with borderline and paranoid personality disorders, 1 with borderline and histrionic personality disorders, and 1 with paranoid, avoid-ant, and dependant personality disorders) and 15 healthy, nonviolent men, reduced whole-brain and temporal lobe volumes and increased putamen volume were found in the patient group (Barkataki et al., 2006). In addition, the violent APD subjects had significantly larger hippocampal volume than a group of 13 men with schizophrenia and a history of violence.

Raine, Lencz, Bihrle, LaCasse, and Colletti (2000) examined the possibility of subtle structural deficits to the PFC, in the absence of discernable lesions, in APD. Subjects consisted of 21 male community volunteers with APD, 34 healthy males, 26 males with substance dependence, and 21 male psychiatric controls matched with the APD group on schizophrenia-spectrum disorders, affective disorders, anxiety disorders, and other personality disorders that do not fall under the category of APD. MRI scans were obtained and volumetric assessments of prefron-tal gray and white matter were conducted. Compared with all other groups, patients with APD showed a reduction in prefrontal gray matter (11% relative to the healthy group, 13.9% relative to the SD group, and 14% relative to the psychiatric controls).

Borderline Personality Disorder

Borderline personality disorder (BPD) is characterized by severe emotional dysreg-ulation and deficits in impulse control, often resulting in turbulent relationships and self-destructive behaviors (Johnson et al., 2003; McCloskey et al., 2005; Zetzsche et al., 2007). Impulsive aggression, typically manifested by assaultive and suicidal behaviors, is a clinical characteristic of BPD (Soloff et al., 2003). Neuroimaging studies of aggression in BPD have focused on areas associated with cognition, affect, and emotional regulation, namely the PFC and limbic areas.

PET neuroimaging during pharmacologic challenge with d,l fenfluramine (FEN) was conducted in five impulsive, self-destructive individuals with BPD to look for disturbances in serotonergic regulation in areas of the PFC associated with regulation of impulsive behavior (Soloff, Meltzer, Greer, Constantine, & Kelly, 2000). Patients were compared with a sample of healthy adults, which included five men and three women. In response to placebo, the healthy group demonstrated increased activity compared with patients in large areas of the PFC, including medial and orbital regions bilaterally, left superior temporal gyrus, and right insular cortex. There were no areas in which patients had greater activity than the healthy sample. In response to the pharmacological challenge, only the healthy group showed increased uptake in the right medial and orbital frontal regions, the left middle and superior temporal gyri, the left parietal lobe, and the left caudate nucleus. Based on these findings, the authors concluded that patients with BPD have diminished response to serotonergic stimulation in areas of the PFC associated with regulation of socially inappropriate behaviors such as impulsive aggression.

In a second study, Soloff and colleagues (2003) used FDG-PET to study glucose metabolism in a community sample of 13 nondepressed, impulsive women with BPD and 9 healthy women. Significant reductions in FDG uptake in the BPD group were found bilaterally in the medial orbital frontal cortex, even when controlling for degree of depression. Measures of impulsivity or impulsive aggression used as a covariate eliminated the groups' differences, supporting the hypothesis that impulsive aggressiveness is related to prefrontal hypometabolism in BPD.

Rusch and colleagues (2007) employed diffusion tensor imaging (DTI) to measure the integrity of inferior frontal white-matter pathways in a community sample of 20 women with BPD and comorbid ADHD, and 20 healthy women matched for age, education, and estimated premorbid intelligence. This study was motivated by the hypothesis that abnormality of pathways in the inferior frontal region are associated with dysfunctional affect regulation, aggression, dissociative symptoms, and impaired neuropsychological functioning in these patients. Although group differences were not observed, integrity of inferior frontal white matter was associated with higher levels of dysfunctional affect regulation, anger-hostility, dissociative symptoms, and general psychopathology in the patient group. The authors concluded that inferior frontal white-matter abnormalities might be linked to key aspects of psychopathology in women with BPD and comorbid ADHD.

Psychopathy

Psychopathy is a construct closely related conceptually to, and frequently (albeit inappropriately) used interchangeably with, APD (Andrade, 2008; Crowe & Blair, 2008; Hare, 1991/2003). APD is more common than the dimensionally defined, higher-order construct of psychopathy as clinically described by Cleckley (1976) and operationalized and empirically validated by Hare (1991/2003). Psychopathy is not currently listed in the *Diagnostic and Statistical Manual–4th Edition (DSM-IV-TR;* APA, 2000) as a diagnosis. The current nomenclature of the *DSM-IV-TR,* which emphasizes the behavioral characteristics of APD as diagnostic criteria, is primarily based on the presence of a pervasive pattern of antisocial behaviors; whereas the criteria for psychopathy are based on combined personality traits and antisocial behaviors (Andrade, 2008; Crowe & Blair, 2008; Hare, 1991/2003; Hare & Neumann, 2008). Fewer than 25% of individuals meeting diagnostic criteria for APD would meet the psychometric cutoffs for psychopathy (Crowe & Blair, 2008). Although rates of APD and psychopathy are higher in prison and forensic samples than in the general population (Hare, 1991/2003), psychopathy assessed using Hare's criteria is estimated to occur in fewer than 20% of inmates with a diagnosis of APD (Hare, 1998). Furthermore, psychopaths receive more convictions for crimes of violence and have a higher incidence of aggressive and violent behaviors while incarcerated than do other male criminals (Hare & McPherson, 1984; Williamson, Hare, & Wong, 1987).

Psychopathy is a concept that is subject to much debate, but it is usually defined as a specific type of personality disorder that has an enduring and distinctive constellation of personality traits and behavioral variables marked by lack of empathy and antisocial behavior. The contemporary construct of psychopathy, typically applied to adults, consists of two major dimensions. One consists of affective and interpersonal traits involving the callous, selfish, and remorseless use of others. The other is related to chronic antisocial behaviors and deviant lifestyle choices (Salekin, Leistico, Trobst, Schrum, & Lochman, 2005; Skeem, Edens, Camp, & Colwell, 2004). Psychopathy has most commonly been assessed with the Revised Psychopathy Checklist (PCL-R) (Hare, 1991/2003).

Psychopathy is one of the most frequently implicated psychiatric conditions in aggressive and violent behavior (Angermeyer et al., 1998). Major advances have been made in the understanding of the neurobiology of psychopathy in the past several years, yet the distribution and extent of neuroanatomical abnormalities underlying the disorder are still poorly understood. It is also unclear whether different dimensions of the construct of psychopathy (e.g., emotional callousness, antisocial behavior) correspond to abnormalities in distinct regions of the brain (see Poythress & Skeem, 2006; Raine & Yang, 2006, for reviews). A common feature of the antisocial behaviors displayed in psychopaths is that they are typically instrumental in nature, that is, directed towards selfish gains, possibly implicating dysfunctional socialization in the etiology of the disorder (Blair, 2003). Psychopathic adults exhibit severe difficulties in both aversive conditioning and instrumental learning necessary for successful socialization. The amygdala, part of the human limbic system, is involved in mediating motivational and incentive responses, plays a critical role in conditioning and learning, and has been implicated in emotional processing, learning, and attention (Nigg & Huang-Pollock, 2003). Nonpsychopathic individuals with acquired lesions of the amygdala commonly show a diminished ability to empathize with the emotions of others (Martens, 2000) and a lack of emotional arousal to negative stimuli (Berntson, Bechara, Damasio, Tranel, & Cacioppo, 2007). Psychopathic adults have been shown to have impediments to processing the fearfulness and sadness of others (Blair, 2001), consistent with psychopathic traits of callousness and lack of empathy, which are possibly related to abnormality of the amygdala, and likely contribute to a lack of empathy (Herba et al., 2007). Therefore, amygdala dysfunction has been implicated as the core neural abnormality in psychopathy (Blair, 2004, 2006; Patrick, 1994).

In a volumetric MRI study, Tiihonen and colleagues (2000) found that reduced amygdala volume was associated with high levels of psychopathy, as measured by the PCL-R, in violent offenders. Raine and colleagues (2004) assessed whether prior findings of a right-greater-than-left structural and functional brain asymmetry in arrested violent criminal offenders generalizes to unsuccessful psychopaths. Hippocampal volume was assessed on structural MRI scans in 23 adult comparison subjects scoring low on the PCL-R, as well as 16 unsuccessful (i.e., convicted) and 12 successful (i.e., no conviction) community psychopaths with high PCL-R scores. Unsuccessful psychopaths were found to have exaggerated structural asymmetry of the anterior hippocampus, right greater than left, relative both to successful psychopaths and comparison subjects, which could not be accounted for by demographic and behavioral confounds (e.g., trauma exposure, schizophrenia-spectrum disorders, head injury, substance use). This finding is consistent with the prior findings of the same hippocampal asymmetry in caught violent offenders during a cognitive activation challenge (Raine et al., 1997). Abnormal anterior hippocampal asymmetries in unsuccessful psychopaths may reflect disruptions in prefrontal hippocampal circuitry, possibly resulting in affect dysregulation, poor contextual fear conditioning, and insensitivity to cues predicting capture.

Two studies to date have used voxel-based morphometry (VBM) to investigate brain structure on MRI scans in relation to psychopthy (de Oliveira-Souza et al., 2008; Müller et al., 2008). This technique allows for the evaluation of the structural integrity of the whole brain simultaneously, as well as identifying regional differences. de Oliveira and colleagues' (2008) sample included 15 adult community psychiatric patients (8 men, 7 women) with high scores on the screening version of PCL (all of which met diagnostic criteria for APD) and 15 matched healthy comparison subjects. The authors were particularly interested in determining whether psychopathy in this mixed diagnostic sample is associated with abnormalities in brain regions that underlie moral conduct and regions previously reported to be abnormal in psychopaths. Results indicated that the worse the score on the interpersonal/affective dimension of psychopathy, the greater the pattern of gray-matter reductions in an interconnected network of frontal-temporal regions that play a critical role in moral sensibility and behavior. Notably, three regions of the PFC that showed gray-matter decreases in relation to psychopathy, the medial and lateral OFC and the frontopolar cortex, had been previously implicated in the regulation of social conduct. Consistent with the above VBM findings, Müller and colleagues' (2008) VBM study found significant reductions in gray matter in frontal and temporal regions, most significantly in the right superior temporal gyrus in their sample of 17 forensic male inpatient psychopaths with high PCL-R scores relative to 17 healthy male volunteers with low PCL-R scores. These two studies suggest that reduced gray-matter volumes in both the frontal and temporal cortex, regions thought to be involved in social functioning, play a role in the pathogenesis of psychopathy. The findings are consistent with the dysfunctional limbic hypothesis of psychopathy.

Functional magnetic resonance imaging has also been used to expound upon prior findings of emotional processing dysfunction and its neurobiological correlates in psychopathy. Using fMRI in a maximum-security prison sample, Kiehl and colleagues examined the neural response to words of neutral and negative valence in eight criminal psychopaths, as determined by high PCL-R scores (> 28/40), compared with eight nonpsychopathic criminals (PCL-R scores <23/40) (Kiehl et al., 2001). During the processing of negative valence words, reduced amygdala and hippocampal response was found in high-relative to low-scoring inmates and a noncriminal comparison group. Furthermore, the criminal psychopaths had a significant reduction in affect-related activity in the rostral and caudal anterior cingulate, posterior cingulate, left inferior frontal gyrus, right amygdala, and ventral striatum. No group differences emerged for the neutral words. Criminal psychopaths also showed reduced affect-related activity compared with non-criminal controls in the left amygdala and parahippocampal gyrus, and bilateral anterior superior temporal gyrus. Interestingly, overactivation in a number of brain regions located outside the limbic system (i.e., left anterior superior temporal gyrus/inferior frontal gyrus, and right inferior frontal gyrus) was observed during the processing of affective stimuli in criminal psychopaths compared with non-criminal and criminal nonpsychopath groups. These results support the hypothesis that criminal psychopathy is associated with abnormalities of the limbic system and frontal cortical regions involved in the processing of affective stimuli. This interpretation is also generally consistent with Hare's (1970) hypothesis that psychopaths suffer from limbic-system dysfunction, which affects their ability to inhibit behaviors that could potentially lead to punishment, as well as with more recent theories of deficient affective processing among adults with antisocial and psychopathic traits such as Damasio's (1994) somatic-marker hypothesis and Blair's (1995) violence-inhibition hypothesis. Thus, psychopaths are likely to display their preferred action or response, such as aggression, despite the potential negative consequences. Indeed, psychopathy is characterized by "an early onset of extremely aggressive behavior that is not tempered by any sense of guilt or empathy with the victim" (Blair, 1995, p. 2).

Functional imaging has also been used to test the hypothesis that psychopathy is associated with abnormalities in semantic processing of linguistic information. Eight criminal psychopaths incarcerated in a maximum-security prison and eight healthy adults with no criminal history performed a lexical decision task during fMRI in which blocks of linguistic stimuli (i.e., visual presentation of either blocks of concrete words and pseudowords, or blocks of abstract words and pseudowords) alternated with a resting baseline condition (Kiehl et al., 2004). Results indicated that psychopathy was associated with significantly slower processing of abstract words and failure to show the expected neural differentiation between abstract and concrete stimuli in the right anterior temporal gyrus and surrounding cortex. When classifying pseudoword stimuli, the psychopaths also responded less accurately than healthy participants. These findings are consistent with prior nonimaging research that observed deficient ability to process abstract word stimuli in psychopathy, and has been interpreted as suggesting abnormal right hemisphere semantic processing of abstract material (Hare & Jutai, 1988; Kiehl, Hare, McDonald, & Brink, 1999).

Traumatic Brain Injury

Aggressive behavior during the acute period after traumatic brain injury (TBI) has been reported to occur in 11–96% of patients (Kim, Manes, Kosier, Baruah, & Robinson, 1999; McKinlay et al., 1981; Silver et al., 2005). After a brain injury, individuals often experience a period of acute agitation and confusion, which may be followed by intermittent, explosive reactive-aggressive outbursts (Silver et al., 2005). It is important to note that while a correlation between TBI and aggression has been demonstrated, a causal relationship indicating that TBI is directly responsible for increased aggression has not been demonstrated. TBI is more common among men who commit acts of domestic violence than among nonviolent men (Elliott, 1982; Rosenbaum et al., 1994), and among individuals with histories of uncontrolled rage (Elliott, 1982). Kavoussi and colleagues (1997) suggest that the increased incidence of brain injury among violent individuals may instead be a result of the increased probability that such individuals would engage in dangerous situations, such as fights, resulting in a TBI. In fact, a preinjury history of aggressiveness, as well as irritability and impulsivity, are considered possible risk factors for post-TBI aggressive behaviors (Silver et al., 2005). As

Kavoussi and colleagues (1997) point out, demonstration of a causal relationship between TBI and aggression would benefit from the consistent identification of aggression-enhancing lesions, that is, individuals with damage to a specific region of the brain consistently exhibit increased aggression.

Grafman and colleagues (1996) examined the relationship between aggression and frontal lobe lesions in 279 Vietnam veterans who had sustained a penetrating TBI. Veterans with TBI were reported to be more aggressive and violent than a sample of 57 non-TBI veterans matched by age, education, and length of deployment. Furthermore, the veterans that had sustained focal ventromedial frontal lobe lesions, as determined by CT scan, exhibited more aggression and violent behaviors than those who sustained lesions in other areas of the brain. In addition, veterans with anterior temporal lobe lesions were more likely to report greater anger and hostility than was observed by their informants; veterans with medio-frontal lesions were reported to have increased aggression and violent behaviors by both self- and informant report; and veterans with focal orbitofrontal lesions were less aware of increased aggression and related behaviors than informants. These findings suggest that lesion location has an impact on the level of awareness one has with respect to aggression and related problems. Lesion size was unrelated to the presence of aggression or violent behavior.

Tateno, Jorge, and Robinson (2003) also found that the presence of aggression was associated with frontal lobe damage. In their study, aggression and associated behaviors were significantly more frequent among trauma patients with TBI than in a comparable group of trauma patients without TBI. Among those studied with a TBI, 33.7% exhibited significant aggressive behaviors during the first six months after their injury. They found that aggressive behavior was associated with the presence of major depression, a history of alcohol or drug abuse, and a significantly higher frequency of aggressive behaviors resulting in legal interventions prior to the TBI. Furthermore, the aggressive TBI group demonstrated a higher frequency of frontal lobe lesions as seen on CT scan, and patients with focal frontal lobe lesions were rated as being more aggressive on the Overt Aggression Scale than those with focal lesions in other brain regions. In contrast, Baguley, Cooper, and Felmingham (2006) found significant, stable levels of aggression in approximately 25% of their TBI sample five years post-discharge, but no significant predictive value of lesion location on CT scan.

Epilepsy

The relationship between epilepsy and aggression has been widely debated among researchers and clinicians (Sbordone, 1993; Trimble & van Elst, 1999; van Elst, Woermann, Lemieux, Thompson, et al., 2000). The prevalence of aggression in patients with epilepsy has been variable across studies, raging from 5–50% (Elliott, 1992; Saver, 2002). Aggression has been most commonly associated with temporal lobe epilepsy (TLE) (Herzberg & Fenwick, 1988), with some patients exhibiting irritable and aggressive behaviors up to several days prior to having a seizure (Sbordone, 1993). In addition, episodic dyscontrol (intermittent explosive disorder) has been reported to be relatively common in patients with complex partial seizures (Elliott, 1982). All aggressive behaviors observed in epilepsy, whether ictal, post-ictal, or interictal, appear to be affective in nature, occurring in the context of high levels of arousal, fear, or anger (Saver, 2002).

It is important to note that most individuals with epilepsy do not exhibit violent or criminal behaviors. Among individuals who engage in repetitive acts of violence, however, the incidence of epilepsy, particularly TLE, has been reported to be greater than in the general public (Elliott, 1992). It is therefore not surprising that early studies implicated TLE as the cause of aggressive behavior (Blake & Grafman, 2004). Given the occurrence of automatisms in seizure disorders, epilepsy has been offered as a rationale for diminished capacity and utilized as a medico-legal defense in violent crimes for nearly 100 years (Sbordone, 1993). As Hawkins and Trobst (2000) note, "The idea that seizures cause uncontrolled violence may be particularly attractive to some individuals facing charges for violent offenses (and their lawyers)" (p. 148).

That TLE should be associated with aggression, at least in some patients, is consistent with the aforementioned role of the limbic system in emotional arousal and responding, and broader frontal lobe-limbic circuitry in decision making and the modulation of innate biological drives (Stuss & Alexander, 2000). The ardent interest in limbic pathology as an etiological explanation for aggression "partially reflects the intuitive connection between a primitive system running amok and apparently senseless violence" (Hawkins & Trobst, 2000, p. 149).

Tonkonogy (1991) studied 23 neuropsychiatric inpatients diagnosed with organic mental syndrome, 14 of whom displayed violent behavior. Five of these fourteen individuals had focal lesions in the anterior-inferior temporal lobe documented by MRI or CT. Although four of the five showed epileptiform activity on an EEG, only one had TLE while the other three had generalized seizures. It was concluded that abnormality of the amygdala or adjacent limbic structures may play a role in violence, along with kindling of preserved limbic structures. Tonkonogy and Geller (1992) reported two cases of craniopharyngiomas and intermittent explosive disorder in which MRI implicated hypothalamic–hypophyseal involvement in the development of aggressive behavior. An early study using CT failed to identify any neuroanatomical differences among 31 patients with TLE classified as either aggressive or nonaggressive, the majority of the aggressive group being classified as minimally violent (Herzberg & Fenwick, 1988).

van Elst and colleagues have conducted several structural MRI studies investigating whether there are neural correlates of aggression in adults with TLE. In their first study, van Elst, Woermann, Lemieux, & Trimble (1999) reported that there was no significant difference in amygdala volume between 24 medically intractable TLE patients with aggression, and 24 without. In a second MRI study, van Elst, Woermann, Lemieux, Thompson, and colleagues (2000) found that among their medically intractable TLE patients with intermittent explosive disorder, 20% had severe bilateral amygdala atrophy, while a subgroup of aggressive patients exhibited left temporal lobe lesions affecting the amygdala and periamygdaloid regions. In total, 44% of their sample with comorbid TLE and intermittent explosive disorder exhibited some evidence of amygdala pathology, albeit of a diverse nature. Notably, evidence did not implicate hippocampal sclerosis in the development of intermittent explosive disorder. Additionally, it was noted that right-sided EEG and MRI abnormalities were less common in those with TLE and aggression, suggesting that dominant hemisphere dysfunction may play a more critical role in the development of intermittent explosive disorder. Finally, no significant relationship between amygdala volume determined by MRI and aggression was observed in a study of 20 healthy participants and male and female patients having TLE, 27 with and 35 without a history of aggressive behavior (van Elst, Woermann, Lemieux, & Trimble, 2000). Other work has used structural MRI and voxel-based morphometry to investigate the brains of patients with both epilepsy and episodes of affective aggression (Woermann et al., 2000). Participants included 35 healthy subjects, 24 patients with TLE and a history of repeated interictal episodes of aggression, and 24 patients with TLE and no previous episodes of aggression. Results revealed decreased gray matter, most markedly in the left frontal lobe, in the group with aggressive episodes as compared with the other two groups.

Criminal Offenders

In a retrospective review of the records of 270 accused murderers undergoing evaluations to establish competency to stand trial and criminal responsibility, Frierson and Finkenbine (2004) found that 29% of the pretrial detainees had a history of TBI with loss of consciousness. Furthermore, structural neuroimaging (i.e., CT or MRI) was abnormal in 18% of the sample, with the most frequent abnormality occurring in the temporal lobe. It should be noted that the neurological examination was within normal limits in 98% of the detainees, that is, most of the detainees were eventually found to be competent to stand trial (93%), criminally responsible (97%), and to have the capacity to conform their behavior to the requirements of the law (96%).

Tiihonen and colleagues (2008) compared regional brain volumes of 26 persistently violent male offenders with APD and substance dependence admitted to a forensic psychiatric hospital for pretrial assessment, and those of 25 healthy males, using MRI volumetry and voxel-based morphometry. All of the offenders had a history of recurrent violent acts, and 23 had a prior conviction for a violent crime. Compared with the healthy group, the violent offenders had larger white-matter volumes in the left cerebellum, and the occipital and parietal lobes bilaterally, as well as larger gray-matter volume in the right cerebellum. Volumes in these regions were not associated with PCL-R scores, substance abuse, psychotropic medications, or global IQ scores. Voxel-based analyses revealed focal and symmetrically bilateral areas of gray-matter atrophy in the postcentral gyri, frontopolar cortex (superior and medial frontal gyrus), and OFC of the violent offenders. Abnormalities were also observed in the left posterior cingulate cortex and the right insula. A subgroup of violent offenders diagnosed as psychopaths, based on the PCL-R, showed generally the same, but more prominent, abnormalities as the offender group as a whole. No significant volume reductions were observed when a subset of 14 nonpsychopathic offenders with APD was compared with psychopathic offenders. Such findings highlight the importance of assessing psychopathy in neuroimaging studies of APD.

Several PET studies have been conducted to investigate neural correlates of violence. In one study, seven subjects with criminal histories of unprovoked violence who completed a medical evaluation associated with legal proceeding were compared with nine healthy subjects (Seidenwurm, Pounds, Globus, & Valk, 1997). The results showed reduced temporal lobe metabolism in the violent offenders during a resting state. Raine and colleagues (1994) studied a heterogenous sample of 22 murderers [schizophrenia ($n = 3$), history of head injury or organic brain damage ($n = 10$), 3 with history of psychoactive substance abuse

($n = 3$), 2 with affective disorder ($n = 2$), epilepsy ($n = 1$), history of hyperactivity and learning disability ($n = 1$), 2 with passive-aggressive or paranoid personality disorder ($n = 2$)] pleading not guilty by reason of insanity (NGRI) and an age- and gender-matched noncriminal sample using PET acquired during performance of a continuous-performance task (CPT). Although no performance difference was observed, suggesting equivalent effort, the murderers showed significantly reduced prefrontal function, especially in the anterior medial cortex and supraventricular superior regions. In a follow-up study (Raine et al., 1997), PET and a CPT task were again employed in a sample of 41 murderers pleading NGRI [schizophrenia ($n = 6$), history of head injury or organic brain damage ($n = 23$), history of psychoactive substance abuse ($n = 3$), affective disorder ($n = 2$), epilepsy ($n = 2$), history of hyperactivity and learning disability ($n = 3$), and passive-aggressive or paranoid personality disorder ($n = 2$)]. In support of their previous findings, the results indicated that the murderers were characterized by reduced glucose metabolism in the bilateral PFC, the posterior parietal cortex (i.e., bilateral superior gyrus and left angular gyrus), and the corpus callosum. Several regions of abnormal asymmetry were also identified, with reduced left-relative-to-right hemisphere activity in the amygdala, hippocampus, and thalamus. The authors concluded that the identified deficits are consistent with theorized biosocial pathways to predatory violence, with: prefrontal deficits resulting in decreased executive functioning, which contributes to aggressive acts; limbic deficits yielding a dysfunctional behavioral inhibition system, impaired formation of conditioned emotional responses and learning, and reduction of autonomic arousal; callosal dysfunction resulting in poor interhemispheric transfer consistent with previously observed lateralized findings in violent individuals; and posterior parietal deficits contributing to the cognitive and social information-processing impairments observed in violent offenders.

Reanalysis of the data from the Raine and colleagues' (1997) study revealed that murderers without any clear psychosocial deprivation during early childhood (i.e., no abuse or neglect) were significantly lower on prefrontal glucose metabolism than murderers with psychosocial deficits and controls (Raine, Stoddard, Bihrle, & Buchsbaum, 1998). The authors argued that the prefrontal deficits found among murderers lacking psychosocial deficits suggest that brain abnormalities provide a relatively stronger predisposition to violence in this group; whereas, offenders from deprived social backgrounds may engage in violence for psychosocial reasons, such as child abuse and domestic disturbances. Further analysis revealed that murderers without psychosocial deficits had reduced OFC functioning in both hemispheres, but particularly the right, which was hypothesized by the authors to be associated with a reduced responsiveness to aversive, emotional activity and possibly an emotionally blunted personality without conscience. Further reanalysis of the data indicated that impulsive, affective murderers relative to healthy subjects had lower prefrontal functioning bilaterally, higher right-hemisphere subcortical functioning, and lower right-hemisphere prefrontal/subcortical ratios. In contrast, predatory murderers had prefrontal functioning that was more equivalent to that of the healthy group, while also having excessively high right subcortical activity (Raine, Meloy, et al., 1998). Findings were viewed as supporting the hypothesis that individuals who commit emotional, impulsive murders are less able to regulate and control aggressive impulses generated from subcortical structures due to deficient prefrontal regulation.

Methodological Limitations of Available Research

The study of brain-behavior relationships underlying aggression and violence is hindered by several challenges. Some of these difficulties are intrinsic to all examinations of brain-behavior relations, whereas others are specific to the study of brain-behavior relations underlying aggression. One of the major difficulties identified in brain-behavior research is that the results of studies carried out in animal models, for obvious ethical reasons, cannot be fully extrapolated and generalized to humans (Karli, 2006). Similarly, most experimental designs are fixed in time and space and yield results devoid of historical context, yet developmental and contextual factors dynamically interact with human behaviors. A limitation specific to research on human aggression relates to personal internal ideological prejudices, which have an impact on the construction of working hypotheses and the interpretation of results (Herzberg & Fenwick, 1988; Karli, 2006). That is, behavior considered aggressive or violent by one observer may be considered situationally appropriate to another.

A concise interpretation of neuroimaging studies of human aggression and violence is difficult due to several methodological limitations. One is the generally small to modest sample sizes employed, which limits the generalization of any significant findings. Perhaps the most fundamental problem lies in the heterogeneity of the samples. There is a lack of consistent definitions for aggression and violence, and of behavioral outcomes, utilized among researchers (Blake & Grafman, 2004; Tateno et al., 2003; Weber, Habel, Amunts, & Schneider, 2008; Zalsman & Apter, 2002). Some researchers classified subjects as aggressive based on psychometric assessments (e.g., Coccaro et al., 2007; Tateno et al., 2003), while others used retrospective surveys or a prior history of violent behaviors resulting in arrest (e.g., Raine et al., 1997; Seidenwurm et al., 1997; Volkow & Tancredi, 1987). Many of the later types of studies do not distinguish between types of violent crimes but instead include perpetrators of various offenses (e.g., attempted homicide, rape, physical assault, arson). Lack of specificity of phenotypic variants is a tremendous hurdle that must be overcome to understand the underlying neurobiology of persons with violent behaviors (Bjorkly, 2006). It has also been suggested that studies should distinguish between impulsive and predatory aggression to ameliorate the current lack of specificity in samples (Bassarath, 2001; Raine & Buchsbaum, 1996). More precise typologies and subtyping of aggressive, violent, and antisocial behaviors are required in future research to more appropriately and specifically connect brain and behavior. In their review of structural and functional neuroimaging studies of violent and nonviolent offenders, Mills and Raine (1994) posited that there may be a relationship between location of brain dysfunction and type of offense, such that frontal lobe dysfunction may be associated with violent offending, temporal lobe dysfunction with sexual offending, and frontal-temporal dysfunction with violent sexual offending.

Heterogeneity of study samples is evident when examining several other relevant variables. Study participants have been recruited from a variety of settings, such as the community, inpatient psychiatric hospitals, maximum-security forensic psychiatric hospitals, maximum-security prisons, and mixed inpatient and outpatient samples. Similarly, a plethora of divergent populations have been studied including Vietnam veterans, individuals with psychiatric and neurological disorders, and criminal offenders. Findings in one population cannot automatically be generalized to other populations. Furthermore, despite valiant attempts to identify homogeneous samples, potentially salient variables, such as heterogeneity of primary psychiatric diagnosis within a given sample of psychiatric patients, have often been neglected. The presence of comorbid alcohol- and substance-use disorders in some studies further confounds interpretation of the results, given the association of these disorders with at least partially overlapping abnormalities in the brain as those reported in association with aggression and violence, brain structure, and function (Weber et al., 2008).

As mentioned previously, there are also important differences between APD and psychopathy that have not been consistently considered in studies of APD. Furthermore, in their review of studies of brain structure in psychopathy, Weber and colleagues (2008) noted that variations among studies in PCL-R cutoff scores used to determine psychopathy present an additional methodological limitation in the literature. Subject-selection bias and group size have also been implicated as a methodological limitation (Grafman et al., 1996).

Another factor rendering comparison of studies difficult is the inconsistent nature of comparison groups used to determine whether a finding is abnormal in aggressive/violent subject samples. Comparison groups have included healthy community volunteers, residential staff, as well as subject groups matched to the aggressive/violent group on as many salient variables as possible with the exception of aggression or violence (e.g., nonaggressive criminals, nonaggressive psychiatric inpatients). The lack of the latter type of comparison group in many studies, especially those involving patient populations, renders it difficult to determine whether the findings are specifically related to aggression/violence.

Methodological divergences in the acquisition, processing, and analysis of neuroimaging data may further contribute to differences in the pattern of intact and abnormal findings (Weber et al., 2008). For example, many functional neuroimaging studies acquired data while participants were resting, while a smaller number of studies have examined brain activation during the performance of a cognitive task. Additionally, it is important to remember that analysis of imaging data involves the use of statistical techniques that are rarely applied uniformly across studies (Brodie, 1996).

Despite the myriad methodological limitations, there is an emerging picture supporting the involvement of certain brain regions in the etiology of aggression and violence. In particular, evidence points most consistently to a role for abnormality of the PFC. Within this region, the OFC and ventromedial subregions have been the most commonly implicated. Furthermore, aggression appears to be associated with abnormality of highly interconnected structures within the frontal lobe and limbic system. It should be noted, however, that the empirical findings to date do not support a simple attribution of aggression of all types and in all populations to a single neuroanatomical region or circuitry. Additionally, all of the brain regions implicated in aggression and violence have also been reported to be abnormal in various clinical samples that are not characterized as aggressive or violent. Thus, further research is needed to determine the specificity of any relationship between the structural and/or functional integrity of a given brain region or circuitry and aggression and violent behavior.

Neuroimaging in the Medical-Legal Context

In many legal cases in the United States, acts of violence have been purported to be secondary to neuropsychiatric disorders, neuroanatomical dysfunction, or both.

Furthermore, human aggression is frequently associated with brain dysfunction in the popular media and among laypersons. The empirical investigation of the neurobiology of human aggression and violence using neuroimaging therefore has significant relevance to neuropsychologists, as well as to other clinicians who are retained by attorneys to evaluate or testify to a defendant's neuropsychiatric condition in an attempt to show the defendant is incompetent to stand trial. Prosecutors may claim certain neuropsychiatric conditions or personality disorders in an attempt to establish future dangerousness as an aggravating factor. As such, there have been increasing attempts, albeit most often rejected, to submit neuroimaging evidence to mitigate criminal responsibility or diminish punishment during sentencing (Husted, Myers, & Lui, 2008; Tancredi & Brodie, 2007). Neuroimaging may be utilized in forensic cases for a variety of reasons, but the most commonly admissible applications include (in order, from most, to least, likely to be admissible) (a) identification of brain structure, (b) characterization of brain functioning, (c) provision of explanation for criminal behavior, or (d) prediction of future behavior based on brain functioning, and lie detection (Pettit, 2007).

As a result of the rapidity of technical advances and the influx of imaging techniques into neuroscience research and the medical field, it is not surprising that there has been an increase in the introduction of neuroimaging data into the courtroom (Brakel, Gonzalez, & Cavanaugh, 1996; Husted et al., 2008; Patel, Meltzer, Mayberg, & Levine, 2007). Historically, courts have accepted the admissibility of structural neuroimaging as proof of brain damage on a fairly routine basis, but the admissibility of functional neuroimaging evidence has been more restricted, given reservations about what can be inferred from such images (Moriarty, 2008). While neuroimaging evidence has been introduced at some level in both civil (e.g., *Hose v. Chicago Northwestern Transp. Co*, 1995; *Lockett v. Anderson*, 2000) and criminal cases (*People of New York v. Weinstein*, 1992; *United States v. Gigante*, 1997), there has been limited success in the introduction of neuroimaging for purposes of establishing insanity or incompetency. Judges have tended to be more open, however, to admitting such evidence in death-penalty hearings (Moriarty, 2008). A court will allow reliable neuroimaging evidence to be admitted only if it benefits the trier of fact in understanding a relevant issue, or if it makes a point at issue more likely to be validated or invalidated (Patel et al., 2007). An expert may testify about scientific knowledge if it will benefit the judge or jury in deciding an issue relevant to the case at hand (Mehr & Gerdes, 2001). Several excellent texts are available for readers interested in more detailed explanations of the issues applicable to the admissibility of neuroimaging and relevant case law (Aharoni, Funk, Sinnott-Armstrong, & Gazzaniga, 2008; Arrigo, 2007; Barth, 2007; Baskin, Edersheim, & Price, 2007; Bigler, 2003; Brakel et al., 1996; Khoshbin & Khoshbin, 2007; Mehr & Gerdes, 2001; Moriarty, 2008; Snead, 2007; Stern, 2001; Witzel, Walter, Bogerts, & Northoff, 2008; Wortzel, Filley, Anderson, Oster, & Arciniegas, 2008).

Given the potential legal implications of aggressive behaviors, the extent to which behavioral dysregulation is related to brain dysfunction has great importance to forensic neuropsychology. Although the application of neuroimaging techniques to the understanding of human behavior is still in its infancy, these techniques have already revolutionized our understanding of the highly complex neural substrate-environment interplay. Although the research examining the relationship between various cognitive domains and structural data is copious compared with functional neuroimaging, the latter techniques are more appropriate for dynamic studies of the brain-behavior relationship (Gur & Gur, 1993), and they have provided neuroscientists and clinicians a means to investigate further how aberrant brain function or structures may be correlated with aggressive behaviors.

Neuroimaging techniques are still evolving, with frequent improvements in data acquisition and image resolution. However, most functional neuroimaging techniques have not yet been accepted for clinical diagnostic purposes and normative data remains elusive (Gur & Gur, 1993; Mobbs, Lau, Jones, & Frith, 2007). Furthermore, research findings based on group data are not always consistent or adequately robust to be reliably applied to individuals (Patel et al., 2007). Despite the reliable detection and classification of several neurological conditions (e.g., neoplasm, multiple sclerosis, stroke) using certain neuroimaging techniques (e.g., CT, MRI), the diagnostic value of neuroimaging for most neurological and all psychiatric disorders has not been firmly established (Gur & Gur, 1993; Ricker, 2005). Although certain structural and functional neuroimaging patterns have emerged in certain sample populations, the diagnostic difficulties inherent in neuroimaging techniques may be best illustrated by the fact that frontal lobe dysfunction has been identified in a myriad of neuropsychiatric conditions, suggesting the possibility that hypofrontality may be a general, nonspecific finding associated with a variety of conditions.

It has been suggested that brain imaging should be applied as a standard forensic practice to exclude organic brain disorders at least, if not more widely, in individuals with antisocial and violent behaviors (Weber et al., 2008). However, methodological limitations, inconsistencies in the literature, and the lack of a pathognomic signature for either antisocial or violent behaviors, either within a given population or across populations, render such ambitious use of neuroimaging problematic. Furthermore, it remains to be determined whether neuroimaging data can be used to predict with a reasonable degree of confidence whether a given individual is likely to behave aggressively or violently in the future. Not surprisingly, therefore, the introduction of neuroimaging findings as forensic evidence is controversial among neuroscientists. When such findings are introduced into legal proceedings, the complexity of the scientific methods and interpretations render it vital that expert testimony be provided by individuals who are actively engaged in neuroimaging work. Although clinicians should recuse themselves from testifying about neuroimaging findings if they are unable to provide the proper legal foundation for their opinions or are not qualified to do so by virtue of knowledge, skill, experience, training, or education, the expert's qualifications and the admissibility of evidence are ultimately determined by the court, because it is the trial judge who serves as the gatekeeper (Klee & Friedman, 2001; Mehr & Gerdes, 2001). The expert must be able to explain the underlying scientific principles of neuroimaging, document that the proper scientific techniques were utilized in obtaining the neuroimaging data, and explain why the particular modality of neuroimaging utilized is scientifically reliable for the purpose it is being used.

The limits of neuroimaging as evidence should be clearly understood by those involved in forensic cases. First and foremost, neuroimaging is not a tool that enables mindreading. Neuroimaging does not reveal the internal thoughts of an individual during the time of an alleged criminal act, nor does it reliably reveal the internal thoughts of an individual during scanning (Mobbs et al., 2007; Yang, Glenn, & Raine, 2008). Second, brain imaging only provides one facet of the complex influences on behavior that may be relevant to understanding why an individual acted in an aggressive or violent manner (Mobbs et al., 2007). Given that aggression is a complex behavior, one should also consider and incorporate additional information, such as relevant medical and psychosocial history, and neuropsychological data, to help elucidate why an aggressive act occurred (Husted et al., 2008; Mehr & Gerdes, 2001). It is also important to remember that interpretation of brain imaging involves some degree of subjectivity (Mobbs et al., 2007), particularly given the lack of well-developed normative data. Also, anatomical landmarks vary significantly among individuals, which may pose difficulties for the legal interpretation of an individual brain scan (Mobbs et al., 2007). As discussed in the above review of neuroimaging studies of aggression, there is not a perfect correlation between brain structure and function and aggression, much less criminal behavior. Thus, the diagnostic and predictive validity of neuroimaging evidence is limited at present (Mobbs et al., 2007). Finally, there is concern that the vivid nature of brain images produced from state-of-the-art neuroimaging may be overwhelming for jurors, causing them to be overly swayed by a perpetrator's alleged brain dysfunction (Mobbs et al., 2007).

Although neuroimaging evidence has become an increasingly utilized tool in the American court system, it is important to remember that neuroscience still has a considerable way to go in fully explaining the neurobiological contribution to criminally aggressive and violent behavior. Although constrained by the aforementioned limitations, neuroimaging can provide some insight into the nature, cause, and behavioral implications of aggression for the court system. Nonetheless, it behooves clinicians and others involved in legal proceedings to introduce neuroimaging data in a scientific and unbiased manner. Enthusiasm for the possibility that neuroimaging will be able to provide insight into our understanding of brain-behavior relationships must be mitigated by an allegiance to the practice of rigorous scientific methodology and an urgency to establish diagnostic utility.

References

Aharoni, E., Funk, C., Sinnott-Armstrong, W., & Gazzaniga, M. (2008). Can neurological evidence help courts assess criminal responsibility? Lessons from law and neuroscience. *Annals of the New York Academy of Sciences, 1124*, 145–160.

Albert, D. J., Walsh, M. L., & Jonik, R. H. (1993). Aggression in humans: What is its biological foundation? *Neuroscience & Biobehavioral Reviews, 17*, 405–425.

Amen, D. G., Stubblefield, M., Carmichael, B., & Thisted, R. (1996). Brain SPECT findings and aggressiveness. *Annals of Clinical Psychiatry, 8*, 129–137.

American Psychiatric Association. (2000). *Diagnostic and statisical manual of mental disorders* (4th ed., text rev.). Washington, DC: American Psychiatric Press.

Anderson, C. A., & Bushman, B. J. (2002). Human aggression. *Annual Review of Psychology, 53*, 27–51.

Anderson, K., & Silver, J. M. (1998). Modulation of anger and aggression. *Seminars in Clinical Neuropsychiatry, 3*, 232–242.

Anderson, S. W., Bechara, A., Damasio, H., Tranel, D., & Damasio, A. R. (1999). Impairment of social and moral behavior related to early damage in human prefrontal cortex. *Nature Neuroscience, 2*, 1032–1037.

Andrade, J. T. (2008). The inclusion of antisocial behavior in the construct of psychopathy: A review of the research. *Aggression and Violent Behavior, 13*, 328–335.

Angermeyer, M. C. (2000). Schizophrenia and violence. *Acta Psychiatrica Scandinavica. Supplementum, 102*, 63–67.

Angermeyer, M. C., Cooper, B., & Link, B. G. (1998). Mental disorder and violence: Results of epidemiological studies in the era of de-institutionalization. *Social Psychiatry and Psychiatric Epidemiology, 33*, 1–6.

Arango, C., Calcedo Barba, A., González-Salvador, T., & Calcedo Ordóñez, A. (1999). Violence in inpatients with schizophrenia: A prospective study. *Schizophrenia Bulletin, 25*, 493–503.

Arrigo, B. A. (2007). Punishment, freedom, and the culture of control: The case of brain imaging and the law. *American Journal of Law & Medicine, 33*, 457–482.

Arthurs, O. J., & Boniface, S. (2002). How well do we understand the neural origins of the fMRI BOLD signal? *Trends in Neurosciences, 25*, 27–13.

Baguley, I. J., Cooper, J., & Felmingham, K. (2006). Aggressive behavior following traumatic brain injury—How common is common? *Journal of Head Trauma Rehabilitation, 21*, 45–56.

Balaban, E., Alper, J. S., & Kasamon, Y. L. (1996). Mean genes and the biology of aggression: A critical review of recent animal and human research. *Journal of Neurogenetics, 11*, 1–43.

Barkataki, I., Kumari, V., Das, M., Hill, M., Morris, R., O'Connell, P., Taylor, P., et al. (2005). A neuropsychological investigation into violence and mental illness. *Schizophrenia Research, 74*, 1–13.

Barkataki, I., Kumari, V., Das, M., Taylor, P., & Sharma, T. (2006). Volumetric structural brain abnormalities in men with schizophrenia or antisocial personality disorder. *Behavioral Brain Research, 169*, 239–247.

Baron, R., & Richardson, D. (1994). *Human aggression* (2nd ed.). New York: Plenum Press.

Barratt, E. S., Stanford, M. S., Kent, T. A., & Felthous, A. (1997). Neuropsychological and cognitive psychophysiological substrates of impulsive aggression. *Biological Psychiatry, 41*, 1045–1061.

Barth, A. S. (2007). A double-edged sword: The role of neuroimaging in federal capital sentencing. *American Journal of Law & Medicine, 33*, 501–522.

Baskin, J. H., Edersheim, J. G., & Price, B. H. (2007). Is a picture worth a thousand words? Neuroimaging in the courtroom. *American Journal of Law & Medicine, 33*, 239–269.

Bassarath, L. (2001). Neuroimaging studies of antisocial behaviour. *Canadian Journal of Psychiatry, 46*, 728–732.

Bechara, A. (2004). The role of emotion in decision-making: Evidence from neurological patients with orbitofrontal damage. *Brain and Cognition, 55*, 30–40.

Bechara, A. (2005). Decision making, impulse control and loss of willpower to resist drugs: A neurocognitive perspective. *Nature Neuroscience, 8*, 1458–1463.

Bechara, A., & van der Linden, M. (2005). Decision-making and impulse control after frontal lobe injuries. *Current Opinons in Neurology, 18*, 734–739.

Bergvall, A. H., Wessely, H., Forsman, A., & Hansen, S. (2001). A deficit in attentional set-shifting of violent offenders. *Psychological Medicine, 31*, 1095–1105.

Berkowitz, L. (1993). *Aggression: Its causes, consequences, and control.* New York: McGraw-Hill.

Berntson, G. G., Bechara, A., Damasio, H., Tranel, D., & Cacioppo, J. T. (2007). Amygdala contribution to selective dimensions of emotion. *Social Cognitive and Affective Neuroscience, 2*, 123–129.

Bigler, E. D. (2003). Neuroimaging in forensic neuropsychology. In A. M. Horton & L. C. Hartlage (Eds.), *Handbook of forensic neuropsychology* (pp. 195–213). New York: Springer Publishing Company.

Bjorkly, S. (2006). Empirical evidence of a relationship between insight and risk of violence in the mentally ill—A review of the literature. *Aggression and Violent Behavior, 11*(4), 414–423.

Blair, R. J. (1995). A cognitive developmental approach to mortality: Investigating the psychopath. *Cognition, 57*, 1–29.

Blair, R. J. R. (2001). Neurocognitive models of aggression, the antisocial personality disorders, and psychopathy. *Journal of Neurology, Neurosurgery and Psychiatry, 71*, 727–731.

Blair, R. J. (2003). Neurobiological basis of psychopathy. *British Journal of Psychiatry, 182*, 5–7.

Blair, R. J. (2004). The roles of orbital frontal cortex in the modulation of antisocial behavior. *Brain and Cognition, 55*, 198–208.

Blair, R. J. R. (2006). Subcortical brain systems in psychopathy: The amygdala and associated structures. In C. J. Patrick (Ed.), *Handbook of psychopathy* (pp. 296–312). New York: Guilford Press.

Blake, P., & Grafman, J. (2004). The neurobiology of aggression. *Lancet, 364*, 12–13.

Brakel, S. J., Gonzalez, E. R., & Cavanaugh, J. L., Jr. (1996). Neuropsychiatry at the courtroom gates: Selective entry or anything goes? *Seminars in Clinical Neuropsychiatry, 1*, 215–221.

Broderick, D. F. (2005). Neuroimaging in neuropsychiatry. *Psychiatric Clinics of North America, 28*, 549–566.

Brodie, J. D. (1996). Imaging for the clinical psychiatrist: Facts, fantasies, and other musings. *American Journal of Psychiatry, 153*, 145–149.

Brower, M. C., & Price, B. H. (2001). Neuropsychiatry of frontal lobe dysfunction in violent and criminal behaviour: A critical review. *Journal of Neurology, Neurosurgery & Psychiatry, 71*, 720–726.

Burgess, J. W. (1992). Neurocognitive impairment in dramatic personalities: Histrionic, narcissistic, borderline, and antisocial disorders. *Psychiatry Research, 42*, 283–290.

Butter, C., Mishkin, M., & Mirsky, A. (1968). Emotional responses towards humans in monkeys with selective frontal lesions. *Physiology and Behavior, 3*, 213–215.

Butter, C., & Synder, D. (1971). Alterations in aversive and aggressive behaviors following orbital frontal lesions in rhesus monkeys. *Acta Neurobiologiae Experimentalis, 32*, 525–565.

Butter, C., Synder, D., & McDonald, J. (1970). Effects of orbital frontal lesions on aversive and aggressive behaviors in rhesus monkeys. *Journal of Comparative and Physiological Psychology, 72*, 132–144.

Buydens-Branchey, L., Branchey, M., Hudson, J., & Fergeson, P. (2000). Low HDL cholesterol, aggression and altered central serotonergic activity. *Psychiatry Research, 93*, 93–102.

Cabeza, R., & Kingstone, A. (2006). *Handbook of functional neuroimaging of cognition* (2nd ed.). Cambridge, MA: The MIT Press.

Cadoret, R. J., Leve, L. D., & Devor, E. (1997). Genetics of aggressive and violent behavior. *Psychiatric Clinics of North America, 20*, 301–322.

Cairns, R. B., & Stoff, D. M. (1996). Conclusion: A synthesis of studies on the biology of aggression and violence. In D. M. Stoff & R. B. Cairns (Eds.), *Aggression and violence: Genetic, neurobiological, and biosocial perspectives* (pp. 337–351). Mahwah, NJ: Lawrence Erlbaum.

Canli, T., Desmond, J. E., Zhao, Z., Glover, G., & Gabrieli, J. D. (1988). Hemispheric asymmetry for emotional stimuli detected with fMRI. *Neuroreport, 9*, 3233–3239.

Cato, M. A., Delis, D. C., Abildskov, T. J., & Bigler, E. D. (2004). Assessing the elusive cognitive deficits associated with ventromedial prefrontal damage: A case of a modern-day Phineas Gage. *Journal of the International Neuropsychological Society, 10*, 453–465.

Chesterman, L. P., Taylor, P. J., Cox, T., Hill, M., & Lumsden, J. (1994). Multiple measures of cerebral state in dangerous mentally disordered inpatients. *Criminal Behaviour and Mental Health, 4*, 228–239.

Chow, T. W., & Cummings, J. L. (1999). Frontal-subcortical circuits. In B. L. Miller & J. L. Cummings (Eds.), *The human frontal lobes: Functions and disorders* (pp. 3–26). New York: Guilford Press.

Cleckley, H. (1976). *The mask of sanity* (5th ed.). St. Louis, MO: Mosby.

Coccaro, E. F., McCloskey, M. S., Fitzgerald, D. A., & Phan, K. L. (2007). Amygdala and orbitofrontal reactivity to social threat in individuals with impulsive aggression. *Biological Psychiatry, 62*, 168–178.

Crowe, S. L., & Blair, R. J. (2008). The development of antisocial behavior: What can we learn from functional neuroimaging studies? *Development and Psychopathology, 20*, 1145–1159.

Damasio, A. R. (1994). *Descartes' error: Emotion, reason, and the human brain*. New York: Avon.

Damasio, H., Grabowski, T. J., Frank, R., Galaburda, A. M., & Damasio, A. R. (1994). The return of Phineas Gage: Clues about the brain from the skull of a famous patient. *Science, 264*, 1102–1105.

Das, M., Barkataki, I., Kumari, V., & Sharma, T. (2002). Neuroimaging violence in the mentally ill: What can it tell us? *Hospital Medicine, 63*, 604–609.

Davidson, L. L., & Heinrichs, R. W. (2003). Quantification of frontal and temporal lobe brain-imaging findings in schizophrenia: A meta-analysis. *Psychiatry Research: Neuroimaging, 122*, 69–87.

Davidson, R. J., Putnam, K. M., & Larson, C. L. (2000). Dysfunction in the neural circuitry of emotion regulation—A possible prelude to violence. *Science, 289*, 591–594.

de Almeida, R. M. M., Ferrari, P. F., Parmigiani, S., & Miczek, K. A. (2005). Escalated aggressive behavior: Dopamine, serotonin and GABA. *European Journal of Pharmacology, 526*, 51–64.

de Oliveira-Souza, R., Hare, R. D., Bramati, I. E., Garrido, G. J., Azevedo Ignácio, F., Tovar-Moll, F., & Moll, J. (2008). Psychopathy as a disorder of the moral brain: Fronto-temporo-limbic grey matter reductions demonstrated by voxel-based morphometry. *Neuroimage, 40*, 1202–1213.

Deckel, A., Hesselbrock, V., & Bauer, L. (1996). Antisocial personality disorder, childhood delinquency, and frontal brain functioning: EEG and neuropsychological findings. *Journal of Clinical Psychology, 52*, 639–650.

Dinn, W. M., & Harris, C. L. (2000). Neurocognitive function in antisocial personality disorder. *Psychiatry Research, 97*, 173–190.

Dolan, M., Deakin, W. J., Roberts, N., & Anderson, I. (2002a). Serotonergic and cognitive impairment in impulsive aggressive personality disordered offenders: Are there implications for treatment? *Psychological Medicine, 32*, 105–117.

Dolan, M., & Fullam, R. (2005). Memory for emotional events in violent offenders with antisocial personality disorder. *Personality and Individual Differences, 38,* 1657–1667.

Dolan, M., & Park, I. (2002). The neuropsychology of antisocial personality disorder. *Psychological Medicine, 32,* 417–427.

Dolan, M. C., Deakin, J. F. W., Roberts, N., & Anderson, I. M. (2002b). Quantitative frontal and temporal structural MRI studies in personality-disordered offenders and control subjects. *Psychiatry Research: Neuroimaging, 116,* 133–149.

Dougherty, D. D., Rauch, S. L., & Fischman, A. J. (2004). Positron emission tomography and single photon emission computed tomography. In D. D. Dougherty, S. L. Rauch & J. F. Rosenbaum (Eds.), *Essentials of neuroimaging for clinical practice.* Washington, DC: American Psychiatric Press.

Dougherty, D. D., Rauch, S. L., & Rosenbaum, J. F. (2004). *Essentials of neuroimaging for clinical practice.* Washington, DC: American Psychiatric Press.

Elliott, F. A. (1982). Neurological findings in adult minimal brain dysfunction and the dyscontrol syndrome. *Journal of Nervous and Mental Disease, 170,* 680–687.

Elliott, F. A. (1992). Violence. The neurologic contribution: An overview. *Archives of Neurology, 49*(6), 595–603.

Eriksson, T., & Lidberg, L. (1997). Increased plasma concentrations of the 5-HT precursor amino acid tryptophan and other large neutral amino acids in violent criminals. *Psychological Medicine, 27,* 477–481.

Eronen, M., Angermeyer, M. C., & Schulze, B. (1998). The psychiatric epidemiology of violent behaviour. *Social Psychiatry and Psychiatric Epidemiology, 33,* 13–23.

Ferris, C. F., Stolberg, T., Kulkarni, P., Murugavel, M., Blanchard, R., Blanchard, D. C., Febo, M., et al. (2008). Imaging the neural circuitry and chemical control of aggressive motivation. *BMC Neuroscience, 9,* 111.

Filley, C. M. (2008). Neuroanatomy for the neuropsychologist. In J. E. Morgan & J. H. Ricker (Eds.), *Textbook of clinical neuropsychology* (pp. 61–82). New York: Taylor & Francis.

Filley, C. M., Price, B. H., Nell, V., Antoinette, T., Morgan, A. S., Bresnahan, J. F., Pincus, J. H., et al. (2001). Toward an understanding of violence: Neurobehavioral aspects of unwarranted physical aggression: Aspen Neurobehavioral Conference consensus statement. *Neuropsychiatry, Neuropsychology, and Behavioral Neurology, 14,* 1–14.

Fishbein, D. H. (1992). The psychobiology of female aggression. *Criminal Justice and Behavior, 19*(2), 99–126.

Fishbein, D. H. (2000). Neuropsychological function, drug abuse, and violence: A conceptual framework. *Criminal Justice and Behavior, 27,* 139–159.

Flashman, L. A., McAllister, T. W., Johnson, S. C., Rick, J. H., Green, R. L., & Saykin, A. J. (2001). Specific frontal lobe subregions correlated with unawareness of illness in schizophrenia: A preliminary study. *Journal of Neuropsychiatry and Clinical Neuroscience, 13,* 255–257.

Fornito, A., Yücel, M., Dean, B., Wood, S. J., & Pantelis, C. (2008, April 23). Anatomical abnormalities of the anterior cingulate cortex in schizophrenia: Bridging the gap between neuroimaging and neuropathology. *Schizophrenia Bulletin,* 1–21.

Fossati, A., Barratt, E. S., Borroni, S., Villa, D., Grazioli, F., & Maffei, C. (2007). Impulsivity, aggressiveness, and DSM-IV personality disorders. *Psychiatry Research, 149,* 157–167.

Foster, H. G., Hillbrand, M., & Silverstein, M. (1993). Neuropsychological deficit and aggressive behavior: A prospective study. *Progress in Neuro-psychopharmacology & Biological Psychiatry, 17,* 939–946.

Fountoulakis, K. N., Leucht, S., & Kaprinis, G. S. (2008). Personality disorders and violence. *Current Opinion in Psychiatry, 21,* 84–92.

Fresan, A., Camarena, B., Apiquian, R., Aguilar, A., Urraca, N., & Nicolini, H. (2007). Association study of MAO-A and DRD4 genes in schizophrenic patients with aggressive behavior. *Neuropsychobiology, 55,* 171–175.

Frierson, R. L., & Finkenbine, R. D. (2004). Psychiatric and neurological characteristics of murder defendants referred for pretrial evaluation. *Journal of Forensic Science, 49,* 604–609.

Friston, K. J., Holmes, A. P., Worsley, K. J., Poline, J. P., Frith, C. D., & Frackowiak, R. S. J. (1995). Statistical parametric maps in functional imaging: A general linear approach. *Human Brain Mapping, 2,* 189–210.

Fullam, R., & Dolan, M. (2006). Emotional information processing in violent patients with schizophrenia: Association with psychopathy and symptomatology. *Psychiatry Research, 141,* 29–37.

Fullam, R., & Dolan, M. (2008). Executive function and in-patient violence in forensic patients with schizophrenia. *British Journal of Psychiatry, 193,* 247–253.

Geen, R. (2001). *Human aggression* (2nd ed.). Buckingham, UK: Open University Press.

Giancola, P. R. (1995). Evidence for dorsolateral and orbital prefrontal cortical involvement in the expression of aggressive behavior. *Aggressive Behavior, 21*, 431–450.

Giancola, P. R., Mezzich, A. C., & Tarter, R. E. (1998). Executive cognitive functioning, temperament, and antisocial behavior in conduct-disordered adolescent females. *Journal of Abnormal Psychology, 107*, 629–641.

Giancola, P. R., Roth, R. M., & Parrott, D. J. (2006). The mediating role of executive functioning in the relation between difficult temperament and physical aggression. *Journal of Psychopathology and Behavioral Assessment, 28*, 211–221.

Giancola, P. R., & Zeichner, A. (1994). Neuropsychological performance on tests of frontal-lobe functioning and aggressive behavior in men *Journal of Abnormal Psychology, 103*, 832–835.

Glicksohn, J. (2002). Criminality, personality, and cognitive neuroscience. In J. Glicksohn (Ed.), *The neurobiology of criminal behavior* (pp. 3-24). Boston: Kluwer.

Goethals, I., Audenaert, K., Jacobs, F., Van den Eynde, F., Bernagie, K., Kolindou, A., Vervaet, M., et al. (2005). Brain perfusion SPECT in impulsivity-related personality disorders. *Behavioural Brain Research, 157*, 187–192.

Goldstein, M. A., & Price, B. H. (2004). Magnetic resonance imaging. In D. D. Dougherty, S. L. Rauch, & J. F. Rosenbaum (Eds.), *Essentials of neuroimaging for clinical practice*. Washington, DC: American Psychiatric Press.

Goyer, P. F., Andreason, P. J., Semple, W. E., Clayton, A. H., King, A. C., Compton-Toth, B. A., et al. (1994). Positron-emission tomography and personality disorders. *Neuropsychopharmacology, 10*, 21–28.

Goyer, P. F., & Semple, W. E. (1996). PET studies of aggression in personality disorder and other nonpsychotic patients. In D. M. Stoff & R. B. Cairns (Eds.), *Aggression and violence: Genetic, neurobiological, and biosocial perspectives* (pp. 219–235). Mahwah, NJ: Lawrence Erlbaum.

Grafman, J., Schwab, K., Warden, D., Pridgen, A., Brown, H. R., & Salazar, A. M. (1996). Frontal lobe injuries, violence, and aggression: A report of the Vietnam Head Injury Study. *Neurology, 46*, 1231–1238.

Gregg, T. R. (2003). Cortical and limbic neural circuits mediating aggressive behavior. In M. P. Mattson (Ed.), *Neurobiology of aggression: Understanding and preventing violence* (pp. 1–20). Totowa, NJ: Humana Press.

Grossman, R. I., & Yousem, D. M. (2003). *Neuroradiology: The requisites* (2nd ed.). Philadelphia: Mosby.

Gur, R. C., & Gur, R. E. (1993). Neurobehavioral and neuroimaging data in the medical-legal context. In H. V. Hall & R. J. Sbordone (Eds.), *Disorders of executive functions: Civil and criminal law applications* (pp. 107–122). Winter Park, MD: PMD Publishers Group.

Hare, R. D. (1970). *Psychopathy: Theory and research*. New York: John Wiley.

Hare, R. D. (1991/2003). *The Hare Psychopathy Checklist-Revised* (2nd ed.). Toronto: Multi-Health Systems.

Hare, R. D. (1998). Psychopaths and their nature: Implications for the mental health and criminal justice system. In T. Millon, E. Simonsen, M. Birket-Smith, & R. D. Davis (Eds.), *Psychopathy: Antisocial, criminal, and violent behavior* (pp. 188–212). New York: Guilford Press.

Hare, R. D., & Jutai, J. W. (1988). Psychopathy and cerebral asymmetry in semantic processing. *Personality and Individual Differences, 9*, 329–337.

Hare, R. D., & McPherson, L. M. (1984). Psychopathy and perceptual asymmetry during verbal dichotic listening. *Journal of Abnormal Psychology, 93*, 141–149.

Hare, R. D., & Neumann, C. S. (2008). Psychopathy as a clinical and empirical construct. *Annual Review of Clinical Psychology, 4*, 217–246.

Hawkins, K. A., & Trobst, K. K. (2000). Frontal lobe dysfunction and aggression: Conceptual issues and research findings. *Aggression and Violent Behavior, 5*, 147–157.

Heaton, R. K., Chelune, G. J., Talley, J. L., Kay, G. G., & Curtis, G. (1993). *Wisconsin Card Sorting Test (WCST) manual, revised and expanded*. Odessa, FL: Psychological Assessment Resources.

Heinrichs, R. W., & Zakzanis, K. K. (1998). Neurocognitive deficit in schizophrenia: A quantitative review of the evidence. *Neuropsychology, 12*, 426–445.

Herba, C. M., Hodgins, S., Blackwood, N., Kumari, V., Naudts, K. H., Phillips, M., Hervé, H., et al. (2007). The neurobiology of psychopathy: A focus on emotion processing. In *The psychopath: Theory, research, and practice* (pp. 253–283). Mahwah: Lawrence Erlbaum.

Herzberg, J. L., & Fenwick, P. B. (1988). The aetiology of aggression in temporal-lobe epilepsy. *British Journal of Psychiatry, 153*, 50–55.

Hess, W. R., & Akert, K. (1955). Experimental data on role of hypothalamus in mechanism of emotional behavior. *Archives of Neurology and Psychiatry, 73*, 127–129.

Hoptman, M. J., Volavka, J., Czobor, P., Gerig, G., Chakos, M., Blocher, J., Citrome, L. L., et al. (2006). Aggression and quantitative MRI measures of caudate in patients with chronic schizophrenia or schizoaffective disorder. *Journal of Neuropsychiatry and Clinical Neurosciences, 18*, 509–515.

Hoptman, M. J., Volavka, J., Weiss, E. M., Czobor, P., Szeszko, P. R., Gerig, G., Chakos, M., et al. (2005). Quantitative MRI measures of orbitofrontal cortex in patients with chronic schizophrenia or schizoaffective disorder. *Psychiatry Research: Neuroimaging, 140*, 133–145.

Hose v. Chicago Northwestern Transp. Co, 70 F.3d 968 (8th Cir. 1995).

Husted, D. S., Myers, W. C., & Lui, Y. (2008). The limited role of neuroimaging in determining criminal liability: An overview and case report. *Forensic Science International, 179*, 9–15.

Jaqust, W. (1999). Neuroimaging and the frontal lobes: Insights from the study of neurodegenerative disorders. In B. L. Miller & J. L. Cummings (Eds.), *The human frontal lobes: Functions and disorders* (pp. 107–122). New York: Guilford Press.

Jezzard, P., Matthews, P. M., & Smith, S. M. (2001). *Functional MRI: An introduction to methods.* New York: Oxford University Press.

Johnson, P. A., Hurley, R. A., Benkelfat, C., Herpertz, S. C., & Taber, K. H. (2003). Understanding emotion regulation in borderline personality disorder: Contributions of neuroimaging. *Journal of Neuropsychiatry and Clinical Neurosciences, 15*, 397–402.

Joyal, C. C., Putkonen, A., Mancini-Marïe, A., Hodgins, S., Kononen, M., Boulay, L., Pihlajamaki, M., et al. (2007). Violent persons with schizophrenia and comorbid disorders: A functional magnetic resonance imaging study. *Schizophrenia Research, 91*, 97–102.

Junginger, J., & McGuire, L. (2004). Psychotic motivation and the paradox of current research on serious mental illness and rates of violence. *Schizophrenia Bulletin, 30*, 21–30.

Kamback, M. (1973). The effects of orbital and dorsolateral frontal cortical ablations on ethanol self-selection and emotional behaviors in monkeys *(Macaca nemestrina). Neuropsychologia, 11*, 331–335.

Kamback, M., & Rogal, R. (1973). The effects of frontal cortical ablations on alcohol selection and emotionality in pigtail monkeys *(Macaca nemistrina). Biological Psychiatry, 7*, 173–177.

Karli, P. (2006). The neurobiology of aggressive behaviour. *Neurosciences, 329*, 460–464.

Kavoussi, R., Armstead, P., & Coccaro, E. (1997). The neurobiology of impulsive aggression. *Psychiatry Clinics of North America, 20*, 395–403.

Khoshbin, L. S., & Khoshbin, S. (2007). Imaging the mind, minding the image: An historical introduction to brain imaging and the law. *American Journal of Law & Medicine, 33*, 171–192.

Kiehl, K. A., Hare, R. D., McDonald, J. J., & Brink, J. (1999). Semantic and affective processing in psychopaths: An event-related potential (ERP) study. *Psychophysiology, 36*, 765–774.

Kiehl, K. A., Smith, A. M., Hare, R. D., Mendrek, A., Forster, B. B., Brink, J., & Liddle, P. F. (2001). Limbic abnormalities in affective processing by criminal psychopaths as revealed by functional magnetic resonance imaging. *Biological Psychiatry, 50*, 677–684.

Kiehl, K. A., Smith, A. M., Mendrek, A., Forster, B. B., Hare, R. D., & Liddle, P. F. (2004). Temporal lobe abnormalities in semantic processing by criminal psychopaths as revealed by functional magnetic resonance imaging. *Psychiatry Research, 130*, 297–312.

Kim, S. H., Manes, F., Kosier, T., Baruah, S., & Robinson, R. G. (1999). Irritability following traumatic brain injury. *Journal of Nervous & Mental Disease, 187*, 327–335.

King, J. A., Blair, R. J. R., Mitchell, D. G. V., Dolan, R. J., & Burgess, N. (2006). Doing the right thing: A common neural circuit for appropriate violent or compassionate behavior. *Neuroimage, 30*, 1069–1076.

Klee, C. H., & Friedman, H. J. (2001). Neurolitigation: A perspective on the elements of expert testimony for extending the Daubert challenge. *NeuroRehabilitation, 16*, 79–85.

Kumari, V., Aasen, I., Taylor, P., ffytche, D. H., Das, M., Barkataki, I., Goswami, S., et al. (2006). Neural dysfunction and violence in schizophrenia: An fMRI investigation. *Schizophrenia Research, 84*, 144–164.

Kwong, K. K., Belliveau, J. W., Chesler, D. A., Goldberg, I. E., Weisskoff, R. M., Poncelet, B. P., et al. (1992). Dynamic magnetic resonance imaging of human brain activity during primary sensory stimulation. *Proceedings of the National Academy of Sciences of the United States of America, 89*, 5675–5679.

Lapierre, D., Braun, C. M. J., Hodgins, S., Toupin, J., Lééveilléé, S., & Constantineau, C. (1995). Neuropsychological correlates of violence in schizophrenia. *Schizophrenia Bulletin, 21*, 253–262.

LeDoux, J. E. (2000). Emotion circuits in the brain. *Annual Review of Neuroscience, 23*, 155–184.

Lee, R., & Coccarro, E. (2001). The neuropsychopharmacology of criminality and aggression. *Canadian Journal of Psychiatry / La Revue canadienne de psychiatrie, 46*, 35–44.

Lezak, M. D., Howieson, D. B., & Loring, D. W. (2004). *Neuropsychological assessment* (4th ed.). New York: Oxford University Press.

Link, B. G., Stueve, A., & Phelan, J. (1998). Psychotic symptoms and violent behaviors: Probing the components of "threat/control-override" symptoms. *Social Psychiatry and Psychiatric Epidemiology, 33*, 55–60.

Lockett v. Anderson, 230 F.3d 695 (5th Cir. 2000).

Logothetis, N. K. (2002). The neural basis of the blood-oxygen-level-dependent functional magnetic resonance imaging signal. *Philosophical Transactions of the Royal Society of London-Series B: Biological Sciences, 357*(1424), 1003–1037.

Martens, W. H. J. (2000). Antisocial and psychopathic personality disorders: Causes, course, and remission—a review article. *International Journal of Offender Therapy and Comparative Criminology, 44*, 406–430.

Mass, R., & Kling, A. (1975). Social behavior in stump-tailed macaques *(Macaca speciosa)* after lesions of the dorsolateral frontal cortex. *Primates, 16*, 239–252.

Mattson, M. P. (2003). Aggression in brain injury, aging, and neurodegenerative disorders. In M. P. Mattson (Ed.), *Neurobiology of aggression: Understanding and preventing violence* (pp. 151–166). Totowa, NJ: Humana Press.

McAllister, T. W., Sparling, M. B., Flashman, L. A., & Saykin, A. J. (2001). Neuroimaging findings in mild traumatic brain injury. *Journal of Clinical and Experimental Neuropsychology, 23*, 775–791.

McCloskey, M. S., Phan, K. L., & Coccaro, E. F. (2005). Neuroimaging and personality disorders. *Current Psychiatry Reports, 7*(1), 65–72.

McKinlay, W. W., Brooks, D. N., Bond, M. R., Martinage, D. P., & Marshall, M. M. (1981). The short-term outcome of severe blunt head injury as reported by relatives of the injured persons. *Journal of Neurology, Neurosurgery and Psychiatry, 44*, 527–533.

Mehr, S. H., & Gerdes, S. L. (2001). Medicolegal applications of PET scans. *NeuroRehabilitation, 16*, 87–92.

Metting, Z., Rodiger, L. A., De Keyser, J., & van der Naalt, J. (2007). Structural and functional neuroimaging in mild-to-moderate head injury. *Lancet Neurology, 6*, 699–710.

Miczek, K. A., de Almeida, R. M. M., Kravitz, E. A., Rissman, E. F., de Boer, S. F., & Raine, A. (2007). Neurobiology of escalated aggression and violence. *Journal of Neuroscience, 27*, 11803–11806.

Miller, M. (1976). Dorsolateral frontal lobe lesions and behavior in the macaque: Dissociation of threat and aggression. *Physiology and Behavior, 17*, 209–213.

Miller, M., & Levine, E. (1977). Effects of orbitofrontal lesions on social behavior in a confined group of stump-tail macaques *(Macaca speciosa)*. *Primates, 18*, 903–912.

Mills, S., & Raine, A. (1994). Neuroimaging and aggression. In M. Hillbrand & N. J. Pallone (Eds.), *The psychobiology of aggression* (pp. 145-158). Binghamton, NY: Haworth Press.

Mobbs, D., Lau, H. C., Jones, O. D., & Frith, C. D. (2007). Law, responsibility, and the brain. *Plos Biology, 5*, 693–700.

Moriarty, J. C. (2008). Flickering admissibility: Neuroimaging evidence in the U.S. Courts. *Behavioral Sciences and the Law, 26*, 29–49.

Müller, J. L., Gänbauer, S., Sommer, M., Döhnel, K., Weber, T., Schmidt-Wilcke, T., & Hajak, G. (2008). Gray matter changes in right superior temporal gyrus in criminal psychopaths. Evidence from voxel-based morphometry. *Psychiatry Research: Neuroimaging, 163*, 213–222.

Müller, J. L., Sommer, M., Wagner, V., Lange, K., Taschler, H., Röder, C. H., Schuierer, G., et al. (2003). Abnormalities in emotion processing within cortical and subcortical regions in criminal psychopaths: Evidence from a functional magnetic resonance imaging study using pictures with emotional content. *Biological Psychiatry, 54*, 152–162.

Narayan, V. M., Narr, K. L., Kumari, V., Woods, R. P., Thompson, P. M., Toga, A. W., & Sharma, T. (2007). Regional cortical thinning in subjects with violent antisocial personality disorder or schizophrenia. *American Journal of Psychiatry, 164*, 1418–1427.

Naudts, K., & Hodgins, S. (2006). Neurobiological correlates of violent behavior among persons with schizophrenia. *Schizophrenia Bulletin, 32*, 562–572.

Nelson, M. D., Saykin, A. J., Flashman, L. A., & Riordan, H. J. (1998). Hippocampal volume reduction in schizophrenia as assessed by magnetic resonance imaging: A meta-analytic study. *Archives of General Psychiatry, 55*, 433–440.

Nelson, R. J., & Trainor, B. C. (2007). Neural mechanisms of aggression. *Nature, 8*, 536–546.

Nigg, J. T., & Huang-Pollock, C. L. (2003). An early-onset model of the role of executive functions and intelligence in conduct disorder/delinquency. In B. B. Lahey, T. E. Moffit, & A. Caspi (Eds.), *Causes of conduct disorder and juvenile delinquency* (pp. 227–253). New York: Guilford Press.

Ogawa, S., Menon, R. S., Kim, S. G., & Ugurbil, K. (1998). On the characteristics of functional magnetic resonance imaging of the brain. *Annual Review of Biophysics & Biomolecular Structure, 27*, 447–474.

Pantelis, C., Barnes, T. R., Nelson, H. E., Tanner, S., Weatherley, L., Owen, A. M., & Robbins, T. W. (1997). Frontal-striatal cognitive deficits in patients with chronic schizophrenia. *Brain, 120*, 1823–1843.

Pantelis, C., Yucel, M., Wood, S. J., Velakoulis, D., Sun, D., Berger, G., Stuart, G. W., et al. (2005). Structural brain imaging evidence for multiple pathological processes at different stages of brain development in schizophrenia. *Schizophrenia Bulletin, 31*, 672–696.

Park, L. T., & Gonzalez, R. G. (2004). Computed tomography. In D. D. Dougherty, S. L. Rauch & J. F. Rosenbaum (Eds.), *Essentials of neuroimaging for clinical practice*. Washington, DC: American Psychiatric Press.

Patel, P., Meltzer, C. C., Mayberg, H. S., & Levine, K. (2007). The role of imaging in United States courtrooms. *Neuroimaging Clinics of North America, 17*, 557–567.

Patrick, C. J. (1994). Emotion and psychopathy: Startling new insights. *Psychophysiology, 31*, 319–330.

People of New York v. Weinstein, 156 Misc152d 134, 591 NYS152d 715 (Sup. Ct. 1992).

Pettit, M., Jr. (2007). FMRI and BF meet FRE: Brain imaging and the federal rules of evidence. *American Journal of Law & Medicine, 33*, 319–340.

Pietrini, P., Guazzelli, M., Basso, G., Jaffe, K., & Grafman, J. (2000). Neural correlates of imaginal aggressive behavior assessed by positron emission tomography in healthy subjects. *American Journal of Psychiatry, 157*, 1772–1781.

Poythress, N. G., & Skeem, J. L. (2006). Disaggregating psychopathy: Where and how to look for subtypes. In C. J. Patrick (Ed.), *Handbook of psychopathy* (pp. 172–192). New York: Guilford Press.

Price, C. J., & Friston, K. J. (2002). Functional imaging studies of neuropsychological patients: Applications and limitations. *Neurocase, 8*, 345–354.

Raine, A., Buchsbaum, M., & LaCasse, L. (1997). Brain abnormalities in murderers indicated by positron emission tomography. *Biological Psychiatry, 42*, 495–508.

Raine, A., & Buchsbaum, M. S. (1996). Violence, brain imaging, and neuropsychology. In D. M. Stoff & R. B. Cairns (Eds.), *Aggression and violence: Genetic, neurobiological, and biosocial perspectives* (pp. 195–217). Mahwah, NJ: Lawrence Erlbaum.

Raine, A., Buchsbaum, M. S., Stanley, J., Lottenberg, S., Abel, L., & Stoddard, J. (1994). Selective reductions in prefrontal glucose metabolism in murderers. *Biological Psychiatry, 36*, 365–373.

Raine, A., Ishikawa, S. S., Arce, E., Lencz, T., Knuth, K. H., Bihrle, S., LaCasse, L., et al. (2004). Hippocampal structural asymmetry in unsuccessful psychopaths. *Biological Psychiatry, 55*, 185-191.

Raine, A., Lencz, T., Bihrle, S., LaCasse, L., & Colletti, P. (2000). Reduced prefrontal gray matter volume and reduced autonomic activity in antisocial personality disorder. *Archives of General Psychiatry, 57*, 119–127.

Raine, A., Lencz, T., Yaralian, P., Bihrle, S., LaCasse, L., Ventura, J., & Colletti, P. (2002). Prefrontal structural and functional deficits in schizotypal personality disorder. *Schizophrenia Bulletin, 28*, 501–513.

Raine, A., Meloy, J. R., Bihrle, S., Stoddard, J., LaCasse, L., & Buchsbaum, M. S. (1998). Reduced prefrontal and increased subcortical brain functioning assessed using positron emission tomography in predatory and affective murderers. *Behavioral Sciences & the Law, 16*, 319–332.

Raine, A., Stoddard, J., Bihrle, S., & Buchsbaum, M. (1998). Prefrontal glucose deficits in murderers lacking psychosocial deprivation. *Neuropsychiatry, Neuropsychology, and Behavioral Neurology, 11*, 1–7.

Raine, A., & Yang, Y. (2006). The neuroanatomical bases of psychopathy: A review of brain imaging findings. In C. J. Patrick (Ed.), *Handbook of psychopathy* (pp. 278–295). New York: Guilford Press.

Rand, M., & Catalano, S. M. (2007). *Criminal victimization, 2006*. Retrieved November 25, 2008, from http://www.ojp.usdoj.gov/bjs/pub/pdf/cv06.pdf

Rasmussen, K., Levander, S., & Sletvold, H. (1995). Aggressive and non-aggressive schizophrenics: Symptom profile and neuropsychological differences. *Psychology, Crime, & Law, 2*, 119–129.

Ricker, J. H. (2005). Functional neuroimaging in forensic neuropsychology. In G. J. Larabee (Ed.), *Forensic neuropsychology: A scientific approach* (pp. 159–181). New York: Oxford University Press.

Rose, S. E., Chalk, J. B., Janke, A. L., Strudwick, M. W., Windus, L. C., Hannah, D. E., McGrath, J. J., et al. (2006). Evidence of altered prefrontal-thalamic circuitry in schizophrenia: An optimized diffusion MRI study. *Neuroimage, 32*, 16–22.

Rosenbaum, A., Hoge, S. K., Adelman, S. A., Warnken, W. J., Fletcher, K. E., & Kane, R. L. (1994). Head injury in partner-abusive men. *Journal of Consulting and Clinical Psychology, 62*, 1187–1193.

Roth, R. M., Flashman, L. A., Saykin, A. J., McAllister, T. W., & Vidaver, R. (2004). Apathy in schizophrenia: Reduced frontal lobe volume and neuropsychological deficits. *American Journal of Psychiatry, 161*, 157–159.

Roth, R. M., Randolph, J. J., Koven, N. S., & Isquith, P. I. (2006). Neural substrates of executive functioning: Insights from functional neuroimaging. In J. R. Dupri (Ed.), *Focus on neuropsychology research* (pp. 1–36). New York: Nova Science Publishers.

Rucco, A. C., & Platek, S. M. (2006). Executive function and language deficits associated wtih aggressive-sadistic personality. *Behavioral and Brain Sciences, 29*, 239–240.

Rusch, N., Weber, M., Il'yasov, K. A., Lieb, K., Ebert, D., Hennig, J., & van Elst, L. T. (2007). Inferior frontal white matter microstructure and patterns of psychopathology in women with borderline personality disorder and comorbid attention-deficit hyperactivity disorder. *Neuroimage, 35*(2), 738–747.

Salekin, R. T., Leistico, A. R., Trobst, K. K., Schrum, C. L., & Lochman, J. E. (2005). Adolescent psychopathy and personality theory—The interpersonal circumplex: Expanding of a nomological net. *Journal of Abnormal Child Psychology, 22*, 445–460.

Saver, J. L. (2002). Aggression. In V. S. Ramachandran (Ed.), *Encyclopedia of the human brain* (pp. 21–42). New York: Academic Press.

Sbordone, R. J. (1993). Epileptic-related executive dysfunction and violent crime. In H. V. Hall & R. J. Sbordone (Eds.), *Disorders of executive functions: Civil and criminal law applications* (pp. 123–133). Winter Park, MD: PMD Publishers.

Scarpa, A., & Raine, A. (2007). Biosocial bases of violence. In D. J. Flannery, A. T. Vazsonyi, & I. D. Waldman (Eds.), *The Cambridge handbook of violent behavior and aggression* (pp. 151–169). New York: Cambridge University Press.

Schneider, F., Grodd, W., Weiss, U., Klose, U., Mayer, K. R., Nägele, T., & Gur, R. C. (1997). Functional MRI reveals left amygdala activation during emotion. *Psychiatry Research: Neuroimaging, 76*, 75–82.

Seguin, J. R., & Zelazo, P. D. (2005). Executive function in early physical aggression. In R. E. Tremblay, W. W. Hartup, & J. Archer (Eds.), *Developmental origins of aggression* (pp. 307–329). New York: Guilford Press.

Seidenwurm, D., Pounds, T. R., Globus, A., & Valk, P. E. (1997). Abnormal temporal lobe metabolism in violent subjects: Correlation of imaging and neuropsychiatric findings. *American Journal of Neuroradiology, 18*, 625–631.

Seidman, L. J., Pantelis, C., Keshavan, M. S., Faraone, S. V., Goldstein, J. M., Horton, N. J., Makris, N., et al. (2003). A review and new report of medial temporal lobe dysfunction as a vulnerability indicator for schizophrenia: A magnetic resonance imaging morphometric family study of the parahippocampal gyrus. *Schizophrenia Bulletin, 29*, 803–830.

Serper, M., Beech, D. R., Harvey, P. D., & Dill, C. (2008). Neuropsychological and symptom predictors of aggression on the psychiatric inpatient service. *Journal of Clinical and Experimental Neuropsychology, 30*, 700–709.

Sestir, M. A., & Bartholow, B. D. (2007). Theoretical explanations of aggression and violence. In T. A. Gannon, T. Ward, & A. R. Beech (Eds.), *Aggressive offenders' cognition: Theory, research, and practice* (pp. 157–178). Hoboken: John Wiley.

Siegel, A., Edinger, H., & Dotto, M. (1975). Effects of electrical stimulation of the lateral aspects of the pre-frontal cortex upon attack behaviors in cats. *Brain Research, 93*, 473–484.

Siegel, A., Edinger, H., & Koo, A. (1977). Suppression of attack behavior in the cat by the prefrontal cortex: Role of the mediodorsal thalamic nucleus. *Brain Research, 127*, 185–190.

Siever, L. J. (2008). Neurobiology of aggression and violence. *American Journal of Psychiatry, 165*, 429–442.

Silver, J. M., Anderson, K. A., & Yudofsky, S. C. (2003). Violence and the brain. In T. E. Feinberg & M. J. Farah (Eds.), *Behavioral neurology and neuropsychology* (2nd ed., pp. 755–762). New York: McGraw-Hill.

Silver, J. M., Yudofsky, S. C., & Anderson, K. E. (2005). Aggressive disorders. In J. M. Silver, T. W. McAllister, & S. C. Yudofsky (Eds.), *Textbook of traumatic brain injury* (pp. 259–277). Washington, DC: American Psychiatric Press.

Skeem, J. L., Edens, J. F., Camp, J., & Colwell, L. H. (2004). Are there ethnic differences in levels of psychopathy? A meta-analysis. *Law and Human Behavior, 28*, 505–527.

Snead, O. C. (2007). Neuroimaging and the "complexity" of capital punishment. *New York University Law Review, 82*, 1265–1339.

Soloff, P. H., Meltzer, C. C., Becker, C., Greer, P. J., Kelly, T. M., & Constantine, D. (2003). Impulsivity and prefrontal hypometabolism in borderline personality disorder. *Psychiatry Research, 123*, 153–163.

Soloff, P. H., Meltzer, C. C., Greer, P. J., Constantine, D., & Kelly, T. M. (2000). A fenfluramine-activated FDG-PET study of borderline personality disorder. *Biological Psychiatry, 47*, 540–547.

Spalletta, G., Troisi, A., Alimenti, S., di Michele, F., Pau, F., Pasini, A., & Caltagirone, C. (2001). Reduced prefrontal cognitive activation associated with aggression in schizophrenia. *Schizophrenia Research, 50*, 135–136.

Stein, D. J., Hollander, E., Cohen, L., Frenkel, M., Saoud, J. B., DeCaria, C., Aronowitz, B., et al. (1993). Neuropsychiatric impairment in impulsive personality disorders. *Psychiatry Research, 48,* 257–266.

Stern, B. H. (2001). Admissibility of PET scan results under Daubert and Kumho Tire. *Trial Lawyer, 24,* 24.

Stuss, D. T., & Alexander, M. P. (2000). Executive functions and the frontal lobes: A conceptual view. *Psychological Research-Psychologische Forschung, 63,* 289–298.

Stuss, D. T., Gow, C. A., & Hetherington, C. R. (1992). No longer Gage: Frontal-lobe dysfunction and emotional changes *Journal of Consulting and Clinical Psychology, 60,* 349–359.

Stuss, D. T., & Levine, B. (2002). Adult clinical neuropsychology: Lessons from studies of the frontal lobes. [Review]. *Annual Review of Psychology, 53,* 401-433.

Swanson, J. W., Holzer, C. E., III, Ganju, V. K., & Jono, R. T. (1990). Violence and psychiatric disorder in the community: Evidence from the Epidemiologic Catchment Area Surveys. *Hospital and Community Psychiatry, 41,* 761–770.

Tancredi, L. R., & Brodie, J. D. (2007). The brain and behavior: Limitations in the legal use of functional magnetic resonance imaging. *American Journal of Law & Medicine, 33,* 271–294.

Tardiff, K. (1998). Unusual diagnoses among violent patients. *Psychiatry Clinics of North America, 21,* 567–576.

Tateno, A., Jorge, R. E., & Robinson, R. G. (2003). Clinical correlates of aggressive behavior after traumatic brain injury. *Journal of Neuropsychiatry and Clinical Neurosciences, 15,* 155–160.

Tehrani, J. A., Brennan, P. A., Hodgins, S., & Mednick, S. A. (1998). Mental illness and criminal violence. *Social Psychiatry and Psychiatric Epidemiology, 33,* 81–85.

Tiihonen, J., Hodgins, S., Vaurio, O., Laakso, M., Repo, E., Soininen, H., Aronen, H. J., et al. (2000, April). *Amygdaloid volumes loss in psychopathy.* Paper presented at the Society for Neuroscience 2000 Annual Meeting, Washington, DC.

Tiihonen, J., Rossi, R., Laakso, M. P., Hodgins, S., Testa, C., Perez, J., Repo-Tiihonen, E., et al. (2008). Brain anatomy of persistent violent offenders: More rather than less. *Psychiatry Research, 163,* 201–212.

Tonkonogy, J. M. (1991). Violence and temporal lobe lesion: Head CT and MRI data. *The Journal of Neuropsychiatry and Clinical Neurosciences, 3,* 189–196.

Tonkonogy, J. M., & Geller, J. L. (1992). Hypothalamic lesions and intermittent explosive disorder. *Journal of Neuropsychiatry and Clinical Neurosciences, 4,* 45–50.

Trimble, M. R., & van Elst, L. T. (1999). On some clinical implications of the ventral striatum and the extended amygdala. Investigations of aggression. *Annals of the New York Academy of Sciences, 877,* 638–644.

United States v. Gigante 989, F. Supp 436, 438 (E.D.N.Y. 1997).

van Elst, L. T., Woermann, F., Lemieux, L., & Trimble, M. R. (2000). Increased amygdala volumes in female and depressed humans. A quantitative magnetic resonance imaging study. *Neuroscience Letters, 281,* 103–106.

van Elst, L. T., Woermann, F. G., Lemieux, L., Thompson, P. J., & Trimble, M. R. (2000). Affective aggression in patients with temporal lobe epilepsy: A quantitative MRI study of the amygdala. *Brain, 123,* 234–243.

van Elst, L. T., Woermann, F. G., Lemieux, L., & Trimble, M. R. (1999). Amygdala enlargement in dysthymia—A volumetric study of patients with temporal lobe epilepsy. *Biological Psychiatry, 46,* 1614–1623.

Volavka, J. (1999). The neurobiology of violence: An update. *Journal of Neuropsychiatry and Clinical Neurosciences, 11,* 307–314.

Volkow, N. D., & Tancredi, L. (1987). Neural substrates of violent behaviour: A preliminary study with positron emission tomography. *British Journal of Psychiatry, 151,* 668–673.

Volkow, N. D., Tancredi, L. R., Grant, C., Gillespie, H., Valentine, A., Mullani, N., Wang, G. J., et al. (1995). Brain glucose metabolism in violent psychiatric patients: A preliminary study. *Psychiatry Research, 61,* 243–253.

Völlm, B., Richardson, P., McKie, S., Elliott, R., Dolan, M., & Deakin, B. (2007). Neuronal correlates of reward and loss in Cluster B personality disorders: A functional magnetic resonance imaging study. *Psychiatry Research, 156,* 151–167.

Völlm, B., Richardson, P., Stirling, J., Elliott, R., Dolan, M., Chaudhry, I., Del Ben, C., et al. (2004). Neurobiological substrates of antisocial and borderline personality disorder: Preliminary results of a functional fMRI study. *Criminal Behaviour and Mental Health, 14,* 39–54.

Völlm, B. A., Dolan, M., Richardson, P., McKie, S., Elliott, R., Williams, S., Anderson, I., et al. (2007). Neurobiological correlates of antisocial personality traits—Research findings and treatment implications. *European Psychiatry, 22,* 14–15.

Wasman, M., & Flynn, J. P. (1962). Directed attack elicited from hypothalamus. *Archives of Neurology,* *6,* 220–227.

Weber, S., Habel, U., Amunts, K., & Schneider, F. (2008). Structural brain abnormalities in psychopaths—A review. *Behavioral Sciences and the Law, 26,* 7–28.

Williamson, S., Hare, R. D., & Wong, S. (1987). Violence—Criminal psychopaths and their victims. *Canadian Journal of Behavioural Science-Revue Canadienne Des Sciences Du Comportement, 19,* 454–462.

Wishart, H. A., Saykin, A. J., & McAllister, T. W. (2002). Functional magnetic resonance imaging: Emerging clinical applications. *Current Psychiatry Reports, 4,* 338–345.

Witzel, J., Walter, M., Bogerts, B., & Northoff, G. (2008). Neurophilosophical perspectives of neuroimaging in forensic psychiatry—Giving way to a paradigm shift? *Behavioral Sciences and the Law,* *26,* 113–130.

Woermann, F. G., van Elst, L. T., Koepp, M. J., Free, S. L., Thompson, P. J., Trimble, M. R., & Duncan, J. S. (2000). Reduction of frontal neocortical grey matter associated with affective aggression in patients with temporal lobe epilepsy: An objective voxel by voxel analysis of automatically segmented MRI. *Journal of Neurology, Neurosurgery & Psychiatry, 68,* 162–169.

Wong, M., Fenwick, P., Fenton, G., Lumsden, J., Maisey, M., & Stevens, J. (1997). Repetitive and non-repetitive violent offending behaviour in male patients in a maximum security mental hospital—Clinical and neuroimaging findings. *Medicine, Science, and The Law, 37,* 150–160.

Wong, M. T. H., Fenwick, P. B. C., Lumsden, J., Fenton, G. W., Maisey, M. N., Lewis, P., & Badawi, R. (1997). Positron emission tomography in male violent offenders with schizophrenia. *Psychiatry Research: Neuroimaging, 68,* 111–123.

Wortzel, H. S., Filley, C. M., Anderson, C. A., Oster, T., & Arciniegas, D. B. (2008). Forensic applications of cerebral single photon emission computed tomography in mild traumatic brain injury. *Journal of the American Academy of Psychiatry and the Law, 36,* 310–322.

Yang, Y., Glenn, A. L., & Raine, A. (2008). Brain abnormalities in antisocial individuals: Implications for the law. *Behavioral Sciences and the Law, 26,* 65–83.

Young, R. M., & Balaban, E. (2003). Aggression, biology, and context: Deja-vu all over again? In M. P. Mattson (Ed.), *Neurobiology of aggression: Understanding and preventing violence* (pp. 191–212). Totowa, NJ: Humana Press.

Zalsman, G., & Apter, A. (2002). Serotonergic metabolism and violence/aggression. In J. Glicksohn (Ed.), *The neurobiology of criminal behavior* (pp. 231–250). Boston: Kluwer.

Zetzsche, T., Preuss, U. W., Frodl, T., Schmitt, G., Seifert, D., Munchhausen, E., Tabrizi, S., et al. (2007). Hippocampal volume reduction and history of aggressive behaviour in patients with borderline personality disorder. *Psychiatry Research: Neuroimaging, 154,* 157–170.

Part II

Ethical/Legal Issues in Neuropsychology

Maximizing Test Security in Forensic Neuropsychology

8

Shane S. Bush
Dorrie L. Rapp
Paul S. Ferber

The legal system requires expert witnesses to disclose the information and materials upon which their opinions are based. This discovery requirement facilitates review by opposing counsel and their experts, and is designed to promote fairness in the legal process and, ultimately, justice in legal decisions. Neuropsychologists who routinely provide services in forensic contexts understand their ethical and legal responsibility to provide copies of their records, when in receipt of proper authorization, to comply with discovery requirements. However, neuropsychologists also understand that there are ethical and legal requirements that restrict their release of certain records, such as test materials and raw test data. These competing ethical and legal requirements pose significant problems for neuropsychologists who want nothing more than to meet all of their ethical and legal responsibilities. The purposes of the present chapter are to (a) present the ethical, legal, and professional requirements and considerations that are involved when neuropsychologists receive requests, subpoenas, or court orders to release test materials and raw data; and (b) provide solutions for neuropsychologists, attorneys, and the courts that both satisfy discovery requirements and promote test security.

Case Example: Notice for Discovery and Inspection

PLEASE TAKE NOTICE that defendants herein, pursuant to Section 3101 et seq. and Rule 3120 of the CPLR, are required to produce and permit discovery, inspection, and copying to be made by plaintiff's physician of the following items, writings, and objects maintained, controlled, and/or supervised by the defendant(s) and/or defendant's agents, servants, and/or employees. In lieu of strict compliance with the terms and conditions of this Notice, the undersigned will accept clearly legible photocopies of said items if received by the undersigned at least five (5) days prior to the return date hereof, together with a letter from defendant's attorney advising as to the completeness of the items provided.

Place of Discovery: [treating neuropsychologist's office]

AND

[plaintiff's attorney's office]

Date of Discovery: [Month XX, XXXX]

Items to be produced relating to the incident that occurred on [date of accident]:

1. Complete copies of all raw and standardized scores, responses to test questions or stimuli, notes concerning statements made by plaintiff and observations of behavior of the plaintiff, and those portions of test materials that include plaintiff responses concerning the testing of the plaintiff [plaintiff's name] by [independent neuropsychologist's name].

PLEASE TAKE FURTHER NOTICE that failure to provide the disclosure will result in a motion to dismiss your defense based on noncompliance with section 394(a)-1.0 of the Administrative Code of the City of City of New York, as per *Blair v. City of New York*. J Clemente, NYLJ March 27, 1986. This is a continuing demand. Your failure to comply will result in our objecting to the introduction of any of such materials in evidence.

This type of correspondence represents one of multiple types of formal or informal requests or demands for neuropsychological records. Although the wording may vary from one request to another, all requests share a common wish for the neuropsychologist to provide copies of records that should typically be released only to those who, by virtue of their education and training, can understand the information, and who, by virtue of their ethical and legal requirements, share a commitment to maintaining test security—that is, other neuropsychologists. Although some requests may appropriately direct the neuropsychologist to provide copies of their test materials and raw test data only to another neuropsychologist, most requests direct the neuropsychologist to provide such records to attorneys or other parties who are not adequately trained to fully understand the information, and who are not bound by the same ethical and legal requirements regarding test security. Neuropsychologists who have not anticipated such requests and are unprepared to address them have much to consider.

Definitions

The ethics code of the American Psychological Association (APA) (2002) serves as the basis for ethical oversight of APA members and for psychologists who are not APA members, but whose state boards for psychology have adopted the code e to define ethical conduct for psychologists in those states. As defined in the APA ethics code, the term *test data* refers to "raw and scaled scores, client/patient responses to test questions or stimuli, and psychologists' notes and recordings concerning client/patient statements and behavior during an examination" (Standard 9.04a). In contrast, the term *test materials* refers to "manuals, instruments, protocols, and test questions or stimuli" (Standard 9.11).

Unfortunately, the separation of test data from test materials is not as clear as the code indicates. For example, although a blank answer sheet is considered a test material, and the examinee's answers are considered test data, a problem emerges when the neuropsychologist writes the examinee's answers on the answer sheet. The problem of physically separating test data from test materials is addressed in Standard 9.04a as follows: "Those portions of test materials that include client/patient responses are included in the definition of *test data*." That is, once test materials have responses written on them, they convert to test data (Behnke, 2003). Thus, test materials, protected under Standard 9.11, are no longer test materials once they have answers written on them, and they no longer enjoy the protection afforded by Standard 9.11. According to the 2002 APA ethics code, it is important to safeguard test protocols, questions, and test stimuli until the neuropsychologist has written the examinee's responses on them—but that requirement is illogical. In contrast to the 1992 APA ethics code that emphasized test security, the 2002 APA ethics code expresses a presumption of release.

The distinction between test data and materials, as defined in the APA ethics code, is in many instances an artificial distinction. For example, with visual reproduction tests or certain memory tests, the responses generated by the examinee (test data) are exactly the same as the test stimuli (test materials) that the neuropsychologist presented to the examinee. Thus, in many instances, the test data *are* *precisely* the test stimuli. In the present chapter we use both terms and take the position that both test materials and test data deserve equal protection under the general rubric of test security.

Interpreting Neuropsychological Test Data

The ability to competently understand neuropsychological test results is obtained over many years of specialized education and training. Answers to test questions, without the neuropsychologist's analysis, are meaningless to, and likely to be misinterpreted by, anyone other than an appropriately trained neuropsychologist.

Courts have recognized that neuropsychological testing is unique, and that the results of such tests can only be understood by specially trained professionals. For example, in *Watts v. the United States* (1977), the appellate court rejected the claim that a psychiatrist is a person qualified to receive psychological test data, because there was no evidence that the psychiatrist had the specialized training necessary to interpret that data. With rare exceptions, attorneys are not qualified to understand or interpret neuropsychological test data, and individual test questions, stimuli, or responses taken out of context can be quite misleading.

The opposing expert neuropsychologist is the appropriate person to receive raw test data in discovery. One expert neuropsychologist can review the opposing expert's report and test data and then inform the retaining attorney about any problems with the administration, scoring, or interpretation of the test results. There is no need for the attorney to have a copy of the raw test data in order to mount an appropriate cross-examination.

Background and Current State of Affairs

Psychologists, neuropsychologists, and others have long considered and debated the situations in which test scores and test materials, including raw test data, should be released (American Psychological Association, 2006; Attix, Donders, Johnson-Greene, Grote, Harris, & Bauer, 2007; Barth, 2000; Behnke, 2003; Bush, 2005; Bush & Lees-Haley, 2005; Bush & Martin, 2006; Erard, 2004; Fisher, 2003; Freides, 1993, 1995; Frumkin, 1995; Greiffenstein & Cohen, 2005; Kaufmann, 2005; Lees-Haley & Courtney, 2000a, 2000b; National Academy of Neuropsychology, 2000, 2003, 2004; Naugle & McSweeny, 1995, 1996; Rapp & Ferber, 1994, 2003; Rapp, Ferber, & Bush, 2008; Rogers, 2004; Shapiro, 2000; Sweet, 1990). Most recent publications reflect an understanding that neuropsychologists have ethical and legal obligations to maintain the integrity and security of the standardized tests upon which important clinical and forensic decisions rest. It is also understood that neuropsychologists are obligated to release raw test data and test materials to meet forensic evidentiary requirements.

Disagreement remains, however, about the steps that should be taken to safeguard raw test data and test materials that are required for discovery purposes. Given the extent of coverage of this topic and the divergence of opinions among scholars and clinicians, neuropsychologists with a personal preference for immediately releasing all records, maximizing test security, or taking some step in between will likely be able to find published material supporting their preference. Generally, less time, effort, and expense are required to immediately comply with requests for raw test data and test materials than to strive to maximize test security. *Our position is that maximizing test security is the ethically and legally preferred course of action and is therefore worth the additional time, effort, and expense.* The following sections provide the rationale for our position and solutions designed to meet the needs of all parties.

Jurisdictional Laws

Experience suggests that courts are more interested in considering relevant laws than in wading through the often contradictory and internally inconsistent psychological ethics. More important, law supersedes ethics. There are multiple legal justifications for neuropsychologists not to release test materials and raw test data to nonpsychologists. Therefore, neuropsychologists wishing to inform the courts about test security may be most successful by presenting the legal issues.

Discovery Law

Upon receipt of proper authorization, the reports of disclosed experts are always provided to opposing counsel. Neuropsychologists freely provide reports in such circumstances. Concerns and reluctance typically arise only when neuropsychologists are asked for, or ordered to provide, test materials and raw test data. Such requests may be embedded, intentionally or unintentionally, in broad requests for "all records."

Rule 26 of the Federal Rules of Civil Procedure (Federal rules of evidence, 1975) broadly defines the scope of discovery in Federal District Courts and in most states. According to Rule 26, litigants are entitled to have access to "any matter, not privileged, which is relevant to the subject matter involved in the pending action" (Federal rules of evidence, 1975, Rule 26[b][1]). Also discoverable are (a) the identity of the opposing side's expert, (b) the subject matter of the expert's expected testimony, (c) the substance of the expert's substantive facts and opinions, and (d) the bases for the expert's opinions. The effect of these requirements on neuropsychology is that all information dealing with the evaluation of the litigant's psychological and neurocognitive functioning is within the scope of discovery. Opposing counsel is entitled to all data underlying the expert's opinion in order to determine the accuracy of testing procedures and scoring, and to evaluate, challenge, or attempt to discredit the expert's opinions.

Opposing counsel may request the neuropsychological expert's records informally via a telephone call or letter, or formally via a *subpoena* or a *subpoena duces tecum*. A subpoena is an order to appear to provide testimony, whereas a subpoena duces tecum is an order to appear and bring specific documents; both types are automatically issued by a court officer upon the request of an attorney. Informal contacts by attorneys can be responded to in kind in an attempt to negotiate a satisfactory solution. However, either type of subpoena must be responded to formally and promptly. In addition to these requests for records from attorneys, judges can issue court orders for testimony or records. Failure to comply with a court order can result in the neuropsychologist being held in contempt of court. Rule 26 recognizes that there may be circumstances that justify limiting discovery, and it specifically allows the court to enter an order limiting the use of, or access to, sensitive information. The neuropsychologist is entitled to protection under Rule 26 (c) as a "person from whom discovery is sought...."

Subpoenas or court orders can be modified or rendered void or invalid (i.e., *quashed*). In some instances, neuropsychologists can discuss the matter directly with opposing counsel and request that a subpoena be quashed. When opposing counsel is not receptive, or when such action is inappropriate, the retaining attorney must make a motion to the court, outlining the reasons justifying the relief (Federal rules of evidence, 1975, Rule 45[c][3]). Rule 26[c][7]); this allows the court to "make any order which justice requires to protect a party or person." Specifically, it empowers the court to "enter an order that a trade secret or other confidential research, development, or commercial information *not be disclosed or be disclosed only in a designated way"* [emphasis added]. Based on Rule 26(c)(7), courts have entered protective orders limiting *who has access to such information* and *how that information can be used* (see, for example, *Quotron Systems, Inc. v. Automatic Data Processing, Inc.*, 1992, cited in Bush, 2005). Courts have even used protective orders to withhold confidential information from attorneys (see, for example, *Digital Equipment Corp v. Micro Technology, Inc.*, 1992, cited in Bush, 2007).

Some litigants and their attorneys believe that the test data generated during a neuropsychological evaluation belongs to the examinee. Although, in some contexts, litigants or their representatives may be entitled to review the data and have it explained to them by the neuropsychologist, the test protocols are the property of the neuropsychologist. Neuropsychologists typically clearly state in their written reports their opinions regarding the forensic issues, as well as the bases for their opinions. Neuropsychologists may, in some forensic contexts, explain to the litigant the evaluation findings and provide the litigant with a copy of the report.

Test Security Laws

There is no federal statutory psychologist nondisclosure privilege regarding test data and test materials. The number of individual states having statutes or regulations providing such psychologist nondisclosure privileges has increased since Rapp and Ferber's (1994) original survey. Eight states (Arizona, Arkansas, California, Illinois, Indiana, Iowa, Maryland, and Minnesota) now have specific nondisclosure privilege statutes, and 10 provide various unique regulatory nondisclosure privileges (Alabama, California, Florida, Georgia, Missouri, New Mexico, Ohio, Oregon, Texas, and Washington), as discussed in detail by Kaufmann (2005). Thus, eighteen states now recognize one or both of the public policy rationales underlying psychologist nondisclosure of test data and test materials to protect the integrity of psychological test materials and safeguard the objectivity and fairness of test interpretation. Each neuropsychologist should be familiar with the statutes and regulations of the state or states in which she or he practices.

Courts in states without nondisclosure statutes or regulations have still recognized the importance of not providing access to psychological test data or test materials in forensic cases as a basic principle of fairness and objective evidence of tort claims used in the courts' search for truth (see the *Legal Decisions* section later in this chapter). Kaufmann (2005) proposed the need for creating a uniform model psychologist nondisclosure privilege through legislation, regulation, or common law. This model would save significant time for both the courts and neuropsychologists by freeing them from having to deal with this issue ad hoc.

Health Insurance Portability and Accountability Act

Some litigants and attorneys are of the opinion that they are entitled to access to neuropsychological records under the Health Insurance Portability and Accountability Act (HIPAA; 1996). However, rights afforded under HIPAA in the context of routine clinical care do not carry over to forensic contexts. HIPAA §Section 164.524(a)(1)(ii) clearly states that information compiled in anticipation of use in civil, criminal, and administrative proceedings is not subject to the same right of review and amendment as is health care information in general (U.S. Department of Health and Human Services, 2003). Therefore, in forensic contexts, HIPAA does not prohibit neuropsychologists from withholding raw test data (Bush, Connell, & Denny, 2006; Connell & Koocher, 2003).

Clinical neuropsychological services provided to patients who have been in motor-vehicle accidents or injured at work occur with reasonable anticipation that the reports and other records will be used in legal proceedings. Thus, records generated in such medico-legal contexts also appear to be exempt from HIPAA's right of review and amendment.

Contractual Obligations

Federal law grants copyright owners (e.g., test publishers) the exclusive right to copy and distribute copyrighted works (17 U.S.C. §§ 106(1) & (3)). Test publishers take precautions to preserve the security of their tests by including nondisclosure provisions in every sale contract and by limiting the sale of tests to those with the appropriate education, training, and ethical foundation to properly use and safeguard the tests. When psychologists purchase tests and test forms, they agree to comply with federal copyright law. For example, when purchasing test materials from Pearson Assessments (PA), the *Terms & Conditions of Purchase* (Pearson Assessments, 2008) state:

> *Tests, inventories, and software offered by PA are protected by various intellectual property laws, including those regarding trade secrets, copyright, and trademarks. Printing or reproducing copyright-protected materials or content, including reproduction of protected test items, scales, scoring algorithms, scoring directions, or other protected content, is prohibited by law and by these Terms. PA software outputs, including but not limited to reports, are protected as trade secrets. TRADE SECRETS ARE NOT PERMITTED TO BE DISCLOSED in response to requests made pursuant to HIPAA (Health Insurance Portability and Accountability Act of 1996) or any other data disclosure law that exempts disclosure of information or documents protected as trade secrets. (See our* HIPAA: Frequently Asked Questions *for additional disclosure information.) Your purchase of protected materials DOES NOT grant You a right to reproduce additional copies of materials or the content or enter protected content onto a computer medium, such as non-PA scoring system or software. However, if You license and use PA software, You may excerpt portions of the output reports, limited to the minimum text necessary to accurately describe Your significant core conclusions, for incorporation into Your written evaluation of the individual, in accordance with Your profession's citation standards, if any. You may not, under any circumstance, copy or reproduce the text of any test question.* [underlined italics added]

Thus, by purchasing psychological and neuropsychological tests, neuropsychologists understand that they are bound by laws governing copyrights and trade secrets. Failure to comply with those laws constitutes a breach of the contract. Thus, a court that compels a neuropsychologist to release test materials and raw test data is ordering the neuropsychologist to commit a breach of the contract with the test publishers. In *Snowden v. Connaught Labs, Inc.* (1991), the court affirmed a magistrate's protective order that was based on the fact that "defendants should not be required to produce documents or records which will require them to violate their contract with [a nonparty]."

Legal Decisions

Although statutory laws provide guidelines for psychological practice in general, such laws frequently do not adequately address the activities of specialties such as neuropsychology. In such instances, case law may provide clarification. In this section we provide examples of relevant case law.

In *Detroit Edison Co. v. National Labor Relations Board (NLRB), 440 U.S. 301* (1979), the U.S. Supreme Court determined that psychologists should not release raw data and psychological test materials to nonpsychologists. Also of interest from this case were the reservations expressed by all of the Supreme Court justices regarding protective orders and potential problems with both inadvertent and intentional wrongful disclosure by the parties that are granted access to the records.

Courts have held that components of the Minnesota Multiphasic Personality Inventory (MMPI) are protected by copyright law (*Applied Innovations v. Regents of the U. of Minn.* [8th Cir. 1989] 876 F.2d 626, 634-636, cited in Bush, 2009). Also, it has been argued (*Carpenter v. Superior Court of Alameda County, 2006*) that standardized tests, such as those designed to evaluate emotional and cognitive functioning, may be copyrighted as secure tests, similar to the Law School Admission Test (LSAT; 2008) (see *Chicago Bd. of Educ. v. Substance, Inc.* [7th Cir. 2003] 354 F.3d 624, 627, cited in Bush 2007), involving the Chicago Academic Standards Exams.

In a more extreme example of withholding raw test data, a New York civil-trial court order denied the defense's expert neuropsychologist access to the plaintiff's expert's neuropsychological raw data, and the decision was reviewed and upheld by a five-judge New York appellate court (*Martinez v. KSM Holding, Ltd.*, 294 A.D.2d 111, [NY App. Div., 2002], cited in Bush, 2007). The court stated that disclosure of the plaintiff neuropsychologist's narrative report fulfilled New York discovery rules because the plaintiff expert was hired solely for the purpose of litigation.

In *Ochs v. Ochs* (2002) a New York court stated that the defendant should not have access to the raw psychological test data used by a forensic psychologist in a child custody dispute. Kaufmann (2005) reported that the court emphasized that disclosure of such material leads to a lengthy and expensive critique of the psychologist's methodology rather than the psychologist's conclusions. The court stated that such lengthy examination of neuropsychological evaluation techniques undermines the effectiveness because responses to item by item analysis would read psychometric test items directly into the public record of the court proceeding and that such disclosure should occur only for circumstances such as deficiency, bias, or other error in the report.

A U.S. District court ruled in *Chiperas v. Rubin* (1998) that neuropsychological test data should not be disclosed to a psychiatrist who did not have the qualifications and training necessary to understand such materials. These cases illustrate an understanding by the courts of the importance of neuropsychological test security and the support of the courts in maintaining test security.

Ethical Requirements and Professional Guidelines

Optimal ethical decision making often involves the review and integration of multiple sources of information. Gathering and reviewing ethical, legal, and professional resources is an important step in ethical decision-making models (see, for example, Bush, 2007; Bush, Connell, & Denney, 2006). In addition to laws, with which practitioners must comply or risk legal penalties, key resources include professional ethics codes, position papers, and scholarly works. Guidelines that promote test security reflect the value of nonmaleficence (Beauchamp & Childress, 2001).

In addition to the positions of the APA ethics code as previously described, a number of other published resources provide guidance to neuropsychologists and others who are seeking answers regarding the dissemination and security of test materials and raw test data. The code *of* conduct *of the Association of State and Provincial Psychology Boards (ASPPB; 2005)*, which governs the professional behavior of psychologists in many states and is a valuable resource for others, provides the following guidance regarding the release of confidential information, "The psychologist may release confidential information upon court order, as defined in Section II of this code, or to conform with state, federal or provincial law, rule, or regulation" (see Section III. F.7).

In 1999, the American Educational Research Association, the American Psychological Association, and the National Council on Measurement in Education jointly published the *Standards for Educational and Psychological Testing (SEPT; 1999)*. *SEPT* Standard 11.7 instructs practitioners that

> Test users have the responsibility to protect the security of tests, to the extent that developers enjoin users to do so....When tests are involved in litigation, inspection of the instruments should be restricted—to the extent permitted by law—to those who are legally or ethically obligated to safeguard test security. (p. 115)

SEPT Standard 11.8 reinforces the responsibility of practitioners to adhere to test copyrights. *SEPT* Standard 11.15 describes the potential for misinterpretation of test data by unqualified persons, the possible unintended negative consequences of inappropriate test use, and the need for examiners to take steps to avoid or minimize negative outcomes that may result from inappropriate test use.

The National Academy of Neuropsychology Policy and Planning Committee Policy and Planning Committee (2003) also recognized the importance of maximizing test security:

> In summary, the National Academy of Neuropsychology fully endorses the need to maintain test security, views the duty to do so as a basic professional and ethical obligation, strongly discourages the release of materials when requests do not contain appropriate safeguards, and, when indicated, urges the neuropsychologist to take appropriate and reasonable steps to arrange conditions for release that ensure adequate safeguards.

Additionally, the *Specialty Guidelines for Forensic Psychologists (SGFP; 1991)*,[1] which are aspirational and reflect "the most desirable and highest-level professional conduct for psychologists when engaged in the practice of forensic psychology," advise that when a forensic psychologist receives a properly served subpoena or court order to release records, the forensic psychologist should comply by making available all records specified in the order unless there is a compelling reason not to do so. The *SGFP* suggest that compelling reasons to object include contractual obligations, federal or state privacy, confidentiality, or privilege regulations, or notice of a counsel's intent to quash or otherwise petition the court to amend or void the subpoena or order for the records. The *SGFP* advise that, when in doubt about an appropriate response or course of action, forensic psychologists may formally notify the drafter of the subpoena of their uncertainty, seek assistance from retaining counsel, retain their own independent counsel, or defer to and request direction from the court or other tribunal.

The APA ethics code and other guidelines recognize that practitioners should strive to resolve conflicts between laws and ethical obligations. If the conflicts cannot be resolved informally, court orders and rules supersede ethical rules of conduct and guidelines.

Ethical issues for attorneys should also be considered. Attorneys who know what tests will be administered and are in possession of test questions and answers from prior cases are well positioned to prepare their clients to attempt to achieve specific results (Faust, Ziskin, & Hiers, 1991; Lees-Haley, 1997; Ziskin & Faust, 1988). In fact, attorneys are advised to coach their clients in this manner, and many attorneys believe that they have an ethical obligation to do so (Wetter & Corrigan, 1995; Youngjohn, 1995). However, the *Model Rules of Professional Conduct* (American Bar Association, 2007) have several provisions that seem to be violated by an attorney's use of protected testing information to coach a client to achieve a specific result. Rule 1.2(d) provides that:

> *A lawyer shall not counsel a client to engage, or assist a client, in conduct that the lawyer knows is criminal or fraudulent, but a lawyer may discuss the legal consequences of any proposed course of conduct with a client and may counsel or assist a client to make a good-faith effort to determine the validity, scope, meaning, or application of the law.* [underlined italics added]

Preparing a client to achieve a result on a neuropsychological test that does not accurately reflect the examinee's true abilities is fraudulent. In addition, Rule 3.3(a)(4) provides that an attorney shall not "offer evidence that the lawyer knows to be false." A lawyer would recognize that Rule 3.3(a)(4) is violated if he or she offers as evidence test results that were known to have been intentionally manipulated and therefore false.

Societal Considerations

The results of neuropsychological evaluations are only valid and reliable if the answers and other responses are not artificially manipulated, which is a risk associated with widespread availability of test materials and raw test data. A person with access to the neuropsychological test questions and other test materials can prepare in advance to answer the questions or respond to stimuli in a way that produces a desired, typically more impaired, result. Maintaining test security decreases the opportunity for examinees to prepare in advance for specific tests. Failure to keep the questions, answers, stimuli, and purposes of each test out of the public domain allows the opportunity for widespread "coaching" and "faking" of test performances, which destroys the validity of the test results in such cases, and ultimately destroys the validity of the tests themselves. Invalid tests are of no use clinically or in forensic contexts (Martelli, Bush, & Zasler, 2003). This situation is analogous to having the Law School Admission Test or the Multistate Bar Examination questions and correct answers freely available.

Additionally, when test validity is compromised, the commercial value of the tests is compromised. Neuropsychological tests are developed by private companies at considerable costs involving financial and human resources over extended periods of time. A significant effect of not safeguarding neuropsychological tests is that the test results may become inadmissible because they would no longer have the validity and reliability required under the *Daubert v. Merril Dow Pharmaceuticals* (1993) standard.

Solutions for Neuropsychologists

Bush (2009) has described the four A's of ethical practice and decision making as *anticipate, avoid, address,* and *aspire.* Neuropsychologists who engage in forensic activities should (a) anticipate and prepare for ethical issues and challenges commonly encountered in their specific practice contexts, (b) strive to avoid ethical misconduct, (c) address ethical challenges when they are anticipated or encountered, and (d) aspire to the highest standards of ethical practice. Pursuit of high ethical ideals, referred to as *positive ethics* (Handelsman, Knapp, & Gottlieb, 2002; Knapp & Van de Creek, 2006), requires clinicians to examine the perspectives and processes that allow maximum adherence to moral principles. However, such efforts can be time- and labor intensive, which are disincentives for some practitioners. Although the pursuit of ethical ideals requires extra time and effort that only a personal commitment to such ideals can support, such a commitment to ethical practice should be made by all neuropsychologists. Frequent review of the four A's of ethical practice and decision making, combined with a personal commitment to positive ethics, promotes sound ethical practice.

Educate Attorneys

Neuropsychologists must recognize from the start that the average attorney is unaware of the need for test security. In fact, many attorneys have been instructed in their continuing legal education programs about how to prepare their clients for independent neuropsychological evaluations, including seeking advanced disclosure of the tests that will be administered (Lees-Haley, 1997). Therefore, neuropsychologists should adopt a position of respectful educator, correcting misconceptions and providing preferable options for meeting discovery requirements and maximizing test security.

Attorneys and courts tend to be more willing to listen to neuropsychologists' concerns about test security and more open to alternative solutions if the problem is properly presented to them. While explaining the legal and ethical issues, it is critical that neuropsychologists demonstrate an appreciation of the importance of the goals of the discovery process. It is also essential that neuropsychologists make clear that the issue has nothing to do with doctor-patient confidentiality, which was waived when the examinee placed his or her mental status at issue in the legal claim. Rather, neuropsychologists should emphasize how neuropsychological tests and their results differ from other medical and scientific tests, and they should stress a collaborative approach to resolving the matter.

Adopt an Active Approach

First, determine the methods that you consider acceptable for resolving requests or orders for test materials and raw test data. Such options may include releasing records only to another qualified expert, requesting a protective order, and requesting a motion to seal the portion of the transcript dealing with specifics of test materials.

Second, send a letter to each referring attorney at the outset, prior to conducting the evaluation, that describes not only the fee agreement and logistics, but also provides a clear statement of how you will handle release of raw test data. Although some attorneys may object to your position, it is best to learn of their objection in advance so that an attempt to resolve the conflict can be made before becoming involved with case. Some attorneys expect a written contract from the neuropsychologist and view such documentation as evidence that the expert is straightforward, organized, and professional.

Third, prepare in advance multiple packets that contain sample protective orders and supporting documents, ready to forward to attorneys upon receipt of an informal request, subpoena, or court order. In addition, forensic neuropsychologists in those states that are currently without specific statutes or regulations regarding nondisclosure of test data and test materials may be well served by working with state psychological associations and legislators to introduce bills that will explicitly define how raw test data and test materials are to be handled, and who is qualified to receive the materials.

Accommodate Discovery Requirements While Avoiding Unnecessary Harm

First, understand that the attorney will obtain the neuropsychological evaluation report and other written notes and records reviewed as part of normal discovery. The neuropsychological report should contain all of the information on which the neuropsychologist's opinions were based, including sources of the patient's history, details of any interviews with third parties, identification of all of the records reviewed and tests used, demographic and other variables that were considered, the interpretation of the raw data results, and the opinions themselves. Thus, disclosure of an appropriate evaluation report provides the attorney with comprehensive discovery.

Second, send a letter to the requesting party that expresses your desire to cooperate, describes the issues of concern, and offers solutions that you consider acceptable (see Appendix for a sample letter). Third, when sending raw test data to the opposing counsel's neuropsychological expert, include a cover letter stating that by accepting the packet of raw test data he or she agrees to maintain test integrity and security and adhere to the test manufacturer's contract regarding copying and dissemination of the records.

Fourth, pursue a protective order and request that records be sealed, returned, or destroyed following conclusion of the case. A protective order should limit access to the test materials and raw test data to qualified neuropsychologists retained by the side seeking discovery. The trial judge has broad discretion in constructing a protective order. The protective order should (a) cover "all test materials and raw test data generated in the case of [patient's name] by [neuropsychologist's name]"; and (b) limit the disclosure of such information "to [name of expert] who is a licensed psychologist or neuropsychologist qualified to administer and interpret such tests, who certifies that he or she will maintain test integrity and security and not further copy or distribute the materials." If the matter reaches the trial stage, the court should also be requested to return, destroy, or seal all parts of the record containing any of the test materials and any exhibits or testimony that make specific reference to any of the test materials. The court order should also prohibit copying of test materials that are not destroyed or returned to the expert at the conclusion of the trial.

Fifth, attempt to determine that the requesting party's designated recipient of the raw test data is actually a qualified neuropsychologist. One suggested strategy is to request and review the opposing expert's curriculum vitae (Bush, 2007). Pursue documentation from the expert designated to receive the raw test data indicating agreement to maintain test security, or at least document expectations of the standard of conduct in a cover letter included with the raw test data being released. The cover letter can be used as evidence of an attempt to resolve the conflicts between laws pertaining to discovery and the ethical and legal obligations to maintain test security.

If the party seeking disclosure of the test data has not disclosed the identity of its expert, the protective order should state: "Raw test data shall be placed in a sealed envelope and delivered to the clerk of the court where the action is proceeding. The clerk shall release the sealed envelope only to the designated licensed psychologist or neuropsychologist who has been determined to be qualified to receive and interpret the test materials." Enclosing a copy of the user qualifications pages from a well-known test catalog with the protective order can facilitate this determination.

To facilitate preparation of the protective order, provide the retaining attorney with a standard prepared motion and documents supporting the legal, contractual, and ethical obligations justifying the request for a protective order. The materials provided to the attorney should address the three categories of information (listed below) courts look to in deciding whether to enter a protective order and what the terms of the order should be. These categories are as follows:

1. Significant harm to individual litigants, the public, and the court's pursuit of truth will result from unrestricted disclosure of the test materials.
2. The significant harm from disclosure can be avoided while still accommodating the opposing side's legitimate need for information to prepare its case.
3. The exact proposed restrictions that the protective order should contain.

Attorneys and the courts tend to appreciate such a methodical, rational, and active approach to meeting the needs of all parties.

Conclusion

Neuropsychologists who provide services in forensic contexts commonly receive requests from colleagues, clients, and attorneys for copies of their test materials and raw test data. Although there are contradictions within and between ethical and legal requirements and guidelines, general bioethical principles, most ethical and professional guidelines, case law, and federal copyright law support the responsibility of practitioners to maintain the security of neuropsychological tests, including raw test data. Neuropsychology, the legal system, and society are best served when neuropsychologists adopt an active, protective, and educational approach to test security and requests for test materials and raw test data. These same parties are also well served when attorneys and courts maintain a willingness to understand the importance of maintaining test security and share the investment in test security for the benefit of society.

Note

1. The *Specialty Guidelines for Forensic Psychologists* (SGFP) (Committee on the Revision of the Specialty Guidelines for Forensic Psychology, 2008) are currently undergoing revision due to advancements in the field since 1991. See http://www.ap-ls.org/links/22808sgfp.pdf for the third draft revision, available online as of February 27, 2008.

References

American Bar Association. (2007). *Model rules of professional conduct.* Chicago: Author. Retrieved September 20, 2007, from http://www.abanet.org/cpr/mrpc/mrpc_toc.html

American Educational Research Association, American Psychological Association, & National Council on Measurement in Education. (1999). *Standards for educational and psychological testing.* Washington, DC: American Educational Research Association.

American Psychological Association. (1992). Ethical principles of psychologists and code of conduct. *American Psychologist, 47*, 1597–1611.

American Psychological Association. (2002). Ethical principles of psychologists and code of conduct. *American Psychologist, 57*(12), 1060–1073.

American Psychological Association. (2006). Strategies for private practitioners coping with subpoenas or compelled testimony for client records or test data. *Professional Psychology: Research and Practice, 37*(2), 215–222.

Association of State and Provincial Psychology Boards. (2005). *Code of conduct for psychologists.* Montgomery, AL: Association of State and Provincial Psychology Boards.

Attix, D. K., Donders, J., Johnson-Greene, D., Grote, C. L., Harris, J. G., & Bauer, R. M. (2007). Disclosure of neuropsychological test data: Official position of Division 40 (Clinical Neuropsychology) of the American Psychological Association, Association of Postdoctoral Programs in Clinical Neuropsychology, and American Academy of Clinical Neuropsychology. *Clinical Neuropsychologist, 21*, 232–238.

Barth, J. T. (2000). Commentary on "Disclosure of tests and raw test data to the courts" by Paul Lees-Haley and John Courtney. *Neuropsychology Review, 10*(3), 179–180.

Beauchamp, T. L., & Childress, J. F. (2001). *Principles of biomedical ethics* (5th ed.). New York: Oxford University Press.

Behnke, S. (2003). Release of test data and APA's new ethics code. *Monitor on Psychology, 34*(7), 70–72.

Bush, S. S. (2005). Differences between the 1992 and 2002 APA ethics codes: A brief overview. In S. S. Bush (Ed.), *A casebook of ethical challenges in neuropsychology* (pp. 1–8). New York: Taylor & Francis/Psychology Press.

Bush, S. S. (2007). *Ethical decision making in clinical neuropsychology.* New York: Oxford University Press.

Bush, S. S. (2009). *Geriatric mental health ethics: A casebook.* New York: Springer Publishing Company.

Bush, S. S., Connell, M. A., & Denney, R. L. (2006). *Ethical practice in forensic psychology: A systematic model for decision making.* Washington, DC: American Psychological Association.

Bush, S. S., & Lees-Haley, P. R. (2005). Threats to the validity of forensic neuropsychological data: Ethical considerations. *Journal of Forensic Neuropsychology, 4*(3), 45–66

Bush, S. S., & Martin, T. A. (2006). The ethical and clinical practice of disclosing raw test data: Addressing the ongoing debate. *Applied Neuropsychology, 13,* 125–136.

Carpenter v. Superior Court of Alameda County (Yamaha Motor Corp., USA), Cal. App. 4th (2006).

Chiperas v. Rubin, No. CIV.A.96-130, 1998 WL 765126 (D.D.C. 1998).

Committee on Ethical Guidelines for Forensic Psychologists. (1991). Specialty guidelines for forensic psychologists. *Law and Human Behavior, 15*(6), 655–665.

Committee on the Revision of the Specialty Guidelines for Forensic Psychology. (2008). *Specialty guidelines for forensic psychology. 3rd official draft.* Available at at www.ap-ls.org/links/22808sgfp.pdf

Connell, M., & Koocher, G. (2003). HIPAA & forensic practice. *American Psychology Law Society News, 23,* 16–19.

Daubert v. Merril Dow Pharmaceuticals, 113 S. Ct. 2786 (1993).

Detroit Edison Co. v. National Labor Relations Board (NLRB*),* 440 U.S. 301 (1979).

Erard, R. E. (2004). A "raw deal" reheated: Reply to comments by Rogers, Fischer, Smith, and Evans. *Journal of Personality Assessment, 82*(1), 44–47.

Faust, D., Ziskin, J., & Hiers, J. (1991). *Brain damage claims: Coping with neuropsychological evidence.* Los Angeles: Law & Psychology Press.

Federal rules of evidence for United States courts and magistrates. (1975). St. Paul, MN: West.

Fisher, C. B. (2003, Jan/Feb). Test data standard most notable change in new APA ethics code. *National Psychologist,* pp. 12–13.

Freides, D. (1993). Proposed standard of professional practice: Neuropsychological reports display all quantitative data. *Clinical Neuropsychologist, 7,* 234–235.

Freides, D. (1995). Interpretations are more benign than data. *Clinical Neuropsychologist, 9,* 248.

Frumkin, I. B. (1995). How to handle attorney requests for psychological test data. *Innovations in Clinical Practice: A Source Book, 14,* 275–292.

Greiffenstein, M. F., & Cohen, L. (2005). Neuropsychology and the law: Principles of productive attorney–neuropsychologist relations. In G. J. Larrabee (Ed.), *Forensic neuropsychology: A scientific approach* (pp. 29–91). New York: Oxford University Press.

Handelsman, M., Knapp, S., & Gottlieb, M. (2002). Positive ethics. In R. Snyder & S. Lopez (Eds.), *Handbook of positive psychology* (pp. 731–744). New York: Oxford University Press.

Kaufmann, P. M. (2005). Protecting the objectivity, fairness, and integrity of neuropsychological evaluations in litigation: A privilege second to none? *Journal of Legal Medicine, 26,* 95–131.

Knapp, S., & Van de Creek, L. (2006). *Practical ethics for psychologists: A positive approach.* Washington, DC: American Psychological Association.

Law School Admission Council. (2008). *Law School Admission Test.* Newtown, PA: Author. Retrieved September 17, 2008, from www.lsat.com/aboutlsac/about-lsac.asp#lsat

Lees-Haley, P. R. (1997). Attorneys influence expert evidence in forensic psychological and neuropsychological cases. *Assessment, 4,* 321–324.

Lees-Haley, P. R., & Courtney, J. C. (2000a). Disclosure of tests and raw test data to the courts: A need for reform. *Neuropsychology Review, 10*(3), 169–175.

Lees-Haley, P. R., & Courtney, J. C. (2000b). Reply to the commentary on "Disclosure of tests and raw test data to the courts."*Neuropsychology Review, 10*(3), 181–182.

Martelli, M. F., Bush, S. S., & Zasler, N. D. (2003). Identifying, avoiding, and addressing ethical misconduct in neuropsychological medicolegal practice. *International Journal of Forensic Psychology, 1*(1), 26–44.

National Academy of Neuropsychology. (2000). Test security: Official position statement of the National Academy of Neuropsychology. *Archives of Clinical Neuropsychology, 15*(5), 383–386.

National Academy of Neuropsychology Policy and Planning Committee. (2003). *Test security: An update: Official position statement of the National Academy of Neuropsychology.* Retrieved February 17, 2004, from http://nanonline.org/paio/security_update.shtm

National Academy of Neuropsychology. (2004). Releasing test materials: Position of the Psychological Corporation. *Bulletin, 19*(1), 1–2, 7–8.

Naugle, R. I., & McSweeny, A. J. (1995). On the practice of routinely appending neuropsychological data to reports. *Clinical Neuropsychologist, 9*(3), 245–247.

Naugle, R. I., & McSweeny, A. J. (1996). More thoughts on the practice of routinely appending raw data to reports: Response to Freides and Matarazzo. *Clinical Neuropsychologist, 10,* 313–314.

Ochs v. Ochs, 749 N.Y.S.2d 650, 656 (N.Y. Gen Term 2002).

Pearson Assessments. (2008). *Trade secrets, copyrights, disclosure and use of unauthorized software.* Retrieved September 18, 2008, from www.pearsonassessments.com/catalog/terms.htm

Rapp, D. L., & Ferber, P. S. (1994, December). Discovery and protective orders relating to raw data in psychological or neuro-psychological testing. *Vermont Bar Journal & Law Digest,* pp. 22–34.

Rapp, D. L., & Ferber, P. S. (2003). To release, or not to release raw test data, that is the question. In A. M. Horton, Jr., & L. C. Hartlage (Eds.), *Handbook of forensic neuropsychology* (pp. 337–368). New York: Springer Publishing Company.

Rapp, D. L., Ferber, P. S., & Bush, S. S. (2008). Unresolved issues about release of test data and test materials. In A. M. Horton, Jr., & D. Wedding (Eds.), *The neuropsychology handbook* (3rd ed., pp. 471–500). New York: Springer Publishing Company.

Rogers, R. (2004). APA 2002 ethic, amphibology, and the release of psychological test records: A counterperspective to Erard. *Journal of Personality Assessment, 82*(1), 31–34.

Shapiro, D. L. (2000). Commentary: Disclosure of tests and raw data to the courts. *Neuropsychology Review, 10*(3), 175–176.

Snowden v. Connaught Labs., Inc., 137 F.R.D. 325, 332 (D. Kan. 1991).

Sweet, J. (1990). Further consideration of ethics in psychological testing: A broader perspective on releasing records. *Illinois Psychologist, 28,* 5–9.

U.S. Department of Health and Human Services. (2003). *Public Law 104-191: Health Insurance Portability and Accountability Act of 1996.* Retrieved November 24, 2003, from www.hhs.gov/ocr/hipaa/

Watts v. the United States, 77–1428, U.S. (Ct. of App., D.C., 1977).

Wetter, M. W., & Corrigan, S. K. (1995). Providing information to clients about psychological tests: A survey of attorneys' and law students' attitudes. *Professional Psychology: Research and Practice, 26,* 474–477.

Youngjohn, J. R. (1995). Confirmed attorney coaching prior to neuropsychological evaluation. *Assessment, 2,* 279–283.

Ziskin, J., & Faust, D. (1988). *Coping with psychiatric and psychological testimony* (4th ed.). Marina Del Rey, CA: Law and Psychology Press.

Appendix 8.1

Sample Response Letter to Request for Raw Test Data

[Professional letterhead]
Date:
[Addressee name and address]
RE: Request for neuropsychological raw test data (test forms)
[To Whom It May Concern:] [Dear Mr./Mrs./Ms./ Surname:] _____

I appreciate the significance of disclosure of important information in litigated matters. However, as detailed in this letter, neuropsychologists have conflicting obligations when they are asked or ordered to release raw test data to anyone other than another neuropsychologist. The three primary issues of concern are as follows:

1. The security of neuropsychological test materials and data is necessary in order to ensure the validity of future examinations. Through the dissemination of test forms and responses, potential examinees may familiarize themselves with the materials and then provide answers that do not reflect their true neuropsychological status. This situation is analogous to making the LSAT questions and answers widely available.
2. Providing raw test data to persons who are not trained to interpret them can result in misuse and misinterpretation of the information and ultimately result in harm to individual litigants, the public, and the court's search for truth. As a result, psychologists have an ethical obligation to release raw test data only to other neuropsychologists who have the education and training to use and interpret the information appropriately.
3. Disclosing test materials to anyone other than another neuropsychologist is a breach of the current contract between the neuropsychologist and the test owners/publishers.

Both legal and ethical obligations to maintain test security are presented in more detail below.

Legal Considerations

In the case of *Detroit Edison Co. v. National Labor Relations Board (NLRB)* 440 U.S. 301 (1979), the U.S. Supreme Court determined that psychologists should not release raw data and psychological test materials to nonpsychologists.

Additionally, when psychologists purchase tests and test forms, they agree to comply with federal copyright law by not copying such materials. For example, when purchasing test materials from Pearson Assessments, the *Terms & Conditions of Purchase* state, "Pearson Products are protected by various intellectual property laws, including trade secrets, copyright and trademarks. Printing or reproducing copyright-protected materials or content...is prohibited by law and by these Terms & Conditions. Pearson software outputs, including but not limited to reports, are protected as trade secrets. Trade secrets are not permitted to be disclosed in response to requests made pursuant to HIPAA or to any other data disclosure law that exempts disclosure of information or documents protected as trade secrets...*The Customer may not, under any circumstance, copy or reproduce the text or graphic image of any test item*" (emphasis added).

Ethical Considerations

The ethics code of the American Psychological Association (2002) states in Standard 9.04, "Psychologists may refrain from releasing test data to protect a client/patient or others from substantial harm or misuse or misrepresentation of the data or the test, recognizing that in many instances release of confidential information under these circumstances is regulated by law." In Standard 9.11, the ethics code further states, "Psychologists make reasonable efforts to maintain the integrity and security of test materials and other assessment techniques consistent with law and contractual obligations, and in a manner that permits adherence to this Ethics Code."

Additionally, Standard 11.7 of the *Standards for Educational and Psychological Testing* (American Educational Research Association, American Psychological Association, National Council on Measurement in Education, 1999) states that test users (psychologists) have a responsibility to protect the security of tests. In litigation, inspection of the instruments should be restricted, to the extent permitted by law, to those who are legally or ethically obligated to safeguard test security (i.e., other psychologists). Standard 11.8 also states that test users have a responsibility to respect test copyrights.

Professional Position Papers

Guidelines published by neuropsychological professional organizations emphasize the importance of maintaining test security and releasing raw test data only to persons who are qualified by education and training to understand the information and who are also bound by ethical and legal requirements to maintain test security. These guidelines are discussed in detail in the following publications:

Attix, D. K., Donders, J., Johnson-Greene, D., Grote, C. L., Harris, J. G., & Bauer, R. M. (2007). Disclosure of neuropsychological test data: Official position of Division 40 (Clinical Neuropsychology) of the American Psychological Association, Association of Postdoctoral Programs in Clinical Neuropsychology, and American Academy of Clinical Neuropsychology. *Clinical Neuropsychologist*, *21*, 232–238.

National Academy of Neuropsychology. (2000). Test security: Official statement of the National Academy of Neuropsychology. *Archives of Clinical Neuropsychology*, *15*(5), 383–386.

National Academy of Neuropsychology Policy and Planning Committee. (2003). *Test Security: An update: Official statement of the National Academy of Neuropsychology.* Available online at http://nanonline.org/paio/security_update.shtm.

Proposed Solutions

1. A summary sheet listing standardized scores for all tests that were administered is appended to the neuropsychological report. This summary sheet should suffice for most purposes. If you do not already have a copy of the summary sheet, a copy will be provided in response to an appropriate request with authorization.
2. Forward the name and contact information of a neuropsychologist to whom the materials can be directly released.
3. Provide a court order stipulating that the test materials and data will be protected in the following ways:

   - no broad circulation
   - no unauthorized copies are made
   - minimal presentation in court
   - protection/sealing of exhibits and court records related to the test materials and raw test data
   - destruction or return of test materials following conclusion of the proceedings

I appreciate your consideration of these issues and your understanding of the importance for the general public of maintaining the security of neuropsychological test materials and raw test data. I look forward to working with you to resolve this issue in a manner that is consistent with my legal, ethical, and professional obligations.

Sincerely,

[Handwritten signature of sender]
[Typed name of sender]

Neuropsychological Evaluations in the Context of Civil Competency Decisions

9

Michael D. Franzen

Introduction

Since the publication of the first edition of this book, the words *competency* and *competency assessment* have taken on a greater range of meaning. The determination and assessment of competency has become a focus in professional training. The American Psychological Association (APA) has delineated core competencies for psychologists in training, as well as competencies for supervisors. Work groups have been formed and guidelines issued for assessing competency of psychologists (Kaslow et al., 2007). Other professional groups have also defined competencies or are in the process of doing so. Although it may seem that the use of the term competency is irrelevant to the current discussion of forensic neuropsychology; in fact all of these uses of the term refer to ecological validity of the assessment methods. All of these uses of the term involve some definition of basic cognitive, psychological, and behavioral skills, and an evaluation of whether an individual in a given situation is able to perform certain tasks. Clinical neuropsychology becomes involved in this evaluation and determination when an objective basis for determination of competency is desired. This is a deviation from the origins of clinical neuropsychology, but it is consistent with larger concerns regarding the ecological validity of test results and the decisions that emanate from use of neuropsychological data.

Clinical neuropsychology has developed largely in a medical context, but it possesses utility in other contexts, including the legal arena. An important facet of legal-neuropsychological assessments is the evaluation of competency. Competency is a legal rather than clinical concept. In a civil, not criminal, context competency includes fiduciary competency (the ability to make decisions regarding the deployment of financial resources), testamentary competency (the ability to sign one's name to legal documents and thereby committing oneself to certain responsibilities), competency to consent to treatment (the ability to make decisions regarding medical disposition), and competency to live independently (the ability to maintain one's own hygiene, safety, and health). Other forms of civil competency that are less formally defined in our legal and social system include driving and responsibility for others, such as the competency required to be a caregiver or teacher. Competency in a criminal context generally involves different issues. There is an area related to competency to consent to treatment in the form of competency to consent to research procedures, whether for reasons of cognitive impairment (Bonnie, 1997) or for reasons of depression (Elliott, 1997). Although this issue has received increasing attention in the literature related to institutional review boards (Hirschfield, Winslade, & Krause, 1997), as yet clinical evaluations have not been involved. There are multiple issues implicated when the question of civil competency is raised. Zaubler, Viederman, and Fins (1996) provide an overview of some of the issues related to psychiatry and the legal realm.

This chapter will provide a brief description of the issues to which clinical neuropsychologists should attend, and a review of selected instruments will be provided to give some idea of the tools available to neuropsychologists. Although competency and commitment are frequently related (Bloom & Faulkner, 1987), this chapter will deal narrowly with the issues specific to competency only. Research in this area has proliferated since publication of the first edition, and this chapter is not meant as an exhaustive review of these studies. Instead, the purpose of this chapter is to alert the reader to the important conceptual and practical considerations in conducting competency evaluations.

Requests for clinical neuropsychologists to conduct competency evaluations reflect at least two distinct sets of concepts and variables. The first set of variables is legal in nature and comprises a consideration of the power of the state to curtail aspects of personal freedom and autonomy under certain circumstances. Included in this realm of variables is the role of the clinical neuropsychologist as an agent of social control The second realm of variables is related to the role of the clinical neuropsychologist as an emissary of the scientific world to the practical, legal world. The clinical neuropsychologist, therefore, must be aware of the legal standards and regulations in force in the venue in which the competency decision is being made.

The curtailment of personal freedom is based on a decision that the greater good, whether for the subject himself or for the individuals in the subject's social environment, would be served by this curtailment. This curtailment of an individual's personal power can be invoked to prevent the harmful consequences of harmful behaviors. For example, to prevent an individual from squandering his financial resources, that person might be relieved of the capacity to spend those resources at will. As Schopp (2001) points out, the issue of determining competency contains a basic conflict between protecting individual liberty and promoting well-being. In fact, there is an a priori presumption of competency, that is, adults are presumed to be competent until there is convincing evidence to the contrary. Furthermore, although a legal proceeding may result in that presumption being revoked, there is a reversible character to the decision such that someone once adjudicated to be incompetent can be later found to be competent.

Competency to Consent to Treatment

Competency to *consent* to treatment is the name by which this set of concepts is known, but in practicality the question is actually competency to *refuse* treatment (Farnsworth, 1990). As long as the patient agrees to treatment, there is no question raised about the competency of the patient, even though at least for psychiatric patients consenting to voluntary hospitalization, this assumption may not be tenable for the majority of patients (Appelbaum, Mirkin, & Bateman, 1981). Another study found that for residents of a nursing home, nearly half were incompetent to give consent for treatment, even though their oral consent had been relied upon in treatment decision implementation (Barton, Malli Orr, & Janofsky, 1996). This form of competency evaluation is a familiar activity among neuropsychologists who work in a psychiatric context. Appelbaum and Roth (1981) discuss the issues related to a psychiatric evaluation of competency to consent to treatment, but the same issues are relevant to an evaluation where the issue of cognitive capacity is in question. As these authors point out, the accuracy and completeness of the information conveyed by the patient should be considered by the clinician, and the stability of the patient's mental status should be evaluated and commented upon.

Objectives

The issues to be addressed include whether the patient understands the need for treatment, whether the patient can explain the possible outcomes of treatment, including side effects, and whether the patient can predict the likely consequences of not getting treatment. Roth, Meisel, and Lidz (1977) describe the relevant content areas as being able to evidence a choice, having an understanding of the outcome, having the choice based on rational reasons, and having the ability to understand (as well as having actual understanding).

Both the cognitive condition and the emotional state of the patient are relevant here. Severe depression may interfere with the capacity to make rational decisions about treatment. A related area is the *advance directive* in which a patient states preferences regarding treatment that may be contemplated in a situation in which the patient is unable to provide consent or even to communicate. In the healthy adult who records advance directives, there is usually no question about his or her mental status. In cases of progressive dementia, however, it may be necessary to document the competency of the patient to make decisions about treatment options and to record those decisions as guidance for surrogate decision makers later in time (Grossberg, 1998).

Although neuropsychological cognitive test data is informative in the evaluation of competency, there is no specific relation between individual tests and competency. Palmer and Savla (2007) reviewed published studies regarding the relationship between cognitive test data and aspects of decisional capacity. They found significant correlations between the two sets of data, but no single cognitive test was found to be preeminently predictive of decisional capacity. Karlawish and colleagues (2008) reported good inter-rater agreement in decisions regarding competency to consent to treatment in a research protocol for Alzheimer's disease clinical trials.

Fiduciary Competency

Fiduciary and testamentary competencies are multifaceted. These are legal decisions, not clinical ones. However, the trier of fact (judge) makes these decisions using information from different sources including clinical sources. The extent to which a given judge relies on the clinical information depends upon the experience and knowledge of the judge in conjunction with the judge's opinion of the clinician. It is incumbent upon the neuropsychologist to represent accurately and dispassionately the status of clinical science in answering the relevant legal questions. It is important to obtain objective information regarding the fiduciary competency of individuals because both the individuals undergoing the evaluations and their informants frequently underestimate the extent of deficits in making financial decisions (Okonkwo et al., 2008). Furthermore, fiduciary competence can decline rapidly under condition of progressive dementia (Martin et al., 2008).

Fiduciary competence requires basic arithmetic skills (or the ability to use a calculator), as well as judgment and problem-solving skills. The upper boundary of fiduciary skill involving the disposition of large sums of money and complicated financial plans is not an issue in these evaluations. Even the most astute manager of his own funds would consult some form of financial advisor in order to optimize the return on his resources. The relevant issue in determining fiduciary competence is whether the patient is allowed to choose or turn down such advisement and whether they possess adequate cognitive skills to understand the likely consequences of certain financial decisions. For example, although the patient may not be able to determine whether the best (most productive) form of investment would be a limited-partnership real estate operation or a stake in a hedge market, the patient would be required to understand that some risk was involved in each undertaking and that writing a check to cover either investment would decrease liquid assets by the same amount. That is, some degree of reasonable knowledge is expected, but not an above-average ability. Okonkwo, Wadley, Griffith, Ball, and Marson (2006) reported that neuropsychological measures of attention and executive function may predict financial competence.

Objectives

The objectives for conducting a fiduciary competency evaluation are (1) to gain an understanding of the financial tasks required of the patient, (2) to obtain a history of recent financial decisions made by the patient and the outcomes, (3) to determine the cognitive skills of the patient required to make the necessary financial decision, (4) to draw reasonable conclusions about the ability of the patient to make reasonable financial decisions in the near future, and (5) to make accurate predictions about the effect of changes in the person's situation or neuropsychological condition (Is the condition static or progressive? Is it reversible?). There are several different domains relevant to the evaluation of financial competence. These include basic money skills, conceptual knowledge related to financial operations, the ability to conduct cash transactions, management of a personal checkbook, ability to read and understand a common bank statement, and ability to make rational decisions related to financial options and plans.

Testamentary Competency

Testamentary competency can be intertwined with fiduciary competency, although it is also possible to separate the two. The complication arises because signing one's name can encumber financial resources. However, there is at least one area in which testamentary competency is separate from financial competency, namely in the capacity to sign a will. A will is signed in the presence of a witness who could theoretically testify later as to the mental state of the patient. But challenges after the fact, especially after the death of the individual involved, are not uncommon. Of course the clinical neuropsychologist can most confidently provide information regarding testamentary competence when an evaluation is requested a priori. Requests for clinical input after the death of the individual require the collection of information from collateral observations and from an examination of the activities and decisions made contemporaneous to the act of signing the document (Spar & Garb, 1997). For a person to be found competent to sign a will (testamentary competence), it is necessary that cognitive skills be reasonably intact, that the person understand the identity of the recipients of the benefits of the will, that the person understand that signing one's name to the will requires the survivors to implement the desires expressed in the document, and to understand that dying while the will is in effect will set in motion a series of events that are irrevocable.

Objectives

The objectives in this situation include (1) to obtain information regarding the cognitive skills of the patient, (2) to obtain a description of the patient's ability to understand the responsibilities and consequences attendant upon signing the document, and (3) to provide a reasonable conclusion regarding the capacity of the individual to commit him- or herself to the exigencies of the contract or document.

General Clinical Model for the Assessment of Civil Competence

Competency evaluations are, in the final measure, clinical evaluations. The purpose is to obtain an accurate depiction of the person's level of cognitive skill and emotional and behavioral functioning, to make reasonable inferences about the likely etiologies of any deficits, and to make valid predictions about extra-test behaviors. There are some differences from a typical evaluation, however. As an initial difference, with the exception of questions of competency to refuse treatment that are initiated by physicians, most competency evaluations are initiated either by family members or by the court. As another important difference, the competency evaluation, more so than any other type of neuropsychological evaluation, will have implications for the civil rights of the patient. Although the neuropsychologist does not make the final competency decision, he contributes to a process that is essentially moral in nature, rather than strictly legal or clinical.

It is important to realize in any form of competency hearing, competency itself is not universal. A person may be competent in one realm and not another, competent in one situation and not another, competent at one time and not another. Therefore the evaluation should be designed with a consideration of which variables would influence the competency of the patient for a given task, and in a given setting. Another important consideration is that cognitive impairment or even dementia does not necessarily indicate that an individual is not competent. However, the presence of dementia increases the probability that an individual may not be competent. Fazel, Hope, and Jocoby (1999) reported that in their sample, 20% of individuals who had been diagnosed with dementia were competent to make decisions regarding advance directives. Although a cognitive evaluation is an important first step in the evaluation of competency, in many cases, the cognitive evaluation alone may not provide sufficient information to make such a determination. The evaluating neuropsychologist must also consider the patient's ability to function in the recent past, the present, and in possible future circumstances (Fountoulakis & Despos, 2008). It is this estimation of future functioning in hypothetical situations that is the most difficult to make—and the most likely to have limitations in inter-rater reliability.

The first step would be to clarify which type of competency is at question. Determining the type of competency will help delineate which neuropsychological content areas are of importance. For example, arithmetic skill would be more pertinent to an evaluation of financial competency than for competency to consent to treatment. Executive functions would play a role in several types of competency, but would be essential in decisions related to independent living.

It would also be important to determine what types of physical limitations are present and how these would interact with the cognitive profile and demands of the task situation. For example, language-based deficits, especially deficits in receptive language skills, would curtail the ability to make reasonable decisions in one's own best interest because of limitations in the accuracy of information received by the patient. Physical impairment would compound the effects of any cognitive deficits related to competency to live independently.

The next step would be to choose instruments with adequate and appropriate normative information. In many, but not all of these situations, geriatric norms would be necessary. Additionally, it would be preferable to use norms that more closely approximate the descriptive characteristics of the patient. For example, for some neuropsychological instruments, norms are available for comparison with subjects living in a nursing home versus subjects living independently. Age and level of education are also important variables to consider. Gender and race may be important in some neuropsychological content areas, especially language-based skills. The most likely relevant content areas for assessment in competency are orientation, attention, memory, communication, perception, and executive functions.

The use of standardized test instruments is not the only component of these evaluations. After determining the cognitive status of the subject, the neuropsychologist should also assess the understanding of the individual regarding the variables surrounding the decision process. In determinations of competency to make medical decisions, the neuropsychologist should interview the subject regarding medical condition and treatment. Can the subject accurately describe the particulars of the diagnosis as well describe the treatments rendered so far? Does the individual understand what future treatment would entail and what the consequences of declining future treatment would be?

The clinical neuropsychologist should clarify the audience/client that will receive the information. For most competency questions, the recipient is a legal authority such as a magistrate or judge. These individuals may have varying degrees of knowledge and familiarity with neuropsychological constructs and terminology. It is important to keep professional jargon to a minimum and to describe the everyday consequences of the assessment results. For example, in reporting a memory impairment related to recalling only 12% of the WMS-III Logical Memory content over the standard delay, the neuropsychologist should be careful to include a statement that the subject will not remember textual or narrative material even if it is repeated once, and multiple repetitions may be necessary to insure that important material is actually encoded.

In addition to knowing the questions to be asked and the patient to be assessed, the neuropsychologist should know how the information is to be used. The clinical neuropsychologist needs to be conversant with the state laws and regulations regarding competency. In some states, for example, only a physician can sign the necessary paperwork to petition for a competency hearing. However, even in those situations, many physicians will not sign the forms without first reviewing the results of cognitive testing.

A second important set of information is the ecological validity of the test instruments chosen, and it should be examined carefully. In many instances, at both ends of the continuum of skill level, ecological validity may be less relevant. A person who scores well into the range of severe dementia is unlikely to possess fiduciary competency. In contrast, a person who scores in the above average range on cognitive measures is unlikely to be found incompetent. It is in the middle ranges, where a person scores in the moderate range of memory impairment and the moderately severe range of executive dysfunction, that it would be important to examine what types of limitations would be empirically supported.

Another facet of the clinical evaluation of competency is obtaining informed consent, which is somewhat different from the concept of consent in treatment or other assessment contexts. The most obvious facet of the evaluation is that the level of cooperation may differ drastically from that found in a typical clinical situation. The evaluation may be court ordered, and the outcome may have untoward effects, from the perspective of the subject. In court-ordered situations, the subject does not have the right to refuse assessment, although certainly, the subject retains control over behavioral aspects of cooperation. Depending upon the results, the person may lose aspects of personal freedom and autonomy. Poythress and colleagues (1999) discuss some of the concepts related to this type of consent in a criminal proceeding. Yet another complicating difference from usual treatment is that obtaining informed consent depends upon an assumption that the person is competent to provide consent when the outcome of the evaluation is a determination that the person does not possess competence to make those decisions and grant that consent. The clinician in those cases must document any information that is provided to the subject and make every effort to provide the information at a level of complexity that can be reasonable understood.

Because older individuals are at greater risk for cognitive impairment, they are frequently the subject of competency evaluations. This requires the use of instruments that have been standardized and empirically evaluated with older individuals. The American Bar Association and the American Psychological Association, jointly, have recently published a useful guide for conducting evaluations of older individuals (American Bar Association & American Psychological Association, 2008). This document provides useful information regarding general considerations as well as specific guidelines for evaluations of competency for medical decisions, sexual consent, and financial, testamentary, driving, and independent living competency. Additionally, the pragmatics of working with the legal system are presented.

An important element in some clinical evaluations for competency is the issue of detecting an exaggeration of impairment. The issue of exaggeration does not usually occur when the patient can be reasonably assumed to be motivated to give the best effort. However, just as in any clinical neuropsychological evaluation, the motivation to give best effort may be less than complete. Not all of these instances involve an individual who is trying to escape responsibility for an action by feigning cognitive impairment. Incomplete effort may also be the result of an individual who is somewhat impaired being evaluated in a context in which he or she fears the consequences of the evaluation and does not trust the health care professional involved. In either case, that of deliberate exaggeration or that of incomplete effort, it is necessary to make some objective evaluation of the level of effort expended by the patient. Wynkoop and Denney (1999) present a case of an attempt to magnify deficits during a pretrial competency evaluation. They suggest techniques that have also been used in general and forensic neuropsychological evaluations.

Review of Relevant Instruments

There are many clinical instruments available to the clinical neuropsychologist conducting a competency evaluation. These include the standardized and familiar tests of memory, attention, abstract problem solving, perception, and emotional functioning. There are also specialized instruments designed to evaluate content areas that would be important in the competency assessments. Golding (2008) provides a good overview of some of the important issues involved.

Competency to Live Alone

Yet another form of competency is related to independent living and the capacity to manage one's finances and personal decisions. Frequently these decisions are made within the context of cognitive testing results and observations regarding the person's performance in the open environment. Because of concerns about the limitations of formal cognitive testing in predicting everyday behavior, new instruments have been developed to evaluate practical skills in a more ecologically valid manner. The Independent Living Scales instrument (Loeb, 1996) is an example of such an instrument. The subscales include Memory/Orientation, Managing Money, Managing Home and Transportation, Health and Safety, and Social Adjustment. Because there is no external criterion for competence, there are no strict cutoff scores. But there are standard scores computed from a sample of 400 independent living adults over the age of 65. Additionally, optimal cutoff scores to separate these individuals from dependent living adults were calculated. It remains to be seen whether these scores and classifications will be accepted in court. Competency to live independently is a complicated construct because it involves many different aspects, including the ability to make personal decisions, understanding risks, the ability to complete activities of daily living, and the ability to take care of the dwelling place.

Instruments to Evaluate Competency to Consent to Treatment

The area of competency to consent to treatment has received the most attention from test developers. Most of the assessment procedures are simple and can be completed at bedside, an important practical consideration. However, the large majority of these instruments have been developed on a certain population, and their generalizability to other populations is unknown. Edelstein and colleagues devised an instrument to evaluate competency to consent to treatment for subjects in a long-term residential care facility (Edelstein, Nygren, Northrop, Staats, & Pool, 1993). This particular instrument combines direct questions with analog assessment of behavioral skills in areas related to competency decisions.

Janofsky, McCarthy, and Folstein (1992) developed the Hopkins Competency Assessment Test (HCAT), which can also be used at bedside. With this instrument, patients are given brief essays to read and are then asked to answer questions derived from the information contained in the essays and related to the issue of consent. Inter-rater reliability was adequate ($r = 0.95$). Validity was assessed by comparison with competency evaluations conducted by a board certified psychiatrist. Using the psychiatrist's ratings as the external criterion and an optimal cutoff point, 100% sensitivity and specificity was achieved in a limited sample of inpatients. Not surprisingly, the Hopkins Test was more accurate than the Folstein Mini Mental State Exam (MMSE) in determining competency.

Another approach to the assessment of competency is to combine measures of cognitive function and measures of competency-related operations. Pruchno, Smyer, Rose, Hartman-Stein, and Henderson-Laribee (1995) report the development of a short assessment instrument that combines the Folstein MMSE with questions regarding two vignettes that are read to the patient. The initial empirical investigation of the instrument indicated 86% accurate classification in a sample of residents of a long-term care facility.

Competency to Consent to Research

Competency to consent to research entails some of the same issues as consent to treatment. Individuals are asked to make decisions regarding sensitive aspects of their life. These decisions have serious implications for safety and health, and are based on complicated technical information. There is considerable concern regarding the competence of average individuals to consent to research such that the federal government has mandated the establishment of Institutional Review Boards (IRBs) to oversee research at hospitals and universities and ensure that study participants are making competent, informed decisions regarding participation in research protocols. There is special concern related to individuals with diminished capacity, and particular attention is paid to the protection of at-risk populations such as children and the elderly. Here the relation between context and competence mediated by facilitation is cast in high relief. Research has investigated the match between the demands of the consent process, as reflected by the reading level of the informed-consent document, and the education level of the potential participant (Christopher, Foti, Roy-Bujnowski, & Appelbaum, 2007). Olver, Whitford, Denson, Peterson, and Olver (2009) developed an interactive CD-ROM to facilitate understanding in patients receiving chemotherapy and to enhance their capacity to provide informed consent.

Competency to Make Medical Decisions

Marson and colleagues have developed an analog assessment instrument that presents the patient with hypothetical situations and then asks questions related to evidence for treatment choice, appreciating the consequences of the choice, providing rational reasons for the choice, and understanding treatment situation and choices. The answers are scored according to a standardized criterion that demonstrated adequate inter-rater reliability in a sample of patients with Alzheimer's disease (Marson, Ingram, Cody, & Harrell, 1995). The greatest single predictor of scores on the instrument developed by Marson was verbal fluency (Marson, Cody, Ingram, & Harrell, 1995). Subsequent research indicated that the four areas and scores could be interpreted as factors of verbal conceptualization and reasoning, and verbal memory (Dymek, Marson, & Harrell, (1999). Further research is needed to determine whether the scores can identify competent and incompetent individuals with diagnoses other than Alzheimer's disease.

The Competency Interview Schedule (Bean, Nishisato, Rector, & Glancy, 1994) is a brief bedside instrument designed to evaluate the competency of an individual to consent to medical treatment. It evaluates the patient's capacity in four areas, i.e., awareness of a choice, ability to understand the issues related to treatment, evidence of a rational reason for the choice, and appreciation of the nature of the situation. It has been reported to have reasonable internal consistency reliability (Cronbach's alpha = 0.96) and inter-rater reliability (intraclass r = 0.79). Initial research indicated that it could distinguish between competent and incompetent patients with low specificity (8%) and high sensitivity (98%).

It was earlier stated that competency to make decisions was situational and could be affected by the amount and type of support available. There is empirical evidence for these characteristics of competency in a study that evaluated the utility of a method to train and enhance the capacity of cognitively limited individuals to make decisions about advance directives related to psychiatric treatment, that is, the ability to make decisions related to giving someone else the power to decide about psychiatric treatment in the event of a debilitating psychiatric illness.

Elbogen and colleagues (2007) reported that in comparison with a treatment as a usual group, individuals assigned at random to a treatment involving meeting with a facilitator improved their capacity to make advance-directive decisions after 1 month. Although much of the focus has been on decisional capacity in older patients with illness leading to dementia, there is also some information related to patients with traumatic brain injury (Dreer, DeVivo, Novack, Krzywanski, & Marson, 2008).

Future Research

The existing assessment instruments are fragmented and frequently pertain only to a narrow population. Future research should focus on the development of broadly applicable, reliable, and valid assessment instruments. In particular, the external validity of the test instruments must be addressed. In this context, external validity would refer to both the relation to decisions made regarding competency independent of the assessment instrument (e.g., by the trier of fact) and to accurate prediction of the patient's ability to perform the relevant tasks accurately. Ecological validity is more of a concern here, perhaps, than in most other areas of clinical neuropsychological assessment.

The other major area of future research is to develop models for the assessment of different types of competency using existing assessment instruments of cognitive function. As a first step in the conceptualization of competency assessments, it would be important to have an agreed taxonomy of the skills necessary for the various forms of competency and the types of instruments that would be necessary to evaluate those skills. Second, research into the degree of impairment necessary to declare that a task is unlikely to be performed adequately would need to be performed. Finally, the cutoff points for the impairment ratings need to be validated against empirical observations of the patients, in the open environment, performing the relevant behaviors.

Conclusions

Competency evaluations carry their own set of values, challenges, and issues. However, this is an area in which clinical neuropsychologists have much to offer, and their contribution to this area of practice can be both challenging and rewarding. The objective evaluation and quantification of behavioral skills is a significant contribution to the legal process of deciding whether to assign culpability to, or restrict the personal freedoms of, individuals who come before the court. Decisions regarding competence are dependent upon information regarding cognitive status, contextual circumstances, extent of support available, and the demands of the particular type of competency process. The neuropsychologist working in this area must be aware of the clinical science supporting the procedures, as well as the legal definitions, regulations, and relevant rulings in the venue being served. Finally, the neuropsychologist must be aware of the significant moral implications of serving as an agent of social control, and must develop a level of comfort working in the adversarial context of our legal system.

References

American Bar Association & American Psychological Association. (2008). *Assessment of older adults with diminished capacity: A handbook for psychologists.* Washington, DC: Author.

Appelbaum, P. S., Mirkin, S. A., & Bateman, A. L. (1981). Empirical assessment of competency to consent to psychiatric treatment. *American Journal of Psychiatry, 138,* 1170–1176.

Appelbaum, P. S., & Roth, L. H. (1981). Clinical issues in the assessment of competency. *American Journal of Psychiatry, 138,* 1462–1467.

Barton, C. D., Malli, H. S., Orr, W. B., & Janofsky, J. S. (1996). Clinicians judgment of capacity of nursing home patients to give informed consent. *Psychiatric Services, 47,* 956–960.

Bean, G., Nishisato, S., Rector, N. A, & Glancy, G. (1994). The psychometric properties of the Competency Interview Schedule. *Canadian Journal of Psychiatry, 39,* 368–376.

Bloom, J. D., & Faulkner, L. R. (1987). Competency determinations in civil commitment. *American Journal of Psychiatry, 144,* 193–196.

Bonnie, R. J. (1997). Research with cognitively impaired subjects: Unfinished business in the regulation of human research. *Archives of General Psychiatry, 54,* 105–111.

Christopher, P. P., Foti, M. E., Roy-Bujnowski, K., & Appelbaum, P. S. (2007). Consent form readability and educational levels of potential participants in mental health research. *Psychiatric Services, 58,* 227–232.

Dreer, L. E., DeVivo, M. J., Novack, T. A., Krzywanski, S., & Marson, D. (2008). Cognitive predictors of medical decision-making capacity in traumatic brain injury. *Rehabilitation Psychology, 53,* 486–497.

Dymek, M. P., Marson, D. C., & Harrell, L. (1999). Factor structure of capacity to consent to medical treatment in patients with Alzheimer's disease: An exploratory study. *Journal of Forensic Neuropsychology, 1,* 27–48.

Edelstein, B., Nygren, M., Northrop, L., Staats, N., & Pool, D. (1993, August). *Assessment of capacity to make financial and medical decisions.* Paper presented at the 101st Meeting of the American Psychological Association. Toronto, CA.

Elbogen, E. B., Sweanson, J. W., Applebaum, P. S., Swartz, M. S., Ferron, J., VanDorn, R. A., et al. (2007). Competence to complete psychiatric advance directives: Effects of facilitated decision making. *Law and Human Behavior, 31,* 275–289.

Elliott, C. (1997). Caring about risks: Are severely depressed patients competent to consent to research? *Archives of General Psychiatry, 54,* 113–120.

Farnsworth, M. G. (1990). Competency evaluations in a general hospital. *Psychosomatics, 31,* 60–66.

Fazel, S., Hope, T., & Jocoby, R. (1999). Dementia, intelligence and the competence to complete advance directives. *Lancet, 354,* 48.

Fountoulakis, N., & Despos, K. (2008). Testamentary and financial competence issues in dementia. In G. Stoppe (Ed.), *Competence assessment in dementia* (pp. 71–75). New York: Springer Publishing Company.

Golding, S. L. (2008). Evaluations of adult adjudicative competency. In R. Jackson (Ed.), *Learning forensic assessment* (pp. 75–108). New York: Routledge.

Grossberg, G. T. (1998). Advance directives, competency evaluation, and surrogate management in elderly patients. *American Journal of Geriatric Psychiatry, 6,* S79–S84.

Hirschfield, R. M. A., Winslade, W., & Krause, T. L. (1997). Protecting subjects and fostering research. *Archives of General Psychiatry, 54,* 121–123.

Janofsky, J. S., McCarthy, R. J., & Folstein, M. F. (1992). The Hopkins Competency Assessment Test: A brief method for evaluating patients. *Hospital and Community Psychiatry, 43*(2), 646–648.

Karlawish, J., Kim, S. Y. H., Knopman, D., van Dyck, C. H., James, B. D., & Marson, D. (2008). Interpreting the clinical significance of capacity scores for informed consent in Alzheimer's disease clinical trials. *American Journal of Geriatric Psychiatry, 16,* 568–574.

Kaslow, N. J., Rubin, N. J., Bebeau, M. J., Leigh, I. W., Lichtenberg, J. W., Nelson, P. D., et al. (2007). Guiding principles and recommendations for the assessment of competence. *Professional Psychology: Research and Practice, 38,* 441–451.

Loeb, P. A. (1996). *Independent Living Scales: Manual.* San Antonio, TX: Psychological Corporation.

Marson, D. C., Cody, H. A., Ingram, K. K., & Harrell, L. E. (1995). Neuropsychological predictors of competency in Alzheimer's disease using a rational reasons standard. *Archives of Neurology, 52,* 955–959.

Marson, D. C., Ingram, K. K., Cody, H. A., & Harrell, L. E. (1995). Assessing the competency of patients with Alzheimer's disease under different legal standards. *Archives of Neurology, 52,* 949–954.

Martin, R., Griffith, H. R., Belue, K., Harrell, L., Zamrini, E., Anderson, B., et al. (2008). Declining financial capacity in patients with mild Alzheimer's disease: A one-year longitudinal study. *American Journal of Geriatric Psychiatry, 16*, 209–219.

Nicholson, R. A., & Kugler, K. E. (1991). Competent and incompetent criminal defendants: A quantitative review of comparative research. *Psychological Bulletin, 109*, 355–370.

Okonkwo, O. C., Wadley, V. G., Griffith, H. R., Ball, K., & Marson, D. C. (2006). Cognitive correlates of financial abilities in mild cognitive impairment. *Journal of the American Geriatrics Society, 54*, 1745–1750.

Okonkwo, O. C., Wadley, V. G., Griffith, H. R., Belue, K., Lanza, S., Zamrini, E. Y., et al. (2008). Awareness of deficits in financial abilities in patients with mild cognitive impairment: Going beyond self-informant discrepancy. *American Journal of Geriatric Psychiatry, 16*, 650–659.

Olver, I. N., Whitford, H. S., Denson, L. A., Peterson, M. J., & Olver, S. I. (2009). Improving informed consent to chemotherapy: A randomized controlled trial of written information versus an interactive multimedia CD-ROM. *Patient Education and Counseling, 74*(2), 197–204.

Otto, R. K., Poythress, N. G., Nicholson, R. A., Edens, J. F., Monahan, J., Bonnie, R.J., et al. (1998). Psychometric properties of the MacArthur Competence Assessment Tool–Criminal Adjudication. *Psychological Assessment, 10*, 435–443.

Palmer, B. W., & Savla, G. N. (2007). The association of specific neuropsychological deficits with capacity to consent to research or treatment. *Journal of the International Neuropsychological Society, 13*, 1047–1059.

Pruchno, R. A., Smyer, M. A., Rose, M. S., Hartman-Stein, P. E., & Henderson-Laribee, D. L. (1995). Competence of long-term care residents to participate in decisions about their medical care: A brief, objective assessment. *The Gerontologist, 35*, 622–629.

Roth, L. H., Meisel, A., & Lidz, C. W. (1977). Tests of competency to consent to treatment. *American Journal of Psychiatry, 134*, 279–284.

Schopp, R. F. (2001). *Competence, condemnation, and commitment*. Washington, DC: American Psychological Association.

Siegert, M., & Weiss, K. J. (2007). Who is an expert?: Competency evaluations in mental retardation and borderline intelligence. *Journal of the American Academy of Psychiatry and the Law, 35*, 346–349.

Spar, J. E., & Garb, A. S. (1997). Assessing competency to make a will. *American Journal of Psychiatry, 149*, 169–174.

Viljoen, J. L., & Roesch, R. (2008). Assessing adolescents' adjudicative competence. In R. Jackson (Ed.), *Learning forensic assessment* (pp. 291–312). New York: Routledge.

Wynkoop, T. F., & Denney, R. L. (1999). Exaggeration of neuropsychological deficit in competency to stand trial. *Journal of Forensic Neuropsychology, 12*, 29–53.

Zaubler, T. S., Viederman, M., & Fins, J. J. (1996). Ethical, legal, and psychiatric issues in capacity, competency, and informed consent: An annotated bibliography. *General Hospital Psychiatry, 18*, 155–172.

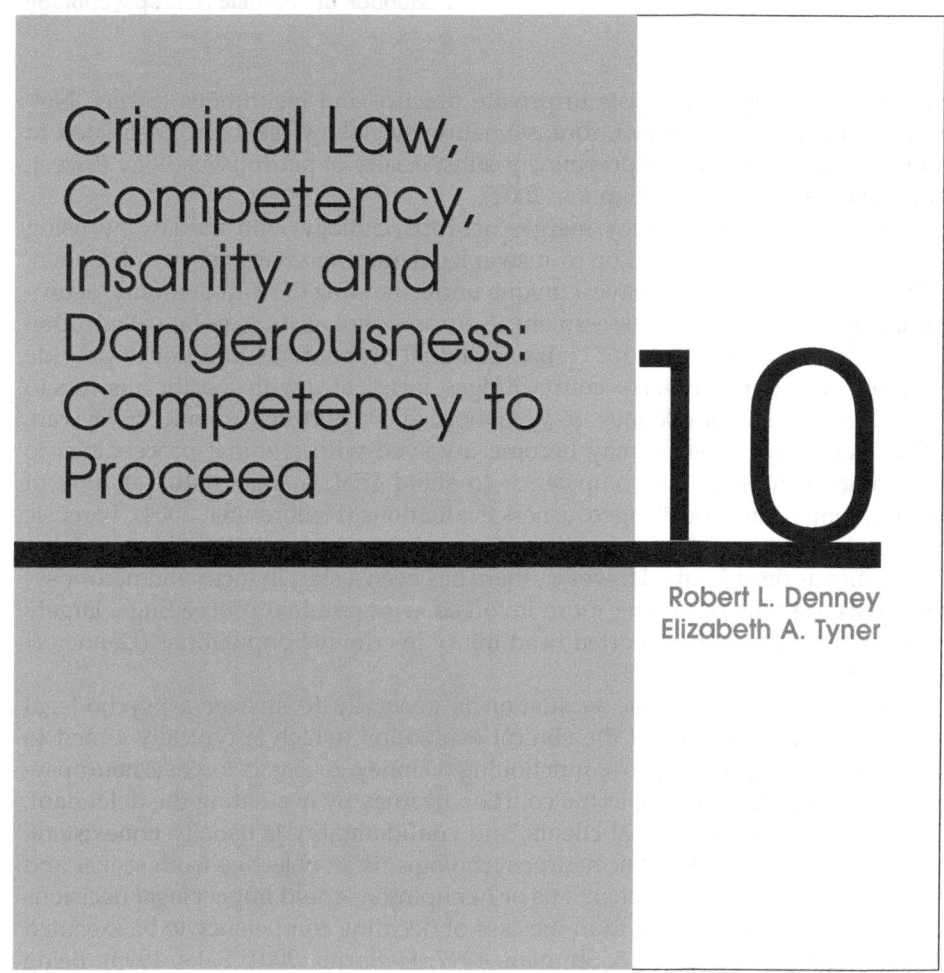

Criminal Law, Competency, Insanity, and Dangerousness: Competency to Proceed

10

Robert L. Denney
Elizabeth A. Tyner

This chapter provides an overview of criminal forensic neuropsychology, which includes discussion of competency, insanity, diminished capacity, and dangerousness. We present each of these issues from the perspective of the forensic neuropsychologist who is seeking to expand his or her practice in the area of criminal forensics.

Forensic Neuropsychology

Forensic neuropsychology is guided by the legal system and, thus, requires a basic understanding of that system's rules, laws, and legal processes. An increasing number of clinical neuropsychologists are performing forensic evaluations (Boake, 2008; Heilbronner, 2004). According to a 2005 professional practice survey of doctoral clinical neuropsychologists, participants revealed that much of their professional activities with adult clients were forensic in nature. Also, according to the survey, law was a frequent referral source for neuropsychological assessments for clinical neuropsychologists in private practice and institutions (Sweet, Nelson, & Moberg, 2006). In fact, forensic neuropsychology has been postulated to emerge in the future as the preeminent subspecialty of neuropsychology (Sweet, King, Malina, Bergman, & Simons, 2002).

Forensic neuropsychology merges neuropsychology with the law by using neuropsychological information to answer legal questions (Greiffenstein & Cohen, 2005). Neuropsychologists have a unique understanding of neuroanatomy, neuropathology, and functional assessment. Neuropsychologists may be called upon as consultants to the courts for civil or criminal proceedings in order to provide the triers of fact, (factfinders—courts, judges, juries, etc.) with specific answers to those legal questions (Denney & Wynkoop, 2000; Pirozzolo, Funk, & Dywan, 1991). Neuropsychologists may become involved with criminal proceedings to determine such issues as competency to stand trial, mental status at time of offense, sentencing, and dangerousness evaluations (Heilbronner, 2004). Forensic neuropsychology, in its infancy, seemed to revolve around civil litigation involving such issues as head injury. However, there has been a shift in focus and neuropsychologists are now becoming more involved with criminal proceedings, largely due to the high rate of purported head injury in criminal populations (Denney & Wynkoop, 2000; Martell, 1992).

The goal of the forensic evaluation is generally to answer a psycho-legal question, unlike the goal of the clinical evaluation, which is typically aimed to alleviate suffering and improve functioning (Denney, 2005a). A forensic neuropsychologist provides a service to the court or attorney by evaluating the defendant; defendants are not the actual clients, and confidentiality is usually nonexistent. In the legal context, a forensic neuropsychologist is an objective truth seeker and consultant to the judicial system. His or her opinions could impact legal decisions and potentially cause harm, as in the case of deciding competency to be executed (Denney, 2005a; Greenberg & Shuman, 1997; Heilbrun, 2001; Saks, 1990). Being mindful of ethical practice is important under all situations, but becomes truly imperative in this arena (see Bush, 2007; Bush, Grote, Johnson-Greene, & Macartney-Filgate, 2008; Grote & Parsons, 2005; Tyson & Sullivan, 2008). We now turn to evaluating competency to proceed, because it is the most common reason neuropsychologists become involved in the criminal judicial system.

Competency

Criminal Competency

In essence, *legal competency* means currently possessing effective knowledge and skills to perform certain functions that pertain to specific legal proceedings. This knowledge requires an understanding of issues such as the nature of proceedings, available options and strategies, and potential risks and outcomes (Denney, 2005a; Denney & Wynkoop, 2000; Reisner & Slobogin, 1990). The concept of legal competency further implies that individuals have a right to make decisions that control their lives, and also acknowledges that some individuals do not have the capacity to make potentially life-altering decisions. In a related manner, it requires the identification of individuals who are incompetent and protects not only their rights, but also the best interests of society (Grisso, Borum, Edens, Moye, & Otto, 2003).

Competency to Stand Trial

The examination of competency is rooted in English common law during the seventeenth century, elements of which were subsequently incorporated into American criminal law (Bardwell & Arrigo, 2002; Frederick, DeMier, & Towers, 2004; Marcopulos, Morgan, & Denney, 2008; Melton et al., 2007; Stafford, 2003). A very significant criminal competency case in the United States arose over 100 years ago in the case of *Youtsey v. United States* (1899). This case involving epilepsy, where memory and judgment were in question, ultimately established competency to proceed as a constitutional right in the United States.

In 1960 the U.S. Supreme Court ruled in a landmark case, *Dusky v. United States*, that a criminal defendant must not only be competent for criminal proceedings, but took *Youtsey* one step further by spelling out the minimal standard required for competency to proceed. Milton Dusky was arrested in 1958 for kidnapping and raping a fifteen-year-old girl. Before trial, he underwent an evaluation to determine if he was competent to stand trial. During the competency hearing, a psychiatrist testified that although Dusky was oriented to time, place, and person, he was still not able to understand the proceedings against him or assist in his defense due to severe mental illness (confused and irrational thinking). The judge concluded that Dusky was competent to stand trial because he was oriented to time, place, and person, and could assist in his defense. Dusky was tried and convicted. On appeal, the U.S. Supreme Court determined that criminal defendants must understand the nature of the proceedings against them and be able to assist in their defense. The Court held that merely being oriented to basics of the environment is not good enough to be considered competent, and thus presented this definition of competency:

> *The test must be whether the defendant has sufficient present ability to consult with his attorney with a reasonable degree of rational understanding and a rational as well as a factual understanding of the proceedings against him. (p. 4.02)*

The *Dusky* requirement established the constitutionally based minimum amount of competency to stand trial for all criminal jurisdictions within the United States. *Dusky* requires a twofold definition of competency, consisting of two prongs and two requirements. One can see that there are two prongs present: (a) capacity to understand the pending legal process (e.g., understanding basic roles of various legal participants such as the judge, attorneys, and jury), and (b) sufficient capacity to assist in a defense. The two requirements are having a *factual* and a *rational* understanding of both prongs. A factual understanding includes the ability to repeat and paraphrase information and incorporate that information into useful legal strategies. A rational understanding encompasses the ability to rationally manipulate that information using reasonably sound judgment and reality testing (Denney, 2005a; Marcopulos et al., 2008; Reisner & Slobogin, 1990).

Also included in the *Dusky* decision is the concept that a defendant have the *present ability* to meet these requirements, which concerns only the current and near future legal proceedings. That is, the *Dusky* standard does not apply to previous mental state during the time of the alleged criminal acts. All state and federal jurisdictions use the *Dusky* standard or a slight adaptation of it to guide proceedings to determine competency to stand trial (Favole, 1983; Grisso et al., 2003; Marcopulos et al., 2008).

Competency is a flexible concept, that is, it is not fixed for any individual (*Kenner v. United States*, 1960). It is not surprising, then, that a defendant could be found incompetent at a certain point in the criminal process, and then later be found competent. This happens quite frequently when dealing with defendants with a serious mental illness such as schizophrenia where treatment with antipsychotic medication often decreases psychosis and restores competency. It can also occur with reversible dementias, mental retardation, and other neurological concerns. Mental-health professionals must recognize this dynamic nature of mental status related to competency. Experts should explain this information to the courts and offer prognostic projections about current mental states and factors that could likely change mental states in the future (Frederick et al., 2004).

Competency can be addressed at any necessary point during the criminal judicial process. It can be dealt with as early as one's initial contact with law enforcement agents or as far along as sentencing or even execution of the person being evaluated (*Seidner v. United States*, 1958). Anyone involved in legal proceedings may raise the question of competency. Trial courts should consider any evidence from previous mental health opinions, or current irrational or concerning behavior. In fact, if there is any bona fide doubt about the defendant's competency, then competency must be evaluated as dictated by *Pate v. Robinson* (1966), and *Drope v. Missouri* (1975). This low standard is based upon the principle that it is better to delay legal proceedings to ensure that a defendant is competent than to try an incompetent defendant and deprive that defendant of their constitutional due process rights.

We have already discussed competency to stand trial, but there are other competencies specific to criminal law, including preconviction competencies (consenting to search or seizure, confession, waiver of right to counsel, waiver of right to trial, refusal of an insanity or other mental state defense, and testifying), and postconviction competencies (ability to be sentenced and executed) (Grisso, 1988; Grisso et al., 2003; Melton et al., 2007). Of the nine competency issues, the most frequently adjudicated is competency to stand trial, which has been referred to as the most important issue in forensic psychology (Bardwell & Arrigo, 2002; Melton et al., 2007), with approximately 60,000 competency evaluations occurring each year in the United States, according to the MacArthur Studies (cited in Melton et al., 2007).

We will briefly present the remaining types of criminal competencies and discuss the specialized contributions that neuropsychologists may provide to these evaluations, with two exceptions: competency to testify is subsumed within competency to stand trial, and competency to consent to search or seizure is rarely addressed by mental health professionals and is closely related to competency to confess. We recommend Melton and colleagues (2007) for a discussion of these issues.

Preconviction Competencies

Competency to Confess

Often in criminal cases, suspects are questioned prior to any arrests or legal proceedings. If these interrogations are not conducted properly, then information obtained during the process could be excluded in court. The Fifth Amendment of the U.S. Constitution affords the right to be free from self-incrimination, and the Sixth Amendment affords the right to legal counsel. The U.S. Supreme Court case *Miranda v. Arizona* (1966) upheld these constitutional rights, which became famously known as *Miranda* rights, that is, the right to remain silent. If a suspect waives the right to remain silent and legal representation, any statements could be used against him or her during criminal proceedings. The Court added that these statements must be provided *voluntarily, intelligently,* and *knowingly.* Subsequent cases have liberally defined these three terms in the context of police deception tactics (Melton et al., 2007).

Colorado v. Connelly (1986) is a U.S. Supreme Court case that pertains to mental disorder and coercion of confessions. In 1983 Francis Connelly confessed to a uniformed officer that he murdered a young girl. Connelly was repeatedly informed of his *Miranda* rights, but continued to provide detailed information of the murder. The police did not observe any symptoms of mental illness. During a preliminary hearing, the defense moved to suppress his confession based upon psychiatric testimony that, prior to his confession, he had ceased taking psychiatric medication for paranoid schizophrenia and that he was "compelled" to confess due to hallucinations from God. The defense asserted that Connelly was unable to freely and rationally choose to waive his rights to silence.

The U.S. Supreme Court held that Connelly's confessions could have been caused by his delusional thinking, but were not caused by police conduct. The Court asserted that no matter the defendant's mental state, confessions not caused by police are admissible in court if they are admissible by state law and if the defendant understood his right to remain silent. The Court concurred with the *Miranda* decision that the waiver of *Miranda* rights must be *knowing, intelligent,* and *voluntary. Miranda* and *Connelly* demonstrate that mental-health professionals can contribute to the issue of competency to make a confession when concerns exist regarding a defendant's knowledge or intelligence.

Competency to Waive Rights to Counsel or to Waive Rights to a Trial

The Sixth Amendment of the U.S. Constitution guarantees protection related to criminal proceedings in federal courts, including the right to a public trial and the right to counsel. The Due Process Clause of the Fourteenth Amendment of the U.S. Constitution provides the same protection for state proceedings. These rights, however, may be denied when a defendant is determined to be incompetent to waive rights to counsel (and act *pro se*) or incompetent to waive rights to a trial (and therefore plead guilty).

In 1993 the U.S. Supreme Court heard *Godinez v. Moran,* a landmark case that resolved inconsistencies between disparate standards for establishing competency to plead guilty and competency to waive counsel. In 1984 Richard Moran was charged with murdering a bartender, a saloon patron, and his ex-wife. After he killed his wife, he attempted suicide by shooting himself in the stomach and attempting to cut his wrists. During his hospital treatment, he confessed to the killings. Later, he pled not guilty. Upon evaluation, he was found competent to stand trial. He later changed his plea to guilty and dismissed his attorney. The trial court concluded that Moran "knowingly and intelligently" waived his right to counsel and "freely and voluntarily" pled guilty. Moran received the death penalty in 1985. Two years later, Moran filed for postconviction relief, stating he was incompetent to represent himself during his proceedings. His appeal was rejected by the trial court, the Nevada Supreme Court, and the U.S. District Court. The Court of Appeals for the Ninth Circuit reversed the decision, citing that under the Due Process Clause of the Fourteenth Amendment, Moran's competency should have been reevaluated before he was allowed to dismiss his attorney and plead guilty.

The U.S. Supreme Court heard the *Godinez* case to determine if the competency standard for pleading guilty and waiving counsel was higher than the *Dusky* competency standard for standing trial (as had been suggested by prior cases). The Court reaffirmed *Dusky* and determined that there is no reason for the standards to differ:

> *The decision to plead guilty, though profound, is no more complicated that the sum total of decisions that a defendant may have to make during the course of a trial, such as whether to testify, whether to waive a jury trial, and whether to cross-examine witnesses for the prosecution. Nor does the decision to waive counsel require an appreciably higher level of mental functioning than the decision to waive other constitutional rights. A higher standard is not necessary in order to ensure that a defendant is competent to represent himself, because the ability to do so has no bearing upon his competence to choose self-representation. (pp. 389–390)*

The U.S. Supreme Court very recently heard the case *Indiana v. Edwards* (2008) to again address if states may constitutionally adopt a higher standard for measuring competency to represent oneself at trial than for measuring competency to stand trial. In 1999, Ahmad Edwards attempted to steal a pair of shoes from a department store in Indiana. He fired a gun at a security officer and wounded a bystander. He was charged with attempted murder, battery with a deadly weapon, criminal recklessness, and theft. His mental condition (due to schizophrenia) became the subject of three competency proceedings and two self-representation requests. In 2004, the trial judge declared Edwards competent to stand trial but not competent to defend himself at trial. Edwards proceeded to trial in 2005 with appointed counsel. He was convicted of all counts by a jury and sentenced to thirty years in prison.

Edwards appealed, stating that the court deprived him of his Sixth Amendment right to self-representation under *Faretta v. California* (1975), and also that there should be no difference in the standards for competence to stand trial and for self-representation under *Godinez*. The Indiana Court of Appeals agreed with Edwards, ruling that because Edwards was found competent to stand trial, the court could not impose upon him a higher competency standard to determine if he could waive his right to counsel. A new trial was ordered. The Indiana Supreme

Court affirmed the Court of Appeal's decision. The U.S. Supreme Court then heard the case.

When reaching its decision, the Court considered information from five submitted *amici* (friend of the court) briefs and its previous decisions in *Dusky, Drope, Faretta,* and *Godinez*. The Court also weighed the autonomy of a defendant with judicial fairness. The Court held that states may deny self-representation "for those competent enough to stand trial," but who have such severe mental illness that renders them "not competent to conduct trial proceedings by themselves." Thus, the Court implied that there are more demands placed upon a defendant who represents him- or herself than on a defendant who participates in trial proceedings with the assistance of counsel. The Court indicated the *Dusky* standard as the minimum requirement, but states may adopt a higher standard for competency to waive the right to counsel because providing counsel actually provides more protection for constitutional rights.

Competency to Refuse an Insanity (or Other Mental State) Defense

In a later section of this chapter we provide a detailed discussion of insanity (also known as sanity, criminal responsibility, or mental state at time of the offense). Here, will we discuss the means of determination whether an individual is competent to refuse an insanity defense. This issue occurs when the facts of the case clearly provide evidence of insanity, but the defendant does not wish to raise an insanity defense. Naturally, the question of whether the defendant is making a competent decision appears. It is then up to the court to determine whether a defendant is competent to make such decisions.

In a District of Columbia Court of Appeals case, *Frendak v. United States* (1979), Paula Frendak was charged with first-degree murder and carrying a pistol without a license. She underwent four competency evaluations and the court ruled she was competent to stand trial. She was found guilty of both charges. Prior to sentencing, the judge ordered a criminal responsibility evaluation to determine her mental state at the time of the offense. The judge overruled her conviction and found her not guilty by reason of insanity, even though she refused to raise the insanity defense at trial. Frendak appealed. The Appeals Court concluded that an insanity plea may not be forced upon a defendant who is competent to stand trial if the defendant intelligently and voluntarily refused the insanity defense.

The court listed five legitimate, rational reasons for which a defendant might reject the insanity defense, including fear of a lengthier confinement in a mental health facility than the potential prison sentence, objection to the type or quality of treatment in a mental health facility, avoidance of the stigma associated with a finding of insanity, desire to avoid lifetime collateral consequences of an insanity acquittal (e.g., the right to vote, serve on a federal jury, obtain a driver's license), and the undermining of his or her political or religious views of the crime. Forensic evaluators should be mindful of these reasons for foregoing an insanity defense when evaluating whether or not a defendant is making an intelligent and voluntary legal decision (Denney, 2005a).

In summary, we have defined criminal competency and presented various types of criminal competencies that are relevant to legal proceedings that occur prior to conviction. We have discussed that according to current law, criminal defendants must have a rational and factual understanding of the nature of the charges against them, and the ability to properly assist in their defense. The concepts of *knowing, intelligent,* and *voluntary* must be evaluated when determining decisional competencies of defendants, including making confessions, representing oneself, pleading guilty, and rejecting an insanity plea. States may employ higher standards of competence for self-representation than for competence to stand trial. We will now discuss criminal competencies that are relevant to postconviction legal proceedings, which place less decision-making demands on criminal defendants.

Postconviction Competencies

Competency to Be Sentenced

A U.S. Court of Appeals for the Sixth Circuit case, *United States v. Liberatore* (1994, 1995), addresses the competency of a defendant to be sentenced. Anthony Liberatore was convicted of racketeering and money laundering in the U.S. District Court for the Northern District of Ohio in 1994. Hours before his sentencing, the defense motioned for a hearing to determine his competency to be sentenced. Liberatore was committed to an inpatient mental health facility and received a neuropsychological evaluation. The mental-health expert diagnosed him with probable primary degenerative dementia of the Alzheimer's type and opined that he was incompetent to be sentenced, due to poor ability to provide proper assistance (difficulty with reasoning defense strategies, and recalling content of previous discussions and speaking, due to memory deficits). However, the trial court concluded that Liberatore's deficits would not necessarily preclude his competency to be sentenced. The court held that when determining competency to be sentenced, an expert must: (a) reveal the defendant's mental capabilities, (b) discern the legal standard of competency, and (c) measure the defendant's capabilities against that standard.

The court noted that although the *Dusky* standard prevailed as the standard for competency to be sentenced, fewer demands are required of a defendant to be sentenced than to stand trial. Therefore, Liberatore's difficulty with reasoning and recall did not render him incompetent to be sentenced. The court considered the difficulty speaking caused by memory problems in light of *Green v. United States* (1961), a case that affords a defendant the right of allocution (to speak on his or her behalf and offer mitigating information at sentencing). The court explained that allocution is not concerned with memory lapse or mild speaking problems. Additionally, the Court ruled that speaking during sentencing required less mental acuity than providing testimony at a trial. The court ruled that Liberatore was competent to be sentenced and the decision was upheld on appeal. Mr. Liberatore died in a prison hospital dementia ward a few years later.

Competency to Be Executed and Waive Death Penalty Appeals

None of the fifty states allow a defendant to be executed if they are considered incompetent to be put to death. This is supported by the Eighth Amendment, which prohibits cruel and unusual punishment. The three cases described below are relevant regarding this issue.

The first is a U.S. Supreme Court case, *Ford v. Wainwright* (1986). In 1974, Alvin Ford was convicted of murder in Florida and sentenced to death. In 1982, while on death row, his mental status deteriorated, and he developed psychosis. He underwent a competency evaluation, per Florida law. There was conflicting opinion on this issue, but the Florida governor (not a judge) determined that Ford was competent to be executed (as per Florida statute). Ford appealed, arguing that Florida's law was unconstitutional and deprived him of due process rights. In a lengthy procedural case, the U.S. Supreme Court held that Florida's law was unconstitutional, and that a person must be competent at the time of execution. The Court did not provide a definition of competency regarding execution, but did reference Florida's standard that an individual should have the capacity to understand the nature of the death penalty and the reason it was imposed. A more specific definition is proposed by Reisner and Slobogin (1990), which states that the condemned must possess a sufficient understanding of any fact that would cause his or her punishment to be unjust or unlawful, and the intelligence to convey that information to the court or defense counsel. This latter definition is in line with the U.S. Supreme Court's ruling that it is unconstitutional to execute individuals with mental retardation (*Atkins v. Virginia*, 2002).

A more recent U.S. Supreme Court case, *Panetti v. Quarterman* (2007), reaffirmed *Ford*. Scott Panetti was sentenced to death in Texas for killing the parents of his estranged wife. Panetti sought appellate review on multiple occasions, to no avail. After an execution date was set, Panetti's defense claimed he was not competent to be executed due to mental illness. Panetti's execution was stayed so that he could be evaluated for competency. Mental health experts concluded that Panetti was malingering to avoid execution. Panetti claimed that the trial court's procedures did not comply with *Ford* procedures. The trial court ruled he was competent to be executed. Panetti returned to a federal district court, where it was ruled that the state courts had not complied with procedural requirements of *Ford*. Relief from execution was denied, however, because Panetti understood the "factual predicate" for his execution, which was enough to be considered competent.

The U.S. Supreme Court heard the case to determine whether it was constitutional to consider Panetti as competent to be executed based upon the decision of the lower courts. The Supreme Court reviewed previous testimony from defense and prosecution experts. Testimony from the defense experts revealed Panetti's delusional beliefs that his execution was a type of spiritual warfare between demonic and angelic forces. Panetti claimed to understand that Texas wanted him executed for the murder he committed, but due to his delusional thinking, he also believed the state wanted him to be executed to stop him from preaching. The experts for the state agreed that Panetti was mentally ill, but opined that his delusions did not make him incompetent. It ruled that the *Ford* standard holds today, and that if a person does not have a rational understanding of the reason for his or her execution, then retribution or deterrence will not be achieved.

When individuals receive the death-penalty, they receive legal representation, including appeals filed on their behalf, regardless of their desire for this to occur. If a prisoner refuses a death-penalty appeal, they are essentially volunteering for their execution. According to Cunningham and Goldstein (2003), it is not rare for death row prisoners to develop mental health problems. Appellate courts, not surprisingly then, request competency evaluations for prisoners who waive rights to their appeals as well (Denney, 2005a). Overall, the standards for being found competent to be sentenced or executed do not differ much from the criteria used to determine competency to stand trial. There should be a factual and rational understanding of the reasons for, and consequences of, sentencing or executing.

Competency Restoration

In most cases, upon being found incompetent, a person will undergo competency restoration treatment. States vary in the amount of time an individual will have for this treatment, which usually occurs in an inpatient mental-health facility. The treatment typically entails administration of psychiatric medication, and group or individual psychotherapy. As we discussed earlier, competency is a dynamic concept, and often incompetent individuals can be restored to competency within a relative short time period. Nevertheless, there are limitations on the length of time an individual may be subjected to this treatment, and there are guidelines for the administration of involuntary medication.

A U.S. Supreme Court case, *Jackson v. Indiana* (1972), is related to the issue of detaining an individual who is found incompetent to stand trial. Theon Jackson was arrested for two misdemeanor robberies (a misdemeanor crime can result in a prison sentence of no more than one year). He was deaf, mute, and mentally retarded. He was found incompetent to stand trial and was committed to a state treatment facility. After well over a year had passed, his counsel requested a new hearing because he had been confined beyond the time he would have served if convicted of the misdemeanor crimes. The U.S. Supreme Court held that a criminal defendant cannot be confined past a reasonable amount of time without additional civil commitment proceedings. If a defendant is found not restorable (not likely to be restored to competency within the foreseeable future), that defendant must be either released or civilly committed (if dangerous to others or their property).

The U.S. Supreme Court case of *Sell v. U.S.* (2003) addresses whether or not individuals who are found incompetent to stand trial can be involuntarily medicated for the sole purpose of restoring competency to stand trial. The Court held that involuntary medication to restore competency to stand trial is acceptable in some circumstances. The Court suggested that in making this determination, trial courts should first consider whether a person is dangerous to self or others, based upon the guidelines set forth in *Washington v. Harper* (1990). If a defendant is deemed dangerous, then trial courts should authorize involuntary medication. Short of dangerousness, the trial court must resolve four separate issues, each affirmatively, to justify involuntary medication. These four issues include: (1) whether there are important government interests (i.e., the seriousness of the crime); (2) whether those interests will be significantly furthered by medication; (3) whether the medication is necessary, with no lesser intrusive alternatives; and (4) whether such medication is medically appropriate.

One particularly thorny issue related to involuntary treatment includes forcing medication on individuals found not competent for execution just to restore their competency to proceed (Denney, 2005a). In *State v. Perry* (1992) the Supreme Court of Louisiana held that it is cruel, excessive, and unusual punishment to "medicate to execute" a prisoner. However, the U.S. Court of Appeals for the Eighth Circuit provided a different view of this concept in *Singleton v. Norris* (2003). This court ruled that it is constitutional to involuntarily medicate a prisoner, even if that prisoner became incompetent on death row, because the state's interest to carry out the sentence outweighed Singleton's liberty interest to be free from psychotropic medication. The U.S. Supreme Court chose not to review the case (*Singleton v. Norris*, 2003), and he was executed in 2004.

Competency Evaluation for the Neuropsychologist

By now it is clear that the determination of competency is a complex process and involves various steps. Grisso and colleagues (2003) proposed five components of legal competency that should guide competency assessments: functional, causal, interactive, judgment, and dispositional. *Functional* relates to the specific abilities, behaviors, beliefs, and capacities directly related to the competency issue and legal situation. The functional component should be assessed through observation and testing to determine whether an individual understands basic legal proceedings and can properly assist his or her attorney with the defense. Identification of symptoms of mental illness and diagnoses are secondary to this determination of functionality. An example of this is determining whether a defendant with mild traumatic brain injury understands potential outcomes of the charges against him or her.

The *causal* component involves identifying and describing the underlying cause of incompetence. An example might include severe memory loss due to normal pressure hydrocephalus that prevents the defendant from recalling court-room happenings. The *interactive* component emphasizes that each legal situation demands specific capabilities, and refers to situational demands and the defendant's ability to meet those particular demands. This is highlighted by the more stringent requirement needed to act as one's own attorney compared with the requirement needed to stand trial with the assistance of counsel.

The *judgment* component refers to making the actual professional determination of competency by deciding if functional deficits preclude the defendant from being able to understand the charges and proceedings or being able to assist in the defense. One must keep in mind that mental-health professionals provide expert opinions, but the trial court (i.e., judge) makes the final determination. The final component, *disposition*, occurs when the defendant is considered incompetent and involves formulating a treatment plan to address deficits in the hope of restoring competency. This last component is important because of the need to have an idea of whether the defendant could be restored to competency and what it might take to accomplish. A relevant example would involve a defendant who was found incompetent to stand trial due to brain injury secondary to a gunshot wound to the head. The trial court ideally needs to know about the natural course of the condition, what would reasonable treatment entail, the probable duration of that treatment, and how likely it would be that the defendant could regain enough abilities to become competent.

Neuropsychologists can draw upon their knowledge of brain-behavior relationships, normal and abnormal cognitive functioning, nervous system functioning, and psychopathology to assist courts with legal questions such as competency to stand trial. In a study of 1,710 criminal defendants referred from U.S. federal courts, 18% were incompetent to stand trial. Defendants with mental retardation were found incompetent 30% of the time, and defendants with organic mental disorder were found incompetent 38% of the time (Cochrane, Grisso, & Frederick, 2001). Another study found that incompetent defendants were commonly diagnosed with schizophrenia, mental retardation, mood disorder, and organic brain disorders (Warren, Fitch, Dietz, & Rosenfeld, 1991). These findings suggest that many incompetent defendants meet criteria for brain disorder, emphasizing the importance for neuropsychologists in forensic evaluations.

Additionally, neuropsychologists can contribute their unique knowledge of symptom validity testing to forensic evaluations (Larrabee, 2005). Individuals involved in criminal proceedings could be tempted to present psychological and neurocognitive deficits to delay or avoid legal consequences (i.e., malinger). It has been estimated that malingering is present in anywhere from 8–21% of evaluations for competency to stand trial (Cornell & Hawk, 1989; Rogers, Salekin, Sewell, Goldstein, & Leonard, 1998; Rogers, Sewell, & Goldstein, 1994; Vitacco, Rogers, Gabel, & Munizza, 2007). Exaggeration of mental illness seems to become more problematic when criminal defendants are evaluated for neurocognitive and memory complaints. Negative response bias rates were detected for approximately 50–70% of 105 presentence male defendants referred for neurocognitive concerns. In that sample, approximately 20% of defendants performed below chance on two-alternative, forced-choice psychological tests (Ardolf, Denney, & Houston, 2006). Denney (2007) took that same set of data and extracted only those defendants who claimed, or had documentation of, mild or moderate closed-head injury. Seventy-three percent performed below cutoffs on two or more measures of negative response bias. These studies demonstrate the need for the neuropsychologists to assess for feigned or exaggerated cognitive problems in criminal defendants. Denney (2007, 2008) provides detailed discussions of this issue, including different psychological tests that may be used to detect malingering or exaggerated cognitive complaints.

Special Competency Issues in Forensic Neuropsychology

Neuropsychologists may provide unique contributions in competency evaluations when the issues of amnesia, traumatic brain injury (TBI), and mental retardation arise. Neuropsychologists have training in memory function and testing that can assist with amnesia claims. Neuropsychologists can contribute their knowledge of TBI severity and sequelae that could impact functioning. Mental retardation, when present, is extremely important in competency determinations. Neuropsychologists have the ability to determine the severity of the retardation and its impact on competency issues.

Amnesia

Criminal defendants may claim memory loss or impairment following the alleged criminal activity. Feigned amnesia should be expected to occur in some forensic evaluations, as a number of studies reveal approximately 30% of criminals assert they cannot remember their crimes (e.g., Cima, Nijman, Merckelbach, Kremer, & Hollnack, 2004; Gudjonsson, Petursson, Skulason, & Sigurdardottir, 1989; Taylor & Kopelman, 1984). The task of teasing out feigned from genuine amnesia, once presumed difficult, is now possible given the advances of neuropsychological research in the areas of test development and symptom validity theory (Denney, 2005a; Marcopulos et al., 2008; Schacter, 1986). Amnesia may be organic and secondary to cerebral dysfunction, psychogenic-based secondary to trauma or other psychiatric conditions, or malingered (Cima et al., 2004).

Because amnesia is commonly claimed and is most likely done so in effort to avoid criminal responsibility, courts have been hesitant to equate amnesia with incompetence (Melton et al., 2007). In the U.S. Court of Appeals for the District of Columbia case, *Wilson v. United States* (1968), the Court held that a defendant with genuine amnesia may be competent, and unless the only way the defense counsel can obtain important evidence is by the defendant's account of the crime, the trial may occur, even if the defendant has no recollection of the crime.

TBI

TBI ranges in magnitude of severity. Mild cases without significant loss of consciousness (with high scores on the Glasgow Coma Scale) usually do not cause lasting cognitive impairment. Postconcussion deficits typically disappear within weeks or months (Mittenberg & Roberts, 2008). Moderate to severe TBI cases are generally followed by lasting cognitive deficits that range from mild to extremely severe, depending upon severity of the injury and neurological impairment (Roebuck-Spencer & Sherer, 2008). Therefore, the more severe the injury, the greater the likelihood that competence could be affected.

Mental Retardation

The U.S. Supreme Court recently overruled *Penry v. Lynaugh* (1989) with *Atkins v. Virginia* (2002), when it held that individuals with mental retardation cannot receive the death penalty. The Court ruled that these individuals may have diminished culpability for criminal actions, but do not warrant exemption from criminal consequences. The Court reasoned that executing a person with mental retardation would constitute "cruel and unusual punishment," and noted that the retribution and deterrence effect of capital punishment was likely not applicable for mentally retarded individuals. The Court also concluded that individuals with mental retardation are confronted with disproportionately high risk of execution because of the increased chance of false confessions, reduced effectiveness of counsel, poor witness capacity, and the wrongful assumption that they lack remorse (due to demeanor).

Mental retardation is an important issue for competency hearings because all competency issues relate to cognitive function. Courts have recognized that mental retardation consists of different levels of severity, and have ruled that mental retardation in and of itself does not meet the *Dusky* standard. The neuropsychologist must evaluate a mentally retarded individual's capacity to factually and rationally understand the charges and the nature of the proceedings, and to properly assist counsel, as well as consider these abilities related to the complexities and demands of the legal case.

Competency Assessment Measures

Melton and colleagues (2007) indicate that psychological testing is not always a necessity, but can contribute significantly to the outcome of a forensic evaluation.

We assert that when neurocognitive concerns arise in a competency evaluation, it is optimal to include neuropsychological testing. We will present below the three most common assessment measures for competency to stand trial (Archer, Buffington-Vollum, Stredny, & Handel, 2006). We refer the reader to Grisso and colleagues (2003) for a detailed description of other competency measures.

The Evaluation of Competency to Stand Trial–Revised (ECST-R) (Rogers, Tillbrook, & Sewell, 2004) was developed in 2004 to assess psycholegal capabilities related to competency to stand trial set forth in *Dusky*. The ECST-R is a semistructured interview that includes 18 items separated into four competency scales. The ECST-R assesses for malingered incompetency to stand trial, with the inclusion of 28 additional items that are separated into five atypical-response style scales. Scoring information from the competency scales is combined with case-specific information (e.g., complexity of particular case, specific impairments) to guide the evaluator into an overall interpretation.

The MacArthur Competence Assessment Tool–Criminal Adjudication (MacCAT-CA; Poythress et al., 1999) was developed based upon research generated by the MacArthur Foundation Research Network on Mental Health and the Law. This instrument is a semistructured interview that can be used before and after adjudication of competence to proceed, and may also be employed to monitor treatment gains of individuals who are involved in competency restoration treatment. The MacCAT-CA has 22 items that are separated into three competency-relevant domains. A vignette is provided to assess the defendant's understanding and reasoning abilities, as applied to a novel criminal situation. Appreciation is evaluated based upon the defendant's current circumstances. The scores assist the administrator in evaluating a defendant's overall abilities.

The Competence Assessment for Standing Trial for Defendants with Mental Retardation (CAST*MR) (Everington & Luckasson, 1992) is a fifty-item instrument designed for use by forensic evaluators when evaluating competency in adult defendants with mental retardation. It is separated into three sections that correspond to *Dusky* criteria. The sections on basic legal concepts and the ability to assist defense include multiple-choice items. The questions on understanding case events are posed in an open-ended format.

Criminal Responsibility

Criminal responsibility, a term used interchangeably with *insanity* (or *sanity*, or even *mental state at the time of the offense*), refers to a determination of mental state during retrospective criminal activity. For instance, a criminal defendant could have been so demented when he stole a bicycle that he may not be held legally responsible for his actions. If brain pathology could have contributed to criminal activity, a neuropsychologist may be asked to perform a criminal-responsibility assessment. The role of the neuropsychologist would be to educate the court or jury, or both, on whether there was any neuropathological cause of altered mental state during the crime that would mitigate or eliminate that individual's culpability. The trier of fact then determines if the individual was insane during the commission of the crime. In the case above, if the defendant were found not guilty by reason of insanity, he would then be excused for the crime.

Insanity is a legal concept that provides understanding to those who cannot be morally blamed for their criminal actions because of some sort of impairment that prevents rational decisions or voluntary actions, or both. Insanity is only one of six categories that may excuse (to some degree) defendants for their crimes. The other five are diminished capacity, intoxication, infancy, entrapment, and duress or coercion (*Congressional Quarterly*, 2005; Yates & Denney, 2008). We will discuss insanity and diminished capacity, and briefly mention intoxication. Coercion could pertain to criminal defendants who falsely believe, because of mental illness, that they are being coerced. If this circumstance were to occur, a mental-health evaluation would likely be guided by insanity or diminished-capacity standards. Entrapment is related to actions of law enforcement individuals, not mental health, and will not be discussed here. We refer the reader to Wynkoop (2008) for an overview of the question of maturation (infancy) as it pertains to neuropsychology in the juvenile justice system.

Criminal acts comprise two aspects: *actus reus* (physical act) and *mens rea* (guilty mind). The determination that a person is criminally responsible for a crime goes beyond the establishment that the act was committed, and requires the demonstration of *mens rea* (Dressler, 2001). The six categories listed above, if affirmed, could preclude an individual from having the *mens rea* for committing a crime.

Insanity

As stated earlier, insanity is a legally defined concept that has changed in meaning over time with statutory development (Yates & Denney, 2008). The U.S. Supreme Court case *Powell v. Texas* (1968) reflects this evolutionary phenomenon. The Court has not ruled the insanity defense to be a constitutional right. Although states vary in their application of its use, most jurisdictions incorporate a version of the M'Naghten (1843) "right/wrong" test (now codified in large part in the federal jurisdiction as part of the Insanity Defense Reform Act IDRA), or a version of the American Law Institute's (1955) Model Penal Code (ALI) standard.

ALI

In 1962, the American Law Institute adopted the Model Penal Code of 1955 to assist legislatures and standardize United States laws. Included in the code is a definition of insanity known as the ALI standard. This standard encompasses two aspects of insanity: cognition and volition. It states that a defendant is insane if, as a result of mental disease or defect, he or she cannot appreciate criminality (or wrongfulness), or conform his or her conduct to the requirements of the law. This definition emphasizes both understanding one's behavior and being able to control one's behavior. The federal system adopted this standard in 1972, and it remains applicable in many states (Yates & Denney, 2008).

IDRA

In 1981 John Hinckley, Jr., shot President Ronald Reagan, his press secretary James Brady, and two law enforcement officers. Experts concluded that he had a delusional disorder causing him to believe that if he assassinated the president, a particular famous actress would be impressed. He was found not guilty by reason of insanity because he was considered to lack the volitional component of the ALI standard. There was significant societal outrage that Hinckley was not going to be criminally punished for his actions. As a result, the Insanity Defense Reform Act (IDRA) was included in the 1984 Crime Control Act.

IDRA currently presides in federal law and the majority of state jurisdictions. This standard redefined insanity to exclude the volitional component and brought it back to close proximity to the M'Naghten (1843) "right/wrong" standard. It required the mental disease or defect to be "severe." IDRA also changed insanity to an affirmative defense, meaning that the defense must prove by clear and convincing evidence that the defendant was insane at the time of the offense in the federal system. Previously the burden was on the prosecution to disprove insanity once the issue was raised. The standard also reflected the view that mental-health experts could exert too much influence over the jury and, consequently, added Federal Rule of Evidence, 704(b), which states that mental-health professionals cannot provide an opinion to the jury on whether a defendant was sane or insane at the time of the offense. IDRA requires that once a federal defendant is acquitted because of insanity, he or she is committed to the U.S. Attorney General's custody for secure hospitalization and treatment. That individual is considered dangerous due to mental illness until the courts determine otherwise.

Neuropsychologists must be knowledgeable about the presiding insanity standards in their practice jurisdictions. Additionally, it is imperative to understand the legal terminology in insanity statutes, such as ability, capacity, nature, quality, and wrongfulness. We refer the reader to Yates and Denney (2008) or Denney (2005b) for a detailed presentation on such definitions.

Many people are surprised to learn that insanity defenses are rarely raised, and insanity acquittals are very infrequent (Silver, Cirincione, & Steadman, 1994; Steadman et al., 1993). The majority of forensic neuropsychological evaluations include neurocognitive problems that are low in severity and do not excuse criminal behavior (Melton et al., 2007; Yates & Denney, 2008). Organic mental disorders are only represented in a small percentage of individuals who raise the insanity defense or are acquitted by reason of insanity. Psychotic or mood disorders are instead more often present in such situations (Cochrane et al., 2001; Denney & Wynkoop, 2000; Melton et al., 2007; Nestor & Haycock, 1997; Rogers & Shuman, 2000; Steadman et al., 1993).

Diminished Capacity

Whereas insanity implies no culpability for criminal actions, diminished capacity refers to decreased (but not excused) responsibility for criminal actions. One common cause of diminished capacity is intoxication (Marlowe, Lambert, & Thompson, 1999). Intoxication could trigger aggression or impulsivity, by interfering with executive functions. This, in turn, could interfere with ability to inform *specific intent*, which is a requisite element of certain criminal activities. Precluding general intent could only occur if an individual were intoxicated to the point of delirium, dissociation, or psychosis (Yates & Denney, 2008). See Keiter (1997) for more information on the intoxication defense.

Similar to intoxication, TBI may cause impulsivity and other problems with poor judgment and reasoning that could render an individual to have diminished capacity (Richardson, 1990). More frequently, however, this issue would be addressed during sentencing as a mitigating factor to lessen punishment, under the concept of *diminished responsibility* (Yates & Denney, 2008).

Criminal Responsibility Assessment

Assessment of criminal responsibility is retrospective and requires a comprehensive evaluation. Information should be obtained pertaining to developmental, educational, social, occupational, medical, psychiatric, and legal history. Investigative materials are absolutely necessary to compare with the defendant's account of the alleged events. Central to this type of evaluation is a detailed interview of the defendant about the events, with special attention given to the time directly preceding and directly following the alleged crime. A current mental-status examination should also be completed. The examiner should consider any information that would suggest that the defendant might not be able to control his or her behavior or understand the nature, consequences, or wrongfulness of the actions involved.

According to a recent survey (Archer et al., 2006), there is only one commonly used measure for criminal responsibility evaluations, the Rogers Criminal Responsibility Assessment Scales (R-CRAS) (Rogers, 1984). This measure contains thirty items relevant to psycho-legal issues of criminal responsibility. The first part of the instrument assists the evaluator with the establishment of degree of impairment at the time of the offense. The second part assists with the generation of an opinion on criminal responsibility, guided by the ALI, Guilty But Mentally Ill, or M'Naghten standards. The test appears to be used infrequently, even by forensic psychologists (Archer et al., 2006).

Dangerousness

Conroy and Murrie (2007) noted that risk assessment is becoming increasingly prevalent in forensic psychology settings. The authors presented a broad risk-assessment model to assist evaluators with predictions of future violence. Their model contains six stages: (a) defining the question, (b) considering normative data and population base rates, (c) considering empirically supported risk and protective factors, (d) considering idiographic risk factors, (e) communicating risk-assessment results, and (f) linking risk assessment to risk management. This model could be helpful for neuropsychologists who are involved in criminal proceedings in evaluating a defendant's future risk for violence, which can be relevant in cases of neurological compromise (Volavka, Martell, & Convit, 1992).

Assessing future risk of violence is also referred to as *assessing dangerousness.* Like competency, dangerousness may be at issue during any stage of criminal proceedings, and it may also arise during detention hearings. In the federal system, dangerousness assessments are almost automatic upon a defendant: (a) being found incompetent to stand trial and not restorable, (b) being found not guilty by reason of insanity, and (c) when a sentenced inmate who is potentially dangerous due to a mental illness reaches the end of his or her sentence. These situations warrant dangerousness assessments because, according to federal law, individuals who are dangerous to others or the significant property of others due to mental illness cannot be released to society. In fact, these individuals could be held in a secure hospital indefinitely if their dangerousness does not subside. When an individual is committed to a secure hospital due to dangerousness, their commitment to that facility becomes a civil legal issue. Nevertheless, evaluators will continue to assess for dangerousness over a fixed period of time and report to the committing court (e.g., annually). Most states follow similar statutory procedures (Denney, 2005b).

Dangerousness assessments have important repercussions. According to Melton and colleagues (2007), "there is no other area of the law in which expert testimony may exert so significant an impact" (p. 299). In a 1983 U.S. Supreme Court Case, *Barefoot v. Estelle*, Dr. James Grigson, without ever meeting the defendant Barefoot, testified that Barefoot was a threat to society because there was a "one hundred percent and absolute chance" that he would commit violent acts in the future. The Court permitted expert testimony even though the defendant had not been personally examined; however, Dr. Grigson provided an opinion that was grossly overstated with enormous implications for Barefoot. Modern practice discourages such crude assessments. Current best-practice predictions of dangerousness are founded in scientific prediction.

Research on risk assessment is vast and mainly concerns prediction. Thus, predictor variables for future violence have been identified and divided categorically. One division includes static versus dynamic factors, and another includes dispositional, historical, contextual, and clinical measures. This latter scheme was incorporated by Monahan and colleagues (2001) with their MacArthur Violence Risk Assessment Study, which was the largest study of community violence prediction to date (Monahan, 2003). Predictor variables from this study included prior violence and criminal behavior, gender (males more likely to invoke serious injury), history of childhood physical abuse, substance abuse coupled with mental illness, anger, suspiciousness and violence thoughts, and living in a high-crime neighborhood. Although their study is a landmark in the prediction of dangerousness, only a few participants had neurological concerns. As a result, neurological compromise and its impact on future, postdischarge violence was not thoroughly assessed.

Neuropathology and Violence

Many parts of the brain are related to behavioral inhibition. Neurobiological factors contribute to aggressive and violent behavior. In the past few decades, technological advances have permitted the neuropsychological study of aggression and violence. Researchers have identified associations between aggression and frontal-lobe dysfunction, executive function deficit, and decreased serotonin, to name a few. We refer the reader to Denney (2005b) and Barr (2008) for more thorough reviews.

Dangerousness Measures

To assess dangerousness, evaluators often use risk-assessment measures that identify individual characteristics. These characteristics have been extensively researched and empirically validated, and do not vary based upon population with regard to incarcerated individuals or individuals housed in psychiatric facilities (secure or general population) (Bonta, Law, & Hanson, 1998; Quinsey, Harris, Rice, & Cormier, 2006). Although there is disagreement regarding the superiority of actuarial over clinical prediction of dangerousness (Odeh, Zeiss, & Huss, 2006; Quinsey et al., 2006; Webster, Hucker, & Bloom, 2002), actuarial prediction has improved with the development of risk-assessment tools (Monahan, 2003). As a result, there is a push in the field of forensic psychology to use these tools for prediction of dangerousness (Quinsey et al., 2006).

Three common measures for assessing risk for future violence are the Psychopathy Checklist–Revised (PCL-R) (Hare, 2003), the Violence Risk Appraisal Guide (VRAG) (Quinsey et al., 2006), and the HCR–20 (Webster, Douglas, Eaves, & Hart, 1997), which will be discussed below.

The PCL-R measures psychopathy and future dangerousness. This measure has been highly praised by researchers and clinicians and has been called the "standard of practice instrument" (Meloy, 2000) and "the gold standard" (Edens, Skeem, Cruise, & Cauffman, 2001). The 20 items are scored based upon collateral information and a semistructured interview. Although it is the gold standard, the PCL-R requires specialized training to perform the interview and also to rate information obtained from records.

The HCR-20 is a 20-item checklist used to assist with future decisions regarding prediction of violence and risk management planning for civilly committed, forensic, and criminal-justice populations. Items are scored based upon collateral information and interviews. This measure yields a probability estimate of future risk within a specific time frame based upon static and dynamic factors that are related to violent behavior. Clinicians can also use this measure to identify treatment goals to reduce the risk of future violence.

The VRAG comprises 20 items that assess for the presence of static, historical items to predict the future risk of offenders' commiting a violent crime within ten years of release into the community. The items are weighted to reflect predictive value, and scores can be separated into nine categories to guide evaluators in estimates of probability of violence by an offender when released. One item measures psychopathy, so this measure includes administration of the PCL-R.

The assessment of future risk for dangerousness is, by necessity, a multidimensional process. Again, we refer the interested reader to Conroy and Murrie (2007). Their model of assessment provides a framework that will prove invaluable for neuropsychologists aspiring to perform risk-assessment evaluations.

Summary

In writing this chapter, we aspired to provide a summary of the core areas with which neuropsychologists must become familiar in order to begin the practice of criminal forensic neuropsychology. We addressed the general issues related to competency to proceed in its various forms. We presented the legal concepts of sanity and diminished capacity, as well as a brief overview of the neurobiology of violence and dangerousness assessment. Any one of these topics could easily span an entire book, so we were, by necessity, brief. We will leave the reader with one last matter that relates to all of the preceding. Neuropsychologists choosing to begin practice in the area of criminal forensics, must fully understand the relevant statutory and case law related to the areas of concern within their practicing jurisdictions. More than once we have seen well-meaning clinical psychologists and neuropsychologists enter the criminal forensic forum without having the correct understanding of the legal definition of competency or sanity within that jurisdiction. Professional ethics demand competency to enter a new area of practice. We would also challenge clinicians to move beyond the basic minimum standards, and strive for truly authentic and exceptional professional competence (Sullivan & Denney, 2008).

References

American Law Institute. (1955). *Model penal code*. Philadelphia: Author.

Archer, R. P., Buffington-Vollum, J. K., Stredney, R. V., & Handel, R. W. (2006). A survey of psychological test use patterns among forensic psychologists. *Journal of Personality Assessment, 87,* 84–94.

Ardolf, B. R., Denney, R. L., & Houston, C. M. (2006). Base rates of negative response bias and malingered neurocognitive dysfunction among criminal defendants referred for neuropsychological evaluation. *Clinical Neuropsychologist, 21,* 899–916.

Atkins v. Virginia, 536 U.S. 304 (2002) 260 Va. 375, 534 S.E.2d, 312, reversed and remanded.

Bardwell, M. C., & Arrigo, B. A. (2002). Competency to stand trial: A law, psychology, and policy assessment. *The Journal of Psychiatry & Law, 30,* 147–269.

Barefoot v. Estelle, 103 S.Ct. 3383 (1983).

Barr, W. B. (2008). Neuropsychological approaches to criminality and violence. In R. L. Denney & J. P. Sullivan (Eds.), *Clinical neuropsychology in the criminal forensic setting* (pp. 238–272). New York: Guilford Press.

Boake, C. (2008). Clinical neuropsychology. *Professional Psychology: Research and Practice, 39,* 234–239.

Bonta, J., Law, M., & Hanson, R. K. (1998). The prediction of criminal and violent recidivism among mentally disordered offenders: A meta-analysis. *Psychological Bulletin, 123,* 123–142.

Bush, S. S. (2007). *Ethical decision making in clinical neuropsychology.* New York: Oxford University Press.

Bush, S. S., Grote, C. L., Johnson-Greene, D. E., & Macartney-Filgate, M. (2008). A panel interview on the ethical practice of neuropsychology. *Clinical Neuropsychologist, 22,* 321–344.

Cima, M., Nijman, H., Merckelbach, H., Kremer, K., & Hollnack, S. (2004). Claims of crime-related amnesia in forensic patients. *International Journal of Law and Psychiatry, 27,* 215–221.

Cochrane, R., Grisso, T., & Frederick, R. I. (2001). The relationship between criminal charges, diagnoses, and psycho-legal opinions among federal defendants. *Behavioral Sciences and the Law, 19,* 565–582.

Colorado v. Connelly, 479 U.S. 157 (1986).

Congressional Quarterly. (2005). Supreme Court Collection., Retrieved October 11, 2005, from http://www.cqpress.com

Conroy, M. A., & Murrie, D. C. (2007). *Forensic assessment of violence risk: A guide for risk assessment and risk management.* Hoboken, NJ: Wiley.

Cornell, D., & Hawk, G. (1989). Clinical presentation of malingerers diagnosed by experienced forensic examiners. *Law and Human Behavior, 13,* 375–383.

Cunningham, M. D., & Goldstein, A. M. (2003). Sentencing determinations in death penalty cases. In I. B. Weiner (Series Ed.) & A. M. Goldstein (Vol. Ed.), *Handbook of psychology: Vol. 11, Forensic psychology* (pp. 407–436). Hoboken, NJ: Wiley .

Denney, R. L. (2005a). Criminal forensic neuropsychology and assessment of competency. In G. L. Larrabee (Ed.), *Forensic neuropsychology: A scientific approach* (pp. 378–424). New York: Oxford University Press.

Denney, R. L. (2005b). Criminal responsibility and other criminal forensic issues. In G. L. Larrabee (Ed.), *Forensic neuropsychology: A scientific approach* (pp. 425–465). New York: Oxford University Press.

Denney, R. L. (2007). Assessment of malingering in criminal forensic neuropsychological settings. In K. B. Boone (Ed.), *Assessment of feigned cognitive impairment: A neuropsychological perspective* (pp. 428–452). New York: Guilford Press.

Denney, R. L. (2008). Negative response bias and malingering during neuropsychological assessment in criminal forensic settings. In R. L. Denney & J. P. Sullivan (Eds.), *Clinical neuropsychology in the criminal forensic setting* (pp. 91–134). New York: Guilford Press.

Denney, R. L., & Wynkoop, T. F. (2000). Clinical neuropsychology in the criminal forensic setting. *Journal of Head and Trauma Rehabilitation, 15,* 804–828.

Dressler, J. (2001). *Understanding criminal law* (3rd ed.). New York: Matthew Bender.

Drope v. Missouri, 420 U.S. 162 (1975).

Dusky v. United States, 362 U.S. 402 (1960).

Edens, J. F., Skeem, J. L., Cruise, K. R., & Cauffman, E. (2001). Assessment of "juvenile psychopathy" and its associations with violence: A critical review. *Behavioral Sciences and the Law, 19,* 53–80.

Everington, C. T., & Luckasson, R. (1992). *Competence assessment for standing trial for defendants with mental retardation: Test manual.* Worthington, OH: IDS Publishing Corporation.

Faretta v. California, 422 U.S. 806 (1975).

Favole, R. J. (1983). Mental disability in the American criminal process: A four-issue survey. In J. Monahan & H. Steadman (Eds.), *Mentally disordered offenders: Perspectives from law and social science.* New York: Plenum Press.

Frederick, R. I., DeMier, R. L., & Towers, K. (2004). *Examinations of competency to stand trial: Foundations in mental health case law.* Sarasota, FL: Professional Resource Press.

Frendak v. United States, 408 A2d 364 (1979).

Ford v. Wainwright, 477 U.S. 399 (1986).

Godinez v. Moran, 509 U.S. 389 (1993).

Green v. United States, 365, U.S. 301 (1961).

Greenberg, S. A., & Shuman, D. W. (1997). Irreconcilable conflict between therapeutic and forensic roles. *Professional Psychology: Research and Practice, 28,* 50–57.

Greiffenstein, M. F., & Cohen, L. (2005). Neuropsychology and the law: Principles of productive attorney-neuropsychologist relations. In G. L. Larrabee (Ed.), *Forensic neuropsychology: A scientific approach* (pp. 29–91). New York: Oxford University Press.

Grisso, T. (1988). *Competency to stand trial evaluations: A manual for practice.* Sarasota, FL: Professional Resource Press.

Grisso, T., Borum, R., Edens, J. F., Moye, J., & Otto, R. K. (2003). *Evaluating competencies: Forensic assessments and instruments* (2nd ed.). New York: Kluwer Academic/Plenum.

Grote, C. L., & Parsons, T. D. (2005). Threats to livelihood of the forensic neuropsychological practice: Avoiding ethical misconduct. *Journal of Forensic Neuropsychology, 4,* 79–93.

Gudjonsson, G. H., Petursson, H., Skulason, S., & Sigurdardottir, H. (1989). Psychiatric evidence: A study of the psychological issues. *Acta Psychiatrica Scandinavica, 80,* 165–169.

Hare, R. D. (2003). *Hare Psychopathy Checklist-Revised (PCL-R): 2nd edition technical manual.* North Tonawand, NY: Multi-Health Systems.

Heilbronner, R. L. (2004). A status report on the practice of forensic neuropsychology. *Clinical Neuropsychologist, 18,* 312–326.

Heilbrun, K. (2001). *Principles of forensic mental health assessment.* New York: Kluwer Academic/Plenum.

Indiana v. Edwards, 866 N.E.2d 252 (2008), vacated and remanded.

Jackson v. Indiana, 406 U.S. 715 (1972).

Keiter, M. (1997). Just say no excuse: The rise and fall of the intoxication defense. *Journal of Criminal Law and Criminology, 87,* 482–520.

Kenner v. United States, 286 F.2d 208 (8th Cir., 1960).

Larabee, G. J. (2005). A scientific approach to forensic neuropsychology. In G. J. Larrabee (Ed.), *Forensic neuropsychology: A scientific approach* (pp. 3–28). New York: Oxford Press.

Marcopulos, B. A., Morgan, J. E., & Denney, R. L. (2008). Neuropsychological evaluation of competency to proceed. In R. L. Denney & J. P. Sullivan (Eds.), *Clinical neuropsychology in the criminal forensic setting* (pp. 176–203). New York: Guilford Press.

Marlowe, D. B., Lambert, J. B., & Thompson, R. G. (1999). Voluntary intoxication and criminal responsibility. *Behavioral Sciences and the Law, 17,* 195–217.

Martell, D. A. (1992). Estimating the prevalence of organic brain dysfunction in maximum-security forensic psychiatric patients. *Journal of Forensic Sciences, 37,* 878–893.

Meloy, J. R. (2000). *Violence risk and threat assessment.* San Diego, CA: Specialized Training Services.

Melton, G. B., Petrila, J., Poythress, N. G., Slobogin, C., Lyons, P. M., & Otto, R. K. (2007). *Psychological evaluations for the courts: A handbook for mental health professionals and lawyers* (3rd ed.). New York: Guilford Press.

Miranda v. Arizona, 384 U.S. 436 (1966).

Mittenberg, W., & Roberts, D. M. (2008). Mild traumatic brain injury and post concussion syndrome. In J. E. Morgan & J. H. Ricker (Eds.), *Textbook of clinical neuropsychology* (pp. 430–436). New York: Taylor & Francis.

M'Naghten's Case, 10 Clark & Finnelly 200 (1843).

Monahan, J. (2003). Violence risk assessment. In I. B. Weiner (Series Ed.) & A. M. Goldstein (Vol. Ed.), *Handbook of psychology: Vol. 11: Forensic psychology* (pp. 527–540). Hoboken, NJ: John Wiley.

Monahan, H., Steadman, H. J., Silver E., Applebaum, P. S., Robbins, P. C., Mulvey, E. P., et al. (2001). In J. Monahan & H. J. Steadman (Eds.), *Violence and mental disorder: Developments in risk assessment.* Chicago: University of Chicago Press.

Nestor, P. G., & Haycock, J. (1997). Not guilty by reason of insanity of murder: Clinical and neuropsychological characteristics. *Journal of the American Academy of Psychiatry and Law, 25,* 161–171.

Odeh, M. S., Zeiss, R. A., & Huss, M. T. (2006). Cues they use: Clinicans' endorsement of risk cues in predictions of dangerousness. *Behavioral Sciences and the Law, 24,* 147–156.

Panetti v. Quarterman, 127 S. Ct. (2007).

Pate v. Robinson, 383 U.S. 375 (1966).

Penry v. Lynaugh, 492 U.S. 302 (1989).

Pirozzolo, F. J., Funk, J., & Dywan, J. (1991). Neuropsychology and its applications to the legal forum. In J. Dywan, R. D. Kaplan, & F. J. Pirozzolo (Eds.), *Neuropsychology and the law* (pp. 1–26). New York: Springer-Verlag.

Powell v. Texas, 392 U.S. 514; L.Ed 2d 1254 (1968).

Poythress, N. G., Nicholson, R., Otto, R. K., Edens, J. F., Bonnie, R. J., Monahan, J., et al. (1999). *The MacArthur Competence Assessment Tool-Criminal Adjudication professional manual.* Lutz, FL: Psychological Assessment Resources.

Quinsey, V. L., Harris, G. T., Rice, M. E., & Cormier, C. A. (2006). *Violent offenders: Appraising and managing risk* (2nd ed.). Washington, DC: American Psychological Association.

Reisner, R., & Slobogin, C. (1990). *Law and the mental health system* (2nd ed.). St. Paul, MN: West.

Richardson, J. T. E. (1990). *Clinical and neuropsychological aspects of closed head injury.* New York: Taylor & Francis.

Roebuck-Spencer, T., & Sherer, M. (2008). Moderate and severe traumatic brain injury. In J. E. Morgan & J. H. Ricker (Eds.), *Textbook of clinical neuropsychology* (pp. 411–429). New York: Taylor & Francis.

Rogers, R. (1984). *Rogers Criminal Responsibility Assessment Scales (R-CRAS) and test manual.* Odessa, FL: Psychological Assessment Resources.

Rogers, R., & Shuman, D. (2000). *Conducting insanity evaluations* (2nd ed.). New York: Guildford Press.

Rogers, R., Salekin, R. T., Sewell, K. W., Goldstein, A., & Leonard, K. (1998). A comparison of forensic and nonforensic malingerers: A prototypical analysis of explanatory models. *Law and Human Behavior, 22,* 353–367.

Rogers, R., Sewell, K. W., & Goldstein, A. (1994). Explanatory models of malingering: A prototypical analysis. *Law and Human Behavior, 18,* 543–552.

Rogers, R., Tillbrook, C. E., & Sewell. K. W. (2004). *The evaluation of competency to stand trial: Revised professional manual.* Sarasota, FL: Psychological Assessment Resources.

Saks, M. J. (1990). Expert witnesses, nonexpert witnesses, and nonwitness experts. *Law and Human Behavior, 14,* 291–313.

Schacter, D. L. (1986). Amnesia and crime: How much do we really know? *American Psychologist, 41,* 286–295.

Seidner v. United States, 260 F.2d 732 (D. C. Cir. 1958).

Sell v. United States, 539 U.S. 166 (2003).

Silver, E., Cirincione, C., & Steadman, J. H. (1994). Demythologizing inaccurate perceptions of the insanity defense: Legal standards and clinical assessment. *Applied and Preventative Psychology, 2,* 163–178.

Singleton v. Norris, 319 F.3d. 1018 (8th Cir., 2003), 124 S. Ct. 74 (2003).

Stafford, K. P. (2003). Assessment of competence to stand trial. In A. M. Goldstein (Series Ed.) & I. B. Weiner (Vol. Ed.), *Handbook of psychology, Vol. 11: Forensic psychology* (pp. 359–380). Hoboken, NJ: John Wiley.

State v. Perry, 610 So.2d. 746 (1992).

Steadman, H. J., McGreevey, M. A., Morrissey, J. P., Callahan, L. A., Robbins, P. C., & Cirincione, C. (1993). *Before and after Hinckley: Evaluating insanity defense reform.* New York: Guilford Press.

Sullivan, J. P., & Denney, R. L. (2008). A final word on authentic professional competence in criminal forensic neuropsychology. In R. L. Denney & J. P. Sullivan (Eds.), *Clinical neuropsychology in the criminal forensic setting* (pp. 391–400). New York: Guilford Press.

Sweet, J. J., King, J. H., Malina, A. C., Bergman, M. A., & Simons, A. (2002). Documenting the prominence of forensic neuropsychology at national meetings and in relevant professional journals from 1990 to 2000. *Clinical Neuropsychologist, 16,* 481–494.

Sweet, J. J., Nelson, N. W., & Moberg, P. J. (2006). The TCN/AACN 2005 "Salary Survey": Professional practices, beliefs, and incomes of U.S. neuropsychologists. *Clinical Neuropsychologist, 20,* 325–364.

Taylor, P. J., & Kopelman, M. D. (1984). Amnesia for criminal offences. *Psychological Medicine, 14,* 581–588.

Tyson, J. A., & Sullivan, J. P. (2008). Ethical issues in criminal forensic neuropsychology. In R. L. Denney & J. P. Sullivan (Eds.), *Clinical neuropsychology in the criminal forensic setting* (pp. 30–54). New York: Guilford Press.

United States v. Liberatore, 546 F. Supp. 569 (N.D. Ohio, 1994).

United States v. Liberatore, 62 F.3d 1418 U.S. App. (1995).

Vitacco, M. J., Rogers, R., Gabel, J., & Munizza, J. (2007). An evaluation of malingering screens with competency to stand trial patients: A known-groups comparison. *Law and Human Behavior, 31,* 249–260.

Volavka, J., Martell, D., & Convit, A. (1992). Psychobiology of the violent offender. *Journal of Forensic Sciences, 37,* 237–251.

Warren, J., Fitch, L., Dietz, P., & Rosenfeld, B. (1991). Criminal offense, psychiatric diagnosis, and psychological opinion: An analysis of 894 pretrial referrals. *Bulletin of the American Academy of Psychiatry and the Law, 19,* 63–69.

Washington v. Harper, 494 U.S. 210 (1990).

Webster, C., Douglas, K., Eaves, D., & Hart, S. D. (1997). *HCR-20: Assessing risk for violence (Version 2).* Vancouver, BC: Simon Frasier University.

Webster, C. D., Hucker, S. J., & Bloom, H. (2002). Transcending the actuarial versus clinical polemic in assessing risk for violence. *Criminal Justice and Behavior, 29,* 659–665.

Wilson v. United States, 391 F.2d 460 (D.C. Cir. 1968).

Wynkoop, T. F. (2008). Neuropsychology in the juvenile justice system. In R. L. Denney & J. P. Sullivan (Eds.), *Clinical neuropsychology in the criminal forensic setting* (pp. 295–325). New York: Guilford Press.

Yates, K. F., & Denney, R. L. (2008). Neuropsychology in the assessment of mental state at the time of the offense. In R. L. Denney & J. P. Sullivan (Eds.), *Clinical neuropsychology in the criminal forensic setting* (pp. 204–237). New York: Guilford Press.

Youtsey v. United States, 97 F. 937, 940 (6th Cir. 1899).

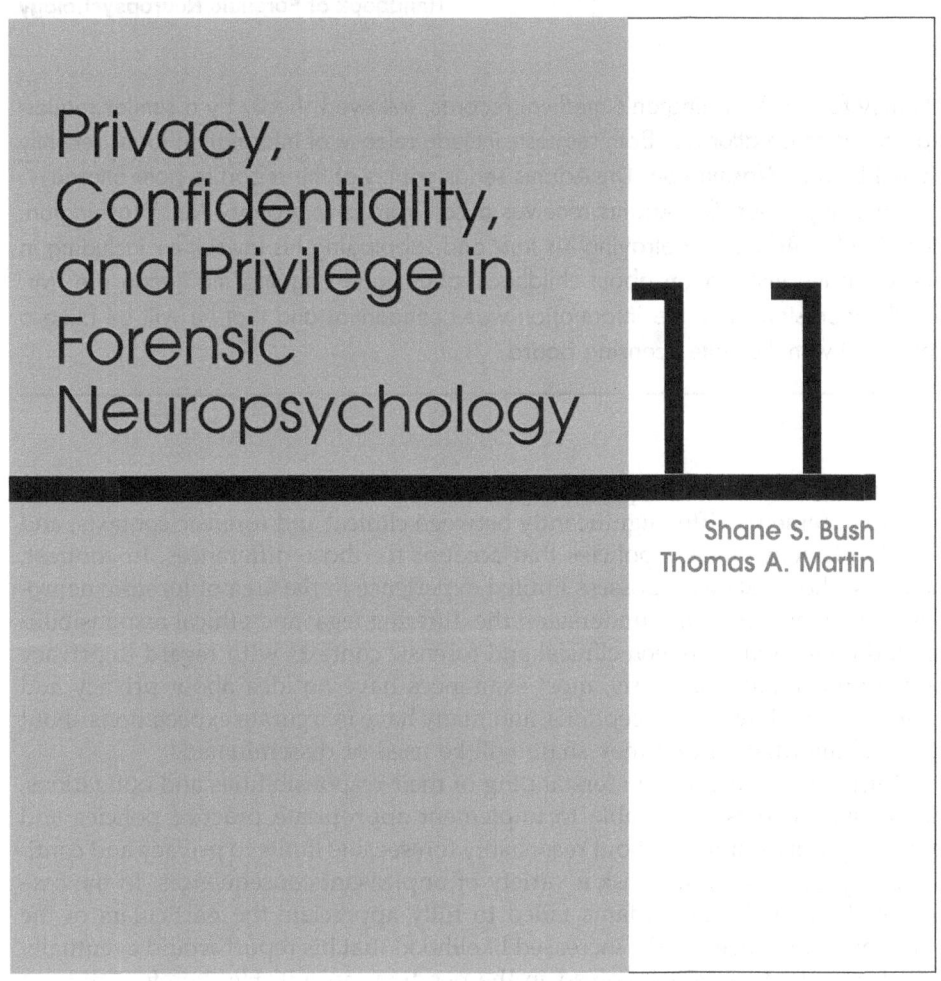

Privacy, Confidentiality, and Privilege in Forensic Neuropsychology

11

Shane S. Bush
Thomas A. Martin

Mr. Washington is referred by his primary medical doctor to Dr. Adams for a neuropsychological evaluation to clarify the nature and extent of his neurocognitive and emotional problems that reportedly emerged following a motor-vehicle accident. The accident occurred 6 months prior to the initial neuropsychological appointment, and Mr. Washington has brought a lawsuit against the driver of the other vehicle.

Upon arrival at Dr. Adams' office, Mr. Washington completes basic paperwork, including no-fault insurance papers and a consent form. The consent form describes Dr. Adams' mandated reporting requirements, such as when statements of danger to oneself or others are made. The consent form also states that a copy of the report will be sent to the referring doctor. Mr. Washington has no questions, and he completes and signs the forms as instructed.

During the clinical interview, Mr. Washington describes his childhood as abusive and states that he has used marijuana daily for many years. The interview and testing are completed in the usual manner, and the report is written and sent to the referring physician. Three months later Dr. Adams receives a request from Mr. Washington's attorney for Mr. Washington's medical records, followed shortly by a similar request from the defense attorney. Both requests include release of information forms recently signed by Mr. Washington. Dr. Adams sends copies of the report to both attorneys.

Two days later, Dr. Adams receives a call from a very angry Mr. Washington, accusing Dr. Adams of betraying his trust and sabotaging his lawsuit by including in the report the information about childhood abuse and ongoing marijuana use. Mr. Washington states that the information was confidential and that he will be filing a complaint with the state licensing board.

Experienced forensic neuropsychologists understand that privacy and confidentiality requirements differ significantly between clinical and forensic contexts, and they implement practice policies that account for those differences. In contrast, neuropsychologists who possess limited experience in the area of forensic neuropsychology may not fully understand the differing legal and ethical responsibilities and obligations between clinical and forensic contexts with regard to privacy and confidentiality. Similarly, most examinees have no idea about privacy and confidentiality laws and exceptions, and many have inaccurate expectations about how the information that they share will be used or disseminated.

Without an adequate understanding of their responsibilities and obligations, neuropsychologists are unable to implement appropriate practice policies and cannot inform examinees about reasonably foreseeable limits to privacy and confidentiality. Therefore, they risk a variety of unpleasant consequences. In the case of Mr. Washington, Dr. Adams failed to fully appreciate the particulars of the situation or to anticipate the increased likelihood that his report would eventually be released to attorneys involved in the pending lawsuit. He therefore did not fully inform Mr. Washington that the information that was conveyed in the context of the neuropsychological evaluation could be disseminated well beyond the referring physician. This oversight was perpetuated by Dr. Adams' routine practice of using a standardized informed consent form that is offered to patients for their signature without the benefit of an interactive process between the patient and a qualified neuropsychologist that would promote appreciation of the particulars of their specific case and a mutual understanding of how the findings would be used and disseminated.

The goals of this chapter are to present the legal, ethical, and practical considerations pertaining to privacy, confidentiality, and privilege in the context of forensic neuropsychological practice, and to offer suggestions for anticipating, avoiding, and addressing related problems. Although the primary focus of this chapter is on privacy, confidentiality, and privilege in the context of forensic neuropsychology, recent publications have addressed these issues in the contexts of clinical neuropsychology (Bush & Martin, 2008) and forensic psychology (Bush, Connell, & Denney, 2006). Readers are reminded that, although some statements and examples regarding privacy and confidentiality are widely applicable, unique variations and exceptions may be encountered in different professional contexts, settings, and jurisdictions, making it important to understand the topic in the specific context of one's own practice and jurisdiction.

Concepts and Definitions

Privacy, confidentiality, and privilege (described in the following sections) are related terms pertaining, in the present context, to the protection of communications from patients to neuropsychologists.

Privacy refers to freedom from unauthorized intrusion into one's life (*Webster's 9th New Collegiate Dictionary*, 1988), including one's thoughts, feelings, beliefs, and experiences (Smith-Bell & Winslade, 1999). Privacy is based on the individual's right to self-determination and the right to be protected from harm—and is, therefore, a core societal value (Behnke, Perlin, & Bernstein, 2003).

Confidentiality is a subset of privacy that represents the responsibility of the neuropsychologist to not disclose information shared by the patient in the professional relationship.

Privilege, a narrower concept than confidentiality, relieves neuropsychologists from having to testify in court about patients' communications. By *invoking privilege*, patients prevent treating neuropsychologists from testifying or releasing records about intimate personal details shared in the context of the professional relationship (Beauchamp & Childress, 2001; Behnke, Perlin, & Bernstein, 2003; Koocher & Keith-Spiegel, 1998). By *waiving privilege*, patients permit treating neuropsychologists to testify or release records in legal proceedings. Thus, privilege is held by patients and is invoked or waived at their choosing. In the absence of a privilege statute or a common-law rule, neuropsychologists can be charged with contempt of court for refusing to testify about information shared by patients in professional contexts (Smith-Bell & Winslade, 1999). Compared with clinical contexts in which neuropsychologists provide clinical evaluations or treatment, there are significant limitations to privacy, confidentiality, and privilege in forensic contexts. This issue is addressed in more depth in subsequent sections of the present chapter.

Legal Considerations

The U.S. Supreme Court has recognized privacy as a constitutional right (*Eisenstadt v. Baird*, 1972; *Griswold v. Connecticut*, 1965; *Hawaii Psychiatric Society v. Ariyoshi*, 1979), with the specific rights and restrictions regarding privacy established at both federal and state levels. However, the protection of sensitive personal information shared by patients has limitations (*Bowers v. Hardwick*, 1985; *Roe v. Wade*, 1973; *Tarasoff v. Regents of the University of California*, 1976; *Whalen v. Roe*, 1976). In forensic neuropsychology, a primary limitation to privacy and confidentiality is inherent in the context of the service. When individuals place their mental state at issue in a legal matter, certain rights are waived in the interest of justice, including the right to privacy of relevant information.

Discovery requirements, as established in the Federal Rules of Evidence (1975), allow the defense (in civil litigation) access to all relevant information, including neuropsychological records. Additionally, in forensic contexts in which neuropsychologists are retained by a third party, such as an attorney, the person being evaluated is not the client. The forensic examiner-examinee relationship differs in important ways from the doctor-patient relationship that exists in clinical contexts (Bush et al., 2005), including control over the release of confidential information.

Typically, the retaining party is the client and the holder of privilege, and is therefore responsible for making decisions regarding the release of information obtained in the course of the neuropsychological evaluation.

In recent years the Health Insurance Portability and Accountability Act (HIPAA) (U.S. Department of Health and Human Services, 2003) has provided increased security of protected health information in clinical contexts. HIPAA is a federal statute that regulates the manner in which patient information is maintained, used, and disclosed. HIPAA's privacy rule governs the privacy of health-care information in clinical contexts. However, HIPAA constraints are limited in forensic evaluation contexts (Connell & Koocher, 2003; Fisher, 2003). Specifically, HIPAA states that information compiled in anticipation of use in civil, criminal, and administrative proceedings is not subject to the same right of review and amendment that is typically afforded to general health-care information (see §164.524(a)(1)(ii)) (U.S. Department of Health and Human Services, 2003). In addition, HIPAA's privacy rule allows health-care providers to disclose protected health information in response to a court order (see §164.524), with disclosure limited to the information explicitly covered by the order.

Ethical Considerations

The ethics code of the American Psychological Association (APA; 2002) and related professional guidelines, for example, the *Standards for Educational and Psychological Testing* (American Educational Research Association, American Psychological Association, & National Council on Measurement in Education, 1999), inform neuropsychologists about their ethical and professional responsibilities regarding privacy and confidentiality.

Although neuropsychologists, like other clinicians, generally have a primary obligation to protect confidential information (see APA Ethical Standard 4.01, Maintaining Confidentiality), Ethical Standard 4.05 (Disclosures) provides guidance regarding the release of confidential information. Specifically, neuropsychologists may disclose confidential information with the appropriate consent of the client, as well as without the consent of the client when mandated by law or where permitted by law for a valid purpose (e.g., to provide needed professional services, obtain appropriate professional consultations, protect persons from harm, or obtain payment). Neuropsychologists have a responsibility to discuss with individuals with whom they have a professional relationship, including examinees and retaining parties, the relevant limits of confidentiality and the foreseeable uses of the information generated from the neuropsychological evaluation (see Ethical Standard 4.02, Discussing the Limits of Confidentiality).

The *Standards for Educational and Psychological Testing* also provide guidance to practitioners related to their obligations and responsibilities during the assessment process. More specifically, Standard 8.2 states, "Where appropriate, test takers should be provided, in advance, as much information about the test, the testing process, the intended test use, test scoring criteria, testing policy, and confidentiality protection as is consistent with obtaining valid responses" (p. 86).

Additionally, consistent with the APA ethics code, the Specialty Guidelines for Forensic Psychology, Draft 3 (Committee on the Revision of the Specialty Guidelines for Forensic Psychology, 2008) state, "A forensic psychologist keeps private and in confidence information relating to a client or a party except so far as disclosure is consented to by the client or required or allowed by law" (see Guideline 10, Privacy, Confidentiality, and Privilege). The Specialty Guidelines further advise:

> *If requested, forensic practitioners provide the retaining party access to, and a mean-ingful explanation of, all information that is in their records for the matter at hand, consistent with the relevant law, applicable codes of ethics and professional standards, and institutional rules and regulations. Forensic examinees typically are not provided access to the forensic practitioner's records without the consent of the retaining party. Access to records by anyone other than the retaining party is governed by legal process, usually subpoena or court order, or by explicit consent of the retaining party (see Guideline 10.03, Access to Information and Guideline 12.06, Provision of Documentation).*

Discussions regarding the parameters of forensic neuropsychological evalua-tions should occur with the retaining party (i.e., the client) and the examinee (typically the examinee is not the retaining party) at the outset of the professional relationship or as soon thereafter as possible. Although formal consent procedures have historically been underutilized during assessment as compared with psycho-therapy sessions (Johnson-Greene & National Academy of Neuropsychology Pol-icy & Planning Committee, 2005), the 2002 APA ethics code underscored the importance of obtaining informed consent as a matter of standard practice prior to initiating testing procedures (see Standard 3.10, Informed Consent and Standard 9.03, Informed Consent in Assessments).

With regard to forensic examinees and medico-legal patients, discussions about privacy and confidentiality typically occur during the informed-consent (or notification-of-purpose, in some contexts) process. Examinees should also be informed in advance about whether they will receive feedback about the results directly from the neuropsychologist (see Standard 9.10, Explaining Assessment Results). When examinees are minors or others who have legal guardians, consent for evaluations must be obtained from the parent or other legal guardian. In the case of minors, it is preferable to obtain consent from both parents whenever possible, rather than solely from the custodial parent when parents are separated or divorced (Rae, Brunnquell, & Sullivan, 2003).

In situations in which examinees have a legal guardian, as well as with legally mandated neuropsychological evaluations, informed consent from the examinee is not required. Nevertheless, in such situations it is typically important for neuro-psychologists to inform or notify examinees of the purpose and nature of the evaluation and to obtain the examinees' assent to participate in the evaluation. Although the APA ethics code (2002) does not specify whether informed consent should be obtained in written or oral format, it is advisable for neuropsychologists to document the consent/assent process whenever possible.

Practical Considerations

While acknowledging the ethical and legal responsibilities of neuropsychologists to discuss the limits of confidentiality with examinees and clients, research suggests that people may have a reduced willingness to disclose personal information when they are informed of the limits to confidentiality (Nowell & Spruill, 1993; Woods & McNamara, 1980). Confronted with the dilemma of providing examinees with information that may ultimately compromise the validity of neuropsychological results (e.g., limits of confidentiality), neuropsychologists must maintain an appropriate appreciation of the collateral and objective evidence that they obtain during their evaluations (e.g., historical records and symptom validity findings).

In contrast to traditional psychotherapy services, most neuropsychological evaluations are performed with the advance knowledge and expectation of all parties that the results will be shared with others (e.g., referring doctor, attorney, family member, school district). Except in cases of severe cognitive impairment, forensic examinees typically have some understanding before entering the neuropsychologist's office that the information collected and the test results generated will be disclosed to other identified parties. Nevertheless, examinees may not fully appreciate all of the limits to confidentiality (Weiss, 1982), including the potential for their personal information to become public record. Examinees may expect more rigorous safeguarding of personal information than actually exists, may become comfortable with the examiner and "forget" the parameters of the forensic evaluation, or may state information "off the record."

Mrs. Jefferson is sent to Dr. Madison for an independent neuropsychological examination following a work-related electrical injury. An appropriate informed-consent process is completed, and the clinical interview is begun. Mrs. Jefferson feels comfortable talking to Dr. Madison about her history, but realizes that some information that she would like to share with Dr. Madison would be harmful to her case. As a result, Mrs. Jefferson says, "Off the record..." and before Dr. Madison can stop her, she blurts out "...my husband knocked me down and I got a concussion the morning before the accident at work, but my attorney told me not to tell you, so don't write it down, OK?" At that point, Dr. Madison reminded Mrs. Jefferson that the usual doctor–patient confidentiality did not exist in this context, that there was no "off the record," and that the information about the concussion would have to be reported. Mrs. Jefferson became sullen and withdrawn and seemed to only half-heartedly engage in the remainder of the examination.

In clinical contexts, when making determinations about what information to disclose and to whom it should be disclosed, two principles should be considered: the *parsimony principle* and the *law of no surprises* (Behnke, Perlin, & Bernstein, 2003). According to the parsimony principle, only the information necessary to achieve the purpose of the disclosure should be released. According to the law of no surprises, all reasonable steps should be taken to inform patients at the outset of the relationship of the circumstances under which disclosure of information to a third party will occur. This principle "is founded upon a clinical truism: You never want your client to be surprised when you disclose confidential information ....disclosure of information should be done together with the client whenever possible" (Behnke, Perlin, & Bernstein, 2003, p. 30).

In the case of Mrs. Jefferson, she was informed and understood at the outset of the examination that all relevant information that she reported would be included in the report. Nevertheless, she, like other examinees, reported information to the independent examiner that she did not want included in a report or otherwise disseminated. Although she prefaced her self-disclosure with the words "Off the record," other examinees, for a variety of reasons, disclose information that they consider personal and private without any indication that they are about to do so. Neuropsychologists in such situations have no obligation to omit such information from their reports. In fact, they are obligated to consider all potentially relevant information in their diagnostic determinations and to document pertinent information in their reports. Certain situations, however (e.g., assessing patients with significant memory impairment), may dictate that neuropsychologists remind examinees, as appropriate, of the limits to confidentiality in the context in which the evaluation is being performed. Consistent with the law of no surprises, such reminders may need to include statements to examinees that the information that they just conveyed and want kept off the record will need to be considered when arriving at conclusions, and may appear in the report.

In the vignette described above, Dr. Madison handled the situation with Mrs. Jefferson appropriately. Although immediately stopping forensic examinees once the words "off the record" are spoken and reminding them of the limits of confidentiality is a preferred course of action, it is not always possible to offer such a reminder prior to the disclosure of information that the examinee wishes to be kept confidential. The negative impact that such a disclosure can have upon an ongoing neuropsychological evaluation highlights the importance of establishing the parameters of confidentiality prior to initiating testing and providing appropriate reminders of these limitations as necessary.

Preparing for and Addressing Ethical Challenges

The ability to prepare for and appropriately address ethical challenges is not obtained by chance; it must be developed. Neuropsychologists who provide forensic services should (1) *anticipate* and prepare for ethical issues and challenges commonly encountered in their specific practice contexts, (2) strive to *avoid* ethical misconduct, (3) *address* ethical challenges when they are anticipated or encountered, and (4) *aspire* to the highest standards of ethical practice. These are the 4 A's of ethical practice and decision making as set forth by Bush (2009). A personal commitment to the 4 A's of ethical practice and decision making promotes sound ethical practice.

Avoiding and resolving ethical dilemmas requires an active approach to ethical practice. Ethical decision making in neuropsychology is facilitated by using a structured decision-making model (Bush, 2007). For more specific application of the model proposed by Bush (2007) to forensic neuropsychology, we have added a new step (Step 3) that takes into account the involvement of the retaining party and the unique relationship with the examinee. Consisting of 9 steps, the proposed model provides a fairly comprehensive and detailed approach to ethical decision making (see Table 11.1).

Like clinical decision making, ethical decision making should be evidence based. As previously presented in this chapter, a variety of ethical and legal

11.1   Ethical Decision-Making Model for Forensic Neuropsychology

1. Identify the problem.
2. Consider the significance of the context, setting, and purpose of the services rendered.
3. Consider obligations owed (e.g., retaining party, examinee).
4. Identify and use ethical and legal resources.
5. Consider personal beliefs and values.
6. Develop possible solutions to the problem.
7. Consider the potential consequences of various solutions.
8. Choose and implement a course of action.
9. Assess the outcome, implement changes as needed, and document the process.

resources are available to inform practitioners about appropriate conduct. Additionally, scholarly publications and experienced, knowledgeable colleagues are important resources to promote ethical decision making. Practitioners need not resort to subjective opinions and "I think" solutions when empirical evidence or reliable resources are available to inform and guide their ethical awareness and decision making. To make sound ethical decisions and determine appropriate courses of professional behavior, forensic neuropsychologists benefit from employing a decision-making model and considering multiple sources of information.

Conclusions and Recommendations

Neuropsychologists providing services in forensic contexts have fundamental ethical and legal responsibilities to inform relevant parties of the foreseeable limits to confidentiality and the anticipated uses of the information obtained. It is advisable for neuropsychologists to clarify issues of privacy and confidentiality with all parties at the outset of the professional relationship. Privacy and confidentiality requirements should be discussed with retaining parties as soon as possible after the initial contact has been made, and with examinees during the informed-consent or notification-of-purpose processes either at or before the initial appointment. Additionally, both the retaining parties and the examinees should be reminded of the extent and limits of confidentiality as needed during the evaluation process. Having examinees describe in their own words their understanding of their privacy and confidentiality rights and any limitations related to the examination, and inviting their questions and feedback, provides an opportunity for further clarification and can help avoid later misunderstandings.

Neuropsychologists practicing in forensic contexts release records and information about examinees in compliance with (a) proper authorization from authorized persons, (b) properly noticed and served subpoenas, and (c) court orders, unless there is a legally valid reason to object to such requests or orders (Committee on the Revision of the Specialty Guidelines for Forensic Psychology, 2008). When questions emerge about an appropriate course of action, practitioners may seek assistance from the retaining party, pursue legal advice from their own attorney, or inform the drafter of the subpoena of their uncertainty about the appropriate course of action.

Neuropsychologists provide valuable services to legal decision makers and to persons involved in litigation (and their representatives). Maintaining an understanding of their ethical and legal responsibilities regarding privacy, confidentiality, and privilege promotes competent practice and allows neuropsychologists to explain their obligations to involved parties. A personal commitment to the 4 A's of ethical practice and decision making and use of an ethical decision-making model further promotes sound ethical practice.

References

American Educational Research Association, American Psychological Association, & National Council on Measurement in Education. (1999). *Standards for educational and psychological testing.* Washington, DC: American Educational Research Association.

American Psychological Association. (2002). Ethical principles of psychologists and code of conduct. *American Psychologist, 57*(12), 1060–1073.

Beauchamp, T. L., & Childress, J. F. (2001). *Principles of biomedical ethics* (5th ed.). New York: Oxford University Press.

Behnke, S. H., Perlin, M. L., & Bernstein, M. (2003). *The essentials of New York mental health law: A straightforward guide for clinicians of all disciplines.* New York: W.W. Norton.

Bowers v. Hardwick, 478 U.S. 186 (1985).

Bush, S. S. (2007). *Ethical decision making in clinical neuropsychology.* New York: Oxford University Press.

Bush, S. S. (2009). *Geriatric mental health ethics: A casebook.* New York: Springer Publishing Company.

Bush, S. S., & Martin, T. A. (2008). Confidentiality in neuropsychological practice. In A. M. Horton, Jr., & D. Wedding (Eds.), *The neuropsychology handbook* (3rd ed., pp. 517–532). New York: Springer Publishing Company.

Bush, S. S., Barth, J. T., Pliskin, N. H., Arffa, S., Axelrod, B. N., Blackburn, L. A., et al. (2005). Independent and court-ordered forensic neuropsychological examinations: Official statement of the National Academy of Neuropsychology. *Archives of Clinical Neuropsychology, 20*(8), 997–1007.

Bush, S. S., Connell, M. A., & Denney, R. L. (2006). *Ethical issues in forensic psychology: A systematic model for decision making.* Washington, DC: American Psychological Association.

Committee on the Revision of the Specialty Guidelines for Forensic Psychology. (2008). *Specialty guidelines for forensic psychology* (3rd draft). Available at http://www.ap-ls.org/links/22808sgfp.pdf

Connell, M., & Koocher, G. (2003). HIPAA & forensic practice. *American Psychology Law Society News, 23,* 16–19.

Eisenstadt v. Baird, 405 U.S. 438 (1972).

Federal rules of evidence for United States courts and magistrates. (1975). St. Paul, MN: West.

Fisher, C.B. (2003, January/February). Test data standard most notable change in new APA ethics code. *National Psychologist,* pp. 12–13.

Griswold v. Connecticut, 381 U.S. 479 (1965).

Hawaii Psychiatric Society v. Ariyoshi, 481 F. Supp. 1028 (D. Hawaii, 1979).

Johnson-Green, D., & The NAN Policy & Planning Committee. (2005). Informed consent in clinical neuropsychology practice: Official statement of the National Academy of Neuropsychology. *Archives of Clinical Neuropsychology, 20,* 335–340.

Koocher, G. P., & Keith-Spiegel, P. (1998). *Ethics in psychology: Professional standards and cases* (2nd ed.). New York: Oxford University Press.

Merriam-Webster, Inc. (1988). *Webster's 9th new collegiate dictionary.* Springfield, MA: Author.

Nowell, E. D., & Spruill, J. (1993). If it's not absolutely confidential, will information be disclosed? *Professional Psychology: Research and Practice, 24,* 367–369.

Rae, W. A., Brunnquell, D., & Sullivan, J. R. (2003). Ethical and legal issues in pediatric psychology. In M. C. Roberts (Ed.), *Handbook of pediatric psychology* (3rd ed., pp. 32–49). New York: Guilford Press.

Roe v. Wade, 410 U.S. 113 (1973).

Smith-Bell, M., & Winslade, W. J. (1999). Privacy, confidentiality, and privilege in psychotherapeutic relationships. In D. N. Bersoff (Ed.), *Ethical conflicts in psychology* (2nd ed., pp. 151–155). Washington, DC: American Psychological Association.

Tarasoff v. Regents of the University of California, 551 P.2d 334 (Cal. 1976).

U.S. Department of Health and Human Services. (2003). *Public Law 104-191: Health Insurance Portability and Accountability Act of 1996*. Retrieved November 24, 2003, from http://www.hhs.gov/ocr/hipaa/

Weiss, B. D. (1982). Confidentiality expectations of patients, physicians, and medical students. *Journal of the American Medical Association, 247*, 2695–2697.

Whalen v. Roe, 429 U.S. 589 (1976).

Woods, K. M., & McNamara, J. R. (1980). Confidentiality: Its effect on interviewee behavior. *Professional Psychology: Research and Practice, 11*, 714–721.

Conflicts of Interest and Other Nettlesome Pitfalls for the Expert Witness

12

Barry M. Crown
H. Scott Fingerhut
Sheryl J. Lowenthal

I will teach you wisdom's ways and lead you in straight paths. If you live a life guided by wisdom, you won't limp or stumble as you run.

—*Proverbs, 4:* 11–12

Introduction

Expert testimony remains big business, and its growing importance in modern litigation cannot be overstated. Indeed, many cases, particularly those involving complex issues of mental states, ability, or causation, often—some would say too often—boil down to battles between experts (Richmond, 1997, p. 485). Not surprisingly, then, for many, "[t]he business of being an expert has become a cottage industry" (*Cordy v. Sherwin-Williams Co.*, 1994, p. 582). Still, in a light far less sinister, it has been said with equal force by others that expert witnesses "play as great a role in the organization and shaping and evaluation of their client's case as do the lawyers" (*Murphy v. A.A. Mathews*, 1992, p. 682; Richmond,

1997, p. 485). In either event, the balance between counsel and their expert witnesses, and the just resolution of causes is a delicate one, to be sure. And although there may be nothing inappropriate per se about the proliferation of expert testimony, there is a strong and steady perception that "[t]rial lawyers are drawn to expert witnesses like moths to light" (Richmond, 2000, p. 909).

The reason for the attraction is manifest. By its very nature, modern litigation calls out to a vast array of properly qualified professionals to testify as experts—to "peer into the past" as well as "predict the future" (Lubet, 1999, p. 465). After all, it is expert testimony that often provides ever-critical reliability (or at least its aura) that enables one party to prevail (Richmond, 2000, p. 909). Consequently, underlying these concerns is the more fundamental notion of access to the courts. Our system of justice, civil and criminal, takes care to foster the ability of rich and poor alike to litigate justifiable claims. Thus, "[o]ne of the paramount goals of the American legal system is to ensure that injured persons have realistic access to the courts" (Parker, 1991, p. 1368).

While "[c]ourts have not stood still in the face of what appears to be an expert witness explosion" (Richmond, 1997, p. 490), the judiciary's focus has remained, in large part, on evidentiary matters of admissibility, reliability, and relevance, especially to prevent dubious scientific evidence from infecting trials (see generally *Daubert v. Merrell Dow Pharmaceuticals, Inc.*, 1993; *Kumho Tire Co. v. Carmichael*, 1999; *Weisgram v. Marley Co.*, 2000; Richmond, 1997, p. 486; Richmond, 2000, p. 909).

With trial courts as gatekeepers, admissibility has been scrutinized not only for scientific information, but for expert testimony based on technical and other specialized knowledge to discern problems posed by unreliable, speculative, misleading, or unfairly prejudicial testimony that should rightly be excluded from the factfinders' view (*Kumho*, 1999, p. 147; Richmond, 2000, p. 910). *Baxter v. Temple* (2008) is also instructive in the application of *Daubert* standards, holding that a neuropsychologist's testimony should have been admitted in a negligence action against defendant apartment lessor's alleged failure to warn of high levels of lead paint, and finding that the testing methodology was based on a generally reliable approach, with no difference in a clinical or forensic context.[1]

In response, in the name of keeping advocacy zealous, and buffered by the availability of ardent cross-examination, attorneys have responded in kind to insist that a party is free to solicit the expert of its choice and to elicit any opinion that suits their theory of the case. Hence, a threefold rationale has developed to keep the playing field even, while recognizing the important role experts play in facilitating justice.

"First, expert testimony which borders on the fantastic, or which is wholly incredible, undermines the integrity of the adversary system" (Richmond, 1997, p. 486). Second, an expert witness should neither be "a party's advocate" nor "the litigation equivalent of hired guns" (Richmond, 1997, p. 486), but rather "an advocate of the truth with testimony to help the court and the jury reach the ultimate truth in a case, which should be the basis of any verdict" (*Selvidge v. United States*, 1995, p. 156). And third, expert witnesses must "merit special attention, because their testimony can be powerful and simultaneously very 'misleading because of the difficulty in evaluating it.' Absent judicial guidance, jurors may 'abdicate their fact-finding obligations' and, instead, simply adopt the opinions of the expert witnesses whose testimony they find persuasive" (Richmond, 1997, p. 487).[2]

Curiously, the field of expert-witness professional ethics and professionalism, and the ramifications of conduct resulting in disqualification, remains rather undeveloped (Lubet, 1999, p. 465). *Professional ethics* typically refers to the "distinct, mandatory responsibilities undertaken by individuals in the course of practicing a trade or calling" (Lubet, p. 465). Because of the obligatory nature of these responsibilities, *breaches* are considered to be those actions that may result in professional discipline, fee forfeiture, or other adverse consequences (Lubet, p. 465). By contrast, the more forgiving term *professionalism* is generally used to "identify admirable, model, or ideal conduct that is generally expected within a given profession—but not absolutely required" (Lubet, pp. 465–466).

To be sure, all expert witnesses are governed by a societal covenant of personal ethics, and all experts must obey court, evidentiary, and procedural rules in their respective jurisdictions (Lubet, 1999, p. 466). "Still, there is no single source that we can look to for a definitive statement of expert witnesses' professional ethics. A few organizations have attempted to draft codes of conduct for expert witnesses, but none have achieved broad acceptance" (Lubet, p. 466). Despite the absence of an established code or other distinct, formal guidance for expert witnesses, this is certainly not to imply an "absence of content-related professional standards" (Lubet, p. 467). Regrettably, though, most seminal authority addressing misconduct still does not arise in the psychiatrist/patient context (Lubet, pp. 466–467).[3]

It is these concerns and issues that this chapter endeavors to survey, in particular, the often overlooked area broadly defined as *conflicts of interest*. In the more formal usage of the term, a conflict of interest arises in connection with public officials, fiduciaries, and their relationship to matters of private interest or gain, i.e., a "clash between public interest and the private pecuniary interest of the individual concerned" (*Black's Law Dictionary*, 1979, p. 271). Stated another way, a conflict of interest is "the circumstance of a public officeholder, corporate officer, etc., whose personal interests might benefit from his or her official actions or influence" (*Webster's College Dictionary*, 1991, p. 285).

For our purposes here, a conflict of interest means not only the breach of a fiduciary relationship between parties, but may also incorporate any number of nettlesome conflicts and pitfalls which expert witnesses should—nay, must—be aware of, from the moment of engagement of their professional services, lest they soon find themselves (along with, perhaps, retaining counsel) unemployed.

"As modern litigation continues its march toward increasing technical complexity, it will become more important to define and understand issues of ethics and professionalism as they relate to expert witnesses" (Lubet, 1999, p. 488). Under this rather large umbrella, this chapter attempts a broad examination for the expert witness, as a primer, and highlights several areas of concern—not only conflicts of interest in the traditional sense, but the related quagmires of compensation, in its various forms, permissible and impermissible alike, as well as the expert's conduct during discovery and trial. The upshot of this analysis is that expert witnesses play a prominent (and proper) role in protecting not just themselves, but both retaining and opposing counsel, and the adversarial system of justice they all serve.

Part I of this chapter examines the important principles that pervade our discussion of the myriad conflicts of interest the expert witness must be vigilant to avoid. In Part II we analyze the standard of review by which courts exercise their inherent power to disqualify expert witnesses. A fundamental understanding of this concept is essential before appreciating the types of conflicts that may result in disqualification. Part III discusses the practices and pitfalls that come under the broad category of conflicts of interest. In particular, we examine first conflicts of interest in their traditional setting—unrelated engagements and the phenomenon known as side switching. Part III will also discuss several related areas of potential concern for experts, namely permissible and impermissible forms of compensation, and the expert's equally important involvement during the discovery process and, ultimately, at trial. Finally, Part IV concludes by addressing experts' co-existent burden of self-preservation in order to ensure that their unique role in the American legal system, and their continuing participation in the process, is preserved.

I: The Expert Witness

There are five overarching principles that bear mentioning at the outset. First, courts are rightfully hesitant to disqualify expert witnesses once they have been retained by counsel at the behest of the client that counsel represents. Second, unlike retained counsel, who must advance a particular cause, experts enjoy a unique independence and objectivity in the American legal system. Third, the treating physician stands on even greater independent footing than the civilian expert, because treatment of the client transforms the expert into a veritable eyewitness, of sorts. Fourth, the expert is nevertheless part of the team for which he or she is engaged, and assists in the presentation of retained counsel's theory of the case. Fifth, because of the nature of the professional engagement, otherwise privileged communications and confidences secured in the expert–client relationship are necessarily vitiated in anticipation of the expert's participation in litigation.

Disqualification Is a Last Resort

First, courts are, and should be, reticent to disqualify expert witnesses. This reticence has one foot in policy, recognizing a public interest, and another in practice, encouraging that reasonable steps be taken to protect confidences and confidential relationships (Richmond, 1997, p. 562). To be sure, courts must take care to "preserve parties' confidences and to prevent a party from profiting by exploiting its adversary's work product" (Richmond, 2000, p. 928). Nevertheless, "disqualification motions have great potential for abuse as a litigation strategy," and judges must be vigilant in "preventing parties from wielding conflict of interest and confidentiality rules as procedural weapons" (Richmond, p. 928).

Thus, "[a]s a matter of policy, courts must balance (1) the need to protect opinion work product and client confidences and maintain the integrity of the judicial process, with (2) the need to ensure that parties have access to qualified expert witnesses who possess useful, specialized knowledge. In conjunction with both elements, courts must be mindful that if experts are too easily disqualified, attorneys and parties 'will be encouraged to engage in a race for expert witnesses holding adverse opinions and...to create some type of inexpensive relationship with those experts in order to conflict them out of cases.' Such behavior threatens the integrity of the judicial process by depriving courts of the benefit of experts' knowledge and insight, and it deprives parties of the assistance of qualified expert witnesses" (Richmond, 2000, pp. 926–927).

Therefore, "[f]rom a practical standpoint, courts should disqualify experts cautiously 'because lawyers seeking to invoke the confidential relationship have the knowledge, experience, and the ability to avoid the conflict[s]'; thus, they rightfully bear the consequence for failing to take appropriate precautions" (Richmond, 2000, p. 927).

Focusing, thus, on the attorney's burden, any attorney seeking to retain the services of an expert and establish a confidential relationship should make this intention unmistakably clear and confirm the same in writing. Thus,

> *The lawyer should include in the engagement letter an explanation of the expert's duty of confidentiality. The lawyer may instruct the expert not to discuss the case with other lawyers or colleagues, although such specificity is not required. Broad confidentiality obligations are the best for all concerned. If the lawyer provides the expert with any materials or communicates with him in writing, work product should be clearly identified. Attorneys should also inquire into the expert's previous employment in order to ferret out potential problems. Before sharing confidential information, counsel should ask potential experts to run formal conflict checks or to make the best inquiry they can in their particular situation. (Richmond, 2000, pp. 927–928)*

Independence and Objectivity

The second important general principle is that, party alliance or affiliation aside, an expert witness enjoys unique independence in an otherwise adversarial legal system. In short, expert witnesses owe no shade of allegiance or undivided loyalty to their employer, as does the employer (the lawyer) to the client (Richmond, 2000, p. 910; Lubet, 1999, p. 474). "While a lawyer is an advocate for his client, an expert witness is supposed to be a source of knowledge and opinions that will aid the trier of fact" (Richmond, p. 910). Thus, expert witnesses are viewed as "independent servants of the court" (Richmond, p. 910).

For this reason, as a rule, experts may accept concurrent engagements for and against the same party, lawyer, or law firm, and may even testify against former clients in successive engagements (Lubet, 1999, p. 474; Richmond, 2000, pp. 910–911). Where an expert's professional freedom is not absolute, however, it is because agency principles come into play to require that the witness "reasonably safeguard client confidences and refrain from trading on confidential information for personal gain or any other improper purpose" (Lubet, p. 472; Richmond, p. 911).

The Unique Double Role of the Treating Physician as an Expert Eyewitness

Distinct from other types of expert witnesses, treating physicians who double as experts present an even more independent front (Richmond, 2000, p. 922). A civilian expert retained solely for litigation purposes may still be considered "part of the litigation team since the expert is oftentimes responsible for developing a party's theory of the case" (*Donovan v. Bowling*, 1998, p. 941). Conversely, consider that "a treating physician is like an eyewitness to an event." Stated another way, "[t]he doctor's opinions are based on facts actually observed, not on the theory of the case developed by people involved in the litigation phase" (Richmond, p. 923). As observed in *Donovan*,

> *First-hand and on-scene observations by a witness, expert or not, should be always and equally accessible to both parties. To allow one party to contact a treating physician and then claim that the treating physician has been retained as a possible expert witness, thereby effectively barring the other party from access to that physician's unique first-hand perspective, would be highly unfair to litigants, regardless of whether the party sits at the plaintiff's or the defendant's counsel table. (Donovan v. Bowling, 1998, p. 941)*

In this fashion, the distinction between counsel and expert, particularly the expert engaged in a client-treatment role, becomes crystallized. The attorney is expected to behave in a biased manner—though not improperly so. The expert, on the other hand, is to "remain objective and independent, both in fact and in appearance" (Parker, 1991, pp. 1371–1372). "The single most important obligation of an expert witness is to approach every question with independence and objectivity" (Lubet, 1999, p. 467). The admissibility of expert testimony is predicated upon the ability of the expert's specialized knowledge to "assist the trier of fact to understand the evidence" (Federal Rules of Evidence, 702). The necessary corollary to this principle is, of course, that the expert's opinion must be "candidly and frankly based upon the witness's own investigation, research and understanding" (Lubet, p. 467). As an objective observer, the expert is called upon to view facts and data "dispassionately, without regard to the consequences for the client" (Lubet, p. 467). Indeed, the truly independent expert "is not affected by the goals of the party for which he or she was retained, and is not reticent to arrive at an opinion that fails to support the client's legal position" (Lubet, p. 467).

Temptation aside, still, no expert witness is an island. Rather, experts must cope with, and work with, lawyers in order to fulfill their function in an adversarial legal system (Lubet, 1999, pp. 469–470). Remember that it is the lawyer's job to be the advocate and to make the best possible argument on behalf of the client in order to win the case (Lubet, p. 468). It is the lawyer who, unlike their expert, does not testify under oath and may often find him- or herself believing that the advance of a particular position will lead to a victory of sorts, "without necessarily believing that the view is correct," and without even having to "convince [them]-self" (Lubet, p. 468). At times, then, a lawyer may indeed be duty bound to make arguments that, although they do not convince that lawyer, might very well convince the factfinder to whom they urge it (Lubet, p. 468). This is the "classic formulation of the advocate's duty...not know[ing] it to be good or bad till the *judge* determines it" (emphasis added) (Boswell, 1887, p. 47; Lubet, p. 468).

Herein lies the inherent clash between the attorney, as advocate, and the expert witness who, to the contrary, has no such latitude in his or her distinct role apart from, not as part of, membership on the litigation team:

> *As a witness testifying under oath, an expert is not entitled to state a position "which does not convince yourself" in the hope that it may convince the judge or jury. The*

entire system of expert testimony rests upon the assumption that expert witnesses are independent of retaining counsel, and that they testify sincerely. Most lawyers understand and accept this on an intellectual level. Still, in the heat of adversary battle, it is not unknown for lawyers to seek to "extend" or "expand" an expert's opinion in just the right direction. This is wrong. It is no more acceptable for a lawyer to attempt to persuade an expert to alter her opinion than it would be to convince an eyewitness to change his account of the facts. (Lubet, 1999, p. 468)

Still an Integral Part of the Team

Recognizing that litigation is often a complex endeavor, and almost always an interactive one, the need for independence and objectivity certainly cannot, and does not, prevent experts from working closely with the lawyers who retain them (Lubet, 1999, p. 469). As long as their respective professional roles are not blurred, "[i]t is entirely legitimate for expert witnesses to cooperate closely with retaining counsel" (Lubet, p. 469). To this end, experts properly may depend on their employers to provide information, explanations, and descriptions about the case, or disregard the same if legally irrelevant or inadmissible; advise of legal standards to be addressed in the formation of the expert's opinion; even convey facts not otherwise readily accessible in the form of reasonable and clearly identified hypothetical questions (Lubet, pp. 469–470).

It is likewise proper for retaining counsel to make suggestions to, or ask questions of, the expert; to seek that the expert reconsider a previous conclusion in light of additional information; to inject pointed questions to ensure the validity of the expert's position; to suggest ways in which the expert's opinion could be solidified; even to assist the expert's preparation for deposition and trial (Lubet, 1999, p. 470).

What is improper is for retaining counsel to pressure the expert to change his or her opinion, or to instruct the expert how to testify (Lubet, 1999, pp. 470–471). Neither may an attorney, as the expert must be aware, "try to stretch a witness's expertise, either as a cost-saving measure or in an effort to broaden the impact of the testimony," as is sometimes their natural impulse to put the expert through such double duty (Lubet, p. 471). So, too, must the expert guard against the slightly more insidious tack of retaining counsel's effort to "induce or inveigle an expert to offer opinions that are truly beyond the scope of his or her expertise," and which, if offered, "put the witness out on a limb that may be sawed off during cross-examination" (Lubet, p. 471).

In the end, "[t]actics aside, experts must be both qualified and independent" (Lubet, 1999, p. 471). "A lawyer must ultimately be willing to take the bad news with the good, and to realize that an expert's opinion may be unfavorable to, or not fully supportive of, the client's position" (Lubet, p. 470). And from this, the silver lining emerges (at least as far as the administrative arms of the justice systems and not too few parties and counsel are concerned):

A lawyer with integrity will normally accept a negative opinion, or even appreciate it, since that may help counsel and client formulate a settlement strategy rather than take a losing case to trial (Lubet, p. 470). It is imperative, therefore, that the expert resolve any such issues by asking this appropriate inquiry: "Either the witness is legitimately able to opine on subject, in which case the engagement proceeds on that basis, or the witness lacks the necessary skills or qualification, in which case the subject is dropped." (Lubet, p. 471)

Diminished Confidentiality

Professional obligations of confidentiality and secrecy are well recognized in both federal and state courts, and the notion of privilege between, among others, husband and wife, lawyer and client, accountant and client, counselor and victim, psychotherapist and patient, even clergy, abounds. The employment of an expert witness, however, necessitates a different result. Notwithstanding the privilege normally accorded private communications, the expert witness must be prepared to heed, expect, and even be compelled to, reveal client confidences. (Lubet, 1999, p. 472). Such is the very nature of the engagement:

> *Forensic evaluation and testimony do not fall within the ordinary practice of most professions. Communications made to a retained witness, for the purpose of facilitating testimony in court, do not fall within the "zone of privacy" necessary for the invocation of an evidentiary privilege. (See, e.g., Federal Rules of Civil Procedure 26(a)(2)(B); Lubet, p. 472)*

For the expert witness, then, the watchword is caution:

> *[E]xpert witnesses should assume that all of their communications, with either the client or retaining counsel, may be subject to disclosure through the process of discovery. Additionally, the witness' research files, work papers, notes, drafts, correspondence, and similar materials may have to be revealed to the attorneys for opposing parties. (Lubet, 1999, p. 472)*

Hence, while in some jurisdictions discovery rules may mitigate against discovery disclosure, "prudence dictates that the [expert] witness presume that her entire file will be an open book" (Lubet, 1999, p. 472). "Because of the complex interplay among professional ethics standards, rules of evidence and discovery, and other laws, it is best to clarify the expectations of confidentiality at the outset of every engagement. According to the ABA Standing Committee on Professional Conduct, a retention letter 'should define the relationship, including its scope and limitations, and should outline the responsibilities of the testifying expert, especially regarding the disclosure of client confidence' " (Lubet, p. 473).

II: The Standard of Review

Life, though lived forward, is often better understood backwards, as mothers and Kierkegaard were wont to say. Thus, a discussion of the legal standard upon which courts exercise their discretion to disqualify expert witnesses is a propos before speaking specifically to the issues of the conflicts of interest that warrant disqualification. Although instances of disqualification are rare, their occasional occurrence has significant ramifications beyond that of terminating the services of a particular expert witness. Indeed, both the expert and the retaining lawyer or law firm are subject to disqualification, fee forfeiture or, even worse—professional discipline.

Federal and state courts alike possess the inherent power to disqualify experts and attorneys. Coffey (2004, pp. 196–197) notes that federal courts' "distinctive jurisprudence" is not anchored upon explicit procedural or ethical rules, or even precedent, but instead on "a series of federal lower court decisions" that have crafted "an expert-disqualification doctrine based on a court's inherent authority to safeguard the integrity of the judicial process and maintain the public's confidence in the court system."

To determine whether the expert witness or the attorney/employer is ripe for disqualification, a two-part test that focuses on the mere appearance of impropriety is generally applied (Richmond 1997, p. 558). The inquiry asks, "[f]irst, was it objectively reasonable for the first party who retained the expert to believe that a confidential relationship existed, [and s]econd, did that party disclose any confidential information to the expert?" (see *Cordy v. Sherwin-Williams, Co.*, 1994, p. 580; *Shadow Traffic Network v. Superior Court*, 1994, pp. 699–700). In addition, "many lower courts have considered a third element: the public's interest in allowing or not allowing an expert to testify" (*Koch Ref. Co. v. Jennifer L. Boudreaux MV*, p. 1181; Lubet, 1997, p. 488, n. 39).

The answers to both primary questions must be affirmative, and the public interest must be compelling, in order to disqualify the witness (Richmond, 2000, p. 913–914). After all, "[i]f the party crying foul should not have reasonably believed that it shared a confidential relationship with the expert, the expert should not be disqualified" (Richmond, p. 914). By the same token, "[i]f neither the complaining party nor its counsel disclosed confidences," or "something akin to attorney-client communications or opinion work product," then "the expert should not be disqualified" (Richmond, p. 914).

Courts which do not apply the "appearance of impropriety" test have opted for a more "careful, precise, and reality based standard" (*Proctor & Gamble, Co. v. Haugen*, 1998, p. 573). To the court in *Haugen* (1998) only "real interference" with work product or similar interests, not the mere appearance of impropriety, should require disqualification of counsel (*Haugen, 1998*), or the enlisted expert witness who was only informally consulted (*Proctor & Gamble, Co. v. Haugen*, 1999, pp. 412–413). *Haugen* (1999) then considered four factors in balancing the relative interests: (1) of paramount import, whether the communication originated in confidence or other privilege that it would not be disclosed; (2) to a lesser degree, whether confidentiality is essential to the full and satisfactory relations between the parties; (3) whether the confidentiality at issue breeds a community sense that the relation ought to be sedulously fostered to the exclusion of production of the evidence; and (4) whether the injury that would occur to the relation by disclosure is greater than the benefit gained for the appropriate resolution of the litigation (*Haugen*, 1999, pp. 413–414; Richmond, 2000, p. 918).

Accordingly, in *Haugen* (1999) the court was not compelled to disqualify an expert witness with whom counsel had only informally consulted. The consultation was informal in that the expert was paid a consultation fee and discussed at length material relevant to the case with counsel. Counsel did not, however, reveal its litigation strategy. Thereafter, counsel did not consult further with the expert or exchange any additional information. No effort was made to contact the expert subsequently, nor was any indication made to prevent the expert from discussing the case with others. As a matter of fact, the expert never considered himself to have been employed by the party, nor did he conduct any research or calculate any data. In sum, there was no evidence to suggest he had been retained as an expert in any capacity. Some two years later, opposing counsel contacted and retained the expert, but took care not to ask him anything about his prior consultation, about which he was fully aware.

In *Haugen* (1998 and 1999), neither present counsel nor the expert were disqualified. Counsel had done nothing to protect its work product, mental impressions, or any of its communications with the expert. Nor did any privilege or basis for disqualification arise as a consequence of the informal consultation with the expert. After all, the expert was not retained, nor had he been privy to any strategic thoughts or impressions. Prior counsel could show no prejudice, nor could it demonstrate that the expert owed any duty of confidentiality. In essence, disqualification would have served only to exclude relevant evidence—something that the court was surely not willing to do for the sake of formality, favoring instead to balance competing interests by permitting the expert's continued participation in the case. (*Haugen*, 1999, p. 434; Richmond, 2000, pp. 918–919).

III: Practices and Pitfalls

It is from this vantage point, and upon engaging the gentle balance of the expert witness as both independent servant of the law and party-agent, that our analysis of the potential problem areas begins.

Traditional Conflicts of Interest

Conflicts of interest involving expert witnesses threaten litigants equally on both sides of a dispute (Richmond, 2000, p. 912). "Parties may consult with *numerous* experts before settling on one who will testify at trial. Those communications are sometimes sensitive and significant, as counsel may have to share their opinion work product or divulge confidential information in order to judge an expert's suitability" (emphasis added) (Richmond, 1997, p. 557). And, of course, circumstances sometimes arise where "a party may also hire consulting experts *unbeknownst* to its adversary" (emphasis added) (Richmond, 1997, p. 557). Parikh (2006/2007, p. 263) also discusses the fact that conflicts happen most often "if the case is against an expert witness they may have hired for their side in another case."

While the independence of the expert witness is an accepted axiom, it is arguable that this independence exists only as an ideal. The public at large, probably most of lawyers' clients, and certainly some members of the bench and bar believe—or urge themselves to believe, in advancing their particular agenda—that "[i]n addition to the bias that naturally results from the selection process, the expert witness is influenced by another form of unconscious bias resulting from partisan associations during trial preparation. It is widely acknowledged that witnesses often participate extensively in trial preparation and are carefully prepared to present only favorable testimony on the stand" (Parker, 1991, p. 1386). Indeed, *[a]ttorneys intent on recovering compensation for their clients often try to instill a favorable bias in the expert and sell them the proposed theory of liability. As a result of such partisan bias, expert witnesses sometimes resort to special-purpose studies, the omission of certain factors, and other manipulations of tests and results in order to support their positions. (Parker, 1991, p. 1386)*

Thus, issues of client loyalty and conflicts of interest predominantly arise in two different contexts: *unrelated engagements*, which ask whether an expert may accept concurrent engagements for and against the same party, and the phenomenon *known as side switching*, in which an expert switches sides in litigation (Lubet, 1999, p. 474).

Unrelated Engagements

As noted previously, the legal and ethical obligations of retained counsel and experts to their clients exist in a distinct tandem. As a matter of legal ethics, it is well established that lawyers may not represent any interest directly adverse to a current client, as in suing and defending the same party (Lubet, 1999, p. 474). Expert witnesses, on the other hand, do not owe that sort of loyalty to their clients:

An expert is not the client's "champion," pledged faithfully to seek the client's goals. Indeed, in many ways the expert's role is precisely the opposite. She must remain independent of the client and detached, if not wholly aloof, from the client's goals. There is no reason that an objective expert could not conclude—and explain—that a party is correct in one case and wrong in another." (Lubet, p. 474)

"Consequently, there is no general ethical principle that prevents an expert from accepting concurrent engagements both for and adverse to the same party," or even testifying adversely to a former client or law firm that had previously retained the expert (Lubet, 1999, p. 474).

Again, it is agency principles that curtail an expert's exercise of absolute freedom in engagement and "imposes an obligation to refrain from exploiting a client's confidences for the benefit of another" (Lubet, 1999, p. 474). An example of this might be an expert's accepting conflicting engagements, "either concurrently or successively, that are *factually related* (emphasis added), since this could risk exploitation or betrayal of a client's confidences" (Lubet, pp. 474–475).

Apart from an actual or case-specific conflict of interest, there exists a more amorphous threat of conflict that might also act to constrain an expert's acceptance of an engagement. Even where there is no threat of revelation of client confidences, or even where the matters requiring an expert's testimony are utterly unrelated, a law firm or client would surely find "discomfort to see their expert turn up on the opposite side of another lawsuit" (Lubet, 1999, p. 475). Indeed, the expert's dual position in such situations may necessarily place the employer in the "troublesome position of having to extol the expert's opinion in one case while attacking it in another" (Lubet, p. 475). The mere existence of this scenario, rather than an actual conflict of interest, creates circumstances that may inure to the expert's professional detriment:

Needless to say, most lawyers would find this situation damaging to the expert's credibility in case one, damaging to the client's position in case two, or both. No doubt, the retaining lawyer would prefer to avoid this dilemma, if possible, even if there is no ethical bar to the expert's actions. (Lubet, p. 475)

Again, as a matter both of courtesy and professionalism, it is best to resolve such issues at the very outset of the engagement. Consequently, "[a] lawyer may reasonable request that the expert refrain from accepting potentially adverse engagements, at least for the duration of the retention. The expert may accept or decline the proposed restriction, or may suggest other terms. The absence of an ethics rule does not prevent the attorney and expert from negotiating a mutually agreeable resolution to what could perhaps become a sticky problem. In any event, a forthright discussion of terms and conditions can prevent the development of an awkward situation down the road" (Lubet, p. 475).

It is common, of course, "for opposing experts to know one another, to be familiar with each other's work, and perhaps to have worked together" (Richmond, 2000, p. 924), thus:

Many experts do not hesitate to call a colleague to inquire about a theory, question data reported in an article, or discuss new methodologies or studies. This is especially true when the experts have forged a personal relationship through service or involvement in professional associations. (Richmond, 2000, p. 924)

Side Switching

The phenomenon commonly known as side switching is well presented in the following query:

Imagine that an expert has been retained by the plaintiff in a lawsuit. The expert conducts her research and arrives at an opinion that is quite unfavorable to the plaintiff, who then discharges the witness. May the expert subsequently testify for the defendant, whose position is supported by the expert's work? (Lubet, 1999, p. 475)

As stated, because of their uniquely independent role, there is no rule per se prohibiting an expert from switching sides in a lawsuit (Lubet, 1999, p. 475). Stated another way, because it is the province of the expert not to join irrevocably with a party, but to "arrive at an independent opinion, it cannot be disloyal for the witness to begin working for one party and end up working for the other" (Lubet, p. 475).

Thus, whether an expert may stray from one camp to another depends ultimately "upon the nature and extent of the relationship between the expert and the original client. In brief, an expert may not switch sides, even following discharge or release, if that would violate the original client's reasonable expectation of confidentiality. This in turn will depend on a number of factors" (Lubet, 1999, pp. 475–476).

The question might be posed another way:

How extensive was the communication between the expert and the client or the client's counsel? Was the expert provided with non-public or privileged information? Did the expert participate in strategy discussions with counsel, or otherwise learn of the client's decision-making strategy? (Lubet, p. 476)

And although courts are likely to apply one of the two analyses previously addressed to weigh these factors, the question turns more often than not on the expert's access to otherwise confidential information (Lubet, p. 476). Such was the case in *English Feedlot, Inc. v. Norden Lab., Inc.* (1993), which demonstrates both that an expert who only participates for a brief while in preliminary discussions with counsel is "free to accept retention from the other side" and that litigants' silence or inconsistent conduct may waive any confidentiality their professional relationship otherwise might bring (Lubet, p. 476).

In the *English Feedlot* case, the defendant tried to disqualify plaintiff's expert and counsel alike. The defense had retained the expert as a veterinary consultant in one matter, and then, some years later, the expert served on behalf of several of defendant's customers, agreeing with their complaints with the defective nature of its vaccines. Between the expert's engagements, he made public his opinions about plaintiff's products, and plaintiff, surprisingly, did not protest or object to "dissemination of this information on 'confidentiality' grounds," essentially acquiescing to the expert's criticisms of their products (*English Feedlot*, 1993, p. 1504; Richmond, 2000, p. 925).

While the court did find that the two shared a confidential relationship, the plaintiff never revealed any confidential information to the expert. And even assuming the plaintiff had revealed confidential information, "the company waived any claims of confidentiality" (Richmond, 2000, p. 925), reasoned as follows;

> *Waiver is the intentional relinquishment of a known right or privilege. "A waiver may be explicit...or it may be implied, as, for example, when a party engages in conduct which manifests an intent to relinquish the right...or acts inconsistently with its assertion." Here, SmithKline repeatedly acquiesced to Brown's public criticism of its products. It is thus inconsistent, after impliedly relinquishing this right, for SmithKline to now assert that [the] information is confidential. There, assuming arguendo SmithKline disclose[d] confidential information to Brown, SmithKline waived its right to assert confidentiality at this late date. (English Feedlot, p. 1504; Richmond, 2000, pp. 925–926)*

And since the expert had not received any confidential information from plaintiff, the expert could not taint defense counsel, his new employer, thus warranting its disqualification either (Richmond, 2000, p. 926).

Waiver may be more subtly imputed, however. For example:

> *[A] party might allow its consulting expert to share information with its testifying expert in order to help the testifying expert shape his opinions. Assuming that confidential information passes from the consulting expert to the testifying expert and the testifying expert considers that information in forming his opinions, the party has likely waived any confidentiality claims otherwise attending its relationship with the consultant. If a consulting expert's work is part of the foundation for another expert's testimony and the sponsoring party does not object to related deposition questions posed to the testifying expert, the party has probably waived any confidentiality arguments. (Richmond, 2000, p. 926)*

"Conversely, an expert who had performed an extensive fact investigation, working closely with counsel, would more likely be barred from switching sides," as set forth in *Wang Laboratories, Inc. v. Toshiba Corp.*, 1991 (Lubet, 1999, p. 476). And, although legal precedent is sparse, an expert who in a rare instance "defects," i.e., either deliberately setting out to switch sides or having been "lured away by opposing counsel"—as opposed to one who is discharged or initially declines an engagement—is surely subject to disqualification, for "[n]ot only is such a witness likely to have compromised confidences, but a defecting witness also creates the appearance of chicanery," and is thus an affront to the fair administration of justice (Lubet, p. 476).

As advised before, "most difficulties can be avoided if there is a frank discussion at the outset of the engagement. A well-drafted retention letter will spell out the expert's duties and the client's expectations concerning confidential information, as well as the expert's options in the event of discharge or release" (Lubet, 1999, pp. 476–477). In *Cordy v. Sherwin-Williams* (1994), for example, the plaintiff was injured riding his bicycle over railroad tracks. In communicating with an engineer as a prospective expert witness, plaintiff's counsel spoke with him over the telephone about ten times, ultimately entering into a retainer agreement. After receiving a host of plaintiff's investigative materials, the expert rendered an oral opinion, though he did not provide a written report.

When the expert subsequently resigned, returning the retainer as well, he was contacted by defense counsel, and despite his revelation that he had indeed been consulted by plaintiff, the expert was hired by the defense and, as a precaution, was instructed not to disclose anything to the defense the expert had learned from his association with plaintiff. The expert ultimately concluded, in a written report, that defendant was not responsible for the accident.

In this instance, the court easily found that plaintiff's counsel rightly concluded that the expert must have shared confidential information with the defense. All in all, the court found that it was "simply not possible" for the expert to "ignore what he learned" from plaintiff's counsel (*Cordy*, 1994, p. 582; Richmond, 2000, p. 915). And the court not only disqualified the expert, but defense counsel as well, because "at the very least, the defense counsel should have contacted Plaintiff's counsel" to investigate or discover the nature of the relationship between the parties (*Cordy*, p. 584). Whether the defense "chose to ignore the warning signs or actually encouraged" the expert's misconduct was of no interest to the court (*Cordy*, p. 584; Richmond, p. 915).

There are other instances where the conflict of interest is between the expert witnesses themselves. The key to whether disqualification is warranted is the degree to which confidential information is shared. Consider, for example, the rather unique case of *Hansen v. Umtech Industrieservice Und Spedition, GmbII* (1996), a products liability action where opposing experts were engaged by the same client. The first expert employed by Umtech assured the corporation that there were no conflicts of interests of concern. This expert then shared client confidences, discussed the case at length, and assessed with counsel the relative strengths and weaknesses of the defendant's position. A letter was subsequently sent to the expert confirming his retention, including a request for confidentiality. In return, the expert faxed a letter identifying documents typically necessary for him to review. However, no one took any action with respect to the fax or "the case in general" (*Hansen*, 1996, p. 2; Richmond, 2000, p. 919).

A short time later, the plaintiff engaged its own expert—from the same firm as the one previously employed by the defendant. The plaintiff's expert ran a computerized conflict-of-interest check which failed to reveal the prior representation because the defendant's expert "had not entered his representation of Umtech on the system" (Richmond, 2000, p. 920). To make matters worse, the defense expert was on vacation at the time the plaintiff sought assistance and therefore was unavailable to properly inform the new expert as to the conflict.

The court disagreed with Umtech that the plaintiff's expert, and his firm, should be disqualified based on its prior relationship with its own expert. It was the uniqueness of the facts of the case—namely, the fleeting memory of the initial expert engaged—that made the court's task less complicated than it otherwise might have been:

> *While [defense counsel] stated that she discussed her analysis of the case, including its strengths and weaknesses, with [its expert], [the expert] has no recollection of the details of that conversation. Additionally, [counsel's] disclosures in connection with the liability phase of the case are not germane to either [the expert's] expertise or expert opinion. Further, [the expert] forgot about the case entirely until the conflict was made known to him by [plaintiff's expert and defense counsel]. It is clear, then, that to the extent that counsel disclosed confidential information, [its expert] did not in any way use that information. Furthermore, and more importantly, [he] never discussed the case with anyone, including [plaintiff's expert]. Suffice it to say that if the expert himself can't remember any of the information, he certainly could not have passed it along to the other expert. (Hansen, 1996, p. 8; Richmond, 2000, p. 920)*

In *Palmer v. Ozbek* (1992) the defendant's expert consulted directly with two of plaintiff's experts for a matter of a few hours. This was their sole contact. Plaintiffs' counsel never communicated directly with the expert, nor did they form a confidential or fiduciary relationship with him. Plaintiffs' experts also did not disclose any trial strategies or confidences; indeed, the only information disclosed was otherwise subject to discovery. Based thereon, the court declined to disqualify the expert (*Palmer*, 1992, p. 68; Richmond, 2000, p. 924). Palmer has been cited as a "well-reasoned" decision, for "[e]xperts' communications with one another should not be punished unless a party's confidences or counsel's work product are revealed. If trial lawyers are concerned about such communications, they must instruct their experts not to discuss their engagement with colleagues" (Richmond, pp. 924–925).

As noted previously, state courts also must resolve conflicts of interests involving experts and whether to disqualify them along with counsel. In *Shadow Traffic Network v. Superior Court*, for example, a California court disqualified the defendant's entire law firm for engaging experts who had been consulted, though not retained, by the plaintiff (Richmond, 2000, p. 921). The defense argued, perhaps understandably so, that it should not be prevented from hiring experts whom the plaintiff chose not to retain—in other words, the plaintiff's communications could not be deemed confidential "as a matter of law" (Richmond, p. 921). Applying the standard two-step disqualification analysis, the court disagreed:

> *[C]ommunications made to a potential expert in a retention interview can be considered confidential and therefore subject to protection from subsequent disclosure...as long as there was a reasonable expectation of such confidentiality. (Shadow Traffic Network v. Superior Court, 1994, p. 700; Richmond, 2000, p. 921)*

Even where opposing counsel is unaware, even through inadvertence of inno-cent oversight, of the dual retention of consulting experts, courts may easily conclude that the whole lot of experts should be disqualified (Richmond, 2000, pp. 921–922). Such was the case in *Mitchell v. Wilmore* (1999), where neither plaintiff nor defendant realized they had engaged the same experts—first, the defense to prepare for deposition, and then the plaintiff, to prepare for trial. Applying the same test, the court agreed with defendant that disqualification was appropriate given its "objectively reasonable belief that their relationship with [the experts] was a confidential one and that the matters discussed would remain inviolate" (*Mitchell*, 1999, pp. 176–177; Richmond, p. 922).

A final consideration, examined by courts to determine whether a party should be allowed to compel the testimony of opposing counsel's former expert, is the availability of other experts on the topic at hand:

> *Courts are unlikely to compel an adversary's former expert to testify where the party seeking to compel the expert's testimony has other available options. The party seeking to compel testimony in that situation cannot claim unfair prejudice if the court precludes the expert's testimony. (Richmond, 2000, pp. 932–933)*

However, it stands to reason that "[i]f a court compels the testimony of a party's former expert, it would not allow the jury to hear that the expert was once employed by the party he is testifying against" (Richmond, 2000, p. 933).

Hence, under a traditional evidentiary balancing test, courts are likely to conclude that "[e]vidence of the prior retention is substantially more prejudicial than probative. Jurors might assume that counsel for the party who first employed the expert is trying to suppress unfavorable evidence by not calling the expert, thus destroying the attorney's credibility. If it appears that jurors may be able to infer how the expert became involved in the case without mention of his prior engagement or if his prior engagement places the party that originally retained him at too great a disadvantage on cross-examination, it may be necessary to exclude the expert's testimony altogether" (Richmond, 2000, p. 933).

Compensation

The expert witness is once again considered to be in a unique context when it comes to the financial aspect of practice. Unlike other witnesses who, although testifying, are traditionally reimbursed only for expenses, an expert is paid a fee for both preparing and testifying in court. It is here where much of the criticism of the use of expert witnesses arises, and the darker side of the business rears its ugly head (Lubet, 1999, p. 477):

> *Litigators regularly shop around for experts to support a partisan theory, rather than accepting a neutral expert who speaks with objectivity. Attorney skepticism of the "so-called impartial educator" is so high, in fact, that many attorneys refuse to employ "an objective, uncommitted, independent expert." (Parker, 1991, pp. 1385–1386)*

Some have even said that

[b]ecause lawyers act as zealous advocates in pursuit of a client's allegedly rightful compensation, "[t]he object is to win" and "[i]n striving to win, lawyers resort to biased interpretations of facts, partial truths, manipulation, and distortion." (Parker, p. 1386)

And often, the

fees to employ necessary expert witnesses constitute substantial litigation expenses and thus potentially act as a bar to effective litigation by litigants who are not wealthy or whose counsel are unable to advance witness fees and absorb them if the case is unsuccessful. (Parker, p. 1368)

It has thus been argued that "[a] major hurdle in obtaining adequate compensation for losses is the prevalence of prohibitively high access fees" (Parker, 1991, p. 1368). The gravamen of the problem is the perception, as well as the fact, of denying a claimant the realistic opportunity to pursue a claim—which is not so much an issue of physical access to courts, but that prohibitively high fees work as an effective bar to recovery just as if a physical barrier had been erected (Parker, p. 1363).

As has been recognized,

[t]he realities of modern medical malpractice may necessitate resort to technical assistance for the education of counsel inexperienced in such litigation, endeavoring to obtain expert witnesses, and marshalling evidence to support the claim. (Parker, 1991, p. 1385). Thus, despite an evidently pervasive fear that "witness shopping" may occur, for the large part, the more rational conclusion is that "the need for competent experts outweigh[s] the possibility of biased testimony" (Parker, p. 1385).

An Exorbitant Fee or a Reasonable Fee?

Not so long ago, a court would not sheepishly extol the ethics of an expert witness, or our perceptions of goodwill, by upholding a contingent fee:

It would be a serious and unwarranted reflection upon the integrity of a physician to say as a matter of law that his testimony was warped or influenced by the fact that, unless a recovery was had, he would not be paid for his services in examining or treating the patient. (Lack Malleable Iron Co. v. Graham, 1912, p. 1018)

The modern experience, however, is altogether differently expressed. Why is this the case? Experts often demand minimum fees for preparation, deposition, and trial testimony "far exceeding that which they would earn were they to charge their regular hourly rate for the actual...time" (Richmond, 1997, p. 566). Furthermore,

Experts may charge the party deposing them an hourly rate exceeding that which they charge the party employing them. Treating physicians may charge expert witness fees far above their regular chargers to their patients, a practice roundly criticized by reviewing courts. (Richmond, p. 566)

And both federal and state courts have long recognized the problems posed by these supposed "abusive fee demands."

Apparently the litigious nature of society has caused litigation participants to forget the adage "an honest day's work for an honest day's pay"...Critics, then, are indeed thankful for the extensive judicial regulation that has come to the fore. (Richmond, 1997, p. 566)

Federal Rule of Civil Procedure 26(b)(4)(C)(i) provides that courts "shall require that the party seeking discovery pay the expert a *reasonable* fee for time spent responding to discovery" (emphasis added). But what is reasonable? How about another test?

Seven factors have been applied by both federal and state courts to evaluate fee reasonableness in light of: (1) the expert's area of expertise; (2) the education and training required to provide the expert the insight which is sought; (3) the prevailing rates of comparable experts; (4) the nature, quality, and complexity of the discovery responses provided; (5) the fee actually being charged to retaining counsel; (6) the fee the expert traditionally charges on related matters; and (7) any other factor likely to be of assistance to the court in balancing the interests implied by Rule 26 (*Jochims v. Isuzu Motors, Ltd.*, 1992, p. 496; Richmond, 1997, p. 567–568). As a consequence, assessing whether a fee is reasonable under such a balancing of interests is rather straightforward.

Still, the often cited decision of *Anthony Abbott Laboratories* (1985) perhaps best illustrates the legal system's frustrations with exorbitant expert witness fees. When the defendant balked at paying one of the plaintiff's key expert's hourly deposition fee, the court, in reducing the fee, waxed so prophetic that we take considerable time here to relate the court's thoughts on the matter:

For a person with little or no discernible overhead, a rate of $420 hourly strikes this court as unconscionable. Based on a standard (40-hour) work week, annualization would produce an income to [the expert] of $840,000 yearly. He may well be a genius in his field, but this court cannot find that even so important and prestigious a profession as medicine has a right to command such exorbitant rewards...There must be some reasonable relationship between the services rendered and the remuneration [sic] to which an expert is entitled; and [the expert's] all-that-the-traffic-will-bear approach falls well outside the outer limits of the universe of rationally-supportable awards.

To be sure, we live in an age where a grown man may be paid a seven figure annual salary to dribble a small round ball. But, the forces of the marketplace are at work in such a situation: not only supply and demand, but the variegated effects of the superstar's presence on attendance, television revenues, and the all-hallowed won/lost record. And, most important, the employer and the employee square off and bargain at arm's length in order to determine an equitable stipend, each with something to lose and something to gain. In the Rule 26(b)(4)(c) context, however, such factors are noticeably absent; the plaintiffs have handpicked the expert, and the defense has neither options nor bargaining power if it desires to obtain the pretrial discovery which the rule permits. Unless the courts patrol the battlefield to ensure fairness, the circumstances invite extortionate fee-setting. (*Anthony Abbott Laboratories*, 1998, p. 464–465; Richmond, 1997, p. 570)

But the court was not done, harkening back to the mainstay of the American legal system:

> *Our citizens' access to justice, which is at the core of our constitutional system of government, is under serious siege. Obtaining justice in this modern era costs too much. The courts are among our most treasured institutions. And, if they are to remain strong and viable, they cannot sit idly by in the face of attempts to loot the system. To be sure, expert witness fees are both the tip of an immense iceberg. But, the skyrocketing costs of litigation have not sprung full-blown from nowhere. Those costs are made up of bits and pieces, and relaxation of standards of fairness threatens further escalation across the board. The effective administration of justice depends, in significant part, on the maintenance and enforcement of a reasoned cost/benefit vigil by the judiciary. (Anthony Abbott Laboratories, 1985, p. 465; Richmond, 1997, p. 570)*

Contingent-Fee Contracts

The American legal system has sought to alleviate the economic barrier preventing access to courts by purportedly prohibitive attorney fees "by allowing claimants to employ counsel on a contingent basis" (Parker, 1991, p. 1363). While an expert is properly paid for his or her testimony, it is utterly impermissible to pay for—let alone foster a legal system predicated upon the use of—testimony bought and paid for on a sliding scale, i.e., dependent upon the outcome of the case. As stated previously, it is the independence of the expert witness that we cherish and hold sacrosanct. Hence, it is a near universal principle that contingent expert witness fees are unethical, and the rationale for the rule is obvious:

> *Such fees are prohibited because they create an unacceptable incentive for the expert to tailor her opinion to the needs or interests of the retaining party. In other words, the expert's independence and objectivity become impaired when payment hinges on the success of the litigation. (Lubet, 1999, p. 477)*

Value Billing

Value billing travels a parallel course, because the fee is determined not by the amount of work actually performed or the "number of hours devoted to the task," but by the "value or benefit conferred by the work" (Lubet, 1999, p. 477). For the expert witness, "value billing can come uncomfortably close to charging on the basis of the content of the testimony" (Lubet, p. 477). It is not only the fact of impropriety, but the appearance of it that must be avoided as well. Thus, for example, an expert's policy of returning fees when the opinion cannot be used by retaining counsel may, at first blush, appear munificent as a cost-cutting grace. The flip side of that coin, however, is the clear result, albeit inadvertent, that the expert receives additional monies when his or her opinion is favorable to the client (Lubet, pp. 477–478). A similar fate might befall an expert who adjusts her hourly rate—either up or down—following the initial research or evaluation of a subject pursuant to an engagement of services (Lubet, p. 478).

Steering clear of such contingencies is rather simple: In order to avoid any undue suggestion, experts should bill "at a constant hourly rate" (Lubet, 1999, p. 478). Then, even when an initial consultation or evaluation leads to a further engagement preparing for deposition or trial, this additional work, while obviously resulting in greater total compensation, is not considered a contingent fee (Lubet, p. 478).

Flat Fees, Minimums, and Retainers

Thankfully, there are several other ethical means by which to arrange fee structures, namely flat fees, minimums, and retainers (Lubet, 1999, p. 478). A flat fee is, as it suggests, a set amount of remuneration for all, or a limited portion, of the engagement.

> *For example, a flat fee could cover the entire engagement all the way through testimony at trial, or it could be determined in stages—perhaps one amount for the initial research and workup, another if a written report becomes necessary, and a final amount for deposition and trial time. (Lubet, p. 478)*

In a similar vein, by charging a minimum fee—usually alongside an hourly assessment—the expert is assured that he or she will be paid a certain amount, irrespective of the amount of work performed (Lubet, p. 478). Finally, a retainer, also known as an advance, traditionally "provides the witness with some or all of her payment at the outset of the engagement, rather than billing exclusively as work is performed" (Lubet, p. 478).

What is critical about each of these fee structures is that in none of them is payment based upon the content of the expert's testimony. For this reason, such financial arrangements are considered by courts to be the flip side of the contingent fee and provide security for experts that they will indeed be compensated for their services (Lubet, 1999, p. 478).

Lock-Up Fees

A final consideration is the lock-up fee (also known as a signing bonus), which essentially represents a nonrefundable payment to the expert at the outset of the engagement of services. The purpose of this fee is "to compensate the witness for agreeing to forego retention by the other parties in the litigation" (Lubet, 1999, p. 478). Here, the expert's uniquely independent role in the legal system rises anew.

There is certainly an element of financial risk in an expert's agreeing to work for one party and receiving client confidences in return. In this instance, as discussed above, the expert may not be permitted to switch sides in the litigation. Imagine the expert's dismay at learning only a short while into the case that his or her opinion is indeed adverse to the client, thus rendering the testimony impotent for the duration of the case for either party. The lock-up fee is an effort to resolve this dilemma "by, in essence, providing the expert with a 'signing bonus' in exchange for agreeing to work exclusively with one client in the matter" (Lubet, 1999, p. 479).

When it comes to retaining counsel, such nonrefundable fee arrangements have been roundly criticized as "oppressive and exploitative," particularly as they affect a client's absolute right to disengage their services (Lubet, 1999, p. 479). The chief objection to the attorney's nonrefundable retainer is that the forfeiture of the retainer creates "a de facto impediment to firing the lawyer" (Lubet, p. 479). Procedural or substantive constructs which chill the free exercise of client rights—constitutional, statutory, or otherwise—are frowned upon. Indeed, these types of signing bonuses have been either banned outright or severely limited, and where they have been used, they have resulted not only in return of monies, but in professional discipline as well (Lubet, p. 479).

Again, the expert witness operates under different constraints from those faced by the attorney. Here, as well, there is an inherent interest in protecting the client from financial loss due to a forced marriage of sorts. Yet, while an expert also may be fired at will by retaining counsel, "no comparable public policy is served" in similarly shielding the client, whose relationship with counsel has been solidified prior to the engagement. The expert is the independent, authoritative source they have solicited to employ (Lubet, 1999, p. 479). Retaining parties should therefore be prepared to accept some risk of cost or penalty in disengaging the services of an expert, whether the expert has performed some or all of the services contracted for. "Consequently, lock-up fees should not be considered unethical when used by expert witnesses" (Lubet, p. 479).

Role During Discovery

An expert's utility to the retaining party is certainly not limited to his or her performance at trial. Indeed, while many cases involve the engagement of expert witnesses, only a small percentage of them actually proceed to trial. Most legal disputes—whether as a sheer consequence of volume or for other more practical reasons—achieve a settlement before the jury reaches a verdict. Therefore, the importance of the role the expert plays in discovery—particularly helping to develop the theory of the case and then advance the cause toward resolution—cannot be overstated. The expert's broad spectrum of involvement is touched upon below.[4]

Communicating With Adverse Counsel

An expert must always remain alert to the potential pitfalls incurred by communicating with lawyers for the opposing party. In order to maintain at least modest vigilance, the expert must know of the distinction between testifying experts and those referred to merely as consulting or nontestifying experts (Lubet, 1999, p. 480). The Federal Rules of Civil Procedure and corresponding provisions in most states limit the right to, and scope of, such contact (Lubet, 1999, p. 480).

> *Although there are limited exceptions, only testifying experts are broadly subject to discovery. Purely consulting experts, other than in extreme circumstances, are exempt from discovery. (Lubet, p. 480; Federal Rules of Civil Procedure 26(b)(4))*

Still, an expert (even a consulting one) cannot turn a blind eye to an impermissible contact. Predictably, most of the discovery rules promulgated to date proscribe conduct by counsel. Thus, most rules probably do not constrain the experts themselves. Once again, it is agency principles which require the expert to take reasonable steps to maintain client confidences (Lubet, 1999, p. 480). The burden is rather simple and straightforward: "A responsible expert, therefore, should notify retaining counsel in the event that she is approached for substantive information by the attorney for an adverse party" (Lubet, p. 480).

Document Production

As discussed herein, the prudent expert, particularly the testifying expert, while keeping client confidences inviolate, knows full well that his or her file may, at some juncture, be subject to full disclosure to the adverse party (Lubet, 1999, p. 480). Whether the expert is testifying or nontestifying, however, the decision whether to turn over materials in discovery is eminently a legal one and the lawyers negotiate this. "Experts are neither expected nor allowed to decide on their own which materials should and should not be disclosed" (Lubet, p. 480).

For the time being, then, for the expert's purposes, the critical obligation—to client, counsel, and court alike—is most obvious:

> *It is unethical, and perhaps even criminal, to conceal or destroy material that has been subpoenaed or requested in discovery. Of course, disclosure may be resisted. There can be objections to discovery and subpoenas may be quashed. But that process nonetheless requires good faith compliance, or at least acknowledgment of the existence of the requested items. (Lubet, 1999, pp. 480–481)*

It is important to note that this limitation is not applicable merely to documents previously requested by the adverse party. As the expert thus abides cautiously by obeying counsel's directives whether to reveal, and if so, the scope of the revelation of otherwise privileged documents or confidences, the expert must take care to "never destroy any item, document, object, photograph, or record for the purpose of concealing it from discovery or obstructing another party's access to evidence" (Lubet, p. 481). This is not to say that in the course of normal housekeeping certain papers and objects may be discarded (Lubet, p. 480). Understandably, this transgression is easiest to discern once the discovery has been requested, and the preservation thereof until the request has been complied with by the expert, or disallowed by the court, is manifest (Lubet, p. 480). It is the matter of concealing materials potentially subject to discovery that is the nefarious undertaking, and should give the expert pause in taking any hasty route which may lead to the imposition of sanctions.

For example, in *House v. Combined Insurance Co.* (1996), a sexual harassment suit, the defendant/insurance company retained a psychiatrist to conduct an independent examination of the plaintiff to discern whether she indeed suffered from emotional distress and subsequently designated that the expert would testify at trial. In preparing for the expert's deposition, the plaintiff sought production of his report in discovery. Likely harboring knowledge that the expert's opinions were adverse to the defense, the defendant then moved for a protective order regarding the report and, though it did not recede from having designated him as an expert witness, it did drop him from its final witness list and apprised the court that it did not intend to call him at trial (Richmond, 2000, p. 930).

The court noted there were "three possible standards to apply when determining whether a party should have access to an adversary's former expert" (Richmond, 2000, p. 930):

The first option is the "exceptional circumstances" standard in Federal Rule of Civil Procedure 26(b)(4)(B), which deals with the consulting experts. The second is a " 'discretionary' or 'balancing' standard," which weighs the "interests of the [discovering] party and the court against the potential for prejudice to the party who hired the expert." The third and most lenient standard is an "entitlement" standard, drawn from a few cases holding that a party is entitled to call an adversary's expert notwithstanding the adversary's opposition. (House v. Combined Insurance Co., 1996, p. 240)

Because the case dealt not with testifying experts, but the "very significant difference from the situation in which an expert has merely been consulted by a party, but never designated as likely to testify at trial," the court rejected the exceptional circumstances standard (*House*, 1996, p. 245), reasoning thus:

Parties should be encouraged to consult experts to formulate their own cases, to discard those experts for any reason, and to place them beyond the reach of an opposing party, if they have never indicated an intention to use the expert at trial. Such a consulted-but-never-designated expert might properly be considered to fall under the work product doctrine that protects matters prepared in anticipation of litigation. (House, p. 245)

"For this reason also, the ability of an opposing party to call a never-designated expert at trial should depend upon a showing of 'extraordinary circumstances' " (*House*, 1996, p. 245).

The court continued:

However, once an expert is designated, the expert is recognized as presenting part of the common body of discoverable, and generally admissible, information and testimony available to all parties. A party's designation of an expert as a witness to be called at trial, even if later revoked, removes the expert from the category of consulting experts who are protected from compelled testimony absent a showing of exceptional circumstances. (House, 1996, p. 245)

When it came to the case at hand, however, the court ultimately applied the intermediate-level discretionary or balancing standard, which best balanced " 'the court's [objective] interest in the proper resolution of the issues' with the parties' interests in presenting their claims and preserving their defenses" (*House*, 1996, p. 246; Richmond, 2000, p. 931). This case demonstrates that the role the "public interest" plays in shaping such decision is significant. Thus, *House* held that the expert's testimony should in fact be presented to the jury to "aid in the proper resolution of the issues" (Richmond, p. 931).

Still, the court placed a logical restriction upon plaintiff's presentation of evidence in order to, as always, keep the playing field as even as possible in the pursuit of the fair administration of justice:

The court was concerned, however, that [the expert's] testimony would unfairly prejudice [the defendant] if the plaintiff was allowed to elicit testimony that [defendant] originally hired the doctor and then dropped him as a witness once his opinions became known. (Richmond, 2000, p. 931)

Therefore, in equity, the court held that the plaintiff could indeed call the expert at trial, "provided that evidence of how he became involved in the case was excluded" (*House, 1996*, p. 248; Richmond, 2000, p. 931).

The court opined that:

"House teaches what should be obvious: a party who hires an expert should do so carefully. The case also illustrates that health-care providers who testify as experts based on independent medical examinations performed under the Federal Rules of Civil Procedure or state court equivalents may be treated differently from other experts." (Richmond, 2000, p. 931)[5]

Depositions

Simply stated, "[a] deposition is pretrial testimony, taken under oath for the purpose of discovering what the witness has to say" (Lubet, 1999, p. 481). There are few ethical pitfalls for the expert to beware of here, "though all the standard issues such as confidentiality, coaching, and candor certainly can and do arise" (Lubet, p. 481). That no judge is present, however, does present a question worthy of note: Should the expert act upon the advice of counsel, received on or off the record, in the face of a contrary directive by opposing counsel? Since local procedures play a large role in directing the expert's response, the more cautious approach is recommended here (Lubet, p. 481). Of course, where the witness has been apprised of more definitive authority, a more precise course of action may be justified.

Conferences between expert witnesses and retained counsel are commonplace during deposition. In days past, it was "considered routine almost everywhere for lawyers to pull aside their witnesses so long as there was no question pending at that particular moment. While most such conferences were no doubt conducted in good faith to clarify a point, to preserve a confidence, or to calm down a nervous witness, they were also the occasion of much abuse. Too many lawyers used off-record conferences to obstruct the deposition, coach the witness, or worse" (Lubet, 1999, pp. 481–482).

Rules governing counsel's right to confer with a witness now vary greatly among jurisdictions. For our purposes, the import of this development was to free the expert from the quandary of facing "a great variety of environments" and not always being able "to count on the lawyers for clear or knowledgeable directions," though it is at them, ironically, that procedural rules are particularly aimed (Lubet, 1999, p. 482). The soundest advice is for the expert to take matters into his or her own, educated hands. Remember that retained counsel is not the expert's counsel (Lubet, p. 485). "The expert is there to provide an independent analysis and opinion. Since the expert is not a party to the case, the expert is not represented by either of the attorneys" (Lubet, p. 485).

Indeed, expert witnesses are rarely, if ever, accompanied by their own attorney at deposition (Lubet, 1999, p. 485). Hence, if adverse counsel does not object to the expert's conferring with retained counsel, there is obviously little reason for concern (Lubet, p. 482). When a disagreement does arise, however—especially those requiring undue revelation of client confidences or responses beyond the scope of expertise—seldom is it "the witness's job to resolve" (Lubet, p. 482). The lawyers are there for something. And unless the expert has "reliable independent knowledge of the jurisdiction's rule, the best approach to this problem is probably to follow the directions of the retaining lawyer" (Lubet, p. 483). Stated more succinctly:

> *Recall that an expert has specific professional obligations to the client, including a duty to take reasonable steps to protect certain confidences. It is the retaining lawyer who speaks for the client, and it is the retaining lawyer who is most knowledgeable about the effect of the deposition upon the client's confidences. Hence, the prudent path is usually to accept the retaining lawyer's understanding of the rules. (Lubet, p. 483)*

This is not to say, of course, that lawyers are infallible (Lubet, 1999, p. 483). No one is. So, if something sounds too good to be true, even if expressed by retained counsel, it probably is. Consequently, "[a]n expert should never violate or disregard a court order, no matter how many assurances are forthcoming from retaining counsel (Lubet, p. 483). More important, even where conferencing is freely allowed, an expert should likewise never permit retaining counsel to dictate or alter the content of her testimony" (Lubet, p. 483). And only "[i]n *extreme* or *extraordinary* circumstances, the expert should consider whether she needs to consult her own attorney" (emphasis added) (Lubet, p. 483).

But what about conflicting directives, where the deposing and retaining lawyers dispute the authority of the expert to reveal a confidence or opinion? Ostensibly, the expert may now be in a bind:

> *Retaining counsel has instructed her not to answer but the deposing lawyer insists threatening court action is she refuses. Which lawyer is right? Which one should the witness believe? Most important, how should the witness respond? (Lubet, 1999, p. 484)*
>
> *Well, it does not take an "expert" to answer this one. Once the cat is out of the bag, so to speak, the damage is already done. Consequently, the expert must always be sensitive to the need to shield privileged information. Once information has been revealed, it may lose its protected nature even if the deposing lawyer was never entitled to it in the first place. (Lubet, 1999, p. 484)*

The better course, then, is for the expert to decline to answer when an impediment arises or an apparent impasse presents itself. After all, there is little downside to a temporary halt in the proceedings. And here, then, is the solution:

> *If the witness improperly declines to answer, the information can always be provided later. Thus, there is relatively little harm in refusing to answer a particular question, pending resolution by the lawyers or a ruling by the court. On the other hand, information can never be retrieved once it has been disclosed. Great damage can be done by ignoring an objection and by proceeding to reply…Thus, in the absence of other factors, the best approach for a witness is to decline to answer questions once*

retaining counsel has objected on the basis of privilege or confidentiality. A polite refusal to answer will preserve the objection so that it may, if necessary, be brought before the court. (Lubet, 1999, p. 484)

For example, a suitable response to a deposing lawyer's admonition that the expert is following his or her lawyer's instructions and refusing to answer the questions may thus be:

"I am not following anyone's instructions, but I decline to answer that question. It is not my job to resolve disputes between counsel about privilege or discoverability" (Lubet, p. 485).

Role at Trial

As litigation enters the trial phase, "the basic principles of professional ethics" continue to govern the expert's conduct (Lubet, 1999, p. 485). There are, however, a few trial-specific issues worthy of mention.

Ex Parte Communications

An *ex parte* communication is one that involves fewer than the total number of parties legally entitled to share it or to be present during the discussion. Thus, as a general rule, "all communication with the court must take place in the presence of all attorneys" (Lubet, 1999, p. 485). Like any other witness or party-agent, the expert witness should take care to avoid any formal or informal private conversation with a judge on any pending matter, even at the appellate level—particularly discussions of "the substance of the case or the content of the witness's testimony" (Lubet, p. 485). This admonition is, indeed, rather straightforward.

Do not think for a moment, however, that the only culprit might be you as the expert witness. "Unfortunately, it also happens that judges seek out witnesses even without legal justification. Perhaps the judge is curious, incautious, or simply unaware of the extent of the rule against *ex parte* communication" (Lubet, 1999, p. 486). Frankly, the reason does not matter very much at all. "*Whatever* the reason, such contact can obviously cause much discomfort for the witness" (emphasis added) (Lubet, p. 486). To be sure, "[m]ost witnesses would *never* presume to question the judge's knowledge of law or ethics" (emphasis added) (Lubet, p. 486). Might the communication therefore be appropriate? After all, "the judge is the judge" (Lubet, p. 486).

It might be argued that alongside the exalted nature of the expert's independent status in the sphere of litigation comes some responsibility considered above and beyond the ken. Foremost, outside of testimony on the witness stand, experts must remain vigilant to avoid such communications—whether with the court or, for that matter, with jurors (Lubet, 1999, p. 486). The expert witness, like any witness, should limit contact with the court or the jury—in the hallway, elevator, or cafeteria—"to a polite smile or greeting," if that. And surely, "[u]nder no circumstances should a witness *ever* discuss a case with a sitting juror" or judge (Lubet, p. 486).

Third-Party Communications

The rules proscribing the expert witness's communications with others during trial, including other witnesses, are rather straightforward as well. More commonly known as the Rule of Sequestration (The Rule), once invoked by one or both of the parties, or by the court on its own motion, normally excludes witnesses from the courtroom while others are testifying (Lubet, 1999, p. 486). The purpose of this rule is to arrive at as pristine a result as possible, i.e., where one witness's testimony is not unduly influenced, tainted, or swayed by another. Obviously, knowledge of other witnesses' testimonies can be gleaned not merely from sitting in the courtroom, but also from discussing prior testimony with them before the expert takes the stand (Lubet, p. 486). Therefore, "[a]n expert should not debrief another witness who has already testified and should not read the transcript of earlier testimony, other than at the direction of trial counsel" (Lubet, p. 487). And remember, even if trial counsel directs you to do so, an insistent bell should go off in your head that you and you alone are ultimately responsible for the candor and tenor of your testimony.

Because of their uniquely independent character in the litigation process, however, expert witnesses are sometimes excepted from this proscription. Therefore, the expert should "always check with retaining counsel before attending the trial as an observer" (Lubet, 1999, p. 486).

When it comes to contact between the expert and retained counsel, particularly contact during trial—including communications during recesses in the witness's testimony—the rules vary from courthouse to courthouse. In some jurisdictions, broad dialogue is permitted; in others, there may be limited, if any, contact once the expert is placed under oath (Lubet, 1999, p. 487). In other jurisdictions, access to speak with the expert is dependent upon where during the expert's testimony the recess is taken, i.e., during, or upon the conclusion of, the witness's direct examination (Lubet, p. 487). Which is the best rule to follow, then? "Needless to say, expert witnesses should determine the applicable rule for the court in question. Whatever the rule, the witness should comply" (Lubet, p. 487).

In most litigation, it does not suit the preferences of the press to seek public commentary by the parties or witnesses. Most cases are, after all, routine. For this reason, trial courts are rarely called upon to enter this forum. There are times, however, when this is not the case. "In the absence of a gag order or secrecy statute, witnesses are free to speak with the press about the trials in which they have participated" (Lubet, 1999, p. 487). Still, an expert's sense of professionalism may, and usually should, cause him or her to think twice before doing so for good reason:

> *Ordinarily, a party to litigation does not retain an expert for the purpose of speaking to the press. The party may not want the case publicized and may not want to risk the exposure of confidences. In this regard, experts should take their cue from retaining counsel. (Lubet, p. 487)*

And the cue from most prudent counsel is, in general, to decline comment, especially in pending litigation. In only the rarest instances will trying the case in the press assist the trier of fact—unless of course that is the expert's particular style. And when it will assist in advancing the course of a case, rest assured that retaining counsel will most likely let the expert know.

Excluded Evidence

As discussed earlier, it is predominantly retained counsel's responsibility to apprise the expert of the information that is available for review, the legal standards to be addressed and, ultimately, where the expert's opinion fits in counsel's theory of the case. However, "[w]ith or without the expert's knowledge, certain evidence may have been ruled inadmissible by the court," either *in limine*, that is, pretrial, or even during the trial itself (Lubet, 1999, p. 487). Trial, after all, is a dynamic, not a static, process. It is therefore incumbent upon counsel to inform the expert of any limitations on his or her testimony to come. And of course, "[o]nce evidence has been ruled inadmissible, either during or before the witness's testimony, it is unethical to sneak it in 'through the back door' " (Lubet, p. 487). Furthermore, the expert, always playing it safe and ethical, once instructed to refrain from revealing certain matters, "should not attempt to blurt out the proscribed information on the pretext of answering an unrelated question" (Lubet, 1999, pp. 487–488).

Conclusion: The Ultimate Burden of Self-Preservation

"It is widely recognized that expert testimony is 'virtually indispensable' in cases where the facts are outside the realm of understanding of lay jurors or judges" (*Natural Soda Prods. v. City of Los Angeles*, 1952, p. 994). Expert witnesses indeed play a prominent role in the American litigation process, but, as discussed, the legal system is ultrasensitive to the potential for abuse given that it bombards triers of fact with potent, scientific testimony, as well as its effect, real or perceived, upon access to courts.

In light of all of the foregoing, and in accord with the legally apt adage that "ignorance is *not* bliss" (Richmond, 2000, p. 928), it is strongly recommended that the expert take it upon him- or herself to ensure both the propriety of the engagement of services and the sanctity of the ensuing agent relationship. From the outset, experts ought to take care "to avoid conduct that contributes to a lack of clarity about the relationship," either with counsel or the opposing party (*Wang Laboratories*, 1991, p. 1250; Richmond, p. 928). Should an expert wish to decline employment, the prudent course is to "express their doubts clearly" (*Wang Laboratories*, p. 1250; Richmond, p. 928). Obviously, "[i]f an expert does not want to share a confidential relationship with a prospective employer, she should decline the engagement" (*English Feedlot, Inc. v. Norden Labs, Inc.* p. 1505; Richmond, at p. 928). And if an expert does not wish to be employed, is unsure about his desire for the employment, or, perhaps most important, does not want to be obligated to maintain client confidences, he or she must take care not to accept information or materials relating to the case altogether (*Wang Laboratories*, p. 1250; Richmond, p. 929). Moreover, in such cases, experts should also "decline a retainer or any other fee advance" (Richmond, p. 929). Finally, where an expert has consulted with a party in a case and is subsequently contacted by another party to the litigation, it stands to reason that it is incumbent upon him or her to "inform the second party of the prior consultation" (*Proctor & Gamble, Co. v. Haugen*, 1999, p. 414; Richmond, p. 929). A conscious effort to observe these simple and straightforward guidelines should serve the expert well in avoiding conflicts of interest that may lead to unanticipated and rather unpleasant results.

Notes

1. In federal courts, six rules of evidence intertwine to govern expert-witness testimony: Rule 104(a) (the trial court's preliminary resolution of questions of admissibility, such as witness competency, privilege, scientific knowledge, and whether the testimony will assist, rather than obfuscate, the trier of fact's effort to understand or determine a fact in issue); Rule 702 (mandating that expert witnesses be qualified to render opinions which clarify issues); Rule 703 (the types of facts and data upon which an expert may base his or her opinion or inference); Rule 705 (permitting the expert to testify in the form of an opinion or inference without necessarily testifying first as to its foundational basis, i.e., in the form of a "naked opinion"); Rule 403 (recognizing the trial court's broad discretion to balance probative value against undue prejudice arising from the admission of evidence); and Rule 704 (permitting an expert to render an opinion as to the ultimate issue in the litigation) (Richmond, 1997, pp. 491–533). Ultimately, it is not the court's function to determine whether an expert's opinions are correct, but "merely whether the bases supporting the conclusions are reliable" (*Joiner v. General Electric Co.,* 1997, p. 533; Richmond, p. 499).

2. Each of these concerns has caused, and continue to cause, increased scrutiny of "professional experts," as ominously summarized thus: Expert testimony often becomes a point of contention in cases in which an expert witness is alleged to be a "professional expert." Professional experts usually are compelling witnesses whose primary function is persuading the jury; the expert's demeanor, personality, and communications skills are far more important than the subject of the expert's testimony. Professional expert witnesses freely change their theories and qualifications to suit their immediate employers...Novel scientific testimony sprouts like weeds. Some scientific testimony borders on the absurd (Richmond, 1997, pp. 487–488). Noted examples include experts specializing in footprint-to-person matching, later debunked as "complete hogwash"; forensic dentistry matching bite marks via ultraviolet light, detectable solely by that single expert; and psychological syndrome evidence—such as child sexual abuse accommodation, rape trauma, and battered-woman, post-traumatic-stress, parental-alienation, and false-memory syndromes, to name a few—which, unlike diseases, "follow no specified temporal course, nor is their pathology clear" (Richmond, p. 488).

3. A prime example, the Model Code of Professional Responsibility, is set forth in three parts: First, Canons, which are statements expressing the standards of conduct to be expected of the professional and embody the general concepts comprising the latter two components of the Code. Second are Ethical Considerations, which are aspirational in nature. And third, Disciplinary Rules, which are mandatory and relate the minimum level of conduct below which no professional can fall lest he or she be subject to discipline (Parker, 1991, p. 1391, n. 6).

4. In addition to the areas addressed herein, an expert's familiarity with procedures embodied in rules such as Federal Rules of Civil Procedure 26 and 37, which discuss, generally, disclosure requirements, rebuttal, and

impeachment testimony, for both testifying and consulting experts alike, is highly recommended (Richmond, 1997, pp. 533–543).

5. Note, however, that "[a] party's designation of an expert to testify at trial does not always entitle an opponent to depose that expert or to call him or her as a witness at trial if the expert switches sides. A party should not be allowed to call an adversary's former expert in an attempt to cure the mistake of not designating its own expert. Nor should a party be allowed to call its adversary's former expert where the expert's testimony is not relevant or is only 'indirectly pertinent'" (Richmond, 1997, p. 931).

References

Anthony Abbott Laboratories, 106 F.R.D. 461 (D. R.I. 1985).

Baxter v. Temple, 949 A. 2d 167 (N.H. 2008).

Black, H. L. (1979). *Black's law dictionary* (5th ed). Eagan, MN: West Publishing.

Boswell, J. (1887). *The life of Samuel Johnson*. New York: Oxford University Press.

Coffey, K., (2004). Inherent judicial authority and the expert disqualification doctrine. *Florida Law Review, 195*, 234–246.

Cordy v. Sherwin-Williams, Co., 156 F.R.D. 575 (D. N.J. 1994).

Daubert v. Merrell Dow Pharmaceuticals, Inc., 509 U.S. 579 (1993).

Donovan v. Bowling, 706 A.2d 937 (R.I. 1998).

English Feedlot, Inc. v. Norden Labs, Inc., 833 F. Supp. 1498 (D. Colo. 1993).

Federal Rules of Civil Procedure 26(a)(2)(B).

Federal Rules of Civil Procedure 26(b)(4).

Federal Rules of Civil Procedure 26(b)(4)(B).

Federal Rules of Civil Procedure 37.

Federal Rules of Evidence 104(a), 702-705.

Hansen v. Umtech Industrieservice Und Spedition, GmbH, No. 95-516 MMS, 1996 WL 622557, at *1 (D. Del. July 3, 1996).

House v. Combined Insurance Co., 168 F.R.D. 236 (N.D. Iowa 1996).

Jochims v. Isuzu Motors, Ltd., 141 F.R.D. 493 (S.D. Iowa 1992).

Joiner v. General Electric Co., 78 F.3d 524 (11th Cir. 1996), *cert. granted*, 117 S.Ct. 1243 (1997).

Koch Ref. Co. v. Jennifer L. Boudreaux MV, 85 F.3d 1178 (5th Cir. 1996).

Kumho Tire Co. v. Carmichael, 526 U.S. 137 (1999).

Lack Malleable Iron Co. v. Graham, 143 S.W. 1016, 1018 (1912).

Lubet, S. (1999). Expert witnesses: Ethics and professionalism. *Georgia Journal of Legal Ethics, 465*, 123–134.

Mitchell v. Wilmore, 981 P.2d 172 (Colo. 1999).

Murphy v. A.A. Mathews, 841 S.W.2d 671 (Mo. 1992).

Natural Soda Prods, Co. v. City of Los Angeles, 240 P.2d 993 (Cal. App. 1952).

Palmer v. Ozbek, 144 F.R.D. 66 (D. Md. 1992).

Parikh, S. (2006/2007). How the spider catches the fly: Referral networks in the plaintiffs' personal injury bar. *New York Law School Review, 56*, 243.

Parker, J., (1991). Contingent expert witness fees: Access and legitimacy. *Southern California Legal Review, 64*, 1363.

Proctor & Gamble, Co. v. Haugen, 183 F.R.D. 571 (D. Utah 1998).

Proctor & Gamble, Co. v. Haugen, 184 F.R.D. 410 (D. Utah 1999).

Richmond, D. R. (1997). Regulating expert testimony. *Missouri Law Review, 62*, 485.

Richmond, D. R. (2000) Expert witness conflicts and compensation. *Tennessee Law Review, 67*, 909.

Selvidge v. United States, 160 F.R.D. 153 (D. Kan. 1995).

Shadow Traffic Network v. Superior Court, 29 Cal. Rptr.2d 693 (Cal. Ct. App. 1994).

Wang Laboratories, Inc. v. Toshiba Corp., 762 F. Supp. 1246 (E.D. Va. 1991).

Webster's college dictionary. (1991). New York: Random House.

Weisgram v. Marley Co., 120 S. Ct. 1011 (2000).

Part III
Practice
Issues in
Neuropsychology

Depositions

13

Lawrence C. Hartlage
Betsy L. Williams

Deposition Basics

A neuropsychologist who examines patients with suspected brain injury, especially an injury of either traumatic or neurotoxic etiology, can expect to be deposed. Even though at the time of the examination of the patient there may be no awareness of any potential forensic involvement, when subsequent legal action is pursued the neuropsychologist may be called for deposition as a witness whose testimony is expected to be favorable to one side (and thus hostile to the opposing side). When examining patients for brain injury of possible traumatic etiology, such as in an automotive or work-related injury, positive findings of the examination can be helpful to the patient (plaintiff) by establishing that damage exists. Conversely, negative examination findings can be helpful to insurers in defending against such claims. Similarly, with neurotoxic exposure, such as to lead paint, if the examination documents brain injury, counsel for the plaintiff alleging brain injury will possibly list you as an expert whose testimony will support his or her case. The defense attorney then would be interested in discrediting or minimizing your findings. Should your examination produce negative evidence of brain injury, the plaintiff's attorney will be interested in challenging or possibly discrediting or minimizing your findings. The deposition serves all these purposes.

Litigants rely on expert testimony in approximately 80% of all civil cases and in approximately 50% of all felony prosecutions (Kline, 1996). Since it is now well recognized that neuropsychological examination can provide the most comprehensive and accurate data concerning how central nervous system insults affect the patient's neurocognitive and neurobehavioral functions, neuropsychologists are the logical expert witnesses to explain to the triers of fact (i.e., the courts) the relationship between an injury to the patient's brain and the effect this injury has—or may be expected to have—on the patient.

Although going through the rigors of preparation for, and the stresses of, being deposed can involve a major interruption in the neuropsychologist's normal schedule, such participation in the legal process represents a professional obligation both to the patient involved and to the legal system in which we practice. A deposition can compel the neuropsychologist to examine his or her own examination practice, especially if the examination at issue involves the use of nonstandardized or out-of-date tests, utilization of only parts of test, or testing in situations in which the patient's English is less than fluent. Justification of examination findings can be challenged and the neuropsychologist should be prepared to defend both the choice of tests and the interpretation of those tests.

Whether the examination is conducted at the request of an attorney for either side, or it is revealed during or after the examination that litigation is planned or underway, the attorney whose case is bolstered or strengthened by the neuropsychological finding will consider the neuropsychologist as *their* witness, and the opposing attorney will consider him or her as *supporting the enemy's side.* The neuropsychologist, of course, is an independent scientist/practitioner whose interest is in the accuracy of the examination data and of the interpretation of those data. The neuropsychologist is not, and must not become, involved in the *us versus them* mindset, even though prior to the deposition there may have been communication with the attorney whose case is strengthened by (or even perhaps based on) neuropsychological examination findings.

Deposition Focus: Discovery

Most commonly, a neuropsychologist will be called to a deposition by the attorney for the defense. If the examination findings confirm the presence of traumatic brain injury from an automotive accident (a finding helpful to the plaintiff's case), the attorney for the defense may wish to conduct the deposition. The typical purpose of this deposition includes several facets that, as described, are for purposes of discovery. This discovery deposition provides the opportunity for the defense attorney to evaluate a neuropsychologist in terms of how he or she would come across to a jury. Issues such as the neuropsychologist's apparent expertise, honesty, candor, and credibility may influence the strategy of one or both sides, and may determine whether the defense attorney wants to rely on or attack the testimony of the neuropsychologist in front of the jury. This can be an important determinant of whether a case is settled or is carried to trial.

During the process of preparation, it is essential that the patient's chart and all records be completely reviewed, and that all scoring be verified as accurate. If the examination was conducted long before the deposition is scheduled, it is advisable to arrange for a brief reexamination, both to update and confirm the findings, and to assess what has occurred in regard to the patient's condition since the initial examination. It is also helpful to contact the attorney(s) involved to determine whether relevant new information has evolved. In any case, it is important to review and be familiar with everything in the record. It may be helpful in preparation for deposition to make a face sheet for handy reference during the deposition containing items in the record arranged in a system meaningful to the individual practitioner. This might include (a) test data and notes corresponding to each successive section of your written report; (b) communications with attorney, including billing; (c) records from other sources such as schools and hospitals; and (d) other data in the record, whether or not it is considered relevant. Separate clusters of related records, fastened with an identifying label, will help provide quick access to sections needed to answer specific questions or address specific requests during the deposition. This system of organization will not only serve to enhance the neuropsychologist's presentation of the case, but also enhance his or her sense of being knowledgeable about the case.

If it is believed, for example, that lateralized brain injury is documented by the examination, it may be helpful to review the test data to list all tests confirming asymmetry in order to have it ready for reference. If it is noted that tests of *hold* abilities (i.e., cognitive abilities resistant to impairment following brain injury) show much more intact functional status than are reflected on don't *hold* measures that are more sensitive to acquired brain injury, having a tabulation of those tests and their comparative scores may be helpful. Another helpful method may be to create a notebook for quick referral with tabbed pages and an index indicating where every test or form is located. Additional tabs can be added to organize new information relevant or potentially relevant to the case. Above all, the expert should know the data; when the patient was seen; which tests were administered and the results of the tests; and the context of any relevant, and even seemingly irrelevant, information, correspondence, or notations in the record. The more readily the patient's record can be reconstructed without referring to notes (e.g., height, weight, handedness, eyeglasses, limping, use of cane or crutches, prominent body piercings, tattoos, or hair, mannerisms, or affective status) the better. Similarly, the more details of the examination you can recall, such as the sequence of tests, special difficulty with a given test, overall findings, clusters of findings, or specific findings, the easier it will be to respond to unexpected questions. Seemingly irrelevant questions regarding things such as if and when breaks were taken and which tests were administered just before break, could be used, for example, as a basis for implying that a low score on a test given just before a break represents fatigue rather than brain damage. The neuropsychologist may be asked to identify each and every piece of paper or notation, and how each relates to the overall professional opinion. As Lord Baden Powell, who founded the Boy Scouts, suggested, and Tom Lehrer immortalized in song, "be prepared."

In the course of the deposition, opposing counsel may adopt a hostile, challenging, or confrontational demeanor to observe how the neuropsychologist reacts; or, conversely, may proceed in a friendly, relaxed manner to enhance the possibility that you may become equally relaxed and thus be more free in making extraneous comments. The focus of the deposition is often to *box you in*, so that there is a possibility that in a subsequent possible trial the opposing counsel will know exactly how you will respond to certain questions. For this reason, a widely accepted maxim for the neuropsychologist in a discovery deposition is to answer the questions, but not reveal more information than is necessary to answer the questions. Tell the truth but do not elaborate beyond the question asked. One reason for this manner of responding is that, in response to the opposing counsel's strategy of not responding to your answer but waiting expectantly, the neuropsychologist often feels compelled to elaborate or explain with additional information that can subsequently be used to impeach that testimony or make an argument against the neuropsychologist, the examination, the conclusions, or the neuropsychologist's thought process in reaching the conclusions. There may be times when the neuropsychologist is pushed for a *yes* or *no* answer even though it would be difficult to respond so succinctly or in such a dichotomous manner. In such instances, the neuropsychologist can simply state, "I cannot answer that question without misleading the court. May I explain?" During the process of cross examination, it is important for the neuropsychologist to be willing to make appropriate concessions. For example, some questions may clearly limit the point that the neuropsychologist wishes to make, but if the question is based on fact, it is important not to argue. It is also important to keep in mind that one cannot hope to always present views in an affirmative way in response to questions on cross examination (Babistski & Mangraviti, 2003).

Effective performance in a deposition may entail more than reflecting competence as a clinician, due to differing criteria typically espoused by the scientist-practitioner psychologist versus the advocate attorney. Such matters as degree of certainty help illustrate this point. To attorneys, the standard of *more probable than not* constitutes sufficient basis for confidence in an opinion, whereas the psychologist may hold to a much higher standard for expressing confidence on an opinion. As a result, scientific conservatism may suggest to the jury that the testimony is weak. For example, while the scientist-practitioner generally evaluates findings in terms of probabilities (e.g., $p < .05$, or the more rigorous $p < .01$), attorneys are more likely to phrase questions in terms of *reasonable (neuropsychological) certainty*. For example, an attorney might ask, "Doctor, can you state with reasonable neuropsychological certainty that the automobile collision on [date] causes the brain injury that you conclude is documented by your examination." The level of probability needed to support an affirmative reply is, in legal terms, *more likely than not* but in scientific terms it would be $> .50$. It must be considered that psychologists are trained to consider all relevant factors (e.g., socioeconomic, educational, environmental, contextual, etc.) resulting in given test findings or outcomes, whereas the legal focus is on a single causation (e.g., Did the wreck cause these problems?).

Although there can be large differences among attorneys concerning how opposing counsel may formulate the discovery deposition focus, the questions may aim at: evaluating the neuropsychologist's qualifications (e.g., education, training, experience, expertise in the type of case at issue); any possible biases (e.g., toward plaintiff versus defense work); and at examining closely the scientific basis for any conclusions reached. The neuropsychologist can expect to be requested to make an up-to-date curriculum vitae (CV) available to the attorney taking the deposition and, in fact, the neuropsychologist's CV may well be submitted as Exhibit 1. Sometimes the attorney taking the deposition may request (or otherwise obtain) a copy of the neuropsychologist's CV well prior to the examination in order to have an opportunity to review it and ask questions about its contents. In this example testimony will involve putative brain injury, so the neuropsychologist may be questioned about which specific aspects of education, training, or experience qualifies him or her to address the topic at hand or which of his or her publications reflect expertise in the subject, and so on. The neuropsychologist's prior publications or professional presentations may be used to indicate a bias (e.g., continuing education presentation to defense or plaintiff's attorneys). Certain topics of scholarship, such as malingering in neuropsychological testing, could suggest a bias that would help either the plaintiff or the defense attorney. The neuropsychologist can expect to be asked to reveal which prior legal cases he or she has provided expert testimony or opinions for, and the names and sides (e.g., plaintiff or defense) of the attorneys involved. In some (e.g., federal) courts, this type of information may need to cover a specific period of years.

The neuropsychologist will quite possibly be seen as biased in favor of the attorneys on one or the other side of the particular case. For example, even though the neuropsychologist was not retained to do the examination by the plaintiff's attorneys, if the majority of the prior involvement with litigated cases included patients in whom he or she documented brain damage, that witness will be considered a *plaintiff's* witness (i.e., having a bias in favor of plaintiff). If the majority of patients the neuropsychologist has examined in litigated cases were found not to have brain injury, he or she would be considered a *defense* expert witness. This characterization of the expert witness as biased in favor of one side or the other based on the proportion of cases done for either plaintiff or defense is most often not accurate as a measure of bias. The incidence of patients with or without brain injury may merely reflect the referral basis of an individual's practice rather than any conscious bias. However, bias is in the mind of the opposing counsel, who may try to use the alleged bias to discredit the neuropsychologist.

The neuropsychologist also may expect questions oriented toward disciplinary action or license suspension, any criminal involvement other than traffic accidents, insurance suits against him or her, or even involvement in other lawsuits not in any way related to neuropsychology.

It is generally a good idea to consider answers carefully before responding, even if the questions appear to be simple and do not involve any ambiguity. There are several reasons for doing this. One is the fact that, for legal reasons, the neuropsychologist's retaining attorney may wish to object to any given question. A too-prompt response deprives the attorney of this option. The second reason is more subtle. If there is a prompt response to most questions, opposing counsel may just try to throw in an apparently innocent question, whose phraseology would render the neuropsychologist's response somewhat different from what was meant. This is especially important when being asked to respond to assumptions. For example, a question involving whether the patient did or did not do or say something on a given date may not be accurate. Given that the neuropsychologist is under oath, whereas the attorney deposing him or her is not, considering a question before answering will give the witness's attorney an opportunity to object (e.g., facts not in evidence) to having the witness answer on the assumption of facts that are not accurate. Additionally, sometimes a questioning attorney will fall into a rhythm of attack, with a prepared sequence of questions directed toward some goal, and if the witness does not respond promptly to such questions, or occasionally takes a longer time than expected, it may help disrupt the timing aimed at leading the witness to some desired goal. Chances are that the attorney deposing the witness has done this sort of thing many, many times and has likely evolved a format for examining witnesses. The witness, by comparison, is a scientist and clinician whose expertise does not lie in depositions. Therefore, careful consideration of answers before responding helps blunt the edge of a well-honed plan of attack and can obviate the likelihood of blurting out something which falls into the category of *I wish I hadn't said that*. Tell the truth but stop after answering.

A few common deposition tactics frequently employed by attorneys who consider a witness's testimony as potentially harmful to their case are worth mention. If the opposing attorney reads from a document and asks the neuropsychologist for a response to what has been read, the witness should ask to see the document before responding and request sufficient time to carefully read and reflect on the document before answering. The witness should not accept the opposing attorney's characterization of his or her prior testimony. Such statements as, "you have earlier testified that…" may well be paraphrased to slightly slant the witness's words into phraseology helpful to the attorney. Occasionally, several such characterizations in a sequence—each slightly distorting what was said—can be used to completely change a witness's testimony. If the neuropsychologist cannot recall exactly what he or she said, or if there is any doubt at all that the statement differs in any way from what was said, the witness should ask to review the court reporter's transcript before responding. The neuropsychologist should avoid agreeing with questions involving *always* or *never* unless absolutely certain that there are no exceptions. The witness will be safer responding to such questions in phraseology like, "In my experience, I have not encountered such situations." If the question is pursued, the witness can add, "I cannot recall any report in the research literature involving such a situation." Responding to broadly phrased questions involving the witness's thought processes in reaching a conclusion can provide the attorney with avenues of attack. Finally, if asked, "Anything else?" the witness is advised not to volunteer answers. A reply such as, "If you have any more specific questions, I will be glad to try to answer them," will suffice. A trick very commonly used in depositions is the question, "Doctor, how much are you being paid for your testimony today?" If the neuropsychologist answers with what he or she is charging, this can be used as evidence that the witness is a hired gun for one side or a neuropsychologist prostitute whose testimony is for sale for a price. The response, "I am being paid for my time away from my practice, not for my testimony," can prevent the witness's response from being used as evidence that he or she will say whatever the retaining attorney wants for a given amount of money. Similarly, the statement "I know you are working for Mr. X (the other attorney), but will you answer a few questions for me?" can be used to establish that you are taking sides or working *for* one side. The witness's response to the effect that he or she is simply providing findings from the examination in an objective manner will help defuse this potential problem.

Although it is not well recognized, and contrary to the maxim of not gratuitously volunteering information to opposing counsel during a discovery deposition, in many cases the attorney whose case is enhanced by (or based on) the neuropsychologist's examination findings and conclusions may use the deposition testimony as a basis for attempting to settle the case outside of court. In such situations, the neuropsychologist's role is quite different, in that explaining or elaborating on the strength of the findings and conclusions (as opposed to keeping mum and not giving more information than absolutely necessary) would be appropriate. Thus, before beginning the deposition, it may be relevant to discuss with the attorney whose case is strengthened by the neuropsychological findings, his or her focus in the deposition. If this focus is toward helping convince the opposition that his or her case is so compelling that it should be settled without further negotiation or litigation, the witness may be encouraged to go beyond barely providing minimal (e.g., *yes* or *no*) responses, and to respond to the questions posed by opposing counsel by elaborating on findings and explaining their implications. In these cases, when the neuropsychologist helps the defense counsel understand that brain injury is present and has exerted an adverse effect on the patient, the patient may be spared further litigation oriented toward claiming no brain damage exists. Conversely, when the examination findings clearly document no evidence of brain damage, the plaintiff's attorney may decide not to continue to claim such damage.

Similar to the deposition situation just described, where the purpose is to put all the cards on the table to help settle the case, is the situation in which the neuropsychologist's deposition will be taken specifically for use at trial. There are a number of reasons for this focus. Perhaps, most commonly, taking a witness's deposition for use at trial—often involving videotaping—can be a way to ensure that the testimony will be available for use at trial, independent of any schedule conflict or travel difficulties that might preclude or limit the witness's availability.[1] Once the deposition is on tape, the attorney who wants to present that testimony to the jury does not need to worry about illness, inclement weather, family problems, or other scheduling issues that might potentially preclude the witness's availability to appear at trial. Further, given that even at the beginning of a trial it is difficult for the attorney to guarantee that any witness will be called at a specific time, or even on a specific day, the neuropsychologist may have a good deal of down time when he or she cannot schedule patients. This is especially problematic if the trial will be located away from the witness's office, such as in another city. In general, trials are held in the jurisdiction where the defendant resides, so that a patient seen in the neuropsychologist's office, who has been injured by a party not from the patient's or the neuropsychologist's locale, may have to go to trial at some location remote from the neuropsychologist's office.

Occasionally the neuropsychologist's deposition for use at trial may be scheduled by the attorney representing the patient to get the attention of the opposing counsel, when the opposing counsel appears to doubt the patient has a case. Because brain injury is usually not obvious and may not be reflected on computerized tomography (CT) scans, emergency room records, or physician notes, the neuropsychologist's deposition may represent the primary scientific basis for the claim. In this instance, the patient's attorney will invite the defense to attend the deposition and question the expert witness.

The neuropsychologist is encouraged to be very clear with the questioning attorney about the specific wording and sequence of the questions that will be asked. Many attorneys have a standard set of questions for medical witnesses, and some of these questions will be irrelevant for neuropsychology. Of special importance, the questions should enable the neuropsychologist to explain neuropsychological examination vis à vis brain damage, and to focus on how the examination of this specific individual confirms or refutes brain injury. Obviously this will not be possible when the neuropsychologist is being deposed by opposing counsel in a discovery deposition where there will be a greater focus on surprising the witness with unanticipated questions for which he or she may not have ready answers.

Whatever the motivation underlying the deposition to be conducted, the witness should be aware that his or her words—and image, if on videotape—will be presented directly to the jury. If the deposition is not videotaped but is read at trial, usually an individual of the same gender as the neuropsychologist will take the stand, be read the question the neuropsychologist was asked, and respond (in his or her place) with the actual responses from the original deposition transcript. If the deposition is to be videotaped—even if it is a discovery deposition where the opposing counsel wants to review the neuropsychologist's demeanor in response to specific questions—it is important to remember that insofar as a jury is concerned, this is the real witness, so the neuropsychologist must appear and act as if actually present in the courtroom.

Frequently opposing counsel will sit or stand in a physical location for questioning that would cause the witness to look away from the camera to face counsel. This positioning has the potential to make the witness appear evasive, if the witness does not remember to look directly into the camera when responding. The neuropsychologist should always face the camera when responding so that he or she appears to be looking at the persons (i.e., jurors) who are being addressed.

The Deposition Book

A practice that helps provide the neuropsychologist with enhanced confidence as an expert in the subject matter at issue—and which may also enhance credibility—involves the compilation and assembly, before each deposition, of a collection of recent scholarly reprints uniquely relevant to the patient and issues involved. A neuropsychologist who is familiar with the deposition process may also wish to include scholarly articles and recent reprints in anticipation of issues that might reasonably be raised by opposing counsel during the course of deposition. A common focus involves neuropsychological sequelae of mild traumatic brain injury and post concussive syndrome, wherein the severity of residual symptoms in neuropsychological impairment may be greater than accident records might suggest. Because the Glasgow Coma Scale often shows little or no impairment at time of injury, it is reasonable to expect skeptical questioning from the defense attorney as to how the Glasgow findings are compatible with later neurocognitive or neurobehavioral findings of brain damage resulting from the injury. Similarly, negative CT findings, questionable brief loss of consciousness, or lack of head bruises or lacerations might reasonably be expected to represent areas of aggressive questioning for the neuropsychologist whose examination documented residual brain injury from such an event. Since these topics can be expected to come up during deposition, appropriate articles or references for the deposition book might include one or two references concerning the relationship between CT findings and neuropsychological findings (Bigler, 2001), the relationship between duration (or presence) of loss of consciousness with neuropsychological outcome (see, for example, Iverson, Lovell, & Smith, 2000; Ruff, Crouch, & Troster, 1994), or the acceleration/deceleration cause of axonal injury independent of specific head trauma (see, for example, Varney & Varney, 1995). If there is reason to expect a need to go into the pathophysiology of acceleration/deceleration injury, it may be wise to add a treatise explaining the topic (see, for example, Bigler, 2001). The neuropsychologist who is not conversant on the topics might wish to include an explanation of the Glasgow Coma Scale and its possible correlates (Balester, Czosnyka, & Chadfield, 2004; Gill, Windemuth, & Steele, 2005; Widget, Bamlex, Marinotum, Manno, & McClelland, 2005). The deposition book will obviously differ from deposition to deposition because each patient or case will present different issues, and the neuropsychologist may wish to have specific reprints available that he or she thinks might have unique relevance to the patient being discussed. If the neuropsychologist glances at the deposition book reprints throughout the deposition before responding to some questions, it is not at all uncommon for opposing counsel to demand that whatever is being referred to be placed into evidence. This can be helpful in that it adds into the official record a good deal of elaboration and support to what the neuropsychologist would have explained from the scientific literature during his or her deposition testimony, and therefore helps augment the scientific basis of that testimony.

Practicalities on the Practice Side

Scheduling a deposition may be a complex affair, in that at least two (opposing) attorneys need to identify a time compatible with the neuropsychologist's schedule in order to specify a date and time for the deposition. This scheduling notice will tend to be issued as an official proceeding of the court to various parties involved. Numerous telephone calls may be exchanged just to schedule the neuropsychologist's deposition. Once scheduled, either party may then choose to *continue* the deposition (i.e., postpone it) for a reason of benefit to them. This may be done with little notice, such as cancellation at 4:30 p.m. Monday of a deposition scheduled for 9:00 a.m. Tuesday, with "to be continued from day to day as needed" phraseology in the deposition notice which precludes any firm scheduling for time following the deposition of at least several hours duration. Thus, not only must the neuropsychologist spend time reviewing extensive records and other information in preparation for this deposition, short notice cancellation may not permit the neuropsychologist to fill the time reserved for the deposition. In such circumstances, loss of time is not inconsequential. Another underlying complication of deposition scheduling involves the not infrequent requests from one side or another for several future dates when the witness would be available for deposition. This may be the last the neuropsychologist will hear about the deposition regarding the dates that have been set aside, with these dates passing without either confirmation or rejection by either side. Either the neuropsychologist will have to try to contact the attorneys as each date approaches to inquire whether the deposition is scheduled, or else reconcile to writing off the days held open at their request. A strategy recommended for minimizing these scheduling problems involves responding when called by an attorney who wants to schedule a deposition with a form letter on the neuropsychologist's letterhead indicating that, upon receipt of a sum to cover a period of professional time and a list of dates and times when all attorneys involved will be available for the deposition, the neuropsychologist will confirm such date. This letter would include the caveat that if the deposition is not held at the mutually agreed time, the payment is forfeited to the neuropsychologist. This has been found to be helpful in preventing waste of the witness's time by frivolous holding of dates open by attorneys or last minute rescheduling of the deposition. An example of such a letter is enclosed (see Appendix 13.1 at the end of this chapter).

In the matter of charges for depositions, many neuropsychologists charge double their usual hourly rate for the time spent in deposition. This is justified on several counts. For one, the neuropsychologist is rarely given a guarantee of when a scheduled deposition will end. Indeed, many standard deposition sub-poena forms include wording to the effect that "commencing at [time] o'clock on given date and continuing from day to day thereafter." Since most opposing attorneys will not box themselves in by guaranteeing how long they will question the neuropsychologist or how long the opposing counsel will cross examine him or her, the witness cannot, with confidence, schedule any patients for the remainder of the day on which the deposition is scheduled, and possibly for a day or two following that. For that reason, it is recommended that the neuropsychologist schedule the deposition to begin early in the day, in the hope the deposition ends that day and to be free the next day, even though this procedure does not provide any absolute assurance. It has been our experience that depositions frequently go into at least 2 days.

Another factor with implications for deposition charges involves the long-term impact on the neuropsychologist's credibility, and even inferences concerning his or her integrity and parentage. To quote from a few attorneys concerning how they approach questions in a deposition, "The strategy is to impeach your testimony and destroy your credibility" (Matson, 1990) or "You deserve to know that many trial attorneys take particular pleasure in knocking out...ignorant experts. I don't just mean from the case at hand. I mean ending their careers..." (Kline 1996) or "Cross examination of an expert witness will resemble peeling of an onion, exposing layer after layer of weakness, error, and fallacy" (Kline, 1996). Further, the neuropsychologist's deposition testimony can, and very likely will, be referred to in other cases in subsequent years as other attorneys with other cases prepare to depose you. We have had numerous questions phrased generally as follows: "Now, Doctor, wouldn't you agree that...?" After expressing some reservation about agreeing with the comment, the attorney will produce with showmanship flourish a deposition from another case, in another state, perhaps a decade or more ago, from which the quote was taken. Thus although the witness's response to questions in a deposition is made in reference to the patient at issue, in the context at hand, that response may later be used in a much more general context to try to impeach the witness or challenge his or her competence. Since the neuropsychologist's phraseology can be used in perpetuity against him or her, charging more for this deposition activity than for interacting with the patient in the office at the time of the neuropsychologist's choosing is certainly defensible. This is the case even though, on occasion, opposing counsel (who usually pays for the deposition) may try to make this seem inappropriate, conve-niently ignoring that it is common practice among attorneys to do exactly that for their own court time.

Records from the neuropsychologist's examination, along with his or her CV, may be expected to be reviewed by opposing counsel during deposition, to serve as basis for the questions asked of the witness. On occasion, the neuropsychologist may be served with a subpoena demanding that he or she produce at deposition other items such as books, manuals, records, or information of any kind on which the witness relied in any way whatsoever in forming an opinion about the patient. This, of course, can raise issues of copyright and other issues, including the neuropsychologist being restricted in proceeding with their appointments and reports because the tools necessary to do the work at hand are not available for an extended length of time. Given that each case is different and that the permutations may have differing implications for copyright, confidentiality, test security, and so on, these topics are covered elsewhere in greater detail.

At some point during the deposition, the neuropsychologist will be asked if he or she wishes to review the deposition. It is usually a good idea for the witness to insist on the opportunity to review and sign the deposition. This is important for a number of reasons. First, it helps to ensure that the phraseology—sometimes involving proper names or psychological tests for neuroanatomic structures—has not been misreported. And, although it is supposedly a routine practice that the witness be provided with a copy of the deposition, he or she cannot always count on receiving one unless there is an insistence on the opportunity to read and sign it. This is very important if the case subsequently goes to trial, because the neuropsychologist can assuredly expect to be questioned about things said in the deposition and will certainly need to be familiar with everything said in that deposition.

As has been pointed out in elaborations on *Daubert* criteria, "Increasingly, proof in civil litigation relies on expert testimony, as the world has gotten more and more complex, so by necessity, has litigation" (Federal Rules of Evidence, 2000). The issue of expertise and scientific validity is often a matter of relevance in the context of a deposition, in that some courts have ruled on issues relating to fixed versus flexible neuropsychological batteries. Some states, as well as many federal jurisdictions, use the *Daubert* criteria for admissibility of scientific evidence (Burszatjn, 1996). Given that, in most cases, there is considerable latitude concerning what is considered scientific, as determined by the judge at issue, these complex issues are the topic of other writings. In general, if an examination was done in a form that is considered acceptable within the general neuropsychological community, the neuropsychologist's conclusions will not be rejected on the basis of any such legal criterion issues. Then, such issues are more apt to be the topic of discussion among attorneys rather than a matter involving your deposition.

Once the deposition has been completed and the participating or observing lawyers have shaken hands and departed—often to meet outside your office and discuss settlement issues, the court reporter has cleared paraphernalia from the office, and the deposition is concluded, it is recommended that the neuropsychologist mentally review his or her performance and note what might have been done differently. Ideally, following each deposition, the neuropsychologist will not only gain more confidence in his or her ability to handle depositions, but will also learn from each deposition possible questionable or unclear aspects of the questions and answers, and determine alternative ways in which to respond. In this manner, both the examination procedure and thinking about the examination results will become sharper and more focused.

Neuropsychologists who wish help in preparing for depositions may wish to consult two works by Babitsky and Mangraviti: *How to Excel During Depositions: Techniques That Work* (1998) or *Cross Examination: The Comprehensive Guide for Experts* (2003).

Note

1. A deposition checklist with helpful preparation tips for videotaped depositions is available at no cost by fax at (508) 540-8304 or by e-mail at http://www.info@seak.com

References

Babitski, S., & Mangraviti, J. J. (1998). *How to excel driving depositions: Techniques that work* (pp. 18–32). Falmouth, MA: S.E.A.K.

Babitski, S., & Mangraviti, J. J. (2003). *Cross examination: The comprehensive guide for experts.* Falmouth, MA: S.E.A.K.

Balester, M., Czosnyka, M., & Chadfield, D. A. (2004). Predictive value of the Glasgow Coma Scale after brain trauma: Change in trends over the past ten years. *Journal of Neurology, Neurosurgery and Psychiatry, 75*, 161–162.

Bigler, E. D. (2001). The lesion(s) in traumatic brain injury: Implications for clinical neuropsychology. *Archives of Clinical Neuropsychology, 58*, 585–593.

Burszatjn, H. (1996). Ethical and effective testimony in the post-*Daubert* era. *Fifth Annual National Expert Witness and Litigation Seminar Conference Handbook.* Falmouth, MA: S.E.A.K.

Federal Rules of Evidence. (2000). Committee Advisory Notes, 702.

Gill, M., Windemuth, R., & Steele, R. (2005). A comparison of the Glasgow Coma Scale to simplified alternative scores for the prediction of traumatic brain injury outcome. *Annals of Emergency Medicine, 45*, 37–42.

Iverson, G. L., Lovell, M., & Smith, S. S. (2000). Does brief loss of consciousness affect cognitive functioning after mild head injury? *Archives of Clinical Neuropsychology, 15*, 643–648.

Klein, M. S. (1996). *How to fight back: The rights and remedies of expert witnesses.* Fifth Annual National Expert Witness and Litigation Seminar, June (77). Falmouth, MA: S.E.A.K.

Matson, J. V. (1990). *Effective expert witnessing* (Document #53). New York: Lewis Publications.

Ruff, R. M., Crouch, J. A., & Troster, A. I. (1994). Selected cases of poor outcome following a minor brain trauma: Comparing neuropsychological and position emission tomography assessment. *Brain Injury, 8*, 297–308.

Steele, I. G., Clement, C. M., & Rowe, B. H. (2005). Comparison of the Canadian CT head scale and the New Orleans criteria in patients with minor head injury. *Journal of the American Medical Association, 296*, 1511–1517.

Varney, N. R., & Varney, R. N. (1995). Brain injury without head injury. Some physics of automobile collisions with particular reference to brain injuries occurring without physical head trauma. *Applied Neuropsychology, 2*, 47–62.

Widget, E. F., Bamlex, W. R., Marinotum, B. V., Manno, E. M., & McClelland, R.L. (2005). Validation of a new coma scale: The four scores. *Annals of Neurology, 58*, 585–593.

Appendix 13.1

Sample Deposition
Request Response Letter

[Your Letterhead]

ATTN: [Name and address of attorney requesting deposition]

RE: Your request that I provide dates for deposition

Dear [Mr./Mrs./Ms. Attorney]:

I shall be glad to cooperate with you in this matter. Professional colleagues involved in similar situations have described problems involving scheduling depositions such as attorneys:

a. Scheduling depositions long in advance, and then canceling on extremely short notice;
b. Scheduling depositions without confirming availability of date with opposing counsel, then canceling;
c. Requesting that I hold open multiple dates for possible deposition scheduling and never notifying me that these dates were not scheduled.

(All of which waste my time)

d. Refusing to pay for deposition charges after deposition has been completed; or
e. Arbitrarily paying some sum randomly chosen by them as representing what my time is worth; or
f. Stopping payment for checks paid for my deposition time.

Accordingly, I have established a policy concerning depositions, which involves the following:

1. If you want to schedule my deposition, you will send a check in the amount of _____ to cover the first 2 hours.
2. Upon receipt of same, I will provide you with an available date, selected by you after confirmation with opposing counsel that same date is available.
3. At termination of deposition, you will pay for any charges of additional time: this may include a charge for reasonable time spent in preparation (e.g. assembly of records and review of same so as to be prepared for questions reasonably anticipated without excessive review of records during deposition). If you cancel deposition after scheduling, the _____ is forfeited as my scheduling charge.

This is provided for your information in an attempt to preclude any misunderstandings.

 Sincerely,

[Your signature]

[Your name typed]

It may be helpful to have a few forms copied in advance, so that all you need to do is fill in the name and address of the requesting attorney, reference the patient, date, and mail.

Neuropsychology in the Courtroom

14

Lawrence C. Hartlage
Bruce H. Stern

Court Decisions Affecting Neuropsychology Testimony in the Courtroom

In addition to earlier rulings that generally reflect an evolutionary trend toward acknowledging the ability of neuropsychologists to provide expert testimony concerning diagnosis and causation of brain injury, a number of court rulings are of relevance to various aspects of contemporary neuropsychological courtroom testimony.

Clinicians as Expert Witnesses in Traumatic Brain Injury Cases

Over the years, there has developed a mythical belief that medical providers and clinicians should not serve as expert witnesses, and that only forensic independent examiners should be permitted to serve as such.

Is there really a difference between clinicians and forensic experts when it comes to testifying in traumatic brain injury (TBI) cases? Should clinicians refrain from acting or serving as expert witnesses? Conversely, should clinicians be encouraged to serve as expert witnesses, and is this conventional wisdom nothing more than a conspiracy by defense forensic experts to limit, or even prohibit, a TBI patient's best weapon at trial (Majestic, 1986)?

A physician, neuropsychologist, or therapist often is asked to testify in a TBI personal injury trial either as a treating doctor, an expert witness, or both (Bigler, 2006). As a treating doctor, that medical professional has obviously provided medical or psychological treatment to the injured plaintiff, and is being asked to provide testimony regarding the treatment that was provided. This witness will be asked to provide his or her opinion of a diagnosis, and often, whether or not the diagnosis and treatment provided was causally related to the trauma involved in the case (Stigliano by Stigliano v. Connaught Laboratories, Inc.). However, questions as to prognosis are often left unasked.

On the other hand, the treating medical provider may be asked to play a dual role, acting not only as a treating doctor, but also providing expert testimony not only regarding diagnosis and causation, but prognosis, the degree of effort given by the patient, as well as other expert questions that may arise in any given specific case (Bianchini, Mathias, & Greve, 2001; Bush et al., 2005; Hartledge, 1975, 1981, 1983, 1995; Larrabee, 2003; Lees-Haley, English, & Glenn, 1991; Slick, Sherman, & Iverson, 1999).

Third, the doctor may be asked to perform a forensic examination, a situation in which the expert has no patient–physician relationship and is requested to review numerous medical, scholastic, and employment records and render expert testimony, often along the same lines as the clinician who is participating in a dual treater–expert role.

In the medical field, the conventional wisdom seems to be that treaters or clinicians should not serve a dual role, acting as both a treating doctor and an expert witness (Reid, 2008). Reid argues that there are five reasons why it is usually inappropriate and a disservice to the court for a doctor or a therapist to assume the dual role of treater and expert witness. The five reasons provided by Reid are:

1. A treatment relationship creates a professional, ethical, and legal (or fiduciary) obligation to act in the patient's best interest both during and after the treatment relationship. Because forensic reports and testimony require objectivity regardless of the patient's wishes or needs, an inherent conflict is created.

2. The clinician who testifies regarding a current or past patient knows, or should know, that he or she is required to act in the patient's interest, and may even have a personal affinity for the patient's viewpoint. This creates a danger of intentional bias.

3. There is a danger of unintended bias toward the patient.

4. Because a treating clinician anticipates reporting to a third party such as a lawyer, court, or insurance company, professional ethics require that this be discussed with the patient as early as it is feasible. This awareness, according to Reid, affects the patient's revelations to the clinician, and thus, the validity of any report or testimony.

5. The clinician's roles in training are not forensic.

An in-depth review of these five reasons fails to support the underlying thesis that clinicians cannot or should not act in this dual role. First, testifying as an expert on behalf of one's patient cannot be seen as failing to act in the patient's best interest, both during and after the treatment relationship. The author's argument that forensic reports and testimony require objectivity is accurate. However, it is naive to believe that forensic experts provide objective testimony, whereas clinicians do not. Bigler correctly recognizes the inherent bias present in forensic work (Bigler, 2006).

This argument was advanced by the defense in the Baxter case, but soundly rejected. The court responded:

Besides Dr. Faust's unsupported opinion that clinical neuropsychologists are not objective examiners because their apparent goal is to advance the patient's interest, nothing in the record indicates that the field of neuropsychology recognizes a relevant distinction between methodologies based upon their use in the clinical setting versus the forensic setting. (Baxter v. Temple, 2008, p. 43)

The recent disclosure exposed by the Center for Public Integrity provides a revelation as to the potential lack of objectivity in defense forensic evaluations. There, it was revealed that defense forensic experts were paid millions of dollars by the welding industry, which had been embattled in litigation over welding fumes containing manganese, a toxic metal, being the cause of numerous plaintiffs' cognitive complaints (Morris, 2008).

Thus, what is the greater fear? A clinician's lack of objectivity in testifying on behalf of his or her patient, or the lack of objectivity of expert forensic witnesses who potentially could distort their research, manipulate their data, and testify falsely on behalf of their defense clients?

Certainly, there is always the issue of intentional or unintentional bias, legitimate issues raised by Reid. However, the harm comes when not acknowledging that this bias may exist. However, the fact that there may be a potential for bias does not automatically rise to the level of an ethical obligation to refrain from testifying as an expert witness.

When an individual is injured and hires an attorney to pursue litigation to obtain compensation, most, if not all, personal injury attorneys advise their clients that they will be requesting and obtaining all medical records, not only relating to the traumatic event and its resultant treatment, but records for all pre-existing medical care, as well as scholastic and employment records. Plaintiffs are also advised that once litigation begins, defense counsel will also request and obtain this same information, which will be shared with insurance adjusters and defense experts. Thus, patients are acutely aware that their treating doctors' medical records will not be private.

Finally, Reid argues that the clinician's role and training are not forensic in nature. There is no formal training for most forensic experts. Rather, in some circumstances, as a result of financial constraints placed upon the medical profession by the insurance industry, doctors have found testifying in forensic matters to be an excellent method to supplement their income. Bigler comments that neuropsychological providers, on average, receive only between 50 and 60% of their hourly charges, whereas forensic services are typically reimbursed fully (Bigler, 2006).

Reid argues that clinicians "often have limited or simplistic views of the legal case and the rules that govern it, making them vulnerable to forensic misunderstanding and, at worst, manipulation by the attorney" (Reid, 2008, p 2). First, what is the role of an expert witness? Should an expert witness be courtroom savvy, or is it really more important that the expert whether a forensic expert or a clinician, comes into court and provides objective testimony outlining his or her opinions and providing a clear and understandable explanation to support those opinions and conclusions?

The final reason Reid advances why clinicians should not serve as expert witnesses has to do with the fact that often clinicians do not obtain full histories or review medical records. Silver and McAllister explain:

> *The forensic evaluation differs in purpose, and thus in practice, from the clinical evaluation. In the usual clinical setting a doctor–patient relationship exists wherein an individual who is suffering from a disorder comes for help with those problems. It is unusual for the clinician to question (at least in the initial phases of treatment) whether or not the patient actually is experiencing those problems or exaggerating their severity.* (Silver & McAllister, 1997, p. 1)

This is certainly a valid criticism, but it is not a sufficient basis to conclude that it is inappropriate and a disservice for a doctor to assume the dual role of a treating doctor and expert witness. It is certainly a recognized problem in the legal profession that "clinicians rarely corroborate patient or case information to the same extent as forensic consultants" (Silver & McAllister, 1997, p.1).

It is for this reason that on many occasions, plaintiff's attorneys will retain a forensic expert. Too often, treating physicians who have not obtained a full medical history and have not reviewed any of the medical records are discredited on cross-examination as a result of their failure to review even the emergency room records generated immediately post-trauma. However, the solution for this deficiency is not to bar the clinician from testifying as an expert witness, but for attorneys to ensure that the clinician has reviewed the appropriate medical, scholastic, and employment records and has obtained a full history prior to calling that clinician as an expert witness.

Third-Party Observers During Neuropsychological Testing

For years, plaintiff attorneys have requested the presence of a third-party observer during orthopedic and neurologic physical examinations. In order to avoid being witnesses at trial, attorneys have retained nurse consultants or other medical professionals to attend defense medical examinations, take notes, and often audiotape the evaluation. More recently, neurolawyers are now requesting the presence of third-party observers during neuropsychological testing. This has created a great deal of controversy between plaintiff's attorneys and the neuropsychological community.

Defense attorneys and insurance companies were slow in retaining neuropsychologists in the defense of TBI cases. Skeptical of their testing, the defense initially retained neurologists and psychiatrists to defend these claims, asserting that neuropsychological testing was subjective and unreliable. As their exposure increased and verdicts returned in favor of plaintiffs, the defense finally began to retain its own neuropsychologists. When plaintiff attorneys requested the presence of a third-party observer, defense neuropsychologists objected, asserting that the presence of a third party would invalidate the results, in that neuropsychological testing was neither normed nor standardized with the presence of a third-party observer, and that the presence of a third-party observer would cause the testee to do poorly on the neuropsychological test.

In 2005, an entire issue of the *Journal of Forensic Neuropsychology* was devoted to research regarding the effects of third-party observer presence. In that journal issue, Lynch reported that in the presence of third-party observers, testees showed impairment on verbal paired associates but not on trail making or finger tapping (Lynch, 2005).

Yantz and McCaffrey found significantly impaired scores on global and verbal memory (MAS) (Yantz & McCaffrey, 2005). A similar result was found when testees were tested in the presence of a video recorder (Constantinou, Ashendorf, & McCaffrey, 2005). Most interestingly, the journal issue contained no research demonstrating that the presence of a third-party observer did not have a significant effect on testing, nor any articles by any neuropsychologist taking a position in favor of the presence of a third party being present during neuropsychological testing.

However, contrary research does exist. In a 2004 doctoral dissertation, Linda S. Lindman investigated the presence of third-party observers during neuropsychological testing (Lindman, 2004). Although earlier studies had examined the effects of third-party observers on memory and learning functioning, Lindman instead chose tests that more clearly required attention and executive functioning. This was done in an effort to more closely approximate the clinical situation in which the tests would have been used in neuropsychological testing. In conducting the study, Lindman selected 75 undergraduate psychology students from Louisiana State University, excluding those with history of moderate or severe brain trauma, illiteracy, neurological disease, clinically elevated level of anxiety, current psychological diagnosis, and current use of psychotropic medications.

Participants were tested using Wechsler digit span and vocabulary subtests, finger-tapping test, controlled oral word association testing, trail-making tests, color word testing, and state-trait anxiety measurement.

The participants were evaluated and broken into three groups: a control group with no third-party observer, a second group involving a third-party observer who sat to the right and behind the testee, and a third group in which the testee was videotaped with the placement of the video recorder identical to the location of the third-party observer in the preceding group.

Lindman hypothesized that subjects being observed during testing with simple tasks would perform as well as those not being observed, that subjects being observed during testing with complex tasks would perform significantly more poorly than those not being observed, that the presence of a third party would negatively affect performance on complex tasks significantly more than the presence of audiovisual recording equipment, and finally, that levels of arousal would be higher for subjects in the observer and audiovisual conditions.

Lindman's hypotheses were based upon the known results of earlier research and published literature. Much to her surprise, the presence of a third-party observer and/or the presence of video recording equipment had no significant effect! Lindman theorized that the reason for her results might be the tests chosen in this study to represent "complex tasks." Lindman wrote:

> *All of these studies found deficits in performance with third-party observation. There is no disagreement with designation of these tasks as complex. However, these tasks represent learning and memory functioning while the tests chosen for the present study more clearly require attention and executive functioning. This was done in an effort to more closely approximate the tests routinely used in neuropsychological testing. As stated earlier, a wide variety of tests comprise a full neuropsychological battery, and memory and new wording are only part of the complete diagnostic examination. (p. 25)*

A second reason or explanation might be that there is no significant effect of observation on performance of complex tasks.

Lindman did acknowledge that there might be limitations in her study. She recognized that the participants, being college-aged students, hardly represent individuals who are referred for neuropsychological testing. Lindman again acknowledged that her tests did not include those of learning and memory. Finally, she indicated that the fact that there was no secondary gain to the testing may have skewed her results.

Position of Professional Organizations

In general, courts tend to support standards of professional practice promulgated by relevant professional organizations (Denney, 2008). Not surprisingly, organizations of clinical and forensic neuropsychologists continually oppose the presence of third-party observers during neuropsychological testing (American Academy of Clinical Neuropsychology, 2001; National Academy of Neuropsychology, 2000). The rationale for excluding third-party observers primarily revolves around the issue of testing validity. The argument expressed is that third-party observation threatens the validity of test results because of nonstandardization procedures (Krauss & Otto, 2007). They argue that neuropsychological testing when normed and standardized did not include the presence of third-party observers. Thus, permitting such a presence is nonstandard procedure and may jeopardize the validity of the testing.

Opponents also point to the numerous research studies cited earlier that call into question the validity of the testee's performance and, therefore, the results. Opponents also argue that the presence of third-party observers threatens the security and integrity of the testing. Finally, because rapport between the testee and test administrator is of paramount importance, the presence of a third party may interfere with this rapport, thus invalidating the results.

This viewpoint is not without its critics. Krauss and Otto (2007) found some of these arguments inconsistent and illogical. For instance, arguing about concerns over observer effects and test standardization that are only to be applied in a specific context (i.e., forensic) although not in others (i.e., treatment) (AACN policy statement, 2001, pp. 433–434). They also point out the inconsistency of the National Academy of Neuropsychology (NAN) statement (1999), which permits third-party observation by a professional or trainee in an educational context, although opposing the presence of a third-party observer during forensic examinations. They also chide the American Academy of Clinical Neuropsychology, which finds it acceptable for psychologists to allow third-party observers in some evaluation contexts, such as criminal evaluations, yet unacceptable during civil forensic examinations (AACN policy statement, 2001, 2007).

Krauss and Otto (2007) point out that although psychological and neuropsychological tests have not been standardized in the presence of third-party observers, they note that psychological and neuropsychological testing was also not standardized or normed during forensic examinations.

Krauss and Otto (2007) recommend either the presence of third parties during interviews or provide alternatives such as taping, and also discourage the presence of third parties (other than psychologist observers) during the administration of standardized, secured testing, but permit the use of psychologist observers or taping. They also recommend the use of third parties whenever necessary to facilitate the psychological examination, and encourage additional research on the effects of third-party observation in the forensic context.

The Legal Response

It is not surprising that plaintiff attorneys question the soundness of opponents' viewpoints to the presence of third parties. First, it is well known that insurance carriers are willing to spend a great deal of money in TBI cases, often paying defense forensic neuropsychologists in excess of $30,000 for one case (Bigler, 2007). Not surprisingly, with so much money to be made, some neuropsychologists have decreased their clinical practice to devote larger portions of their time to defense forensic practice. Plaintiff attorneys also point out that some of the neuropsychologists involved in the research related to the effects of the presence of third parties devote over 90% of their forensic practice to representing insurance companies and manufacturers in the defense of personal injury TBI claims.

Finally, some plaintiff attorneys may view this opposition as a wall erected by defense neuropsychologists to inhibit plaintiffs' attorneys from being able to properly prepare a cross-examination.

Legal Cases

The issue of the presence of third-party observers during neuropsychological testing has been the subject of many legal decisions. Not surprisingly, the courts have been inconsistent. Some courts permit the presence of third-party observers, either by statute or case law. In other jurisdictions it is forbidden, whereas other courts take a middle approach, examining the issue on a case-by-case basis, usually requiring good cause.

For example, in *Langfeldt-Haaland v. Saupe Enterprises, Inc.* (1989), after the defendant requested a defense medical examination, the plaintiff's attorney requested permission to have his attorney present and to record the examination. The court granted the defendant's motion compelling the plaintiff to submit to the examination, but denied the plaintiff's request to permit counsel to be present and to tape-record the examination. On appeal to the Alaska Supreme Court, that court ruled that a party in a civil litigation had the right to have his attorney present during an examination by a physician hired by his opponent. After examining the various viewpoints of the parties as well as contrasting decisions in other states, the court ruled:

> In our view, those cases which allow the examinee's attorney to be present are the more persuasive. The Rule 35 examination is part of the litigation process, often a critical part. Parties are, in general, entitled to the protection and advice of counsel when they enter the litigation arena. An attorney's protection and advice may be needed in the context of a Rule 35 examination, and we see no good reason why it should not be available. We align Alaska with those authorities which allow plaintiff's counsel to attend and record, as a matter of course, court-ordered medical examinations in civil cases. (p. 18)

A similar result was handed down in New York (*Jessica H. ex rel. Arp v. Spagnolo*, 2007). There, the plaintiff, by her mother, commenced a lawsuit to recover damages for injuries sustained as a result of her child's exposure to lead paint while residing in an apartment owned by defendants. The trial court denied the defendant's motion to preclude all third-party observers from attending the neuropsychological examination of the plaintiff to be conducted by the defendant's expert doctor. In upholding the trial court's decision to permit the observation, the New York Appellate Court commented:

> We conclude that the Court properly allowed plaintiff's attorney to observe the neuropsychological examination. A party is entitled to be examined in the presence of his or her attorney or other representative so long as that person does not interfere with the conduct of the examinations unless the defendant makes a positive showing of the necessity for the exclusion of such an individual. Here, defendants failed to meet their burden of establishing that the presence of the attorney or other representative will impair the validity and effectiveness of the neuropsychological examination. (p. 335)

A contrary result was decided in *Cabana v. Forcier* (2001); there, the defendant filed a motion requiring the plaintiff to submit to psychological testing by the defendant's expert. The plaintiff countered by requesting permission to attend the mental examination of his client during administration of the formal neuropsychological testing by the defendant's expert. The Federal District Court denied the plaintiff's request, finding that the clear majority of federal court cases have refused to permit third-party observers at Rule 35 (IME) examinations.

Explaining its decision, the court ruled:

> (1) The special nature of the psychiatric examination requires direct and unimpeded one-on-one communication without external interference or atrusion; (2) in contrast to depositions and other forms of discovery, Rule 35 expert examinations are not intended to be adversarial; (3) fairness dictates if the defense counsel cannot be present when a plaintiff is interviewed by a psychiatrist who will testify at trial on his behalf, then plaintiff's counsel cannot be present when plaintiff is examined by defendant's expert psychiatrist; and (4) any concerns with distortions or inaccuracies by the examining psychiatrist can be addressed through traditional methods of impeachment and cross-examination. (p. 234)

Similarly, in *Hertenstein v. Kimberly Home Healthcare, Inc.* (1999), the Federal District Court once again denied the plaintiff attorney's request for the presence of a third person or a mechanical recording device. The plaintiff had requested permission to tape record her examination, contending that the defendant's expert was not neutral, as the defendant had engaged him to advance interests. The plaintiff suggested that a tape recording would ensure that the scope and manner of the examination was proper, and expressed concern that an unsupervised examination would be transformed into a defacto deposition. The court rejected the plaintiff's arguments, finding that the plaintiff had neither the right to have counsel present nor the right to mechanically record the examination.

The decision in *Bacallao v. Dauphin* (2007) represents an excellent example of the case-by-case approach used by the Florida courts. In Florida, a party seeking to exclude a third-party observer from a compulsory medical examination during discovery must provide a case-specific reason why their presence would disrupt the examination, and prove at an evidentiary hearing that no other qualified physician could be located in the area who would be willing to perform the examination under such circumstances. At the hearing, the defendant's expert neuropsychologist, Dr. Bonnie Levin, testified that third parties, including the plaintiff's counsel, should not be allowed to attend the examination and that the examination should not be taped. She testified that the presence of a third party as well as video or audio taping of the examination would be disruptive, would potentially affect the validity of the examination, would compromise test security by releasing confidential test material to the general public, and violated professional and ethical obligations. Dr. Levin did concede that there were others in private practice who would be willing to conduct the examination with a third-party observer for financial reasons. Relying on published literature in the area of neuropsychology as well as Dr. Levin's testimony, the trial court granted the defendant's request to prohibit any third-party observations, including video or audio recording.

On appeal, the Appellate Court recited Florida law that requires the parties seeking to exclude a third-party observer to provide a case-specific reason why the trial court should deny the plaintiff's right to have a third party present. Citing two prior decisions, the Appellate Court found that a neuropsychologist's testimony regarding his or her standards of practice, references to test, and conclusory statements that a third party's presence would render an examination invalid do not constitute case-specific reasons to exclude a third party from a medical examination. Thus, under Florida law, it is necessary for a defendant, in objecting to a third-party observer, to carry the burden of showing, in that specific case, why there should not be a third-party observer present.

Noteworthy is that none of the reported cases cite the published research to support their decisions, suggesting that in most cases, the research is either not being provided to the court or the court had decide to use other factors upon which to reach a decision.

The Future

Although neuropsychologists have weathered the attack on whether they are competent to give expert medical testimony, and neuropsychology appears to have

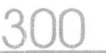

weathered various Daubert attacks (Fisher, 1994), nonetheless neuropsychologists and the field of neuropsychology as it applies to forensic cases, may face an uncertain future.

Because traditional neurodiagnostic tests, such as the computed tomography (CT) scan and magnetic resonance imaging (MRI), lack the sensitivity to the depth of brain injury in patients with acquired mild TBI, neuropsychology in the past has proven to be the only objective way to document and measure TBI and its residual impairments. However, with the advent of new diagnostic tests, such as diffuse tensor imaging and functional MRI (fMRI), the role of neuropsychological testing as the gold standard in the diagnosis of TBI may be in jeopardy. It very well may be that these new diagnostic tests will become the future gold standard, and that neuropsychological testing will be used not to diagnose brain injury, but rather to demonstrate the behavioral impairments resulting from that brain injury.

However, the field of neuropsychology also faces a greater threat in forensic settings. Defense forensic neuropsychologists who are paid thousands and thousands of dollars by insurance and manufacturing companies may be seen as likely to have their opinions influenced by financial considerations. In situations in which forensic neuropsychologists earn all of their income from defense cases, the forensic neuropsychologists are likely to be under a degree of pressure to produce opinions that will ensure financial survival. That is not to say that every forensic neuropsychologist who works for the defense will produce biased opinions. As professionals, all forensic neuropsychologists have a professional responsibility to render evidence-based opinions, and the expectation is the majority of defense forensic neuropsychologists will uphold their professional responsibilities. Nonetheless, every field may have a few members who are less than exemplary. The expectation of the court is that forensic neuropsychologists will be providing unbiased opinions regardless of which side the forensic neuropsychologist is working for, and unprofessional forensic neuropsychologists who provide biased opinions because they are paid large sums of money would threaten to destroy the field of forensic neuropsychology. Unless forensic neuropsychology opinions are seen as unbiased by financial considerations, then the question is why should forensic neuropsychology testimony be admitted in court? If forensic neuropsychology is seen as biased, then the courts will likely be less apt to admit forensic neuropsychology testimony and an important resource to the courts for fair judicial decision would be lost to the courts. Another threat to the future of forensic neuropsychology is the methodology used to form forensic neuropsychology opinions.

In order for neuropsychological testimony to be admitted into our courts under a Daubert standard (Fisher, 1994; Larvie, 1994), a party must show that such testing has gained widespread acceptance by the particular scientific community as well as other technical considerations. To survive future technical challenges, forensic neuropsychologists will need to aspire to the very highest psychometric standards in selection and use of neuropsychological testing in the forensic area. Failure to uphold high professional and psychometric standards will call into question the validity of neuropsychological testing and reduce future reliance by the courts on forensic neuropsychology testimony.

Neuropsychological Research and Literature

Ever since the Rules of Evidence liberalized and modernized the use of learned treatises, the use of medical literature to support one's theories or to cross-examine an adversary's experts has proven helpful (*Jacober v. Saint Peter's Medical Center*, 1992; N.J.R.E. 803(c)(18), 2006). Although this liberalization was a welcomed change to the stifling old rule, which, in reality, prevented the use of learned treatises, new issues regarding the validity of medical research mandates that the trial attorney now research not only one's opponent's experts, but investigate the authors of those learned treatises that will be relied upon by one's adversary.

Previously, one could only use a learned treatise during cross-examination if, and only if, the defense expert acknowledged that the learned treatise was authoritative. Should the expert fail or refuse to acknowledge such authoritativeness, the attorney was precluded from using the learned treatise to cross-examine that expert. Federal Rules of Evidence, 803(c)(18) states:

> To the extent called to the attention of an expert witness upon cross-examination or relied upon by the expert in direct examination, statements contained in published treatises, periodicals or pamphlets on a subject of history, medicine or other science or art, established as a reliable authority by testimony or by judicial notice. If admitted, the statements may not be received as exhibits, but may be read into evidence or, if graphics, shown to the jury. (p. 256)

According to one state commentary:

> The adoption of this rule represents a change in practice by allowing the use of learned treatise evidence even if an expert witness fails to acknowledge that it is authoritative, so long as the reliability of the authority is established by other testimony or by judicial notice. Using learned treatises to cross-examine an expert can have a significant impact in attacking the credibility of an expert witness. Jurors are used to the battle of experts that takes place every day in our courtrooms. However, when jurors are confronted by the opinion of a paid expert witness and then presented with medical literature published by an impartial non expert author or researcher, jurors have a natural tendency to adopt and believe what is written and published in medical and scientific journals. (New Jersey Supreme Court Committee, 1991, p. 23)

Since then, the rule change use of learned treatises has become a customary part of trials. However, is what is published in these journals always trustworthy? What are the biases that these published authors bring to any specific issue? Who or what was the funding source(s) behind the research? Could the published research be biased toward a particular point of view?

For quite some time, the medical and scientific communities have been concerned about the financial relationships between authors and researchers and the pharmaceutical community (DeAngeles & Fontanarosa, 2008). This has led many scientific journals, such as *Journal of the American Medical Association* and *The New England Journal of Medicine*, as well as others, to establish stringent disclosure requirements to enhance the integrity of medical publications.

However, a recent study in the April 21, 2008, issue of *Journal of the American Medical Association* highlights that the deception continues, nevertheless. Clinical trial manuscripts related to Rofecoxib were authored by sponsor employees, but often attributed first authorship to academically affiliated investigators who did not always disclose industry financial support. Review manuscripts were often prepared by unacknowledged authors, who worked for the industry, and subsequently authorship was falsely attributed to academically affiliated investigators who often did not disclose industry financial support or that the actual authors of the publication worked for the industry (Ross, Hill, Egilman, & Krumholz, 2008). Citing from other sources, the authors noted that ghostwriting was demonstrated in 13% of researched articles, 10% of review articles, 6% of editorials, and 11% of Cochrane reviews; other research has found similar rates.

Writing in that same issue of *Journal of the American Medical Association*, DeAngelis and Fontanarosa reveal:

> *The articles by Ross and colleagues and by Psaty and Kronmal [Psaty, B.M., & Kronmal, R.A. Reporting mortality findings in trials of Rofecoxib for Alzheimer's disease or cognitive impairment: A case study based on documents from Rofecoxib litigation, JAMA. 2008; 299 (15); 1813-1817] document how one company, Merck and Co., Inc., apparently manipulated dozens of publications to promote one of its products. But make no mistake—the manipulation of study results, authors, editors and reviewers is not the sole purview of one company. (p. 1833)*

Ghostwriting and financial support by industry is not limited to the pharmaceutical industry. Recent financial disclosures in litigation disclose that such practices also exist in the field of forensic neuropsychology. Such unprofessional practices threaten to destroy the integrity of neuropsychological research and the use of neuropsychological research in the forensic area if steps are not taken to police this unethical behavior by the fields of neuropsychology.

The Center for Public Integrity just released a shocking story disclosing that researchers were paid millions of dollars by the welding industry, which has been embattled in litigation over whether welding fumes contain manganese, a toxic metal that specialists suggest causes Parkinsonism. According to the Center, lawsuits against the welding industry have been ongoing since the 1970s. The welding products industry has consistently argued that there were no reliable scientific data to prove that welding fumes cause the Parkinson-like syndrome known as Parkinsonism.

Recently, in December (2008), U.S. District Judge Kathleen O'Malley, who has been handling hundreds of these cases, ordered both sides to fully disclose payments made by any of the parties to researchers. Court documents obtained by the Center for Public Integrity demonstrate that the welding companies pay more than $12.5 million to 25 organizations and 33 researchers, virtually all of whom have published papers dismissing the connection between welding fumes and workers' ailments. Most of the money, $11 million, was spent after the litigation achieved critical mass in 2003; attorneys for the welders, meanwhile, spent about half a million.

This supports the concerns expressed by Bigler, who has been severely critical of forensic neuropsychologists who may be influenced by financial concerns and the effect that large payments for favorable testimony may be having on forensic neuropsychology (Bigler, 2007). In an article published in the *Archives of Clinical Neuropsychology*, Bigler (2006) exposed the positions being taken by defense forensic neuropsychologists in TBI litigation. Criticizing the reliance on defense-oriented articles published in the Archives, Bigler notes that if taken at face value, "[reliance on these articles] would have excluded all of the so-called flexible neuropsychological tests, approaches, and comprehensive additional norms—including age, education, and demographically adjusted norms"(p. 504).

Further acceptance of this literature also ignores the other clinical neuropsychology practice methods used by neuropsychologists in a comprehensive neuropsychological evaluation involving interview of the patient and significant others with knowledge of the patient, observation of the patient's behavior, and review of relevant educational, medical, criminal justice and other records, including clinical reports by other professionals.

Finally, Bigler raised serious concerns about the amount of financial incentive paid by defense insurance carriers and corporate defendants to forensic neuropsychologists. Bigler raises the important concern that the financial incentives paid to forensic neuropsychologists may increase the potential for biased opinions being provided to the courts.

Bigler, in an open letter to the editor, writes what he calls "the extravagant income, unreasonable and improper charges being made in neuropsychological evaluations done in the name of forensic neuropsychology in cases of individuals with acquired brain injury" (Bigler, 2004, p. 8). There, Bigler called for a public forum to set guidelines and standards for reasonable compensation within forensic neuropsychology. Bigler stated that these guidelines are desperately needed, because what is occurring has the potential to undermine the entire process of neuropsychological assessment and consultation in the evaluation of patients with acquired brain injury. Bigler believes that unreasonable financial compensation is undermining some of the research in TBI as it relates to neuropsychological outcome, and is having a damaging effect on patients with brain injury and also on the future of the field of forensic neuropsychology.

The Neuropsychologist in the Courtroom

Jurors do not represent a professionally trained body of experts maintained by the courts to evaluate evidence. Rather, they are drawn from the ranks of the general population and are assigned the tasks producing judgments about complex phenomena, concerning which they typically had little, if any, prior expertise.

An important contribution that the neuropsychologist can make in the courtroom involves the education of the court in such matters as the definition of neuropsychology and how neuropsychology can provide information of relevance to judgments the jury must make (Hartlage & DeFilippis, 1983; Hartlage & Green, 1971; Hartlage & Long, 1978; Hecaen, 1962; Kixmiller, Briggs, Hartlage, & Dean, 1993; Milner, 1954). Just as a good teacher educates students by making complex matters understandable, so can the neuropsychologist help the jury put into perspective the concept underlying neuropsychological assessment, the tools and the procedures used, and the implications of findings for decisions the jury must make. It has been said that the best way to present forensic neuropsychological evidence is by means of testimony that does not sound like testimony, but more like education (Hartlage, 1993).

Presenting neuropsychological data in a seamless flow takes preparation, but can help jurors feel they are being guided along intriguing paths to knowledge. For this purpose, educational aids can help serve as guidelines. Displays of the brain or other visual aids may be helpful in some cases, and sometimes handouts containing illustrations or outlines of the main points may be appropriate (Chalfant & Scheffelin, 1969). If you plan to use any such aids, they must be approved by the opposing attorney: they will likely be objected to if not pre-approved before your testimony. Even though the aids planned for use in educating the jury may be commonly available items, such as a model or picture of the brain, opposing counsel may be counted on to move to suppress it as inadmissible if it is not reviewed before you are allowed to refer to it.

An advantage to using such aids is that they become an exhibit available to jurors, on which they may rely in reaching a conclusion. Technically, having such an aid available can help highlight a point you consider important or want to emphasize: breaking the monotony of questions and answers by leaving the witness box to point out something on a picture or model can help with enhancing the jurors' attention. For some jurors, one picture may be worth ten thousand words. Having available some form of visual aid or handout summarizing a high point of your testimony may provide a way to help overcome problems, such as explaining a difficult neuropsychological concept to the jury (or some jurors). Unlike your students or interns, who may be unclear about some part of your presentation, but whom you can help by using previously shared knowledge, with the jury, there is typically no preexisting shared knowledge on which you can rely. Accordingly, it is important to carefully build a relevant fund of information for the jury, into the context of which findings from the patient may be placed into focus. Again, unlike students or interns for whom you can provide illustrations, examples, or possibly sample cases, in the courtroom you can only answer questions. You must make certain the attorney questioning you provides you the opportunity you need to answer in a clear and comprehensive manner.

Although before testifying, it is important to be thoroughly familiar with such phenomena as base rates, validity, and reliability issues, such matters are typically not likely to be very compelling to jurors (Gouvier, Hayes, & Smiroldo, 1998; Gouvier, Uddo-Crane, & Brown, 1998). Some experienced neuropsychologists choose not to discuss such areas during direct examination, so that if cross-examination addresses them, the juror can be bored by the focus of opposing counsel, while remembering the down-to-earth practical presentation in direct examination. Jurors, all being human beings living in a real world of relationships, can identify with the patient as a human being, and can appreciate how the presence or absence of brain injury will or will not alter such relationships and interactions. (Hartlage, 1993).

After this direct examination phase, which normally you will have prepared for and which should not present any surprises, the attorney whose case is adversely affected by your opinion will have the opportunity to try to minimize any adverse effects of your testimony to his or her case by cross-examination.

Although the prospect of being cross-examined in court may be viewed by forensic neuropsychologists who have not yet been so summoned to court as a potentially traumatic experience, in actuality, the experience may be more benign than that in a deposition: whereas in a deposition, part of opposing counsel's strategy may be to determine how well you handle stress or aggressive questioning, in a court room, the jury is watching, and (most, but not certainly all) attorneys tend to be careful not to provoke the jury in anger toward them and sympathy for the witness. Similarly, in a deposition, although opposing counsel may delve into minutia and apparently minor details in order to discover some issues in which your knowledge is weak, in the court room, the attorney will not want to run the risk of alienating the jurors by diverting attention to such minor, potentially boring parts, nor by weakening his/her case by pursuing time developing apparently arcane or overly technical points. Indeed, if opposing counsel becomes too aggressive, he or she runs the risk of being admonished by the judge, so that in a courtroom you can generally expect somewhat less hostile cross-examination than might prevail in a deposition setting.

Those readers who have carefully considered the points concerning preparation and testimony as detailed in the depositions chapter will, for the most part, find few new challenges in the courtroom setting. A couple of minor issues offer slight differences in courtroom practice: in general, anything you take with you to the witness chair may be demanded by opposing counsel, and attention to this before entering the courtroom can prevent possible problems. Second, because your role in the courtroom is to educate the jury, you may want to have examples readily at hand, or even (in consultation with the attorney who called you) a visual depiction or two of a point you believe will enhance your testimony. In general, instructional materials at the level appropriate to the introductory brain–behavioral relationship are most helpful (Hartlage, 1993).

If there are particular problems with which a patient has demonstrated special difficulty on examination, it may be helpful to have a very brief videotaped segment of the examination illustrating this difficulty. In this context, it is also most helpful to relate how a specific deficit or constellation of deficits relates to difficulty in real-life educational, socio-personal, or vocational settings.

Some years ago, in the context of a mnemonic list titled *Neuropsychological-Legal Testimony from A to Z*, Hartlage (1993) was prepared to assist neuropsychologists in preparing for testimony. Interestingly, after more than a decade and a half, the points still are relevant, and were reprinted in the first edition of this *Handbook*.

References

American Academy of Clinical Neuropsychology (AACN). (2001) Policy statement on the presence of third-party observers in neuropsychology assessment. *Clinical Neuropsychologist, 15*, 433–439.

Bacallao v. Dauphin, 963 So. 2d 962 (Fla. App. 3 Dist. 2007).

Baxter v. Temple, 949 A. 2d 167 (NH 2008).

Bianchini, K. J., Mathias, C. W., & Greve, K. W. (2001). Symptom validity testing: A critical review. *Clinical Neuropsychologist, 15*(1), 19–45.

Bigler, E. D. (2004). An open letter to the editors of *Brain Injury Professional*. *Brain Injury Professional, 3*(4), 8–9.

Bigler, E. D. (2006). Can author bias be determined in forensic neuropsychology research published in *Archives of Clinical Neuropsychology*? *Archives of Clinical Neuropsychology, 21*, 503–508.

Bigler, E. D. (2007). A motion to exclude and the "fixed" version "flexible single" battery in "forensic" neuropsychology: Challenges to the practice of clinical neuropsychology. *Archives of Clinical Neuropsychology, 22*, 45–51.

Bush, S. S., Ruff, R. M., Troster, A. T., Barth, J. T., Koffler, S. P., Pligram, N. H., et al. (2005). Symptom validity assessment: Practice issues and medical necessity in policy planning conferences. *Archives of Clinical Neuropsychology, 20*, 419–427.

Cabana v. Forcier, 200 F.R.D. 9, 12 (D. Mass. 2001).

Chalfant, J. C., & Scheffelin M. A. (1969). *Central processing dysfunction in children: A review of research.* Bethesda, MD: U.S. Department of Health, Education, and Welfare.

Constantinou, M., Ashendorf, L., & McCaffrey, R. J. (2005). Effects of a third-party observer during neuropsychological assessment: When the observer is a video camera. *Journal of Forensic Neuropsychology, 4*(2), 39–48.

DeAngelis, C. D., & Fontanarosa, P. B. (2008). Impugning the integrity of medical science—The adverse effects of industry influence. *Journal of the American Medical Association, 299*(15), 1833–1835.

Denney, R. L. (2008, June). *Foundations of neuropsychological assessment for the criminal courts.* Three-hour workshop presented at Contemporary Issues in Forensic Pssychology, Workshop Series of the American Academy of Forensic Psychology, San Antonio, TX.

Fisher, D. (1994). Daubert v. Merrell Dow Pharmaceuticals: The Supreme Court gives federal judges the keys to admissibility of expert scientific testimony. 395 *San Diego Law Review,* 141.

Gouvier, W. D., Hayes, J. S., & Smiroldo, B. B. (1998). The significance of base rates test sensitivity, test specificity, and subjects' knowledge of symptoms in assessing TBI sequelae and malingering. In C. Reynolds (Ed.), *Detection of malingering during head injury litigation* (pp. 56–79). New York: Plenum.

Gouvier, W. D., Uddo-Crane, M., & Brown, L. (1998). Base rates of postconcussional symptoms. *Archives of Clinical Neuropsychology, 3,* 273–278.

Hartlage, L. C. (1975). Neuropsychological approaches to predicting outcome of remedial educational strategies for learning disabled children. *Pediatric Psychology, 3*(3), 23.

Hartlage, L. C. (1981). Clinical application of neuropsychological data. *School Psychology Review,* 10(3), 362–366.

Hartlage, L. C. (1983). The evolution of professional neuropsychology. *Bulletin of the National Academy of Neuropsychologists, 3,* 3–4.

Hartlage, L. C. (1993). Neuropsychological legal testimony from A to Z. *Independent Practitioner,* 13, 229–230.

Hartlage, L. C. (1995). Neuropsychological complaint base rates in personal injury, revisited. *Archives of Clinical Neuropsychology, 10,* 279–280.

Hartlage, L. C., & DeFilippis, N. (1983). History of neuropsychological assessment. In C. J. Golden & P. T. Vicente (Eds.), *Foundations of clinical neuropsychology* (pp. 1–23). New York: Plenum.

Hartlage, L. C., & Green, J. B. (1971). EEG differences in children's reading, spelling and arithmetic ability. *Perceptual and Motor Skills, 32,* 133–134.

Hartlage, L. C., & Long, C. J. (1978). Development of neuropsychology and a professional psychological specialty: History and credentialing. In C. R. Reynolds & E. Fletcher-Jansen (Eds.), *Handbook of clinical child psychology* (2nd ed., pp. 3–16). New York: Plenum.

Hecaen, H. (1962). Clinical symptomatology in right and left hemiplegic lesions. In U. B. Mountcastle (Ed.), *Interhemispheric relations and cerebral dominance.* Baltimore: Johns Hopkins Press.

Hertenstein v. Kimberly Home Health Care, Inc., 189 F.R.D. 620, 628-634 (D. Kan. 1999).

Jacober v. Saint Peter's Medical Center, 128 N.J. 475 (1992).

Jessica H. ex rel. Arp v. Spagnolo, 41 A.D.3d 1261, 839 N.Y.S.2d 638 N.Y.A.D. 4 Dept. (2007). *Journal of Forensic Neuropsychology.* (2005). 4(2).

Kixmiller, J. S., Briggs, J. R., Hartlage, L. C., & Dean, R. S. (1993). Factor structure of emotional and cognitive behaviors for normals and neurological impaired patients. *Journal of Clinical Psychology,* 49(2), 233–241.

Krauss, D., & Otto, R. (2007, August). *Do observers belong in the testing room?* Paper presented at the annual meeting of the American Psychological Association.

Langfeldt-Haaland v. Saupe Enterprises, Inc., 768 P.2d 1144 (Alaska 1089).

Larrabee, G. J. (2003). Exaggerated MMPI-2 symptom report in personal injury litigants with malingered neurocognitive deficit. *Archives of Clinical Neuropsychology, 18,* 673–686.

Larvie, V. (1994). Evidence: Admissibility of scientific evidence in federal courts. Daubert v. Pharmaceuticals, 1135. Ct. 2786. 29. *Lane & Wafer Law Review,* 275.

Lees-Haley, P. R., English, L. T., & Glenn, W. J. (1991). A fake bad scale on the MMPI-2 for personal injury claimants. *Psychological Reports, 68,* 203–210.

Lindman, L. S. (2004). *The effect of observational method and task complexity on neuropsychological test performance.* Retrieved January 21, 2008, from http://etd.lsu.edu/docs/available/etd-07072004-191224/unrestricted/Lindman_dis.pdf

Lynch, J. K. (2005). Effect of a third party observer on neuropsychological test performance following closed head injury. *Journal of Forensic Neuropsychology, 4*(2), 17–26.

Majestic A. L. (1986). Amici Curia, North Carolina Psychological Association. N. Carolina Court of Appeals, Horne v. Goodson.

Milner B. (1954). Intellectual function of the temporal lobes. *Psychological Bulletin, 51,* 42–62.

Morris, J. (2008, July/August). Toxic smoking mirrors. *Mother Jones.*

N.J.R.E. 803(c)(18). (2006). *Federal rules of evidence: Learned treatises provision.*

Reid, W. H. (2008). The treatment-forensic interface. *Journal of Psychiatric Practice, 14,* 122–125.

Ross, J. S., Hill, K. P., Egilman, D. S., & Krumholz, H. M. (2008). Guest authorship and ghostwriting in publications related to rofecox: A case study of industry documents from rofecoxib litigation. *Journal of the American Medical Association,* 299(15), 1800–1812.

Silver, J. M., & McAlister, T. W. (1997). Forensic issues in the neuropsychiatric evaluation of a patient with mild traumatic brain injury. *Neuropsychiatric Practice and Opinion, 9*, 19–21.

Slick, D. J., Sherman, E. M. S., & Iverson, G. L. (1999). Diagnostic criteria for malingering cognitive dysfunction: Proposed standards for clinical practice and research. *Clinical Neuropsychologist, 13*, 545–561.

Stigliano by Stigliano v. Connaught Laboratories, Inc., 140 N.J. 305, 658 A.2d 715 (NJ 1995).

Yantz, C. L., & McCaffrey, R. J. (2005). Effects of a supervisor's observation on memory test performance of the examinee: Third-party observer effect confirmed. *Journal of Forensic Neuropsychology, 4*(2), 27–38.

Forensic Neuropsychological Assessment of Members of Minority Groups: The Case for Assessing Hispanics

15

Raquel Vilar-López
Antonio E. Puente

Majority individuals of well-developed countries represent no more than 10% of the world population. In this global context, neuropsychology has been almost exclusively directed to the study of world minorities.

—A. E. Puente and A. Ardila

Introduction

Forensic neuropsychology has experienced spectacular growth recently (Bigler, 2006; Heilbronner, 2004; Sweet, King, Malina, Bergman, & Simmons, 2002). Nevertheless, studies about forensic assessment of minority groups are practically nonexistent. In this chapter, we will review different factors that should be considered when evaluating ethnic and racial minorities, focusing on Hispanics as an example.

We decided to focus on this group because it constitutes the fastest growing ethnic minority in the United States, and by 2050, the U.S. Hispanic population is projected to comprise one quarter of the nation's total population (U.S. Bureau of the Census, 1997). Considering that referrals for neuropsychological evaluations among ethnic minorities are growing (Echemendia & Harris, 2004), it is highly probable that every neuropsychologist in the forensic arena will face the assessment of several Hispanics during his/her career. Further, the combination of linguistic and cultural variations pose unique challenges that could serve as a paradigm for other neuropsychologists of a majority group attempting to evaluate those from non-majority groups.

Hispanic Definitions and Demographic Variables

Merriam-Webster's Collegiate Dictionary (2009) defines *Hispanic* as "relating to the people, speech, or culture of Spain and Portugal, or Latin America," whereas the *Diccionario de la Lengua Española* (2001) (*The Dictionary of the Spanish Language*) defines the same word as "pertaining to Spain or the nations of Latin America." Thus, depending on the definition, Portugal could be included or not as a Hispanic country. What is important to underscore is that Hispanic is *not* a race, but an ethnic group (Ardila, Rodríguez-Menéndez, & Rosselli, 2002; Puente & Ardila, 2000) comprised of multiple races such as Caucasian, Black, Mongolian, or mixtures thereof (U.S. Census Bureau, 1999). Language variations, cultural characteristics, heritage, behavioral patterns, country of origin and residence, cultural and educational level, socioeconomic status (SES), and so on, make Hispanics a very heterogeneous group. By 2005, the Hispanic population reached 41.8 million people, becoming the largest minority in the United States (U.S. Census Bureau, 2006). Most of them have Mexican origin (63%, according to the U.S. Census Bureau, 1999), but their geographical distribution is uneven across the country (Cubans in south Florida, Puerto Ricans in New York, Mexicans in Texas and California) (Puente & Ardilla, 2000).

Performing Forensic Evaluations With Spanish Speakers

Studies demonstrating the superiority of Anglos performing neuropsychological tests when compared with ethnic minorities are abundant (Agranovich & Puente, 2007; Ardila & Keating, 2007; Arnold, Montgomery, Castaneda, & Longoria, 1994; Baird, Ford, & Podell, 2007; Boone, Victor, Wen, Razani, & Pontón, 2007; Byrd et al., 2006; Byrd, Touradji, Tang, & Manly, 2004; Coffey, Marmol, Shock, & Adams, 2005; Demsky, Mittenberg, Quintar, Katell, & Golden, 1998; Diehr, Heaton, Miller, & Grant, 1998; Norman, Evans, Miller, & Heaton, 2000; Patton, Duff, Schoenberg, Mold, Scott, & Adams, 2003; Ross, Lichtenberg, & Christensen, 1995; Rosselli, Ardila, Salvatierra, Marquez, Matos, & Weekes, 2002; Schwartz et al., 2004; Whitfield et al., 2000). Those differences are generalized to all cognitive domains (perception, attention, spatial abilities, memory, executive functions) and not limited to verbal tasks, as traditionally thought. Nevertheless, the reasons underlying such differences remain elusive, though it is of interest that Anglos comprise almost all, if not all, of the authors of major neuropsychological tests. Variables that are considered most important to those from a well-educated and compensated stratum of the majority group generally use that information to make up test themes and items. For example, time is of the greatest essence in Anglo cultures, but of much less value in Hispanic ones.

A host of variables have been proposed as mediators of such findings that professionals should take into account when assessing an individual belonging to an ethnic minority. The consideration of such variables could completely change the conclusions and recommendations of a report. Thus, they are especially important on forensic cases because of the repercussion those reports could have for the individual being assessed (including the death penalty as an extreme situation).

Education

Hispanics, compared with Americans, have a low educational attainment (both living in and out of the United States) (Puente & Ardila, 2000). Low levels of formal education are very frequent among immigrants, but very few studies analyze the performance of such individuals on psychometric tests. Most neuropsychological norms erroneously consider people with fewer than 8 years of education a homogenous group, despite the fact that educational effect represents a negatively accelerated curve, tending toward a plateau (thus, differences between 0 and 3 years of education are highly significant, between 3 and 6 can be lower, and so on, with virtually no differences between, for example, 12 and 15 years of education). Given this fact, considering individuals with less than 8 or 10 years of education as a homogeneous group is a big mistake (Ardila, 2007). Neuropsychological performance tends to be extremely poor in illiterates in most cognitive domains. Psychometric testing instruments significantly penalize illiterates because of the undertraining of the abilities included in most tests, and the lack of familiarity with and difficulties in understanding the testing situations, among others (Ardila & Rosselli, 2007), and practitioners should consider all this information in their reports. Nevertheless, educational level is not related to everyday problem solving (Cornelious & Caspi, 1987), so forensic neuropsychologists should provide special attention to this aspect when evaluating illiterate individuals.

Research in the last decade or so has demonstrated that it is more appropriate to consider the quality of the education, and not the number of years of formal education, when evaluating minority groups (Byrd, Sanchez, & Manly, 2005; Byrd, Touradji, Tang, & Manly, 2004; Cosentino, Manly, & Mungas, 2007; Manly, Byrd, Touradji, & Stern, 2004; Manly, Jacobs, Touradji, Small, & Stern, 2002). Because minorities have less opportunity due to their social situation (racism, poverty, etc.), the reasons for obtaining fewer years of education could be different from those in the dominant group. On the other hand, different countries have different education levels. Thus, quality of education seems a better option. A test devised to measure this variable with Hispanics is the Word Accentuation Test (WAT; Del Ser, Gonzalez-Montalvo, Martinez-Espinosa, Delgado-Villapalos, & Bermejo, 1997).

Acculturation

Acculturation is the individual's ability to understand and maneuver outside of the culture in which he or she was raised and with which he or she is most familiar

(Berry, 1997). Consistent with the heterogeneity of Hispanics, acculturation is very variable in this group, but patterns of behavior, as well as beliefs and values of Hispanics living in the United States, tend to become progressively more similar to traditional middle-American standards (Ardila, Rodriguez-Menéndez, & Rosselli, 2002). Acculturation level was related to the performance on different neuropsychological tests, such as the Halstead-Reitan Battery (Arnold, Montgomery, Castenada, & Longoria, 1994), the Wisconsin Card Sorting Test (Coffey et al., 2005), Vocabulary and Similarities subtests (Razani, Murcia, Tabares, & Wong, 2007), Boston Naming Test, FAS, and Digit Span (Boone et al., 2007), Trail Making Test, and Stroop and Auditory Consonant Trigrams (Razani, Burciaga, et al., 2007). Thus, this variable should be considered when assessing minority individuals, because its control will improve the diagnostic accuracy of neuropsychological assessment.

To assess acculturation, we should consider the identification with the culture of origin (Hispanic) and the identification with the host culture (North American) in several aspects of the individual's lifestyle (i.e., food, recreational activities, values, and customs) (Ward & Kennedy, 1994), as well as language (English as first or second language, age at which English was learned), residency (number of years residing in the United States), and education (number of years educated in the United States) (Boone et al., 2007).

Two examples of acculturation measures that could be used with Hispanics are the Marin Acculturation Scale (English and Spanish versions) (Marin & Marin, 1991), and the Acculturation Rating Scales for Mexican Americans, 2nd Edition (Cuellar, Arnold, & Maldonado, 1995).

Language and the Use of Interpreters

To determine the language of the assessment, Pontón has proposed a decision tree that is briefly reviewed here: whether the patient is monolingual, the decision is clear, and the individual should be evaluated in his/her language. Nevertheless, if the patient is bilingual, a formal assessment of the proficiency should be done, and level of acculturation and educational background (years of education in the United States) should be taken into account. If the patient is not a monolingual Spanish speaker, has a low English proficiency, or has a medium or low acculturation and was educated in a Spanish-speaking culture, a bilingual neuropsychologist should conduct the assessment (Pontón, 2001; Ponón & Corona-LoMonaco, 2007).

The use of interpreters should be avoided whenever possible for several reasons: the addition of a third person changes the dynamics of the standard neuropsychological assessment (Wong, Strickland, Fletcher-Janzen, Ardila, & Reynolds, 2000), rapport is decreased and subtleties will be missed (Puente & Ardila, 2000), and their use invalidates the tests being administered (Melendez, 2001). The referral to bilingual neuropsychologists, when necessary, is highly desirable, and recommended by the American Psychological Association (APA, 1991, 2002). Nevertheless, doing so seems unrealistic, considering that the estimated number of bilingual or bicultural neuropsychologists is fewer than 50 some years ago (Puente & Ardila, 2000), and that number has not increased by much. Federal courts require the interpreter to pass a proficiency examination to be employed, but no such requirement exists for neuropsychologists, so this is left to his/her own judgement. The tendency to overestimate our linguistic competency is remarkably frequent among neuropsychologists, so professionals conduct assessments in Spanish who are not qualified to do so (of course, with their best intention). Professionals are advised that those assessments violate the *Guidelines for Providers of Psychological Services to Ethnic, Linguistic, and Culturally Diverse Populations* (APA, 1991), as well as the *Standards for Education and Psychological Testing* (American Educational Research Association [AERA], American Psychological Association [APA], & National Council on Measurement in Education [NCME], 1999). In chapter 9, they address the critical problems facing interpreters. Standard 9.11 considers this issue and the readers of this chapter ought to be familiar with that language, as well as being cognizant of the ongoing revision of those standards. Among other things, they mention the importance of understanding not just the language, but the culture of the individual being tested. Indeed, being bicultural is much more involved and complex than simply being bilingual. In essence, literal translations often miss the cognitive or emotional equivalence that is the hallmark of an appropriate evaluation. In addition, there is the problem that sometimes an appropriate linguistic and cultural translation still does not match the conceptual goal intended by the author of the original test. The Hispanic Neuropsychological Society, together with the National Academy of Neuropsychology, recently agreed, after much study, to a position paper that addresses these issues (Judd et al., 2009).

When an appropriate referral is not possible, it is important to consider several recommendations for minimizing the damage of using interpreters (Melendez, 2001; Wong et al., 2000):

- Inquire about professionals with experience translating psychological interactions.
- Interview various interpreters before selecting one (taking into account their backgrounds, but also their appearances, attitudes, and social ease).
- The interpreter should be fluent in the dialect of the patient and familiar with the specific culture of the region the patient is from.
- The interpreter should conduct the examination, and not be just a player (the more discreet and self-effacing, the better).
- The neuropsychologist should spend a preparation/training session with the interpreter to explain to him/her the basic neuropsychological assessment principles (i.e., no verbal or nonverbal help or cues should be provided, verbatim instructions and responses are required, confidentiality issues, etc.), and to review the tests and materials that will be used in the examination (so the instructions, lists of words, etc., will flow fluently during the assessment).

Even when following all these recommendations, the use of interpreters was never included on the standardization of neuropsychological instruments, and their use introduces an unknown amount of error in the assessment. This should be noted on the report, and interpretations of the results when using interpreters should be extremely cautious.

Bilingualism

Bilingualism is a very complex concept, influenced by a wide range of variables that make its exact determination almost impossible. Some of these variables considered crucial to its determination are: age and sequence of acquisition, method of acquisition, schooling language, contexts of the two languages, patterns of use of the two languages, personal and social attitudes toward each language, and individual differences in verbal abilities (Ardila, 1998).

It is probable that different degrees of bilingualism are related differently to each of the cognitive domains. Nowadays, there are no studies that investigate the understanding of the relation of bilingualism and cognitive status, so under- or over-estimation of cognitive abilities is possible when assessing bilinguals. For example, it was stated that Spanish–English bilinguals may be at a disadvantage when using either language, because using either Spanish or English testing materials and norms penalize these bilinguals (Ardila et al., 2002; Puente & Ardila, 2000; Ardila et al., 2000). On the other hand, bilinguals seem to possess better executive function skills, compared with monolinguals (Bialystock, 1999). It is possible that future imaging studies will allow better understanding of the relation between bilingualism and cognitive results (i.e., De Bleser et al., 2003, demonstrated different brain activation in bilinguals, compared with monolinguals).

Socioeconomic Status

Hispanics living below the poverty level exceed by far the non-Hispanic white population in such a condition. Low SES is linked to variables such as lack of appropriate nutrition, which has been associated with brain dysfunction and altered neuropsychological results (Llorente, 2008).

When SES is controlled, studies show that differences between ethnicities often disappeared. As an example, Armengol (2002) studied the effect of SES in children from Mexico City, showing that low-SES children achieve a significantly lower performance on the Stroop, compared with high-SES children. On the other hand, the performance of bilingual children in Massachusetts from low-SES backgrounds was close to that of low-SES children in Mexico City, whereas values obtained by high-SES Mexican children were equivalent to the normative data in American children. Due to its possible impact on neuropsychological measures, SES of the patient should be always contemplated in the report.

Other Cultural Factors

According to Ardila (2005, 2007), some cultural values that are not universal underlie psychometrically oriented cognitive testing, and help to explain why members of the culture in which the test was developed obtain the highest scores:

  ■ There is a one-to-one relationship between an examiner and an examinee who have never met before and will not meet again.
  ■ One must consider the background or situational authority of the examiner.
  ■ The idea is that the examinee will perform at his/her best level of effort.
  ■ Testing is done in an isolated environment; it is a private and intimate situation that may be quite inappropriate in many cultures.
  ■ The examiner uses a stereotyped and formal language. The examinee is not allowed to talk about himself or herself, the examination is far from a

normal social relationship and usual conversation. For Hispanics, the personal relationship with the examiner may be more important than the test results. In fact, Mexicans, compared with Americans, place greater emphasis on being simpatico (friendly, charming, caring) versus being efficient (Diaz-Guerrero, 1993), and acquiescence and trying to please the examiner was found to be more important than the task itself for some groups (Perez-Arce, 1999).

■ The idea that the examinee must perform as quickly as possible; for many cultural groups, including Hispanics, speed and quality are seen as contradictory. Speed, competitiveness, and high productivity are important cultural values in literate Anglo-American society, but not in other cultural groups. For example, cooperation and social abilities are very important for Hispanics (being "educated" implies good social skills, and not educational attainment), whereas competitiveness is viewed with suspicion (Puente & Ardila, 2000).

■ The examiner may ask questions that are perceived as a violation of privacy. Intellectual testing may be perceived as a kind of humiliating situation and disrespectful of privacy in Latin America.

■ The use of specific testing elements (figures, blocks, pictures) and strategies (memorize meaningless information) that are not easy to understand for some cultural groups.

Cultural relevance (meaningfulness) is another important variable in cross-cultural assessments (Puente & Ardila, 2000). In fact, it has been demonstrated that an execution of a particular cognitive task might require the involvement of different constellations of brain structures, depending on relevance of the task to one's cultural background (Golden & Thomas, 2000). All these cultural factors, and the degree to which they are influencing the results of a neuropsychological testing in a specific individual, are very difficult to detect and understand for an examiner who is not familiar with the culture of the examinee. Also, Hispanics frequently do not feel totally comfortable with English-speaking examiners (Ardila et al., 2002), and the "distance" (e.g., gender, age, ethnicity) between the examiner and the examinee may impact the results of the testing situation (Ardila & Keating, 2007). Thus, the reasons for referring Hispanic individuals to Hispanic neuropsychologists go far beyond language factors.

What Tests Can We Use With Hispanics?

We often assume that simply translating the test or obtaining an interpreter resolves the barriers posed in evaluating Spanish-speakers. In reality, the situation is complex.

The Problems of Translating Tests

It is not uncommon for practitioners to merely use idiosyncratic translated tests when faced with a cross-cultural assessment. This method is not only completely erroneous and invalid, but also unethical, according to the *Standards for Educational and Psychological Testing* (American Educational Research Association, American

Psychological Association, National Council on Measurement in Education, 1996). Somebody translating a test assumes that language is the only barrier to a valid assessment in such minority cases (Wong et al., 2000), forgetting the multitude of factors that influence the differences found in cognitive tests between different ethnic groups (see the last section).

Puente and Ardila (2000) highlighted some of the main problems involved in the translation of tests. In the first place, appropriate translation and adaptation of a test is a very complex endeavor that requires the balance of bilinguals familiar with the different dialects and language variations of the subgroups of the population at hand, so the final version could be considered standard language for all members of the population (i.e., Hispanics from Spain, Argentina, Colombia, Mexico, etc.). In the second place, cultural meaningfulness should always be considered, because items literally translated to another culture may have different relevance (i.e., the beaver or an igloo are not as familiar to a Hispanic as they are to a North American), or even make no sense (i.e., "it's raining cats and dogs" makes no sense in Spanish), resulting in differences in performance. Even more important, cognitive equivalence should be addressed (i.e., in the tests requiring digits in the Wechsler Adult Intelligence test [WAIS], is the task to remember a single-digit number or a single-digit number with a specified number of syllables? The numbers 1, 4, 5, 7, 8, and 9 have two syllables in Spanish and only one in English, so is the memorization of digit series equivalent?).

Even when adequate translations are conducted, psychometric properties of the test in the new language need to be determined before considering the test a good tool (Pontón & Ardila, 1999; Ardila et al., 2002; Wong et al., 2000).

The Problem of Adequate Norms

Several authors have pointed out the problems and caveats of developing race-based norms (Ardila, 2007; Brickman, Cabo, & Manly, 2006; Gasquoine, 1999; Manly, 2005; Manly et al., 2002, 2004; Manly & Echemendia, 2007; Pedraza & Mungas, 2008), based on several ideas. First, race is a social or political construct, lacking a genetic or biological base (Helms, Jernigan, & Mascher, 2005; Manly et al., 2004), and explains little about the variations of test scores from group to group (Brickman et al., 2006). Second, the thousands of languages and cultures (including mixtures of them) make impossible the endeavour of developing race-specific norms for all of them (Ardila, 2007; Brickman et al., 2006). Also, it has been pointed out that race could be deconstructed in factors such as those exposed in the previous section (level and quality of education, acculturation, language usage, etc.), responsible for the differences found between ethnic groups on cognitive measures (i.e., Manly et al., 2002; Razani, Murcia, et al., 2007; Touradji, Manly, Jacobs, & Stern, 2001). It is our hope that future studies will determine the specific weight of different cultural factors, so norms could be stratified according to them. Nevertheless, the current situation is far from that.

On the other hand, several authors conclude that separate norms for different ethnic groups could be an appropriate resource, because they increase the sensitivity and specificity of neuropsychological measures in detecting cognitive impairment, and thus the accuracy of diagnosis (Agranovich & Puente, 2007; Ardila, 1995; Lucas et al., 2005; Manly, 2005; Nabors, Evans, & Strickland, 2000; Wong et al., 2000).

Currently, most neuropsychological tests do not have norms for Hispanics (Pedraza & Mungas, 2008), and it is not uncommon to find clinicians scoring Hispanic protocols with norms designed for the United States mainstream (White English-speaking, middle-class subjects with a high school or college level of education) (Ardila et al., 2002), leading to drawing inferences and making erroneous conclusions (Uzzell, 2007). Furthermore, recent research contradicts the traditional assumption that Caucasian norms can be used with Hispanics who speak English as a first language. Both Boone et al. (2007) and Razani, Burciaga, et al. (2007) demonstrated that minorities who spoke English as a first versus second language performed comparably to each other and worse than Anglo-Americans on neuropsychological measures. Once again, studies point out that neuropsychological results are not just a question of language.

Some authors have made the effort to make lists of neuropsychological tests with norms for Hispanic speakers (Ardila et al., 2002; Boone et al., 2007; Llorente & Weber, 2008; Pontón, 2001; Pontón & Corona-LoMonaco, 2007; Poreh, 2002; Salazar, Pérez-García, & Puente, 2007). Considering all of them, we present a list of tests with references that could serve as a guide for clinicians facing the assessment of Hispanic adults (see Table 15.1).

The selection of appropriate norms will depend on the question at hand. Thus, descriptive and diagnostic uses should be differentiated (Manly & Echemendia, 2007). The use of English norms to assess a Hispanic patient can be adequate if, for example, we need to establish the understanding of indications of and explanations about the legal system given in English.

When trying to diagnose brain damage, neuropsychologists interpreting test results should always consider whether age, education, acculturation, specific cultural background, language level, country of origin, region of residence, and SES are similar for the person being assessed and the comparative normative group. It is clear that is not appropriate to compare a 25-year-old Mexican with a master's degree obtained in North Carolina with an elder sample obtained with Puerto Ricans residing in New York. Obviously, all of them are Hispanics, but each situation is substantially different. In this regard, it is noteworthy that the majority of research on the neuropsychological assessment of Hispanics has used elderly, poorly educated, Spanish-speaking participants, resident in the United States for more than 15 years (Gasquoine, 2001). Thus, heterogeneity of Hispanics is not reflected in the available norms.

Detection of Limited Effort in Hispanics

Detection of less-than-optimal effort in minorities is extremely complicated, fundamentally because of the lack of studies in this area. Nevertheless, the forensic assessment would not be complete if the possibility of deception is not considered.

Malingering is the "intentional production of false or grossly exaggerated physical or psychological symptoms" (*Diagnostic and Statistical Manual of Mental Disorders, Fourth Edition* [*DSM-IV*]; American Psychiatric Association, 1994) with the aim of getting an external goal, such as an economic reward or avoiding work. According to the *DSM-IV*, clinicians should suspect malingering if the individual is facing a medico-legal evaluation, if the referred complaints are discrepant with the objective findings, if a lack of cooperation is observed from the patient, and

15.1 Available Tests With Norms for Hispanics

Tests	References
Batería Neuropsicológica en Español	Artiola-i-Fortuny, 2000; Artiola-i-Fortuny, Hermosillo-Romo, Heaton, & Pardee, 1999
Batería Woodcock-Muñoz: Pruebas de Aprovechamiento-R	Woodcock & Muñoz-Sandoval, 1996a
Batería Woodcock-Muñoz: Pruebas de Habilidad Cognitiva-R	Woodcock & Muñoz-Sandoval, 1996b
Batería-III	Woodcock & Muñoz-Sandoval, 2005
Beck Depression Scale	Sanz & Vázquez, 1991
Benton Visual Form Discrimination	Campo & Morales, 2003
Benton Visual Retention Test	Jacobs et al., 1997
Bilingual Verbal Ability Tests	Muñoz-Sandoval, Cummins, Alvarado, & Ruef, 1998
Block Design	Taussig, Henderson, & Mack, 1992; Pontón, Satz, Herrera, Ortiz, Urrutia, Young, et al., 1996
Boston Naming Test	Ardila, Rosselli, & Puente, 1994; Kohnert, Hernández, & Bates, 1998; Loewenstein, Rubert, Arguelles, & Duara, 1995; Pontón et al., 1996
Cancellation Test	Ardila et al., 1994
Cognistat, Spanish Version	Kiernan, Mueller, & Langston, 1998
Color Trails	Pontón et al., 1996
Controlled Word Association Test	Manly et al., 1998
Design Fluency	Delgado, Guerrero, Goggin, & Ellis, 1999
Digit-Span	Ardila et al., 1994; Olazaran, Jacobs, & Stern, 1996; Pontón et al., 1996; Loewenstein et al., 1995
Direct Assessment of Functional Status	Loewenstein, Ardila, Rosselli, Hayden, Duara, Berkowitz, et al., 1992
Fuld Object Memory	Loewenstein et al., 1995
General Ability Measure for Adults	Naglieri & Bardos, 1997
Geriatric Depression Scale	Zamanian, Thackrey, Starrett, Brown, Lassman, & Blanchart, 1992
Mattis Dementia Rating Scale	Taussig et al., 1992
Minnesota Multiphasic Personality Inventory-2	Gómez-Maqueo, León-Guzmán, & Medina-Mora, 2003
Mini Mental Status Examination	Ardila et al., 1994; Bird, Canino, Stippec, & Shrout, 1987; Escobar, Burman, & Marno, 1986; Gurland, Wilder, Cross, Teresi, & Barret, 1992; Mungas, Marshal, Weldon, Haan, & Reed, 1996; Ostroski-Solís, López-Arango, & Ardila, 2000; Taussing et al., 1992; Taussing & Pontón, 1996
Multilingual Aphasia Exam-Spanish	Rey & Benton, 1991
NEUROPSI	Ostrosky, Ardila, & Rosselli, 1997
Neuropsychological Screening Battery for Hispanics	Pontón et al., 1996; Pontón, Gonzalez, Hernandez, & Igareda, 2000; Pontón, 2001
Non-Verbal Reasoning Test Series	Ostrosky, Ardila, & Roselli, 1997

(continued)

Table 15.1 *(continued)*

Tests	References
Paced Auditory Serial Addition Test	Diehr et al., 1998
Raven's Standard Progressive Matrices	Pontón et al., 1996
Rey-Osterrieth Complex Figure	Ardila, Rosselli, & Rosas, 1989; Ardila et al., 1994; Ardila & Rosselli, 2003; Ostrosky-Solís, Jaime, & Ardila, 1998; Pontón et al., 1996
Serial Verbal Learning	Ardila et al., 1994
Spanish English Verbal Learning	Gonzalez, Mungas, & Haan, 2002
Stroop Test	Golden, 1978: Spanish adaptation by TEA ediciones, 2001
Token Test	Ardila et al., 1994
Trail Making Test	Rosseli & Ardila, 1996
Verbal Fluency	Ardila et al., 1994; Loewenstein et al., 1995; Pontón et al., 1996
Wechsler Adult Intelligence Scale	Wechsler, 1997: Spanish adaptation by TEA ediciones, 1999
Wechsler Memory Scale	Ardila et al., 1994; Demsky et al., 1998; Loewenstein et al., 1995; Ostrosky-Solís et al., 2000
WHO-UCLA-Auditory Verbal Learning Test	Pontón et al., 1996
Wisconsin Card Sorting Test	Artiola-i-Fortuny & Heaton, 1996; Artiola-i-Fortuny & Mullaney, 1998; Mejia, Pineda, Alvarez, & Ardila, 1998; Rey, Feldman, Rivas-Vaz-quez, Levin, & Benton, 1999; Rosselli & Ardila, 1996
Woodcock Language Proficiency Battery-Revised, Spanish Form	Woodcock & Muñoz-Sandoval, 1993

if the individual presents antisocial personality disorder. The only study that tested this model was done by Rogers (1990) in a criminal forensic sample. The author found that the criterion of two or more indices had a false positive rate of approximately 80%, showing the ineffectiveness of the *DSM-IV* model. Rogers (1997) affirms that this vision is congruent with a "criminological" model. As an alternative, Rogers proposed the "adaptive" model, according to which the probability of malingering is higher when the evaluation context is perceived as adverse, personal risk is very high, and other alternatives do not seem available. This model could be especially applicable with ethnic minority individuals, who tend to perceive the legal system and the concept of justice from a negative point of view (established to benefit those in a powerful/dominant situation), who had suffered discrimination and negative experiences because of being part of a minority, and who may have the necessity of "making themselves be heard" (Poreh, 2002), that could lead to an exaggeration of symptoms. These sociocultural factors should be considered when assessing malingering in Hispanics, who could perceive malingering as the only way to get what they deserve.

Due to the problems and flaws detected on the *DSM-IV* concept of malingering, different authors have proposed alternative diagnostic criteria (Faust & Ackley, 1998; Greiffenstein, Baker, & Gola, 1994; Prigatano, Smason, Lamb, & Bortz, 1997; Slick, Sherman, & Iverson, 1999; Teichner & Wagner, 2004). Slick et al.'s proposal about malingered neurocognitive dysfunction has been widely used in malingering research, and it has a great clinical utility and could be applied with Hispanics, with an extra-careful consideration for the criteria of probable response bias.

The Study of Inconsistencies

There is a consensus in accepting inconsistencies as the key to detecting malingering. Larrabee (2000) expressed this idea, stating that everything on the assessment should make "neuropsychological sense," and Reynolds (1998) affirmed that malingering detection has three components: congruence, congruence, and congruence. Inconsistencies potentially useful in detecting malingering in minority groups could be produced by:

- Test results from the same domain (i.e., in two tests of verbal memory, the individual appears as severely impaired in one and between normal levels in another one; recall is better than recognition)
- Test results from different domains; results do not coincide with known neuropsychological patterns (i.e., attention is better than memory)
- Test results from different assessments (on a repeated administration of a test, the individual obtains a result significantly different from the first time)
- Test results and the expected results attending to the documented damage (a patient with neuroimaging findings on the left hemisphere obtained higher scores with the right hand on the Finger-Tapping Test)
- Test results and the observed behavior or activities of daily living (i.e., a patient obtained scores indicative of severe memory problems on several tests, but arrives alone on time to the neuropsychological assessment, remembers what he had for breakfast, and does not need any help to live independently)
- Test results and reliable collateral informers (i.e., the patient obtained very poor neuropsychological results, but his boss reports the individual working properly in his administrative position after the supposed brain damage)
- The reported and documented history (i.e., the patient states she was in coma for two days, but her reports indicate her lack of consciousness lasted five minutes)
- The reported symptoms (internal inconsistency in the symptom presentation that do not correspond to any known syndrome)
- The reported symptoms and the observed behavior
- The reported symptoms and the information obtained from reliable collateral informers.

Despite the agreement considering inconsistencies as an important construct, this approach has received little attention from an empirical perspective. Some studies have demonstrated the utility of the test–retest approach with the Halstead Reitan battery (Reitan & Wolfson, 1995, 1997), Victoria Symptom Validity Test (Strauss et al., 2000, 2002), and the Dot Counting Test and Digit subtest (Strauss et al., 2002), but generally, the assessment of the inconsistencies relies on the clinical opinion of the neuropsychologist. No studies proved the utility of this approach with minorities.

The Use of Tests of Effort

Tests of effort could be divided into two broad groups:

1. Floor effect. These tests rely on very basic cognitive abilities with items that should be passed by nearly everyone. The most extended test that uses this approach is the Rey 15-Item Test (see Lezak, Howieson, & Loring, 2004). Other examples are the Dot Counting Test (Boone et al., 2002), or the b test (Boone, Lu, & Herzberg, 2002).

2. Forced-choice tests or symptom validity testing. The use of these tests is recommended by the National Academy of Neuropsychology to assess the patients' effort (Bush et al., 2005), and its contribution to the forensic evaluations is considered very valuable (O'Bryant, Duff, Fisher, & McCaffrey 2004; Tombaugh, 1996). It is the most employed and studied method to detect cognitive malingering (Gervais, Rohling, Green, & Ford, 2004). These tests relied initially on binomial distribution: as there are only two choices, malingerers can be detected if the failure rate significantly exceeds chance level (50%). In other words, if someone selects the correct responses significantly below the chance level because that person knows the correct responses and intentionally decides to select the incorrect ones, that person may be malingering. The Digit Memory Test (Hiscock & Hiscock, 1989) or the Portland Digit Recognition Test (Binder, 1990) use this approach. Nevertheless, this criterion has been considered too stringent and unnecessary, so other tests have established cut-off points under the chance level, such as the Test of Memory Malingering (Tombaugh, 1996), Victoria Symptom Validity Test (Slick, Hopp, Strauss, & Thompson, 1997), Computerized Assessment of Response Bias (Allen, Conder, Green, & Cox, 1997), or the Word Memory Test (Green, Allen, & Astner, 1996). These tools are considered an exception to malingering tests because of their high sensitivity (Slick, Sherman, & Iverson, 1999; Willison & Tombaugh, 2006). For excellent reviews of this method, see Bianchini, Mathias, and Greve (2001) and chapter 6 of this book.

Binomial distribution is a mathematical and universal concept that, from a theoretical point of view, could be applied to any individual (including minorities). Furthermore, if these tests are measuring effort and not ability, there is no reason for them to change systematically with respect to age, education, gender, or variables related to neurologic damage (Boone, Lu, & Herzberg, 2002). In fact, several studies have shown that there is no correlation between malingering tests and demographic or neurological variables (Constantinou & McCaffrey, 2003; Grote et al., 2000; Haber & Fichtenberg, 2006; Macciocchi, Seel, Alderson, & Godsall, 2006; Rees, Tombaugh, & Boulay, 2001; Teichner & Wagner, 2004; Tombaugh, 1996). The problem with the below-chance-level is that, despite its excellent specificity, its sensitivity is unacceptably low (Bender & Rogers, 2004; Gervais et al., 2004; Guilmette, Hart, & Giuliano, 1993; Guilmette, Hart, Giuliano, & Leininger, 1994; Greiffenstein et al., 1994; Hiscock, Branham, & Hiscock, 1994; Holmquist & Wanlass, 2002; Martin, Bolter, Todd, Gouvier, & Niccolls, 1993; Martin, Hayes, & Gouvier, 1996; Rose, Hall, & Szalda-Petree, 1995; Slick, Hopp, Strauss, Hunter, & Pinch, 1994). Thus, the majority of the malingering ethnic minority individuals assessed with these tests would be undetected.

The rest of the tests (both those following the floor-effect approach and the forced-choice tests with cut-off scores under the chance level) are not appropriate for use with minorities, because their sensitivity and specificity have not been studied in such populations. The only studies in this regard were done with Spaniards, and demonstrated that the Victoria Symptom Validity Test and the Test of Memory Malingering, and to a lesser degree, the Dot Counting Test, obtained results very similar to the original populations, whereas the Rey 15-Items Test obtained very poor results (Vilar-López et al., 2007; Vilar-López, Gómez-Rio, Santiago-Ramajo, Rodriguez-Fernandez, Puente, & Pérez-García, 2008; Vilar-López, Gómez-Río, Caracuel-Romero, Llamas-Elvira, & Pérez-García, 2008). Nevertheless, other studies are necessary in order to demonstrate the applicability of such tests to other groups (i.e., Mexican or Puerto Ricans residing in the United States).

The Final Decision

As a result of the lack of empirical data, malingering diagnoses in minority cases depend on the clinical judgment of the professional. In this judgment, we should conduct a careful examination of the individual's history before the damage (birth and developmental, as well as medical, school, work, legal, military, mental health, or substance abuse records), during the incident, if there is one (e.g., witness reports), and in the present time (medical, neurological, psychological reports). All this information should be considered to interpret our neuropsychological evaluation (interview and tests results), always paying special attention to the cultural issues relevant to the specific case.

Special Issues in Forensic Evaluations

Despite forensic neuropsychology being considered an area of clinical neuropsychology, there are some differences between clinic and forensic evaluations that make them substantially different (Bush & NAN Policy & Planning Committee, 2005). Denney & Wynkoop (2000) highlight the following:

1. Although the relationship established in clinical assessment is based on collaboration and confidence, forensic evaluations are frequently considered adverse. This is especially important with Hispanic individuals. For them, opening up to a stranger is abnormal, mental issues are a very private matter, and intellectual or cognitive testing is perceived as aversive (Puente & Ardila, 2000). Thus, it is extremely important to make very clear the terms of our relationship to the individual, the goal of the evaluation, and explain in advance the different steps of the process to diminish the anxiety level of the individual.

2. The alliance of forensic neuropsychologists is with the truth, and not with the patient. Again, this aspect has a special relevance to Hispanics, for whom establishing a good rapport with the professional is a fundamental issue. Transparency, establishing a natural environment, and sincerity are key elements to obtaining reliable information from Hispanics.

3. Forensic evaluations require more information sources and, thus, more time and attention to details. In fact, these assessments are the longest in clinical

neuropsychology (Sweet, Peck, Abramowitz, & Etzweiler, 2002). Even more time will be necessary with Hispanics. A structured interview is recommended, given the possibility of missing important elements because of the complexities associated with cultural issues.

Who Should Conduct a Forensic Neuropsychological Assessment of a Hispanic Patient?

On the first hand, the qualified professional should be a certified clinical neuropsychologist (through The American Board of Clinical Neuropsychology or The American Board of Professional Neuropsychology) with an appropriate knowledge of the area pertinent to the specific case at hand (i.e., traumatic brain injury, dementia, etc.), and possess an adequate knowledge of forensic psychology, being familiar with the American Academy of Forensic Psychology and the *American Law Society's Specialty Guidelines for Forensic Psychologists* (Committee on Ethical Guidelines for Forensic Psychologists, 1991, 2008), and of the legal aspects relevant for the specific case. On the other hand, the clinician should be proficient in the patient's language, or make a referral to another professional whenever possible (APA, 1991; Llorente & Weber, 2008; Melendez, 2001). Also, cultural expertise or competence at the individual level is essential for the clinician who is working with cross-cultural populations (APA, 1992, 2002, 2003). Education and training programs are essential to get that competence (APA, 2003; Brickman et al., 2006; Fastenau, Evans, Johnson & Bond, 2002; van Gorp, Myers, & Drake, 2000), but there is much to work on in this regard.

Conclusions and Recommendations

Forensic evaluations of minorities constitute one of the most difficult challenges in clinical neuropsychology. When facing such a challenge, clinicians should consider:

1. Their proficiency in the patient's language and their knowledge of the patient's culture. If the appropriate language of the assessment is not English, or if the clinician is not sufficiently familiar with the culture of the individual, referral to a bilingual and bicultural neuropsychologist is the best option. If this is not possible, consultation with such professionals is indispensable. The use of interpreters should be avoided, if possible.
2. Using tests appropriately adapted and including studies about psychometric properties for the patient's group.
3. Using demographically matched norms.
4. Considering cultural issues in every phase of the process (interview, assessment, test interpretation, etc.).
5. Fulfilling their professional responsibility to be up-to-date on the literature and scientific advances on minority research.
6. Clearly stating all the variables possibly influencing test results (test version, selected norms, cultural issues, use of interpreters, etc.) on the report. Be cautious with the interpretation of the results.

7. Reviewing other types of information, such as records review, functional assessment of the patient, interviews with the patient and collateral people (family, friends, coworkers...), and so on. Because of limited tests and norms for minorities and their limitations, these other types of information are especially important.

Despite the growing research in the last few years and the remarkable efforts of some researchers, many more studies are necessary in the field of cross-cultural neuropsychology, and specifically, on cross-cultural forensic neuropsychology. The development of these areas will be beneficial not only for ethnic minorities, but for the progress of clinical neuropsychology as a whole.

References

Agranovich, A. V., & Puente, A. E. (2007). Do Russian and American normal adults perform similarly on neuropsychological tests? Preliminary findings on the relationship between culture and test performance. *Archives of Clinical Neuropsychology, 22,* 273–282.

Allen, L. M., Conder, R. L., Green, P., & Cox, D. R. (1997). *CARB '97 manual for the computerized assessment of response bias.* Durham, NC: CogniSyst.

American Educational Research Association, American Psychological Association, & National Council on Measurement in Education. (1999). *Standards for educational and psychological testing.* Washington, DC: American Psychological Association.

American Psychiatric Association. (1994). *Diagnostic and statistical manual for mental disorders* (4th ed.). Washington, DC: American Psychiatric Press.

American Psychological Association. (1991). *Guidelines for providers of psychological services to ethnic, linguistic, and culturally diverse populations.* Washington, DC: APA Office of Ethnic and Minority Affairs.

American Psychological Association. (1992). Ethical principles of psychologists and code of conduct. *American Psychologist, 48,* 45–48.

American Psychological Association. (2002). Ethical principles of psychologists and code of conduct. *American Psychologist, 57,* 1060–1073.

American Psychological Association. (2003). Guidelines on multicultural education, training, research, practice, and organizational change for psychologists. *American Psychologist, 58,* 377–402.

Ardila, A. (1995). Directions of research in cross-cultural neuropsychology. *Journal of Clinical and Experimental Neuropsychology, 17,* 143–150.

Ardila, A. (1998). Bilingualism: A neglected and chaotic area. *Aphasiology, 12,* 131–134.

Ardila, A. (2005). Cultural values underlying cognitive test performance. *Neuropsychology Review, 15,* 185–195.

Ardila, A. (2007). The impact of culture on neuropsychological performance. In B. P. Uzzell, M. Pontón, & A. Ardila (Eds.), *International handbook of cross-cultural neuropsychology* (pp. 23–44). Mahwah, NJ: Lawrence Erlbaum.

Ardila, A., & Keating, K. (2007). Cognitive abilities in different cultural contexts. In B. P. Uzzell, M. Pontón, & A. Ardila (Eds.), *International handbook of cross-cultural neuropsychology* (pp. 109–125). Mahwah, NJ: Lawrence Erlbaum.

Ardila, A., Rodríguez-Menéndez, G., & Rosselli, M. (2002). Current issues in neuropsychological assessment with Hispanics/Latinos. In F. R. Ferraro (Ed.), *Minority and cross-cultural aspects of neuropsychological assessment* (pp. 161–179). Lisse, The Netherlands: Swets & Zeitlinger.

Ardila, A., & Rosselli, M. (2003). Educational effects on the ROCF performance. In J. Knight & E. Kaplan (Eds.), *Rey-Osterrieth complex figure handbook* (pp. 271–281). New York: Psychological Assessment Resources.

Ardila, A., & Rosselli, M. (2007). Illiterates and cognition: The impact of education. In B. P. Uzzell, M. Pontón, & A. Ardila (Eds.), *International handbook of cross-cultural neuropsychology* (pp. 181–198). Mahwah, NJ: Lawrence Erlbaum.

Ardila, A., Rosselli, M., Ostroski-Solís, F., Marcos, J., Granda, G., & Soto, M. (2000). Syntactic comprehension, verbal memory, and calculation abilities in Spanish-English bilinguals. *Applied Neuropsychology, 7,* 3–16.

Ardila, A., Rosselli, M., & Puente, A. E. (1994). *Neuropsychological evaluation of the Spanish speaker*. New York: Plenum Press.

Ardila, A., Rosselli, M., & Rosas, P. (1989). Neuropsychological assessment in illiterates: Visuospatial and memory abilities. *Brain and Cognition, 11*, 147–166.

Armengol, C. G. (2002). The Stroop test in Spanish: Children's norms. *Neuropsychologist, 16*, 67–80.

Arnold, B., Montgomery, G., Castaneda, I., & Longoria, R. (1994). Acculturation and performance of Hispanics on selected Halstead-Reitan neuropsychological tests. *Assessment, 1*, 239–248.

Artiola-i-Fortuny, L. (2000). *Manual de normas y procedimientos para la Batería Neuropsicológica en Español*. Lisse, The Netherlands: Swets & Zeitlinger.

Artiola-i-Fortuny, L., & Heaton, R. K. (1996). Standard versus computerized administration of the Wisconsin Card Sorting Test. *Clinical Neuropsychologist, 10*, 419–424.

Artiola-i-Fortuny, L., Hermosillo-Romo, D. H., Heaton, R. K., & Pardee, R. E. (1999). *Manual de normas y procedimientos para la Batería Neuropsicológica en Español*. Tucson, AZ: mPress.

Artiola-i-Fortuny, L., & Mullaney, H. (1998). Neuropsychological comparisons of Spanish-speaking participants from the U.S.-Mexico border region versus Spain. *Journal of the International Neuropsychological Society, 4*, 363–379.

Baird, A. D., Ford, M., & Podell, K. (2007). Ethnic differences in functional and neuropsychological test performance in older adults. *Archives of Clinical Neuropsychology, 22*, 309–318.

Bender, S. D., & Rogers, R. (2004). Detection of neurocognitive feigning: Development of a multi-strategy assessment. *Archives of Clinical Neuropsychology, 19*, 49–60.

Berry, J. W. (1997). Immigration, acculturation, and adaptation. *Applied Psychology, 46*, 5–68.

Bialystock, E. (1999). Cognitive complexity and attentional control in the bilingual mind. *Cognitive Development, 70*, 636–644.

Bianchini, K. J., Mathias, C. W., & Greve, K. W. (2001). Symptom validity testing: A critical review. *Clinical Neuropsychologist, 15*, 19–45.

Bigler, E. D. (2006). Can author bias be determined in forensic neuropsychology research published in *Archives of Clinical Neuropsychology*? *Archives of Clinical Neuropsychology, 21*, 503–508.

Binder, L. M. (1990). Malingering following minor head trauma. *Clinical Neuropsychologist, 4*, 25–36.

Bird, H. R., Canino, G., Stippec, M. R., & Shrout, P. (1987). Use of the Mini-Mental State Examination in a probabilistic sample of a Hispanic population. *Journal of Nervous and Mental Diseases, 175*, 731–737.

Boone, K., Lu, P., & Herzberg, D. S. (2002). *The b Test. Manual*. Los Angeles: Western Psychological Services.

Boone, K. B., Lu, P., Back, C., King, C., Lee, A., Philpott, L., et al. (2002). Sensitivity and specificity of the Rey dot counting test in patients with suspect effort and various clinical samples. *Archives of Clinical Neuropsychology, 17*, 625–642.

Boone, K. B., Victor, T. L., Wen, J., Razani, J., & Pontón, M. (2007). The association between neuropsychological scores and ethnicity, language, and acculturation variables in a large patient population. *Archives of Clinical Neuropsychology, 22*, 355–365.

Brickman, A. M., Cabo, R., & Manly, J. J. (2006). Ethical issues in cross-cultural neuropsychology. *Applied Neuropsychology, 13*, 91–100.

Bush, S. S., & NAN Policy & Planning Committee. (2005). Independent and court-ordered forensic neuropsychological examinations: Official statement of the National Academy of Neuropsychology. *Archives of Clinical Neuropsychology, 20*, 997–1007.

Bush, S. S., Ruff, R. M., Tröster, A. I., Barth, J. T., Koffler, S. P., Pliskin, N., et al. (2005). Symptom validity assessment: Practice issues and medical necessity. *Archives of Clinical Neuropsychology, 20*, 419–426.

Byrd, D. A., Miller, S. W., Reilly, J., Weber, S., Wall, T. L., & Heaton, R. K. (2006). Early environmental factors, ethnicity, and adult cognitive test performance. *Clinical Neuropsychologist, 20*, 243–260.

Byrd, D. A., Sanchez, D., & Manly, J. (2005). Neuropsychological test performance among Caribbean-born and U.S.-born African American elderly: The role of age, education and reading level. *Journal of Clinical and Experimental Neuropsychology, 27*, 1056–1069.

Byrd, D. A., Touradji, P., Tang, M. X., & Manly, J. J. (2004). Cancellation test performance in African Americans, Hispanic, and White elderly. *Journal of the International Neuropsychological Society, 10*, 401–411.

Campo, P., & Morales, M. (2003). Reliability and normative data for the Benton visual form discrimination test. *Clinical Neuropsychologist, 17*, 220–225.

Coffey, D. M., Marmol, L., Schock, L., & Adams, W. (2005). The influence of acculturation on the Wisconsin card sorting test by Mexican Americans. *Archives of Clinical Neuropsychology, 20*, 795–803.

Committee on Ethical Guidelines for Forensic Psychologists. (1991). Specialty guidelines for forensic psychologists. *Law and Human Behavior, 15*(6), 655–665.

Committee on the Revision of the Specialty Guidelines for Forensic Psychology. (2008). *Specialty guidelines for forensic psychology third official draft.* Retrieved February 27, 2008, from www.ap-ls.org/links/22808sgfp.pdf

Constantinou, M., & McCaffrey, R. J. (2003). Using the TOMM to evaluate children's effort to perform optimally on neuropsychological measures. *Child Neuropsychology, 9*, 81–90.

Cornelious, S. W., & Caspi, A. (1987). Everyday problem solving in adulthood and old age. *Psychology of Aging, 2*, 144–153.

Cosentino, S., Manly, J., & Mungas, D. (2007). Do reading tests measure the same construct in multiethnic and multilingual older persons? *Journal of the International Neuropsychological Society, 13*, 228–236.

Cuellar, I., Arnold, B., & Maldonado, R. (1995). Acculturation ratings scale for Mexican Americans-II: A revision of the original ARSMA scale. *Hispanic Journal of Behavioral Sciences, 17*, 275–304.

De Bleser, R., Dupont, R., Postler, J., Bormans, G., Speelman, D., Mortelmans, L., et al. (2003). The organisation of the bilingual lexicon: A PET study. *Journal of Neurolinguistics, 16*, 439–456.

Del Ser, T., Gonzalez-Montalvo, J., Martinez-Espinosa, S., Delgado-Villapalos, C., & Bermejo, F. (1997). Estimation of premorbid intelligence in Spanish people with the Word Accentuation Test and its application to the diagnosis of dementia. *Brain and Cognition, 33*, 343–356.

Delgado, P., Guerrero, G., Goggin, J. P., & Ellis, B. B. (1999). Self-assessment of linguistic skills by bilingual Hispanics. *Hispanic Journal of Behavioral Sciences, 21*, 31–46.

Demsky, Y. I., Mittenberg, W., Quintar, B., Katell, A. D., & Golden, C. J. (1998). Bias in the use of standard American norm with Spanish translations of the Wechsler Memory Scale—Revised. *Assessment, 5*, 115–121.

Denney, R. L., & Wynkoop, T. F. (2000). Clinical neuropsychology in the criminal forensic setting. *Journal of Head Trauma Rehabilitation, 15*, 804–828.

Diaz-Guerrero, R. (1993). Mexican ethnopsychology. In U. Kim & J. W. Berry (Eds.), *Indigenous psychologies: Research and experience in cultural context* (pp.44–55). Newbury Park, CA: Sage Publications.

Diccionario de la Lengua Española. (2001, 22nd ed.). Retrieved February 3, 2009, from http://buscon.rae.es/draeI/SrvltConsulta?TIPO_BUS=3&LEMA=hispano

Diehr, M. C., Heaton, R. K., Miller, W., & Grant, I. (1998). The paced auditory serial addition task (PASAT): Norms for age, education and ethnicity. *Assessment, 5*, 375–387.

Echemendia, R. J., & Harris, J. G. (2004). Neuropsychological test use with Hispanic/Latino populations in the U.S.: Part II of a national survey. *Applied Neuropsychology, 11*, 4–12.

Escobar, J. I., Burman, R., & Marno, M. (1986). Use of the Mini-Mental State Examination (MMSE) in a community population of mixed ethnicity: Cultural and linguistic artifacts. *Journal of Nervous and Mental Diseases, 174*, 607–614.

Fastenau, P. S., Evans, J. D., Johnson, K. E., & Bond, G. R. (2002). Multicultural training in clinical neuropsychology. In F. R. Ferraro (Ed.), *Minority and cross-cultural aspects of neuropsychological assessment* (pp. 345–371). Lisse, The Netherlands: Swets & Zeitlinger.

Faust, D., & Ackley, M. A. (1998). Did you think it was going to be easy? Some methodological suggestions for the investigation and development of malingering detection techniques. In C. R. Reynolds (Ed.), *Detection of malingering during head injury litigation* (pp. 1–54). New York: Plenum Press.

Gasquoine, P. G. (1999). Variables moderating cultural and ethnic differences in neuropsychological assessment: The case of Hispanic Americans. *Clinical Neuropsychologist, 13*, 376–383.

Gasquoine, P. G. (2001). Research in clinical neuropsychology with Hispanic American participants: A review. *Clinical Neuropsychologist, 15*, 2–12.

Gervais, R. O., Rohling, M. L., Green, P., & Ford, W. (2004). A comparison of WMT, CARB, and TOMM failure rates in non-head injury disability claimants. *Archives of Clinical Neuropsychology, 19*, 475–487.

Golden, C. J. (1978). *Stroop color and word test. A manual for clinical and experimental uses.* Wood Dale, IL: Stoelting.

Golden, C. J., & Thomas, R. B. (2000). Cross-cultural application of the Luria-Nebraska neuropsychological test battery and Lurian principles of syndrome analysis. In E. Fletcher-Janzen, T. L. Strickland, & C. R. Reynolds (Eds.), *Handbook of cross-cultural neuropsychology* (pp. 305–315). New York: Kluwer Academics/Plenum Publishers.

González, G., Mungas, D., & Haan, M. (2002). A verbal learning and memory test for English and Spanish-speaking older Mexican-American adults. *Clinical Neuropsychologist, 16*, 439–451.

Gómez-Maqueo, E. L., León-Guzmán, M. I., & Medina-Mora, M. E. (2003). *Uso e interpretación del MMPI-2 en español.* Mexico City, México: El Manual Moderno.

Green, P., Allen, L., & Astner, K. (1996). *The word memory test: A user's guide to the oral and computer-administered forms. U.S. version 1.1.* Durham, NC: CogniSyst.

Greiffenstein, M. F., Baker, W. J., & Gola, T. (1994). Validation of malingered amnesia measures with a large clinical sample. *Psychological Assessment, 6,* 218–224.

Grote, C. L., Kooker, E. K., Garron, D. C., Nyenhuis, D. L., Smith, C. A., & Mattingly, M. L. (2000). Performance of compensation seeking and non-compensation seeking samples on the Victoria symptom validity test: Cross-validation and extension of a standardization study. *Journal of Clinical and Experimental Neuropsychology, 22,* 709–719.

Guilmette, T. J., Hart, K. J., & Giuliano, A. J. (1993). Malingering detection: The use of a forced-choice method in identifying organic versus simulated memory impairment. *Clinical Neuropsychologist, 7,* 59–69.

Guilmette, T. J., Hart, K. J., Giuliano, A. J., & Leininger, B. E. (1994). Detecting simulated memory impairment: Comparison of the Rey fifteen-item test and the Hiscock forced-choice procedure. *Clinical Neuropsychologist, 8,* 283–294.

Gurland, B. L., Wilder, D. E., Cross, P., Teresi, J., & Barret, V. W. (1992). Screening scales for dementia: Toward a reconciliation of conflicting cross-cultural findings. *International Journal of Geriatric Psychiatry, 7,* 105–113.

Haber, A. H., & Fichtenberg, N. L. (2006). Replication of the test of memory malingering (TOMM) in a traumatic brain injury and head trauma sample. *Clinical Neuropsychologist, 20,* 524–532.

Heilbronner, R. L. (2004). A status report on the practice of forensic neuropsychology. *Clinical Neuropsychologist, 18,* 312–326.

Helms, J. E., Jernigan, M., & Mascher, J. (2005). The meaning of race in psychology and how to change it. *American Psychologist, 60,* 27–36.

Hiscock, C. K., Branham, J. D., & Hiscock, M. (1994). Detection of feigned cognitive impairment: The two-alternative forced-choice method compared with selected conventional tests. *Journal of Psychopathology & Behavioral Assessment, 16,* 95–110.

Hiscock, M., & Hiscock, C. K. (1989). Refining the forced-choice method of detection of malingering. *Journal of Clinical and Experimental Neuropsychology, 11,* 967–974.

Holmquist, L. A., & Wanlass, R. L. (2002). A multidimensional approach towards malingering detection. *Archives of Clinical Neuropsychology, 17,* 143–156.

Jacobs, D., Sano, M., Albert, S., Schofield, P., Dooneief, G., & Stern, Y. (1997). Cross-cultural neuropsychological assessment: A comparison of randomly selected, demographically matched cohorts of English and Spanish-speaking older adults. *Journal of Clinical and Experimental Neuropsychology, 19,* 331–339.

Judd, T., Capetillo, D., Carrion-Baralt, J., Marmol, L. M., San Miguel-Montes, L., Navarrete, M. G., et al. (2009). Professional considerations for improving the neuropsychological evaluation of Hispanics: NAN education paper. *Archives of Clinical Neuropsychology, 24*(3), 127–136.

Kiernan, R. J., Mueller, J., & Langston, W. (1998). *Cognistat (neurobehavioral cognitive status examination. López, E., versión Español).* Fairfax, CA: Northern California Neurobehavioral Group.

Kohnert, K., Hernández, A., & Bates, E. (1998). Bilingual performance on the Boston naming test: Preliminary norms in Spanish and English. *Brain and Language, 65,* 422–440.

Larrabee, G. J. (2000). Forensic neuropsychological assessment. In R. D. Vanderploeg (Ed.), *Clinician's guide to neuropsychological assessment* (pp. 301–335). Mahwah, NJ: Lawrence Erlbaum.

Lezak, M. D., Howieson, D. B., & Loring, D. W. (2004). *Neuropsychological assessment* (4th ed.). New York: Oxford University Press.

Llorente, A. M. (2008). Hispanic populations: Special issues in neuropsychology. In A. M. Llorente (Ed.), *Principles of neuropsychological assessment with Hispanics: Theoretical foundations and clinical practice* (pp. 47–56). New York: Springer Science.

Llorente, A. M., & Weber, D. (2008). The neuropsychological assessment of the Hispanic client. In A. M. Llorente (Ed.), *Principles of neuropsychological assessment with Hispanics: Theoretical foundations and clinical practice* (pp. 121–135). New York: Springer Science.

Loewenstein, D. A., Ardila, A., Rosselli, M., Hayden, S., Duara, R., Berkowitz, N., et al. (1992). A comparative analysis of functional status among Spanish- and English-speaking patients with dementia. *Journal of Gerontology, 47,* 389–394.

Loewenstein, D. A., Rubert, M. P., Arguelles, T., & Duara, R. (1995). Neuropsychological test performance and prediction of functional capacities among Spanish-speaking and English-speaking patients with dementia. *Archives of Clinical Neuropsychology, 16,* 75–88.

Lucas, J. A., Ivnik, R. J., Willis, F. B., Ferman, T. J., Smith, G. E., Parfitt, F. C., et al. (2005). Mayo's older African Americans normative studies: Normative data for commonly used clinical neuropsychological measures. *Clinical Neuropsychologist, 19,* 162–183.

Macciocchi, S. N., Seel, R. T., Alderson, A., & Godsall, R. (2006). Victoria Symptom Validity Test performance in acute severe traumatic brain injury: Implications for test interpretation. *Archives of Clinical Neuropsychology, 21,* 395–404.

Manly, J. J. (2005). Advantages and disadvantages of separate norms for African Americans. *Clinical Neuropsychologist, 19,* 270–275.

Manly, J. J., Byrd, D. A., Touradji, P., & Stern, Y. (2004). Acculturation, reading level, and neuropsychological test performance among African American elders. *Applied Neuropsychology, 11,* 37–46.

Manly, J. J., & Echemendia, R. J. (2007). Race-specific norms: Using the model of hypertension to understand issues of race, culture, and education in neuropsychology. *Archives of Clinical Neuropsychology, 22,* 319–325.

Manly, J. J., Jacobs, D. M., Sano, M., Bell, K., Merchant, C. A., Samall, S. A., et al. (1998). Cognitive test performance among nondemented elderly African Americans and Whites. *Neurology, 50,* 1238–1245.

Manly, J. J., Jacobs, D. M., Touradji, P., Small, S. A., & Stern, Y. (2002). Reading level attenuates differences in neuropsychological test performance between African American and White elders. *Journal of the International Neuropsychological Society, 8,* 341–348.

Marin, G., & Marin, B. V. (1991). *Research with Hispanic populations.* Newbury Park, CA: Sage.

Martin, R. C., Bolter, J. F., Todd, M. E., Gouvier, W. D., & Niccolls, R. (1993). Effects of sophistication and motivation on the detection of malingered memory performance using a computerized forced-choice task. *Journal of Clinical and Experimental Neuropsychology, 15,* 867–880.

Martin, R. C., Hayes, J. S, & Gouvier, W. D. (1996). Differential vulnerability between postconcussion self-report and objective malingering tests in identifying simulated mild head injury. *Journal of Clinical and Experimental Neuropsychology, 18,* 265–275.

Mejia, S., Pineda, D., Alvarez, L., & Ardila, A. (1998). Individual differences in memory and executive function abilities during normalaging. *International Journal of Neuroscience, 95,* 271–284.

Melendez, F. (2001). Forensic assessment of Hispanics. In M. O. Pontón & J. León-Carrión (Eds.), *Neuropsychology and the Hispanic patient* (pp. 321–340). Mahwah, NJ: Lawrence Erlbaum.

Merriam-Webster Collegiate Dictionary. (2009). Retrieved February 3, 2009, from http://www.merriam-webster.com/dictionary/Hispanic

Mungas, D., Marshall, S. C., Weldon, M., Haan, M., & Reed, B. R. (1996). Age and education correction of Mini-Mental State Examination for English and Spanish-speaking elderly. *Neurology, 46,* 700–706.

Muñoz-Sandoval, A. F., Cummins, J., Alvarado, C. G., & Ruef, M. L. (1998). *The bilingual verbal ability tests (BVAT).* Itasca, IL: Riverside Publishing, Houghton-Mifflin.

Nabors, N. A., Evans, J. D., & Strickland, T. L. (2000). Neuropsychological assessment and intervention with African Americans. In E. Fletcher-Janzen, T. L. Strickland, & C. R. Reynolds (Eds.), *Handbook of cross-cultural neuropsychology* (pp. 31–42). New York: Kluwer Academics/Plenum Publishers.

Naglieri, J. A., & Bardos, A. N. (1997). *General ability measure for adults.* Minneapolis, MN: National Computer Systems, Inc.

Norman, M., Evans, J., Miller, W., & Heaton, R. (2000). Demographically corrected norms for the California verbal learning test. *Journal of Clinical and Experimental Neuropsychology, 22,* 80–94.

O'Bryant, S. E., Duff, K., Fisher, J., & McCaffrey, R. J. (2004). Performance profiles and cut-off scores on the Memory Assessment Scales. *Archives of Clinical Neuropsychology, 19,* 489–496.

Olazaran, J., Jacobs, D., & Stern, Y. (1996). Comparative study of visual and verbal short term memory in English and Spanish speakers: Testing a linguistic hypothesis. *Journal of the International Neuropsychological Society, 2,* 105–110.

Ostrosky, R., Ardila, A., & Rosselli, M. (1997). *Neuropsi: Un eXámen neuropsicológico breve en español.* Mexico City, México: Bayer.

Ostrosky-Solís, F., Jaime, R. M., & Ardila, A. (1998). Memory abilities during normal aging. *International Journal of Neuroscience, 93,* 151–162.

Ostrosky-Solís, F., López-Arango, G., & Ardila, A. (2000). Sensitivity and specificity of the Mini-Mental State Examination in a Spanish-speaking population. *Applied Neuropsychology, 7,* 47–60.

Patton, D., Duff, K., Schoenberg, M., Mold, J., Scott, J., & Adams, R. (2003). Performance of cognitively normal African Americans on the RBANS in community dwelling older adults. *Clinical Neuropsychologist, 20,* 873–887.

Pedraza, O., & Mungas, D. (2008). Measurement in cross-cultural neuropsychology. *Neuropsychology Review, 18,* 184–193.

Pérez-Arce, P. (1999). The influence of culture on cognition. *Archives of Clinical Neuropsychology, 14,* 581–592.

Pontón, M. O. (2001). Research and assessment issues with Hispanic populations. In M. O. Pontón & J. León-Carrión (Eds.), *Neuropsychology and the Hispanic patient* (pp. 39–58). Mahwah, NJ: Lawrence Erlbaum.

Pontón, M. O., & Ardila, A. (1999). The future of neuropsychology with Hispanic populations in the U.S. *Archives of Clinical Neuropsychology, 14,* 565–580.

Pontón, M. O., & Corona-LoMonaco, M. E. (2007). Cross-cultural issues in neuropsychology: Assessment of the Hispanic patient. In B. P. Uzzell, M. Pontón, & A. Ardila (Eds.), *International handbook of cross-cultural neuropsychology* (pp. 265–282). Mahwah, NJ: Lawrence Erlbaum.

Pontón, M. O., González, J. J., Hernández, I., & Igareda, J. (2000). Factor analysis of the Neuropsychological Screening Battery for Hispanics (NeSBHIS). *Applied Neuropsychology, 7,* 32–39.

Pontón, M. O., & León-Carrión, J. (2001). The Hispanic population in the United States: An overview of sociocultural and demographic issues. In M. O. Pontón & J. León-Carrión (Eds.), *Neuropsychology and the Hispanic patient* (pp. 1–13). Mahwah, NJ: Lawrence Erlbaum.

Pontón, M. O., Satz, P., Herrera, L., Ortiz, F., Urrutia, C. P., Young, R., et al. (1996). Normative data stratified by age and education for the neuropsychological screening battery for Hispanics (NeSBHis): Initial report. *Journal of the International Neuropsychological Society, 2,* 96–104.

Poreh, A. (2002). Neuropsychological and psychological issues associated with cross-cultural and minority assessment. In F. R. Ferraro (Ed.), *Minority and cross-cultural aspects of neuropsychological assessment* (pp. 329–343). Lisse, The Netherlands: Swets & Zeitlinger.

Prigatano, G. P., Smason, I., Lamb, D. G., & Bortz, J. J. (1997). Suspected malingering and the Digit Memory Test: A replication and extension. *Archives of Clinical Neuropsychology, 12,* 609–619.

Puente, A. E., & Ardila, A. (2000). Neuropsychological assessment of Hispanics. In E. Fletcher-Janzen, T. L. Strickland, & C. R. Reynolds (Eds.), *Handbook of cross-cultural neuropsychology* (pp. 87–104). New York: Kluwer Academics/Plenum Publishers.

Razani, J., Burciaga, J., Madore, M., & Wong, J. (2007). Effects of acculturation on tests of attention and information processing in an ethnically diverse group. *Archives of Clinical Neuropsychology, 22,* 333–341.

Razani, J., Murcia, G., Tabares, J., & Wong, J. (2007). The effects of culture on WASI test performance in ethnically diverse individuals. *Clinical Neuropsychologist, 5,* 1–13.

Rees, L. M., Tombaugh, T. N., & Boulay, L. (2001). Depression and the test of memory malingering. *Archives of Clinical Neuropsychology, 16,* 501–506.

Reitan, R. M., & Wolfson, D. (1995). Consistency of responses on retesting among head-injured subjects in litigation versus head-injured subjects not in litigation. *Applied Neuropsychology, 2,* 67–71.

Reitan, R. M., & Wolfson, D. (1997). Consistency of neuropsychological test scores of head-injured subjects involved in litigation compared with head-injured subjects not involved in litigation: Development of the retest consistency index. *Clinical Neuropsychologist, 11,* 69–76.

Rey, G., & Benton, A. (1991). *Examen de afasia multilingue (multilingual aphasia examination-Spanish).* Iowa City, IA: AFA Associates.

Rey, G. J., Feldman, E., Rivas-Vazquez, R., Levin, B. E., & Benton, A. (1999). Neuropsychological test development and normative data on Hispanics. *Archives of Clinical Neuropsychology, 14,* 593–601.

Reynolds, C. R. (1998). Common sense, clinicians, and actuarialism in the detection of malingering during head injury litigation. In C. R. Reynolds (Ed.), *Detection of malingering during head injury litigation* (pp. 261–286). New York: Plenum Press.

Rogers, R. (1990). Models of feigned mental illness. *Professional Psychology: Research and Practice, 21,* 182–188.

Rogers, R. (1997). *Clinical assessment of malingering and deception* (2nd ed.). New York: Guilford Press.

Rose, F. E., Hall, S., & Szalda-Petree, A. D. (1995). Portland digit recognition test-computerized: The measurement of response latency improves the detection of malingering. *Clinical Neuropsychologist, 9,* 124–134.

Ross, T. P., Lichtenberg, P. A., & Christensen, B. K. (1995). Normative data on the Boston naming test for elderly adults in a demographically diverse medical sample. *Clinical Neuropsychologist, 9,* 321–325.

Rosselli, M., & Ardila, A. (1996). Cognitive effects of cocaine and polydrug abuse. *Journal of Clinical and Experimental Neuropsychology, 18,* 122–135.

Rosselli, M., Ardila, A., Salvatierra, J., Marquez, M., Matos, L., & Weekes, V. (2002). A cross-linguistic comparison of verbal fluency test. *International Journal of Neuroscience, 112,* 112–156.

Salazar, G. D., Pérez-García, M., & Puente, A. E. (2007). Clinical neuropsychology of Spanish speakers: The challenges and pitfalls of a neuropsychology of a heterogeneous population. In B. P. Uzzell, M. Pontón, & A. Ardila (Eds.), *International handbook of cross-cultural neuropsychology* (pp. 283–302). Mahwah, NJ: Lawrence Erlbaum.

Sanz, J., & Vázquez, C. (1991). Fiabilidad, validez y datos normativos del Inventario para la Depresión de Beck. *Psicothema, 10*, 303–318.

Schwartz, B. S., Glass, T. A., Bolla, K. I., Stewart, W. F., Glass, G., Rasmussen, M., et al. (2004). Disparities in cognitive functioning by race/ethnicity in the Baltimore memory study. *Environmental Health Perspectives, 112*, 314–320.

Slick, D., Hopp, G., Strauss, E., & Thompson, G. (1997). *The Victoria Symptom Validity Test.* Lutz, FL: PAR.

Slick, D. J., Hopp, G., Strauss, E., Hunter, M., & Pinch, D. (1994). Detecting dissimulation: Profiles of simulated malingerers, traumatic brain-injury patients, and normal controls on a revised version of Hiscock and Hiscock's Forced-Choice Memory Test. *Journal of Clinical and Experimental Neuropsychology, 16*, 472–481.

Slick, D. J., Sherman, E. M. S., & Iverson, G. L. (1999). Diagnostic criteria for malingered neurocognitive dysfunction: Proposed standards for clinical practice and research. *Clinical Neuropsychologist, 13*, 545–561.

Strauss, E., Hultsch, D. F., Hunter, M., Slick, D. J., Patry, B., & Levy-Bencheton, J. (2000). Using intraindividual variability to detect malingering in cognitive performance. *Clinical Neuropsychologist, 14*, 420–432.

Strauss, E., Slick, D. J., Levy-Bencheton, J., Hunter, M., MacDonald, S. W. S., & Hultsch, D. F. (2002). Intraindividual variability as an indicator of malingering in head injury. *Archives of Clinical Neuropsychology, 17*, 423–444.

Sweet, J. J., King, F. H., Malina, A. C., Bergman, M. A., & Simmons, A. (2002). Documenting the prominence of forensic neuropsychology at national meetings and in relevant professional journals from 1990 to 2000. *Clinical Neuropsychologist, 16*, 481–494.

Sweet, J. J., Peck, E. A., Abramowitz, C., & Etzweiler, S. (2002). National Academy of Neuropsychology/ Division 40 of the American Psychological Association practice survey of clinical neuropsychology in the United States, Part I: Practitioner and practice characteristics, professional activities, and time requirements. *Clinical Neuropsychologist, 16*, 109–127.

Taussig, I. M., Henderson, V., & Mack, W. (1992). Spanish translation and validation of a neuropsychological battery: Performance of Spanish and English speaking Alzheimer's disease patients and normal comparison subjects. *Clinical Gerontologist, 11*, 95–108.

Taussig, I. M., & Pontón, M. O. (1996). Issues in neuropsychological assessment for Hispanic older adults: Cultural and linguistic factors. In G. Yeo & T. D. Gallagher (Eds.), *Ethnicity and the dementias* (pp. 165–179). Washington, DC: Taylor & Francis.

Teichner, G., & Wagner, M. T. (2004). The test of memory malingering (TOMM): Normative data from cognitively intact, cognitively impaired, and elderly patients with dementia. *Archives of Clinical Neuropsychology, 19*, 455–464.

Tombaugh, T. N. (1996). *Test of memory malingering, TOMM.* New York/Toronto: MHS.

Touradji, P., Manly, J. J., Jacobs, D., & Stern, Y. (2001). Neuropsychological test performance: A study of non-Hispanic White elderly. *Journal of Clinical and Experimental Neuropsychology, 23*, 643–649.

U.S. Bureau of the Census. (1997). *Census facts for Hispanic heritage month* (Press release CB97-fs. 10, issued 9/11/97).

U.S. Bureau of the Census. (1999). *United States census 2000: Race, Hispanic origin, and ancestry: Why, what and how.* Washington, DC: U.S. Department of Commerce.

U.S. Bureau of the Census. (2006). *2005 American community survey data profile highlights.* Retrieved February 3, 2009, from http://factfinder.census.gov/servlet/ACSSAFFFacts?_event=&geo_id= 01000US&_geoContext=01000US&_street=&_county=&_cityTown=&_state=&_zip=&_lang=en& _sse=on&ActiveGeoDiv=&_useEV=&pctxt=fph&pgsl=010&_submenuId=factsheet_1& ds_name=null&_ci_nbr=null&qr_name=null® = null%3Anull&_keyword=&_industry=

Uzzell, B. P. (2007). Grasping the cross-cultural reality. In B. P. Uzzell, M. Pontón, & A. Ardila (Eds.), *International handbook of cross-cultural neuropsychology* (pp. 1–21). Mahwah, NJ: Lawrence Erlbaum.

Van Gorp, W. G., Myers, G. F., & Drake, E. B. (2000). Neuropsychology training: Ethnocultural considerations in the context of general competency training. In E. Fletcher-Janzen, T. L. Strickland, & C. R. Reynolds (Eds.), *Handbook of cross-cultural neuropsychology* (pp. 19–27). New York: Kluwer Academic/Plenum Publishers.

Vilar-López, R., Gómez-Río, M., Caracuel-Romero, A., Llamas-Elvira, J. M., & Pérez-García, M. (2008). Use of specific malingering measures in a Spanish sample. *Journal of Clinical and Experimental Neuropsychology, 30*, 710–722.

Vilar-López, R., Gómez-Río, M., Santiago-Ramajo, S., Rodriguez-Fernandez, A., Puente, A. E., & Pérez-García, M. (2008). Malingering detection in a Spanish population with a known-groups design. *Archives of Clinical Neuropsychology, 23*, 365–377.

Vilar-López, R., Santiago-Ramajo, S., Gómez-Río, M., Verdejo-García, A., Llamas-Elvira, J. M., & Pérez-García, M. (2007). Detection of malingering in a Spanish population using three specific malingering tests. *Archives of Clinical Neuropsychology, 22*, 379–388.

Ward, C., & Kennedy, A. (1994). Acculturation strategies, psychological adjustment, and sociocultural competence during cross-cultural transitions. *International Journal of Intercultural Relations, 18*, 329–343.

Wechsler, D. (1997). *Wechsler adult intelligence scale* (3rd ed.). San Antonio, TX: Harcourt Assessment.

Whitfield, K. E., Fillenbaum, G. G., Pieper, C., Albert, M. S., Berkman, L. F., Blazer, D. G., et al. (2000). The effect of race and health-related factors on naming and memory. *Journal of Aging and Health, 12*, 69–89.

Willison, J., & Tombaugh, T. N. (2006). Detecting simulation of attention deficits using reaction times tests. *Archives of Clinical Neuropsychology, 21*, 41–52.

Wong, T. M., Strickland, T. L., Fletcher-Janzen, E., Ardila, A., & Reynolds, C. R. (2000). Theoretical and practical issues in the neuropsychological assessment and treatment of culturally dissimilar patients. In E. Fletcher-Janzen, T. L. Strickland, & C. R. Reynolds (Eds.), *Handbook of cross-cultural neuropsychology* (pp. 3–18). New York: Kluwer Academics/Plenum Publishers.

Woodcock, R. W., & Muñoz-Sandoval, A. F. (1993). *Woodcock language proficiency battery-Revised, Spanish form* (Suppl. manual). Chicago: Riverside.

Woodcock, R. W., & Muñoz-Sandoval, A. F. (1996a). *Batería Woodcock-Muñoz: Pruebas de aprovechamiento-revisada (Woodcock-Johnson III test of achievement)*. Chicago: Riverside.

Woodcock, R. W., & Muñoz-Sandoval, A. F. (1996b). *Batería Woodcock-Muñoz: Pruebas de habilidad cognitiva-revisada (Woodcock-Johnson test of cognitive ability-revised)*. Chicago: Riverside.

Woodcock, R. W., & Muñoz-Sandoval, A. F. (2005). *Batería III*. Itasca, IL: Riverside.

Zamanian, K., Thackrey, M., Starrett, R. A., Brown, L. G., Lassman, D., & Blanchart, A. (1992). Acculturation and depression in Mexican American elderly. *Clinical Gerontologist, 11*, 3–4.

When Change Matters: Objective Methods for Measuring Change in Neuropsychology Test Scores

16

Ronald D. Franklin

Introduction

The use of neuropsychological evaluation in legal settings has a well established, if controversial, history (Faust, Ziskin, & Hiers, 1991). Forensic assessments commonly include comparisons of current with past performance, current with predicted performance, or concurrent performance with other measures. Assessment results are then interpreted as evidence of malingering, brain injury, or competency (Larrabee, 2005). In each situation, the neuropsychologist must determine whether changes in scores have real meaning, or whether they are due to systematic or random variation. He must then describe how the change relates to the case at hand. The ethical neuropsychologist understands that similar score differences may have meaning or relevance in some situations and not others. In order for changes in test scores to matter, they must diagnose disorder, predict outcome, and offer ecological validity while reflecting a meaningful and modified performance that: (a) affects the patient's quality of life, (b) accurately measures change in ability, or (c) has important financial consequences. Two or all of these situations can coexist.

Changes in Quality of Life

Few will argue that failing abilities or the financial hardships associated with medical treatment can change one's quality of life; however, more subtle changes in the various aspects of one's life experience can also occur even if obvious ability changes and dire financial catastrophe are not imminent. For many "normal" adults, the putative diagnosis of dementia initiates a cascade of reactions that can include making a will, planning for nursing home care, postponing vacations, or abandoning planned financial gifts to children. Likewise, the diagnosis of "brain damage" can precipitate levels of fear, anxiety, and depression that become more debilitating than physical injury. If the neuropsychologist opines "significant" ability loss based on score differences that fluctuate within the range of probable error but suggest mild statistical significance, the patient may experience iatrogenic quality-of-life changes.

Changes in Ability

Clinicians versed in the interpretation of Gaussian distributions often forget that the bell curve is three dimensional rather than two dimensional. In neuropsychology, the "third" dimension of time is parsed by grouping control and clinical samples into age cohorts. It is easy for us to forget that scores along the tails of distributions become rectangular as we construct cohort groups near the extremes. Classical statistical inference assumes that normative (control) samples exclude individuals having disabilities comparable to those of our patient, and that clinical samples include individuals having disabilities comparable to those of our patient. We infer that our patient is unlike individuals in the normal group, and similar to individuals in the clinical group. Readers who have benefited from conducting behavioral research on rats and other animals will appreciate that a group of genetically homogenous animals experiencing the exact same injury often present very different patterns of behavior from one another pre- and post-lesion. Human behavior, however, is much more complex than the behavior of laboratory animals. Because all that we can objectively evaluate is behavior, apparent change in ability can occur when controls having our patients' problems are present in the normative sample and not represented in the clinical sample. There are arguably no tests in psychology or neuropsychology capable of consistently and reliably diagnosing discrete disability. Measuring multiple abilities simultaneously is the rule, rather than the exception. Accurate inference of disorder, disability, or recovery is dependent upon the expertise of the evaluator rather than the predictive accuracy of our tests.

Financial Consequences

Persons of working- and middle-class backgrounds who have "good" insurance can face financial ruin following head injury, yet many (if not most) of the people I have been involved with who file civil suits have a history of financial distress that predates his/her legal claim. Concerns of "secondary gain" and "malingering" are so common that attorneys routinely challenge the efficacy of evaluations that do not include one or more measures of dissimulation.

To understand when change has relevant meaning, the neuropsychologist must test multiple hypotheses. Traditional methods for hypothesis testing rely on classical statistical theory and null hypothesis inference. The classical model never "proves" or "confirms," it only "rejects." That is to say, classical theory tells us what we do not have rather than what we have. There is an alternative hypothesis testing model known as Bayesian statistical theory that can, under proper circumstances, tell us what we have. This chapter will consider relevant research emerging from the rich neuropsychology literature that addresses changes in observed scores over time as they relate to helping us understand the situation at hand.

In a more-than-three-decade professional career that has involved the reviewing of thousands of reports, I have no recollection of seeing a psychological or neuropsychological evaluator report calculations of change scores in clinical practice. I have frequently observed reference to score changes as well as causative opinions regarding those changes. This practice leads me to believe that evaluators are more likely to rely on informal visual inspection heuristics than to take time out of a busy schedule for painstaking statistical calculations. For this reason, I have included in this chapter a section on the visual inspection of psychological data in the belief that application of a systematic approach to heuristic analysis is preferable to an idiosyncratic one.

The emerging literature addressing Bayesian predictive models offers great promise to neuropsychology. Although both classical and Bayesian methods are technologies of past centuries, new discoveries using Monte Carlo methods, with or without the use of Markov chains, allow Bayesian methods to leapfrog their classicist cousins (Crawford & Garthwaite, 2007). Consequently, Bayesian methods in general, and forensic applications in particular, may be the best hope for progress in diagnostic inference ever introduced to neuropsychology.

In this chapter, I will briefly explore all three approaches, starting with the longest established and recognized methods, proceeding to those methods most widely practiced, and ending with the most recent techniques. For convenience, I reference these approaches as *Linear*, *Visual*, and *Bayesian*, respectively.

Linear Approaches to the Identification of Meaningful Change

Linear approaches include those statistical tools psychologists associate with Null Hypothesis Statistical Tests (NHST). NHST in psychology is particularly prone to confirmation bias (see Faust, Ziskin, & Hiers, 1991; Nickerson, 1998). For this reason, the evaluation of change must include clearly defined and well-organized hypothesis testing (Franklin, 2003). Table 16.1 offers questions that are appropriate for hypothesis testing using linear statistical modeling.

Richard Bost, Frances Wen, and Michael Basso (2005) organize methods for evaluating individual change appropriate to linear statistical models into four strategies based upon data type, frequency distribution, base rate changes, and confidence intervals (CIs). Methods include the Reliable Change Index (RCI), an RCI that has been adjusted to consider known biasing effects of practice and

16.1 Evaluative Hypothesis for Neuropsychological Assessment

Do findings represent a change from prior function?

Do findings represent a change since initial diagnosis?

Do findings indicate additional improvement is likely?

If additional improvement is likely, do findings suggest which interventions may benefit the patient?

Are scores above or below expectations given the known error?

To what extent might error affect scores?

16.2 Clinical Concerns Appropriate for Linear Models

Model	Clinical Concern
RCI	Is the patient's score above or below that expected from normal variation described in the standardization sample?
RCI-*m*	Is the patient's score above or below that expected from normal variation and known bias described in the standardization sample and subsequent research?
BR	Do the observed differences in the patient's second evaluation exceed the score predicted from the first evaluation?
MR	Do the observed differences in the patient's second evaluation exceed the score predicted from the first evaluation after considering related factors such as education and gender?

regression toward the mean (RCI-*m*), Bivariate regression (BR), and multivariate regression (MR). Clinical concerns appropriate to each of these models appear in Table 16.2.

Reliable Change Index

First reported in 1986 by Christensen and Mendoza, then modified in 1991 by Jacobson and Traux, the Reliable Change Index (RCI) answers the clinical question: *Is the patient's score above or below that which is expected from the normal variation described in the standardization sample?* Later adapted by Chelune, Naugel, Lüders, Sedlak, and Awad (1993), a modified method also considers how the patient's score varies from normal when the evaluator considers known bias. Consequently, the revised clinical question becomes: *Is the patient's score above or below that which is expected from normal variation and known bias described in the standardization sample and subsequent research?* Statistics that have been employed in the attempt to draw inferences concerning change in an individual include practice effect, standard error of estimate (SE_E), standard error of differences (S_{diff}), *test–retest reliability* (r_{12}), the statistical property of regression to the mean, standard-error-of-the-measurement (SE_M), standard error of prediction (SE_P), and standard error of the estimate of regression (SE_{reg}). Chelune's discussion, therefore, addresses both the RCI and RCI-m as discussed by Bost et al.

Chelune (2003) describes five formulations for calculating change reliably: the observed distribution of differences, reliable change, practice-adjusted reliable change, modified practice-adjusted reliable change (RCI-m), and reliable change using the standard error of prediction. Complete discussion of these methods is beyond the scope of this chapter, and readers who are interested in a thorough historical review should read his original paper. Here, I limit discussion to the RCI-m incorporating the standard error of prediction because it includes earlier measures and provides the best single example of this model.

The RCI-m calculates S_{diff} from the standard errors of test–retest using the following formula as recommended by Iverson (Chelune, p. 134):

$$>S_{diff} = [(SE_{M1})^2 + (SE_{M2})^2]^{1/2}](1)$$

in which SE_{M1} and SE_{M2} come from their respective test and retest SE_M.

The *standard error of prediction*, adapted from Garrett (1958), relies on the standardized beta coefficient of the regression (r_{12}) and the standard deviation of the observed retest scores (SD_Y).

$$SE_P = SD_Y * (1-r_{12})^{1/2} (2)$$

Table 16.3 presents Iverson's formula as it is expressed within an Excel® spreadsheet (available from the author) using the formula [= SQRT((SE_{M1} * SE_{M1}) + (SE_{M2} * SE_{M2}))], in which $SE_{M\ Test\ 1}$ calls SE_{M1} and $SE_{M\ Test\ 2}$ calls SE_{M2}. The second function (SE_P) becomes [$SD_{Test\ 2}$ * SQRT(1-(corrected r_{12} * corrected r_{12}))], in which SD is the observed retest standard deviation, and corrected r_{12} is the standardized beta coefficient taken from the publisher's technical manual. Table 16.3 compares current scores (white text on dark shading) with meaningful values calculated using both S_{diff} and SE_P. Data provided in the *WAIS-III/WMS-III Technical Manual* (The Psychological Corporation, 1997, p. 55) appear in black type on shaded cells. Results show that scores from Logical Memory I and Logical Memory II are neither meaningfully high nor low on the second testing when compared with the first testing. Keep in mind that Excel rounds to one decimal in this spreadsheet, so corrected r_{12} values appearing in the table are not the same as those appearing in the technical manual; however, only the display is affected, and calculations are derived from technical manual entries.

Standardized Regression-Based Change Scores

Because practice effects are difficult to model using RCI, Sawrie (2002) recommends the use of a regression-based approach. Research suggests that practice effects vary, and the magnitude of that variance is influenced by the time between tests (Rapport, Brines, Axelrod, & Theisen, 1997). McSweeny, Naugle, Chelune, and Lüders (1993) show that norms can be created from regression equations that control not only regression effects, measurement error, and practice effects, but also demographic and practice magnitude differences. Regression scores use base-

16.3 Meaningful Change in WMS III Index Scores

	Logical Memory I		Logical Memory II	
	Test 1	Test 2	Test 1	Test 2
Current Results	13.0	10.0	10.0	10.0
Mean	9.6	11.3	9.9	12.1
SD	2.8	3.1	2.9	3.0
SEM	1.3	1.4	1.4	1.5
Test–retest				
Practice Effects		1.7		2.2
Corrected r12		0.8		0.8
Sdiff		1.9		2.0
95% CI		3.7		4.0
Upper CI		16.7		14.0
Lower CI		9.3		6.0
Test 2 meaningfully high?	FALSE		FALSE	
Test 2 meaningfully low?	FALSE		FALSE	
SEP		1.9		1.9
95% CI		3.6		3.8
Upper CI		16.6		16.8
Lower CI		9.4		6.2
Test 2 meaningfully high?		FALSE		FALSE
Test 2 meaningfully low?		FALSE		FALSE

line and control subjects to obtain predicted retest scores. The regression approach uses scores from sample administrations taken on two occasions. From these data, an equation is created that predicts scores at retest from scores at initial testing. This equation can then be used with an individual case to provide a predicted retest score from his/her initial test score. This predicted score is then compared with the score he or she actually obtained. Although the sample used to generate the equation is often a healthy control sample, it need not be. Indeed, "special populations" of the type included in technical manuals for tests work as well. Two models are available—bivariate standardized regression-based change scores (SRB_b) and multivariate (SRB_m). Calculations for these models can be complex and technical, so interested readers should peruse Crawford and Garthwaite (2006, 2007) for that purpose. Multiple models for comparing obtained with predicted scores have been proposed, but I prefer the method proposed by Crawford and Garthwaite (2006) because it provides the best-documented control of Type-1 error to date, and remains relatively stable with small sample sizes. Software for employing these techniques along with the original articles describing their use can be downloaded at the time of writing from http://www.abdn.ac.uk/~psy086/dept/regbuild.htm.

Research has demonstrated the effects of test–retest practice on numerous neuropsychological instruments (Basso, Lowery, Ghormley, & Bornstein, 2001; Basso, Bornstein, & Lang, 1999; Barr, 2003). Empirical research conducted by

16.4 Comparison of RCI and SRB

	RCI	SRB
Practice Effects	Limited to poor control	High control possible
Sample Size	Requires large N	Workable with small N
Null Hypothesis	Observed vs. measured scores	Observed vs. predicted scores
Demographic Effects	Static	Variable

Theisen, Rapport, Axelrod, and Brines (1998) shows that normal adults do not continually improve performance, but reach maximum effect following one retesting. Similar results were found in older subjects by Ivnik, et al. (1999). The effect of time between trials on subsequent performance remains unanswered. I once evaluated a prisoner using the same WAIS edition with a lapse of 14 years between the first and second administrations. He scored in the borderline range on the first administration and in the very high average range on the second administration. Suspecting that imprisonment had not made him any smarter, I met with him a few days later, informing him that his score on the second test was much better. He confessed that after the first testing, some day he would take the test again and decided that it might have bearing on his parole. Consequently, he reconstructed as much as he could remember of the test and spent the next decade practicing similar motor skills and looking up answers to recalled verbal items.

RCI and SRB models are not equivalent. Table 16.4 contrasts the models in terms of their treatments of practice effects, sample size, null hypothesis, and demographic effects.

Bivariate Model

The bivariate model (SRB_b) addresses the clinical question of whether the observed differences in the patient's second evaluation exceed the score predicted from the first evaluation. SRB_b predicts performance primarily from earlier (baseline) test scores by building regression equations using known relationships. Data can be obtained from normal (Crawford, 2004; Heaton & Marcotte, 2000) or clinical populations (Chelune et al., 1993). Other data could be used as well, including demographic variables, such as age, gender, education and socioeconomic status. More typically, neuropsychologists use multiple demographic variables with multivariate (SRB_m) models.

Multivariate Model

An SRB_m is sometimes referred to as a vector model or vector case (Crawford & Garthwaite, 2006). Here, the clinician is concerned with the patient's score exceeding acceptable variation from predicted scores, as it might be influenced by multiple factors, such as age, education, and gender. An important point worth remembering is that demographic effects can impact scores and changes in scores in different ways. Consider age as an example. Performance declines with age on many neuropsychological tests. Age can also impact the extent to which performance improves as a consequence of practice effects. Some tasks may be less affected by prior exposure than others, and other tasks may improve more. Both of these circumstances can be incorporated by including age in the regression equation.

Advantages of SRB

One central question for many neuropsychological evaluations is how far does positive change exceed practice effects? Also, are improvements in cognitive function due to intervention effects? Well-designed SRB models address these problems by factoring in known practice and intervention effects.

Criticisms of SRB

As in most statistical analyses, we must remain mindful of Babbage's (1864) admonition, "if you put into the machine wrong figures, will the right answers come out?"(p. 1). Many tests used in neuropsychology have poor or unknown external validity. As a general rule, if the specificity of a test is unknown, consider it "wrong figures." Also, the effects of some covariates (e.g., age) are curvilinear rather than linear, so if their distributions are unknown or uncorrected, the regression equation will mislead.

General Criticisms of Linear Models

Recall from introductory statistics the admonition that, one cannot infer causation from correlation Other problems associated with NHST also apply to both SRB and RCI models. Most problematically, neither test provides a statement of "truth." Also, obtaining a small p-value may have neither theoretical nor practical significance, and does not measure magnitude of effect (Nickerson, 2000).

In recent years, major test publishers have begun providing multiple standardization samples for both "normal" and "abnormal" populations. Many also provide important base-rate and error statistics. Unfortunately, comparable data are not available for all tests, and the age cohorts across tests published by the same company do not consistently correspond with one another. When "special population" norms exist, the sample sizes are often so small, particularly within a given age cohort, that they cannot possibly include examples of all variants of the disorder. For these and other reasons, evaluators often incorporate "process" information within their "clinical judgment." In doing so, they may use process heuristics derived from an informal visual inspection of test data. The following section reviews methods that have proven useful in reducing subjective aspects of visual analysis.

Visual Analysis Approaches to the Identification of Meaningful Change

In the literature of behavioral psychology and applied behavior analysis, there is a rich tradition of visual analysis of graphed data in single-case studies (Franklin,

Gorman, Beasley, & Allison, 1997). Single-case evaluation strategies typically require larger numbers of observations than are generally available to neuropsychologists, although exceptions may occur in settings in which multiple daily observations are possible, such as trauma and rehabilitation settings. There are five methods that can be adapted to neuropsychological assessment, four of which (i.e., Least Squares Regression, Split-Middle Method, Resistant Trend Line, and Nonlinear Trends) rely on regression methods similar to those described above. One additional technique, Non-Overlapping CIs, shares similarities with RCI.

Least Squares Regression

Jaccard and Becker (1990) proposed incorporating linear regression with visual analysis in order to reduce judgment error in trend analysis. Figure 16.1 compares obtained with predicted scores taken from a series of Wechsler Memory Scales, Visual Memory 2 Subtest Scores plotted in conjunction with upper and lower 95% CIs. The measure taken at age 74 falls slightly below the lower confidence interval of the predicted score using this method.

This graph, along with others presented in this work, is constructed from standard Excel functions. Table 16.5 shows the data organization. Predicted scores come from a separate spreadsheet, Regression Equations, that performs functions similar to Regbuild Software (Crawford & Garthwaite, 2007). Upper and lower CIs are based on standard error estimates of predicted scores. All Excel examples, as well as construction instructions, are available from the author on request.

Meaning

This graph implies that our patient scored lower than his predicted score on two of four observations, with much weaker than expected performance on the final evaluation. Regardless of any putative effects that practice may have had, the last observation is far enough below expectation to suggest that it may not be due to error. Qualitative information documented during the assessment may offer insight regarding the effects of motivation, fatigue, or some other process on this performance. However, the evidence supporting the deficit is weak because the final score is so near the lower confidence interval that, were we to superimpose CIs around the observed score, they would overlap completely.

Split-Middle Method

The split-middle method divides data sets into two sections, providing median scores for each section (Med 1 and Med 2), with each median containing two data points (Figure 16.2). Comparison occurs between these median scores. Table 16.6 provides Excel functions with the first and last columns calculating median scores, =@median(E1:G1) and =@median(I1:L1), respectively, for C1 and N1. The split-middle technique is more conservative than least squares, because our patient's score remains within the 95% CI bands.

Meaning

Like the least squares example, the split-middle provides a falling trend line. It implies that continued testing will eventually produce performance that is far

16.1

Illustration of least squares, comparing obtained (score) with predicted score as they are bound by the upper and lower 95% CI.

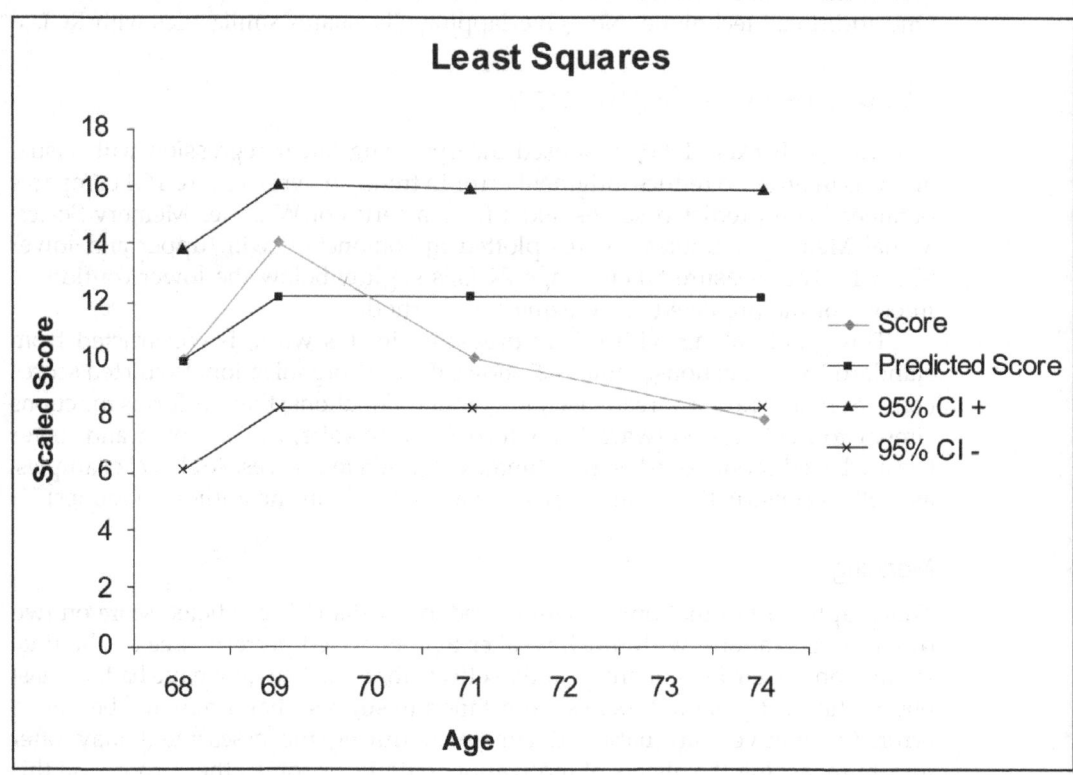

16.5 Excel Organization for Least-Squares Graphing

	A	B	C	D	E	F	G	H	I
1	Score		10.00	14.00		10.00			08.00
2	Predicted Score		10.00	12.17		12.17			12.17
3	95% CI +		13.84	16.01		16.01			16.01
4	95% CI −		06.16	08.33		08.33			08.33
5	Age		68	69	70	71	72	73	74

16.2

The split-middle arrangement of obtained score, predicted score, and corresponding CIs.

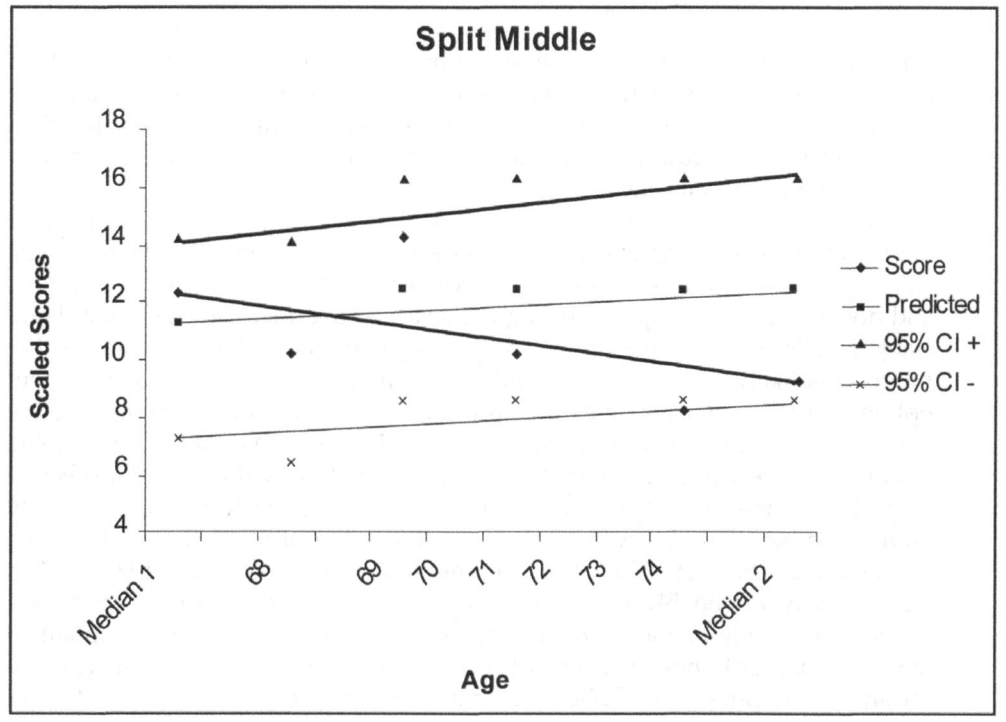

16.6 Split-Middle Data Organization

	A	B	C	D	E	F	G	H	I	J	K	L	M	N
1	Score		12		10		14		10			8		9
2	Predicted Score		11		10		12		12			12		12.17
3	95% CI +		14		14		16		16			16		16.01
4	95% CI –		7		6.2		8		8			8.3		8.33
5	Age		Med 1		68		69	70	71	72	73	74		Med 2

enough below the predicted score to produce deficient scores. However, this presentation indicates that the patient's current functioning remains within the CI boundaries, so additional testing is necessary to determine whether the plotted trend continues.

Resistant Trend Line

When larger data sets are available, as might occur in rehabilitation settings, then calculation of a resistant trend line is possible. This method is the same as the split-middle described previously, but divides data into three groups rather than two. Grip strength could be measured three times each day during inpatient rehabilitation, for example.

Longer data series, such as the one displayed in Figure 16.3, also provide opportunity for inferring maximum medical improvement (MMI). The trend line shows progressive improvement in therapy during the last portion of treatment, and documents an asymptote during the last four treatment sessions. Serial and stable results such as these are typically interpreted as evidence that no further progress is likely unless current conditions change. When additional treatment options exist, a pattern such as this indicates progression of intervention to the next level of difficulty is appropriate. Otherwise, it implies that continuing ongoing treatment is likely to be unproductive. Other heuristics used in visual inspection analysis that may be appropriate to neuropsychology include low variability within and between observation phases and stability of trend line as described by Parson and Baer in 1978 (cited in Franklin, Allison, & Gorman, 1997, p. 136). Readers may reasonably question the appropriateness of heuristics that were developed outside of the normative assessment model that is most familiar to neuropsychologists; however, the utility of these heuristics in many applied behavior analysis applications implies they have some value in the absence of other more robustly demonstrated methods.

Meaning

The resistant trend line design corresponds with three distinct phases of treatment recovery. Initially, recovery progresses quickly during phase 1, stalls during phase 2, and demonstrates the most rapid gains during phase 3. The stability observed during the last four observations may aid in establishing discharge criteria. As is customary in visual graphing, I have added vertical phase lines, each showing a separate phase of treatment associated with each median block, which clearly demonstrates the phases of recovery commonly seen during rehabilitation when the patient initially avoids treatment or participates inconsistently. As the patient feels stronger and responds more consistently (phase 2), the rate of improvement increases and then shows rapid progress during the final treatment phase.

Nonlinear Trends

Trauma centers provide opportunities for obtaining repeated daily screenings with cognitive instruments, such as the Mini-Mental State Exam (MMSE) or the Galveston Orientation and Amnesia Test (GOAT). Figure 16.4 shows data taken

16.3

An example of the resistant trend line across three treatment blocks using grip strength as the dependent variable.

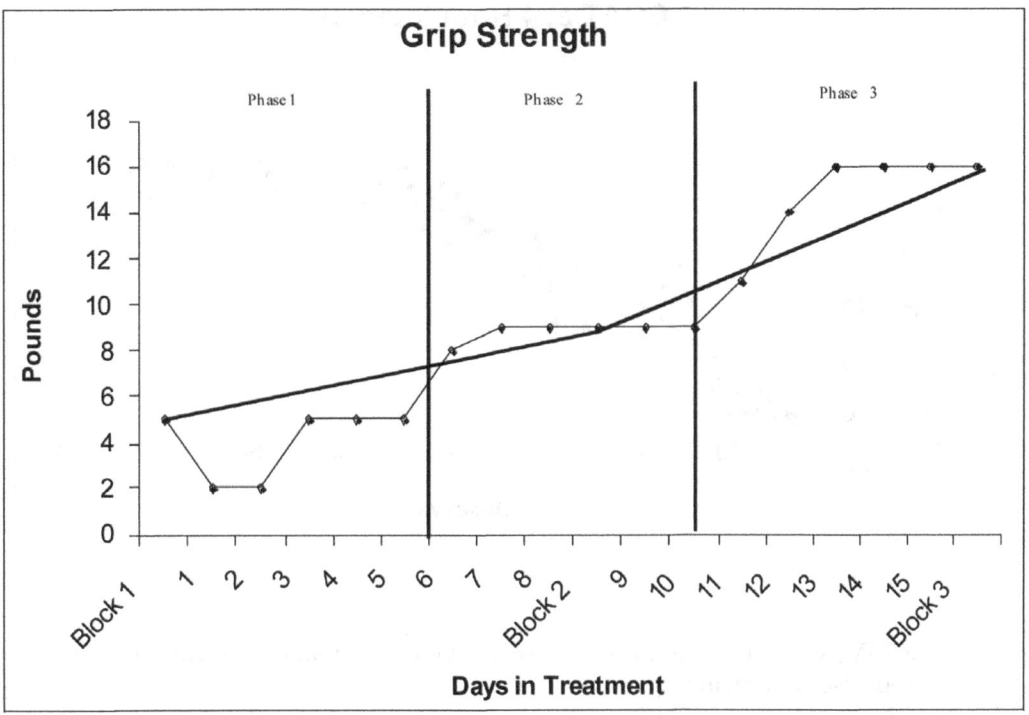

from a trauma unit every 4 hours for 12 days and displayed with a polynomial (order 6) trend line. Bars displayed above and below the data points indicate bands of standard error in measurement.

Meaning

Scores below 66 indicate defective performance, with borderline function interpreted when scores are between 66 and 75. Clinicians sometimes discontinue administration of the GOAT once the patient scores above 75. So long as the patient progresses adequately, this rule may have value, but continued evaluation following one "pass" score offers the evaluator greater confidence that the patient will not be discharged prematurely. A different interpretation of "meaningful" is necessary for patients who continue presenting defective scores day in and day out. Both the hospital and treating physicians benefit from reduced exposure to litigation when written policies establish standing procedures for patients failing to progress. In these situations, scores presenting a trend line that is stable within

16.4

Demonstration of the nonlinear trend, plotting GOAT scores at 4-hour intervals.

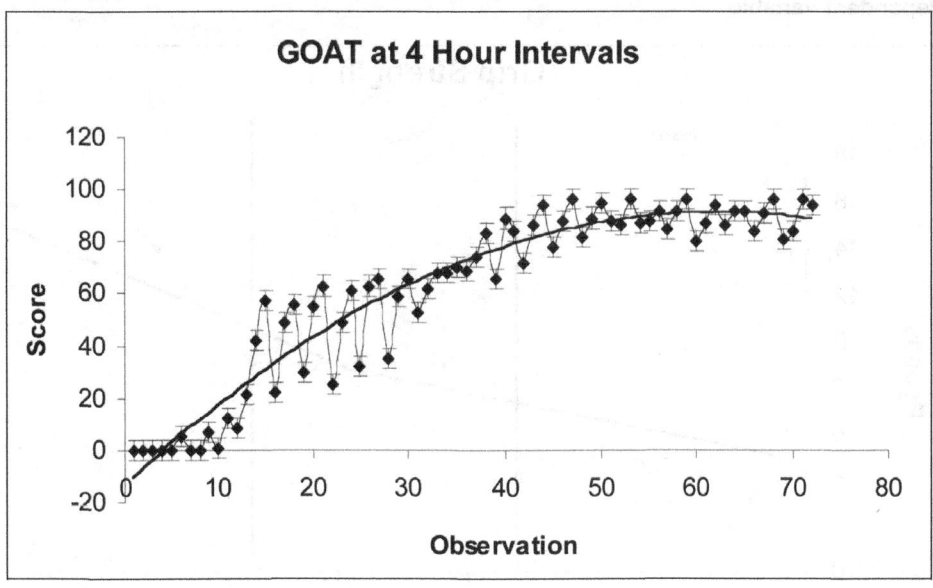

the SEM, yet below the normal score, provide data that are useful for evidence-based discharge planning.

Nonlinear tread analysis may also be of value in comparing the progress of a single patient with standardized recovery curves. Figure 16.5 contrasts a patient's recovery from stroke with the mean recovery curve calculated from eight patients described by Ward, Brown, Thompson, and Frackowiak (2003). The Excel Test function can also provide a probability statement of the comparison ($p = 0.018655$). Table 16.7 provides a look at GOAT observations for the nonlinear trend, and Table 16.8 shows an Excel arrangement for recovery curve comparison.

Meaning

Figure 16.5 clearly shows that the defendant's recovery was below expectations by day 20 post-stroke. At no time thereafter did performance return to within the lower 95% CI. By day 200, his performance was falling in relation to expected recovery patterns.

Nonoverlapping Confidence Intervals

Figure 16.6 compares obtained with predicted scores, showing their corresponding 95% CIs. The hatched squares mark overlap. The larger the overlap, the less confidence one has that observed scores vary significantly from predicted scores.

16.5

Recovery curve analysis of recovery, comparing the performance of a single patient with a group recovery mean and ± 1 standard deviation scores from the group mean.

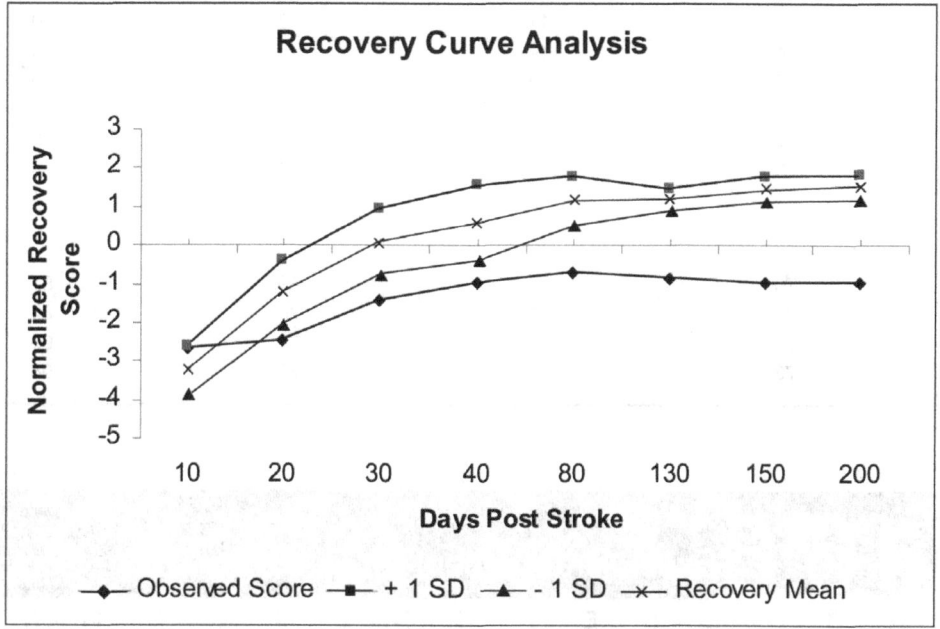

The greatest confidence occurs where no overlap is present. Table 16.9 shows an Excel table for evaluating confidence intervals.

Were scores for the final actual period lower, as presented in Table 16.10, then the final contrast would show a nonoverlapping interval (Figure 16.7). Here, the shaded square marks do not overlap. Large areas of non-overlap offer increasing evidence that the difference between actual and predicted scores was not due to chance.

This far, we have considered a variety of numeric and graphic methods for demonstrating that the differences observed between sets of data were not due to chance. Unfortunately, the hypothesis testing inherent to all of these methods is incapable of telling us whether these scores were due to head trauma, infarct, aging, or some biological process. Bayesian methods, however, have this capability.

Bayesian Approaches to the Identification of Meaningful Change

Bayesian analysis is relatively obscure in neuropsychology, even though Bayes (1763) described the methods long before Fisher popularized "classical" or "fre-

16.7 GOAT Observations for Nonlinear Trend

	A	B	D
1	Time	Observation	GOAT
2	7	1	0
3	11	2	0
4	14	3	0
5	18	4	0
6	22	5	0
7	1	6	5
8	7	7	0
.	.	.	.
.	.	.	.
.	.	.	.
70	14	69	81
71	18	70	84
72	22	71	96
73	1	72	94

16.8 Excel Arrangement for Recovery Curve Comparison

A	B	C	D	E	F	G	H	I	J	K	L	M	N	O
1		Patient										+σ	−σ X	σ
2	Days post	1	2	3	4	5	6	7	8	s				
3	10	-4	-4	-4	-3	-4	-4	-2	-3	-3	-2.7	-3.9	-3.3	0.6
4	20	-1	-1	0	-1	-2	-2	-2	-2	-3	-0.5	-2.1	-1.3	0.8
5	30	-1	0.9	1	1	-1	0	-1	-0	-2	0.89	-0.9	0	0.9
6	40	1	0.9		1	2	0	-1	0	-1	1.52	-0.5	0.5	1
7	80	2			1	2	1	1	1	-1	1.69	0.5	1.1	0.6
8	130		0.9	1	2		2	1	1	-1	1.42	0.85	1.1	0.3
9	150			1	2	1	2	2	1	-1	1.72	1.11	1.4	0.3
10	200	2	1.2	1				2	1	-1	1.77	1.09	1.4	0.3
11														
12	0.0186554					t test p								

quentist" models. R. L. Thorndike recommended in 1986 (p. 54) that psychology adopt Bayes methods for test interpretation. Bayesian statistics address the highly relevant question: "If Bobby scores in the brain damage range on a test, what is the probability that he is brain damaged?" Alternatively, classical statistical theory answers a different question: "If 60% of the patients with Bobby's score are brain-

16.6

Nonoverlapping CI analysis showing considerable overlap of CIs between predicted and observed scale scores.

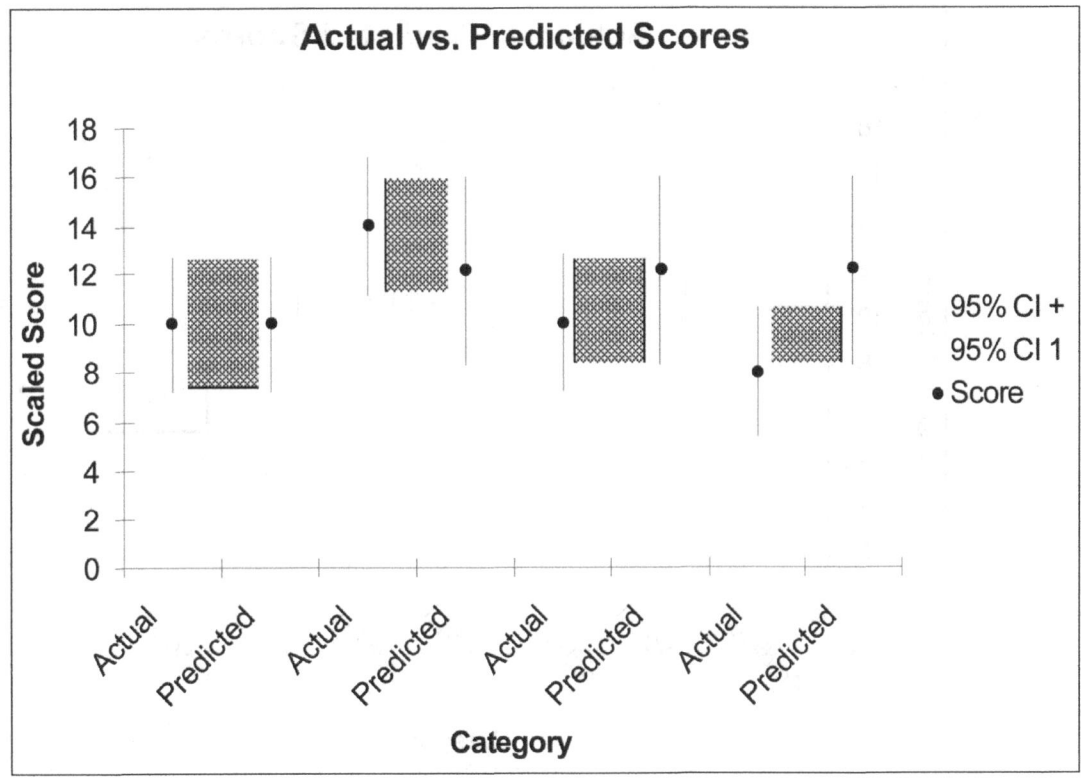

16.9 Excel Table for Evaluating Confidence Intervals

	A	B	C	D	E	F	G	H
1	Actual	Predicted	Actual	Predicted	Actual	Predicted	Actual	Predicted
2	12.7	12.7	16.8	16.01	12.82	16.01	10.63	16.01
3	7.2	7.2	11.2	8.33	7.18	8.33	5.37	8.33
4	10	10	14	12.17	10	12.17	8	12.17

16.7

Nonoverlapping CI analysis where no overlap occurs between actual and predicted scores on one score pair.

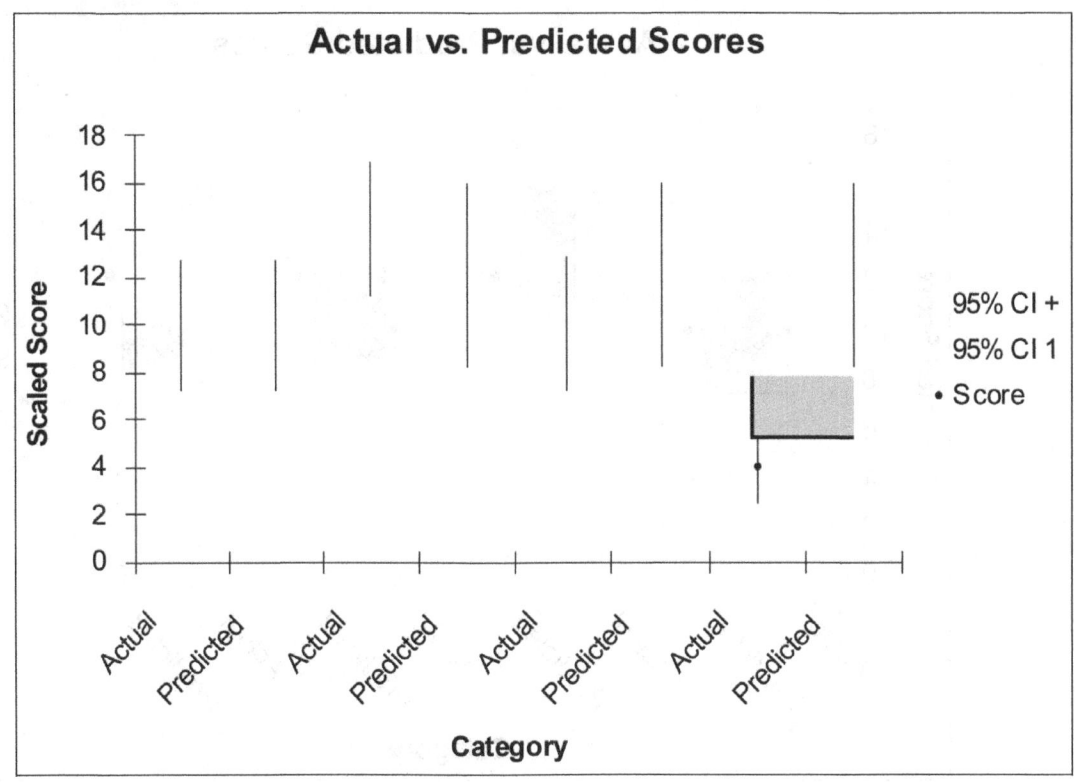

16.10 Excel Table Showing Reduced Actual Results in the Final Observation Period

	A	B	C	D	E	F	G	H
1	Actual	Predicted	Actual	Predicted	Actual	Predicted	Actual	Predicted
2	12.7	12.7	16.8	16.01	12.82	16.01	5.1	16.01
3	7.2	7.2	11.2	8.33	7.18	8.33	2.5	8.33
4	10	10	14	12.17	10	12.17	4	12.17

16.11 Comparison of Bayesian and Classical Analysis in Neuropsychology

	Bayesian Analysis	Classical Analysis
Probability	Direct measure	Estimated measure
Extreme Scores	Appropriate, Low Type I Error	High Type I Error
p-value estimate	Exact point for abnormality	Estimate of testing error
Testing dissociations	Rigorous	Weak
Estimate of abnormality	Interval estimate	No interval estimate

damaged, what is the probability that Bobby is brain-damaged?" (Franklin & Allison, 1992). Although many neuropsychologists seek test measures having high sensitivity, Bayes' rule shows that increases in specificity entail the largest increases in positive predictive value (Franklin & Krueger, 2003).

The primary distinction between these methods arises from their treatment of statistical parameters. Classical models view statistical parameters as unknown but fixed, whereas Bayesian models treat them as random variables having their own probability distributions. Crawford and Garthwaite (2007) note that frequentist and Bayesian approaches can at some times, produce different results, and at other times, the same results. Reassurance is greatest when convergence occurs, regardless of the evaluator's preference for one approach over the other. Nonetheless, the Bayesian analysis provides five advantages to neuropsychologists, as described in Table 16.11.

Bayesian inference provides a mechanism for incorporating base rates in the diagnostic decision-making process. Dawes (1988) cautions against base-rate neglect, warning that it leads to overconfidence, which has been attributed to a variety of fallible judgmental heuristics. Garb and Schramke (1996) argue that judgments improve when clinicians are vividly reminded of the relevance of base rates. The primary diagnostic goal involves obtaining the joint occurrence of a positive test result with the presence of a given disorder. Statistically, this is represented by the sensitivity of the test multiplied by the base-rate of the disease that is then multiplied by the total number of cases. Because patients in clinical settings are rarely sampled randomly, clinical sampling bias likely increases the *available* base rate. Bayesian analysis can independently assess the sampling bias of the tests at hand, thereby providing clinical practitioners with more accurate decision-making tools.

Bayesian methods incorporate prior knowledge, such as base rate, into the distribution. So long as prior knowledge is quantifiable, the method improves prediction. While conducting three experiments, John Crawford and Paul Garthwaite (2007) showed how Bayesian methods can be used for neuropsychological applications.

The first experiment used a Bayesian approach for detecting impairment in a single case. Crawford and Garthwaite (2002) compared Bayesian methods with th regression equations (C&H), and with classical z-score theory. Both Bayesian and C&H models produced perfect convergence; however, the z-score exaggerated the level of abnormality and inflated Type-I errors. Crawford and Garthwaite (2002) demonstrated that both frequentist CIs and Bayesian interval estimates were nonsymmetrical, as occurs in a non-central t-distribution. In contrast with the frequentist model, the Bayesian approach need not concern itself with the distribution parameters, whereas statistical machinations were necessary to get around the distribution with the frequentist model. Both methods produced higher variability in point estimates as the sample size of the control sample became extreme. Systematic bias occurred in the frequentist model, exaggerating abnormality of the z score when the normative sample was small. The Bayesian method did not present this systematic bias. CIs for the classical model were nonsymmetrical around the point estimate, whereas the Bayesian credible interval showed a "true level of abnormality" (p. 348). Both CIs and credible intervals provided interval estimates of ± 95%.

The second experiment compared score differences taken from two different tests, as observed in a single case, with scores of control subjects. They provided two examples in this experiment—a comparison of scores from the same individual taken at different points in time and dissociations. They demonstrated that, if the error or uncertainty that is associated with estimating parameters in sample data were not incorporated into the formula, high percentages of normal subjects were incorrectly classified as impaired when evaluations used dissociations. Earlier formulas ignored uncertainty altogether, such as those proposed by Payne and Jones (1957). Comparisons of performance on tests having different means, standard deviations, and normative samples using z score comparisons produced very high Type-I error rates (>25%) unless comparisons occurred between very large normative samples. Bayesian and frequentist methods estimated the abnormality of clinical scores equally well when comparing *unstandardized* differences between test scores; however, findings were not equivalent when they compared *standardized* differences between test scores. Point estimates deviated considerably in the comparisons when normative sample sizes were small or moderate. Bayesian models, however, produced more conservative estimates. More importantly, unlike classical statistics, the Bayesian inferential model was capable of directly evaluating the proportion of the control population that would obtain a score more extreme than an identified patient. Authors concluded that, "the Bayesian test will provide a more rigorous means of testing for a strong dissociation than any of the available frequentist methods"(p. 10) . They presented four advantages of Bayesian methods over classical methods as derived from the second experiment. First, Bayesian methods directly evaluated probability rather than estimating it. Second, they provided a more conservative estimate of abnormality. Third, the probability value offered an exact point estimate of the abnormality of the difference. Fourth, Bayesian methods produced an interval estimate of the abnormality.

Experiment three compared Type-I errors occurring in frequentist and Bayesian methods. Bayesian methods produced Type-I error rates that were lower than those produced by frequentist methods.

Despite the obvious advantages that Bayesian analysis offers to neuropsychology, the necessary theoretical background and mathematical calculations required present a barrier to many practitioners who would otherwise adopt it. In order to assist the clinician, Crawford and Garthwaite created three excellent software

16.8

Data-entry screen for DIFFBAYES.

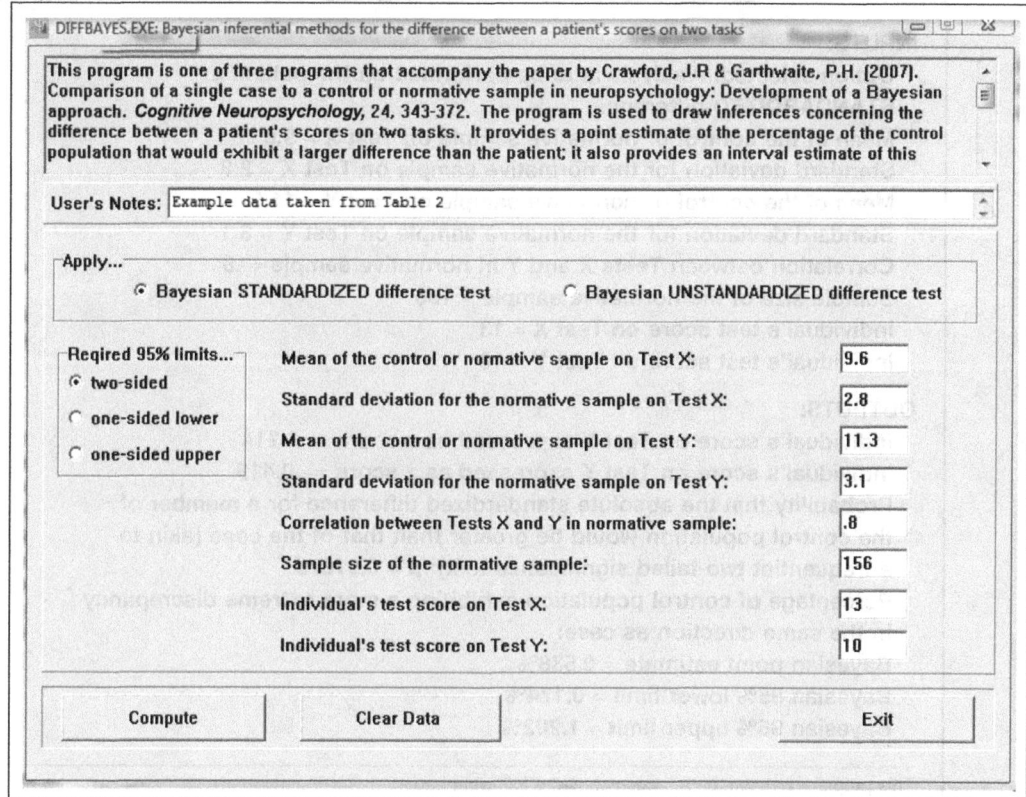

programs, *DiffBayes*, *DissocsBayes*, and *SingleBayes*, from their experiments. These programs allow practitioners who may be unfamiliar with mathematical aspects of Bayesian theory to benefit from their research.

DiffBayes

DiffBayes compares a case's difference against the difference in controls. The program calculates either an unstandardized or standardized difference test and produces a two-tailed probability, point estimate of abnormality, and 95% Bayesian credible interval for this percentage. Data in the following screen capture (Figure 16.8) come from Table 16.2. Clicking on "Compute" produces an output (Figure 16.9) that can be written to a text file for editing and pasting into reports.

16.9

Data printout of DIFFBAYES using data presented in Figure 16.8.

INPUTS:

Option selected: Analysis is to be performed on the patient's STANDARDIZED difference

Mean of the control or normative sample on Test X = 9.6

Standard deviation for the normative sample on Test X = 2.8

Mean of the control or normative sample on Test Y = 11.3

Standard deviation for the normative sample on Test Y = 3.1

Correlation between Tests X and Y in normative sample = .8

Sample size of the normative sample = 156

Individual's test score on Test X = 13

Individual's test score on Test Y = 10

OUTPUTS:

Individual's score on Test X expressed as z score = 1.214

Individual's score on Test Y expressed as z score = −0.419

Probability that the absolute standardized difference for a member of the control population would be greater than that of the case (akin to a frequentist two-tailed significance test): p = 0.01076

Percentage of control population exhibiting a more extreme discrepancy in the same direction as case:

Bayesian point estimate = 0.538%

Bayesian 95% lower limit = 0.174%

Bayesian 95% upper limit = 1.202%

This program was written to accompany the following paper:
Crawford, J.R., & Garthwaite, P.H. (2007). Comparison of a single case to a control or normative sample in neuropsychology: Development of a Bayesian approach. *Cognitive Neuropsychology, 24*, 343-372. User's Notes: Example data taken from Table 2.

DissocsBayes

DissocsBayes implements criteria for dissociations by testing for deficit on two tasks and then testing the standardized difference. Results show whether the patient meets criteria for strong association (i.e., poor performance on both tasks) or dissociation (i.e., poor performance on one task). A screen capture of the data entry screen appears in Figure 16.10, again using data taken from Table 16.2. The output (Figure 16.11) provides both frequentist and Bayesian interpretations of entered data.

SingleBayes

SingleBayes conducts an analysis of deficit and produce one- and two-tailed Bayesian *p*-values, a point estimate of the abnormality of the score, and a 95%

16.10

Data-entry screen for DISSOCSBAYES.

DISSOCSBAYES.EXE: Bayesian criteria for dissociations in single-case studies

This program is one of three programs that accompany the paper by Crawford, J.R & Garthwaite, P.H. (2007). Comparison of a single case to a control or normative sample in neuropsychology: Development of a Bayesian approach." Cognitive Neuropsychology, 24, 343-372. The program is used to apply Bayesian criteria for dissociations in single-case studies in which the scores of a patient on two tasks are compared to those of a control sample. (The program tests for a strong dissociation and a dissociation, putatively classical). The

User's Notes: Example data from Table 2

Apply...

○ Bayesian criteria for dissociations   ● Combined Bayesian / frequentist criteria for dissociations

Mean of the control or normative sample on Test X:	9.6
Standard deviation for the normative sample on Test X:	2.8
Mean of the control or normative sample on Test Y:	11.3
Standard deviation for the normative sample on Test Y:	3.1
Correlation between Tests X and Y in normative sample:	.8
Sample size of the normative sample:	156
Individual's test score on Test X:	13
Individual's test score on Test Y:	10

Compute	Clear Data	Exit

Bayesian credible interval on the percentage. Data in the example (Figure 16.12) again originate in Table 16.2. Results of the analysis appear in Figure 16.13.

As in all analyses of this type, the evaluating neuropsychologist must interpret the meaning from the numbers. Future iterations of Bayesian models will, hopefully, include multiple distributions of "prior knowledge" in their formulations. At the time of writing, these programs could be downloaded at no charge from www.abdn.ac.uk/~psy086/dept/BayesSingleCase.htm.

Summary

The concept of identifying change in psychology as meaningful is relatively new to the field (Christensen & Mendoza,1986; Jacobson & Truax, 1991). Early adoption of this notion in neuropsychology was limited to tests having large normative samples and well-understood statistical properties, principally the Wechsler intel-

16.11

Printed output for DISSOCSBAYES.

INPUTS:
  Option selected: Apply combined Bayesian / frequentist criteria for dissociations
  Mean of the control or normative sample on Test X = 9.6
  Standard deviation for the normative sample on Test X = 2.8
  Mean of the control or normative sample on Test Y = 11.3
  Standard deviation for the normative sample on Test Y = 3.1
  Correlation between Tests X and Y in normative sample = 0.8
  Sample size of the normative sample = 156
  Individual's test score on Test X = 13
  Individual's test score on Test Y = 10

OUTPUTS:
  Individual's score on Test X expressed as z score = 1.214
  Individual's score on Test Y expressed as z score = −0.419

CRAWFORD & HOWELL'S (1998) TEST FOR A DEFICIT ON TASK X:
  Significance test: $t = 1.210$, $df = 155$, p (one-tailed) = 0.11398
  Estimated percentage of control population (+95% CI) obtaining a lower score than the patient on Task X = 88.6018% (95% CI = 84.2812% to 92.2219%)
  Dissociations criterion: The patient does not meet the criterion for a deficit on Task X

CRAWFORD & HOWELL'S (1998) TEST FOR A DEFICIT ON TASK Y:
  Significance test: $t = −0.418$, $df = 155$, p (one-tailed) = 0.33826
  Estimated percentage of control population (+95% CI) obtaining a lower score than the patient on Task Y = 33.8257% (95% CI = 28.0135% to 39.9353%)
  Dissociations criterion: The patient does not meet the criterion for a deficit on Task Y

BAYESIAN TEST (BSDT) ON THE DIFFERENCE BETWEEN THE PATIENT'S STANDARDIZED SCORES ON X AND Y:
  Probability that the absolute difference for a member of the control population would be greater than that of the patient (akin to a frequentist two-tailed significance test): $p = 0.01076$
Percentage of control population exhibiting a more extreme discrepancy in same direction as patient:
  Bayesian point estimate (+ 95% CI) = 0.538% (95% CI = 0.1738% to 1.2024%)
  Dissociations criterion: The difference between the patient's standardized scores is statistically significant on the BSDT

FREQUENTIST TEST (RSDT) ON THE DIFFERENCE BETWEEN THE PATIENT'S STANDARD-IZED SCORES ON X AND Y: RSDT t value = 2.560, $df = 155$, p (two-tailed) = 0.01144
  Dissociations criterion: The difference between the patient's standardized scores is statistically significant on the frequentist RSDT

OVERALL RESULT OF APPLYING COMBINED BAYESIAN/FREQUENTIST CRITERIA FOR A DISSOCIATION:
  The patient does not fulfill the criteria for either a strong or classical dissociation.

This program was written to accompany the following paper:
Crawford, J. R., & Garthwaite, P. H. (2007). Comparison of a single case to a control or normative sample in neuropsychology: Development of a Bayesian approach. *Cognitive Neuropsychology, 24,* 343-372. User's Notes: Example data taken from Table 2.

16.12

Data-entry screen for SINGLEBAYES.

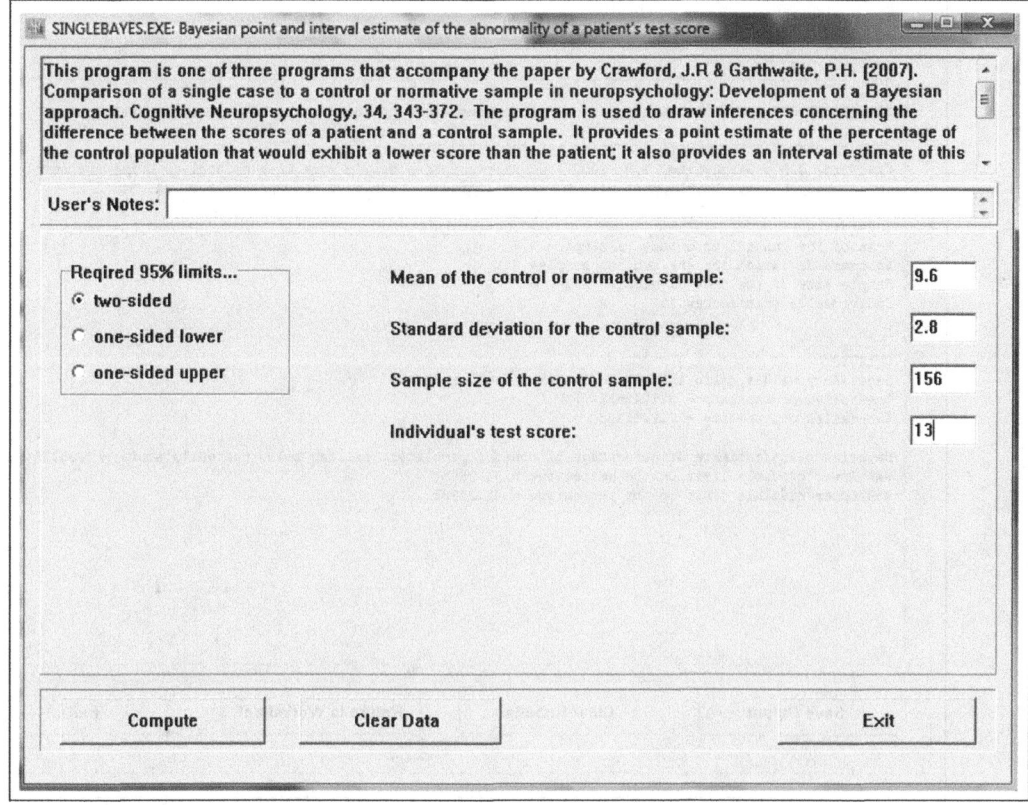

This program is one of three programs that accompany the paper by Crawford, J.R & Garthwaite, P.H. (2007). Comparison of a single case to a control or normative sample in neuropsychology: Development of a Bayesian approach. Cognitive Neuropsychology, 34, 343-372. The program is used to draw inferences concerning the difference between the scores of a patient and a control sample. It provides a point estimate of the percentage of the control population that would exhibit a lower score than the patient; it also provides an interval estimate of this

User's Notes:

Reqired 95% limits...
- ⦿ two-sided
- ○ one-sided lower
- ○ one-sided upper

Mean of the control or normative sample: 9.6

Standard deviation for the control sample: 2.8

Sample size of the control sample: 156

Individual's test score: 13

| Compute | Clear Data | Exit |

ligence and memory scales (Chelune et al., 1993). The effects of practice, statistical regression, and other forms of known error were accounted for using the RCI process. By 1993, regression models were being explored as an alternative to RCI (McSweeny et al., 1993; Charter, 1996). Basso et al. (1999) extended the boundaries of test measures by evaluating executive function in patients at 12-month intervals. That same year, Ivnik, Smith, Lucas, Petersen, Boeve, Kokmen, and Tangalos explored normal variance in older adults four times during a two-year interval. Both authors concluded that when practice effects occurred, their statistically significant impact appeared during the second testing, but did not progress meaningfully thereafter. The first attempt at documenting meaningful change in an entire battery appeared in 2006 when Woods, Childers, Ellis, Guaman, Grant, and Heaton adapted RCI technology to an eight-battery examination of normal and HIV-infected clinical samples. Crawford and Garthwaite (2004) presented a

16.13

Printed report for SINGLEBAYES.

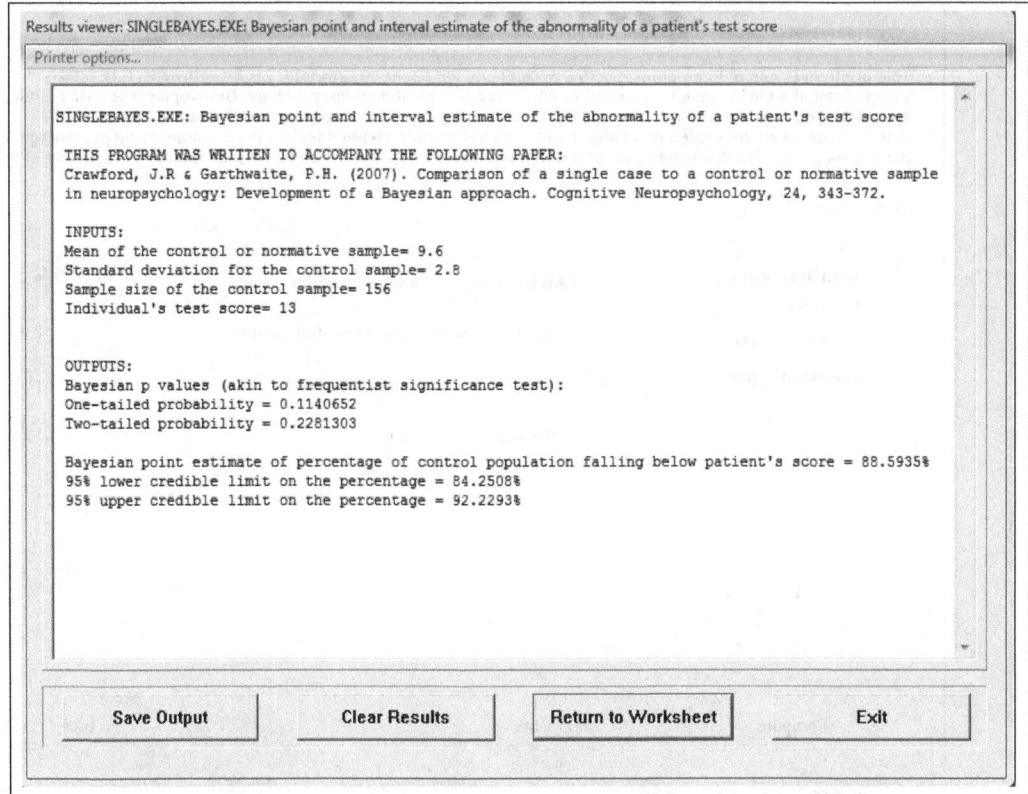

Results viewer: SINGLEBAYES.EXE: Bayesian point and interval estimate of the abnormality of a patient's test score

Printer options...

```
SINGLEBAYES.EXE: Bayesian point and interval estimate of the abnormality of a patient's test score

THIS PROGRAM WAS WRITTEN TO ACCOMPANY THE FOLLOWING PAPER:
Crawford, J.R & Garthwaite, P.H. (2007). Comparison of a single case to a control or normative sample
in neuropsychology: Development of a Bayesian approach. Cognitive Neuropsychology, 24, 343-372.

INPUTS:
Mean of the control or normative sample= 9.6
Standard deviation for the control sample= 2.8
Sample size of the control sample= 156
Individual's test score= 13


OUTPUTS:
Bayesian p values (akin to frequentist significance test):
One-tailed probability = 0.1140652
Two-tailed probability = 0.2281303

Bayesian point estimate of percentage of control population falling below patient's score = 88.5935%
95% lower credible limit on the percentage = 84.2508%
95% upper credible limit on the percentage = 92.2293%
```

| Save Output | Clear Results | Return to Worksheet | Exit |

method for comparing a patient's scores with those of a control sample. They also used regression equations for comparing predicted with obtained scores (2006).

All of the RCI and regression models are built around classical statistical theory, or a statistical theory that requires testing against null and alternative hypotheses. Since Faust, Ziskin, and Hiers published *Brain Damage Claims: Coping with Neuropsychological Evidence* in 1991, clinicians have generally avoided referring to classical statistics in practice, and particularly, in court. Instead, many have relied on a variety of visual inspection heuristics. Visual inspection is well established in psychology, but those methods used in behavior analysis rarely appear in psychological reports. This chapter considers five applied behavior analysis techniques that have particular relevance to neuropsychology; Least Squares Regression, Split-middle Method, Resistant Trend Line, Nonlinear Trends, and Non-overlapping CIs. Each of these tools can be combined with one or more classical statistical models.

16.12 Advantages Offered by Bayesian Analysis

Bayesian analysis makes use of all of the information in the data.

All parts of inquiry, including prior distributions, are included in the model.

Bayesian analysis requires less attention be given to the mathematical requirements of the model, such as normality of distribution, skewness, sampling, etc.

Awkward problems encountered in sampling theory, such as CIs and estimators, do not arise.

Bayesian models consider ignorance as a form of prior knowledge.

More recently, Bayesian statistical methods have become a focus of interest (Crawford & Garthwaite, 2007). Although Bayesian methods are new to many clinical neuropsychologists, they actually predate classical statistical theory. For years, the applicability of Bayes' Theorem to general problems of scientific inference has been questioned (Box & Tiao, 1973, p. 12). Much of the controversy originated in how the differing methods thought of "prior knowledge." Classical statistical theory ignores prior knowledge completely by focusing exclusively on the "here-and-now" as it is represented in normalized distributions. Table 16.12 presents Box and Tiao's view of the advantages that Bayesian analysis brings to scientific inquiry.

At the heart of Bayesian theory is the likelihood function, which tells us that the probability distribution is proportional (indicated by the symbol "~") to the likelihood of an event multiplied by the prior distribution of the event.

$$\text{Posterior distribution} \sim \text{likelihood} * \text{prior distribution} \quad (3)$$

The prior distribution can include ignorance, an accumulation of prior knowledge, or some combination of the two. Several types of non-test historical information are typically included in the inferential process. The loss of consciousness, duration of coma, substance-abuse history, and a history of special education serve as examples. Also, there are process markers, such as those used in the inductive approach to diagnosis (Luria & Majovski, 1977) that are better suited to the Bayesian approach.

Conclusions

It may be reasonable to assume that "normal" behavior is adequately modeled by a bell-shaped curve; however, making that same assumption for "abnormal" populations may not be as reasonable. The term "abnormal" implies behavior, health conditions, and the like that are decidedly aberrant. As Luria and Majovski (1977) intimate, we should not expect methods that were designed around a normal model paradigm to work just as effectively elsewhere. What is more, reliance on population average may not be an appropriate standard of comparison in any case, because it does not directly apply to individuals.

Bayesian methods allow for modeling abnormal behavior that is free from most of the statistical assumptions that create interpretative problems for neuropsychologists. In particular, their ability to incorporate prior knowledge into a testable paradigm offers our best method to date for quantifying process, medical, and historical information within hypothesis testing; however, their clinical utility remains largely unexplored for several reasons. First, few graduate clinical programs teach them. Second, calculations can be much more complex than those typically used in clinical practice. Third, methods for defining and understanding prior knowledge are only now emerging.

Those who earn their living by the administration and interpretation of psychological tests often complain that they have experienced gradual, and occasionally precipitous, declines in reimbursement for their services. Some attribute this to increasing amounts of practitioners claiming expertise in neuropsychological methods. Others refute this opinion, noting that advances in imaging techniques undermine medical reliance on neuropsychology. Yet, attorneys and collaborative-minded medical practitioners appreciate expertly administered and interpreted neuropsychological evaluations, because of the ability of these evaluations to describe the functioning of patients in behavioral terms. Missing pieces of the neuropsychology puzzle remain (e.g., measures that accurately diagnosis disorders, accurately predict outcome, and offer ecological validity). Change matters when fluctuations in test scores address these concerns as they relate to ability, performance, or income.

Using extant techniques, tests only tell us when change does not matter. Bayesian analysis is capable of helping us understand when change truly addresses ecological validity and diagnostic efficacy, yet the challenges in developing these models are huge. Cooperative efforts will be necessary between test publishers, clinicians, and researchers. Fortunately, tools now exist that make collaboration of this type possible, if parties accept a Web-based scheme for scoring and interpreting tests that is managed by an independent not-for-profit organization willing to protect propriety rights of publishers and compensate participants fairly. Advances in the prediction of outcomes are possible with further development of recovery curves specific to focal injuries and clearly defined diseases.

Web-Based Test Scoring and Interpretation

A major concern of clinical neuropsychologists is the cost of tests, scoring software, and test materials. They want the ability to compare scores from the tests of a variety of publishers with analysis of these tests vis-á-vis predictive and diagnostic heuristics. Researchers need data, and test publishers need to protect their investment in printing and development. All of these interests can be addressed simultaneously through a Web-based scoring and interpretation system. Normative data from all test publishers would be maintained on-line, as would clinician scoring and interpretive software.

The system would work for clinicians by allowing one-stop scoring and interpretative assistance with any test they might need. It would allow them to purchase test materials inexpensively as they need them, so they could afford to maintain test inventories large enough to address unique and rare circumstances. They would be able to use the most current tests at a reasonable cost. Clinicians would pay per use, improving their cash flow and reducing financial loss due to test obsolescence.

Test publishers would receive royalties for every administration. They could distribute test materials and protocols less expensively and minimize research and development costs. Because data from *all* administrations of a test would be available, they could develop more specific and better targeted standardization cohorts. Access to test results from clinicians would allow publishers to develop more effective products at lower cost, thereby increasing their profit margins.

Researchers would benefit from participation because they could mine huge databases containing raw and scaled scores from tests administered worldwide. From these resources, it would be possible to develop Bayesian and other forms of inference that would not only answer questions of clinical and academic interest, but also provide fodder for theory development and verification.

Development of Recovery Curves for Specific Injury Types

There are two sides to the recovery curve issue. The first side references untreated patients. We need to understand what happens when people who have experienced head injury, dementia, or other disorders with neuropsychological sequels receive no treatment. Few of us would withhold intervention from patients for experimental reasons, yet there are thousands of patients diagnosed with these disorders who receive no treatment for a variety of reasons. Many can be identified, but few are followed by health care systems. If governments are unwilling or unable to provide tracking, then professional and business interests need to fill this gap. With the number of personal computers growing rapidly worldwide, on-line tracking using patient or caregiver data entry may now be possible. Many of the untreated patients I see during disability evaluations are untreated because they cannot afford treatment. They, or their caregivers, independently seek "in-home" treatments through Internet or library research. If the testing clearinghouse mentioned earlier were established, it could also provide patient access and track outcome.

The second side of recovery curves considers clinical populations. Standards for evaluating and reporting patients' progress at crucial times during their recoveries must be established. Efforts have been made in this regard for some types of injuries (Acker, 1982), but their impact has been limited by geographic isolation, inconsistent sampling, and inconsistent testing practices. The Centers for Disease Control maintain reporting protocols for infectious disorders, so why not establish reporting protocols for neuropsychological and traumatic disorders, as well? Professional associations, certifying authorities, and publishers of psychological tests have some responsibility in this regard.

Acknowledgment

The author gratefully acknowledges John R. Crawford, College of Life Sciences and Medicine, King's College, University of Aberdeen for his thoughtful review and commentary.

References

Acker, M. D. (Ed.). (1982). *Head injury rehabilitation project: Final report*. San Jose, CA: Santa Clara Valley Medical Center.

Babbage, C. (1864). *Passages from the life of a philosopher* (p. 67). London: Longman.

Barr, W. B. (2003). Neuropsychological testing of high school athletes: Preliminary norms and test-retest indices. *Archives of Clinical Neuropsychology, 18*, 91–101.

Basso, M. R., Bornstein, R. A., & Lang, J. M. (1999). Practice effects on commonly used measures of executive function across twelve months. *Clinical Neuropsychologist, 13*(3), 283–292.

Basso, M. R., Lowery, N., Ghormley, C., & Bornstein, R. A. (2001). Practice effects on the Wisconsin card sorting test–64 card version across 12 months. *Clinical Neuropsychologist, 15*(4), 471–478.

Bayes, T. (1763). An essay toward solving a problem in the doctrine of chance. *Philosophical Transactions of the Royal Society, 53*, 370–418.

Bost, R. H., Wen, F., & Basso, M. R. (2005, August). *Detecting significant change in individual patients using RCI or regression*. Paper presented at the annual convention of The American Psychological Association, Washington, DC.

Box, G. E. P., & Tiao, G. C. (1973). *Bayesian inference in statistical analysis*. New York: John Wiley.

Charter, R. A. (1996). Revisiting the standard error of measurement, estimate, and prediction and their application to test scores. *Perceptual and Motor Skills, 82*, 1139–1144.

Chelune, G. H. (2003). Assessing reliable neuropsychological change. In R. D. Franklin (Ed.), *Prediction in forensic and neuropsychology* (pp. 123–148). Mahwah, NJ: Lawrence Erlbaum.

Chelune, G. H., Naugle, R. I., Lüders, H., Sedlak, J., & Awad, I. A. (1993). Individual change after epilepsy surgery: Practice effects and base rate information. *Neuropsychology, 7*, 41–52.

Christensen, L., & Mendoza, J. L. (1986). A method of assessing change in a single subject: An alteration of the RC index. *Behavior Therapy, 17*, 305–308.

Crawford, J. R. (2004). Psychometric foundations of neuropsychological assessment. In L. H. Goldstein & J. E. McNeil (Eds.), *Clinical neuropsychology: A practical guide to assessment and management for clinicians* (pp. 121–140). Chichester, UK: Wiley.

Crawford, J. R., & Garthwaite, P. H. (2002). Investigation of the single case in neuropsychology: Confidence limits on the abnormality of test scores and test score differences. *Neuropsychology, 24*, 343–372.

Crawford, J. R., & Garthwaite, P. H. (2004). Statistical methods for single-case studies in neuropsychology: Comparing the slope of a patient's regression line with those of a control sample. *Cortex, 40*, 533–548.

Crawford, J. R., & Garthwaite, P. H. (2006). Comparing patients' predicted test scores from a regressive equation with their obtained scores: A significance test and point estimate of abnormality with accompanying confidence limits. *Neuropsychology, 20*(3), 259–271.

Crawford, J. R., & Garthwaite, P. H. (2007). Comparison of a single case to a control or normative sample in neuropsychology: Development of a Bayesian approach. *Cognitive Neuropsychology, 24*(4), 343–372.

Dawes, R. M. (1988). *Rational choice in an uncertain world*. San Diego, CA: Harcourt Brace.

Faust, D., Ziskin, J., & Hiers, J. B. (1991). *Brain damage claims: Coping with neuropsychological evidence*. Los Angeles: Law and Psychology Press.

Franklin, R. D. (2003). Neuropsychological hypothesis testing. In R. D. Franklin (Ed.), *Prediction in forensic and neuropsychology* (pp. 65–88). Mahwah, NJ: Lawrence Erlbaum.

Franklin, R. D., & Allison, D. B. (1992). The Rev.: An IBM BASIC program for Bayesian test interpretation. *Behavior Research Methods, Instruments & Computers, 24*(3), 491–492.

Franklin, R. D., Allison, D. B., & Gorman, B. S. (Eds.). (1997). *Design and analysis of single-case research*. Mahwah, NJ: Lawrence Erlbaum.

Franklin, R. D., & Krueger, J. (2003). Bayesian inference and belief networks. In R. D. Franklin (Ed.), *Prediction in forensic and neuropsychology* (pp. 65–88). Mahwah, NJ: Lawrence Erlbaum.

Franklin, R. D., Gorman, B. S., Beasley, T. M., & Allison, D. B. (1997). Graphical display and visual analysis. In R. D. Franklin, D. B. Allison, & B. S. Gorman (Eds.), *Design and analysis of single-case research* (pp. 119–158). Mahwah, NJ: Lawrence Erlbaum.

Garb, H. N., & Schramke, C. J. (1996). Judgment research and neurological assessment: A narrative review and meta-analysis. *Psychological Bulletin, 120*, 140–153.

Garrett, H. E. (1958). *Statistics in psychology and education*. New York: Longmans, Green.

Heaton, R. K., & Marcotte, T. D. (2000). Clinical neuropsychological tests and assessment techniques. In F. Boller & J. Grafman (Eds.), *Handbook of neuropsychology* (2nd ed., Vol. 1, pp. 27–52). Amsterdam: Elsevier.

Ivnik, R. J., Smith, G. E., Lucas, J. A., Petersen, R. C., Boeve, B. R., Kokmen, E., et al. (1999). Testing normal older people three or four times at 1- to 2-year intervals: Defining normal variance. *Neuropsychology, 13*(1), 121–127.

Jaccard, J., & Becker, M. A. (1990). *Statistics for the behavioral sciences.* Belmont, CA: Wadsworth.

Jacobson, N. S., & Truax, P. (1991). Clinical significance: A statistical approach to defining meaningful change in psychotherapy research. *Journal of Consulting & Clinical Psychology, 59*(1), 12–19.

Larrabee, G. J. (Ed.). (2005). *Forensic neuropsychology: A scientific approach.* New York: Oxford Press.

Luria, A. R., & Majovski, L. V. (1977). Basic approaches used in American and Soviet clinical neuropsychology. *American Psychologist, 32*(11), 959–968.

McSweeny, A., Naugle, R. I., Chelune, G. J., & Lüders, H. (1993). T scores for change: An illustration of a regression approach to depicting change in clinical neuropsychology. *Clinical Neuropsychologist, 7*(3), 300–312.

Nickerson, R. S. (1998). Confirmation bias: A ubiquitous phenomenon in many cases. *Review of General Psychology, 2*(2), 175–220.

Nickerson, R. S. (2000). Null hypothesis significance testing: A review of an old and continuing controversy. *Psychological Methods, 5*(2), 241–301.

Payne, R. W., & Jones, G. (1957). Statistics for the investigation of individual cases. *Journal of Clinical Psychology, 13*, 115–121.

The Psychological Corporation. (1997). *WAIS-III/WMS-III technical manual.* San Antonio, TX: Author.

Rapport, L. J., Brines, D. B., Axelrod, B. N., & Theisen, M. E. (1997). Full scale IQ as mediator of practice effects: The rich get richer. *Clinical Neuropsychologist, 11*(4), 375–380.

Sawrie, S. M. (2002). Analysis of cognitive change: A commentary on Keith et al. (2002). *Neuropsychology, 16*, 429–431.

Theisen, M. E., Rapport, L. J., Axelrod, B. N., & Brines, E. B. (1998). Effects of practice in repeated administrations of the Wechsler memory scale revised in normal adults. *Assessment, 5*(1), 85–92.

Thorndike, R. L. (1986). The role of Bayesian concepts in test development and test interpretation. *Journal of Counseling & Development, 65*, 54–65.

Ward, N. S., Brown, M. M., Thompson, A. J., & Frackowiak, R. S. J. (2003). Neural correlates of motor recovery after stroke: A longitudinal fMRI study. *Brain, 126*(11), 2476–2496.

Woods, S. P., Childers, M., Ellis, R. J., Guaman, S., Grant, I. & Heaton, R. K. (2006). A battery approach for measuring neuropsychological change. *Archives of Clinical Neuropsychology, 21*(1), 83–89.

Estimation of Premorbid IQ

17

Robert J. McCaffrey
Jana L.Vanderslice-Barr

Introduction

This chapter traces the historical and current practices involved in the assessment of premorbid intellectual ability. The evolution of measures developed to estimate premorbid intellectual functioning will be discussed, and current techniques and the related research will be described.

The measurement of premorbid ability has primarily focused on the estimation of prefunctioning IQ. In an excellent special edition of the *Archives of Clinical Neuropsychology* published in 1997, the issue of the estimation of premorbid functioning was reviewed. Karekan (1997) reviews the inherent flaws in using clinical judgment to estimate premorbid functioning, and proposed several alternative approaches; this opinion is further supported by research indicating that IQ estimates based on clinical judgment were significantly off from a true measurement assessed by a well-validated IQ test (Crawford, Millar, & Milne, 2001). Extensive research has demonstrated that clinical judgment is inherently flawed for a variety of reasons, including the variability of information across clinicians used to determine the premorbid functioning of patients. Decisions based on the outcome of statistical or actuarial methods surpass those based upon clinical judgment alone. Unfortunately, there is no standardized method of estimating premorbid IQ, so clinicians must choose from a variety of methods, not all of which are equivalent, when attempting to estimate the premorbid intellectual functioning of a patient.

Various methods to estimate premorbid IQ have been proposed in the literature, including measurement of current intellectual performance, the use of demographic information and/or actuarial and regression equation techniques, and the use of reading tests. These approaches to determining premorbid intellectual ability may be categorized into either direct or indirect methods (Lezak, Howieson, & Loring, 2004). The direct method for estimating premorbid IQ includes evaluating standardized testing performance from educational/vocational testing, school achievement records, and other test scores from the patient's *pre*injury/ illness status. Unfortunately, these direct methods rely upon data that although domain-specific (e.g., IQ), may not be useful depending upon other factors. For example, an Otis-Lennon IQ obtained in elementary or middle school may not be used to reliably estimate the premorbid IQ of the same individual at age 25, because childhood IQ to adulthood IQ may vary as much as ± 20 points (Lynch & McCaffrey, 1997). More commonly, the estimation of premorbid intellectual functioning relies upon an indirect method, which may include the evaluation of data sources obtained *post*-injury/illness, for example, patient demographic factors, actuarial-based estimates, and the use of complex regression equations, each of which has its strengths and weaknesses. Regardless of the method(s) selected by the clinician, it is only possible to estimate the extent of any decline in IQ following an acquired brain insult.

Methods for estimation of premorbid intellectual functioning originate from the early 20th century. Discussion surrounding methods to quantify "mental deterioration" began shortly after Binet's development of the first test of intelligence in 1905 (Hothersall, 1995). Pressey and Cole (1918) examined 157 "feebleminded," 67 "dementia praecox," and 55 "chronic alcoholic" subjects using A Point Scale for Measuring Mental Ability, developed by Yerkes, Bridges, and Hardwick (1915), which was standardized on unimpaired subjects. The Pressey and Cole (1918) study was conducted to determine whether these impaired groups could be differentiated from each other according to their test performance. The evaluation administered was based on the presumption that at each age, an unimpaired individual has obtained a certain level of intellectual ability. Therefore, an unimpaired, average person would be expected to obtain a numbered score that was roughly equivalent to his/her current age. Pressey and Cole (1918) suggested a number of points that would indicate that a patient should be considered to fall within a certain group (feeble-minded, deteriorating psychoses). The score proposed as a cut-off for group diagnosis was reported by the researchers to enable a 70% probability of correctly differentiating between a feeble-minded or deteriorating (dementia, alcoholic, psychotic) patient. Essentially, this was one of the first studies to develop and evaluate the use of a standardized method for use in clinical settings to identify and diagnose significant cognitive deterioration.

Babcock (1930) was the first to develop and use a scale solely for the estimated measurement of mental deterioration. Babcock administered this measure to 164 unimpaired and 75 paretic, 33 nonimproving paretic, and 42 improving paretic subjects. The full test, including administration instructions, can be found in Babcock's original publication (Babcock, 1930). In a brief review of the available research methods used in examining cognitive deterioration, Babcock stated, "None of them have an estimate of the former intelligence level of the deteriorated subjects, nor give any indication as to how much failure or success may be due to innate pre-deteriorated capacity" (p. 1).

Following the publication of her scale in 1930 for the measurement of mental deterioration, Babcock later stated that the "important practical result is the difference between the individual's normal intelligence and his present efficiency. The former is obtained by the vocabulary test, the latter by a series of efficiency tests which really estimate the power of abstract thinking (Fleming, 1943, p. 2). Interestingly, the Babcock Story Recall Test (Babcock & Levy, 1940), which was one test in the battery of measures Babcock used in the initial development of the Babcock Deterioration Scale, is still being used by some neuropsychologists (Cao, Ferrari, Patella, Marra, & Rasura, 2007; Horner, Teichner, Kortte, & Harvey, 2002).

Subsequent to the work of Babcock (1930) and Babcock and Levy (1940), Shipley (1940) developed a self-administered scale intended to detect intellectual impairment and deterioration. The Shipley-Hartford Retreat Scale (Shipley, 1940) is a short test, which consists of a vocabulary and an abstract reasoning measure. The vocabulary measure was proposed to be insensitive to cognitive decline following impairment, whereas the abstract reasoning portion was included as a measure sensitive to deterioration (Yates, 1956). The full test, including administration instructions, can be found in the original publication (Shipley, 1940).

In 1958, Wechsler published his "Deterioration Quotient." Briefly, Wechsler's Deterioration Quotient was calculated by contrasting subject performance on four "hold" subtests (information, vocabulary, picture completion, and object assembly) with four "don't hold" subtests (Similarities, Digit Span, Digit Symbol, and Block Design). Essentially, "hold" subtests, according to Wechsler, were an accurate measure of premorbid intellectual functioning, as he believed performance on these measures does not deteriorate. Performance on the "don't hold" subtests, he believed, was susceptible to intellectual decline (Wechsler, 1958).

The "Best Performance Method" essentially entails selecting the individual subject's highest test score(s) or highest functioning abilities in everyday life as the basis for estimation of premorbid IQ. According to research conducted by Mortensen, Gade, and Reinisch (1991), this approach grossly overestimates IQ scores, and may lead to errors in the expectation of level of performance of unimpaired subjects and those with diffuse cerebral atrophy on neuropsychological tests.

Current Measures of Premorbid IQ

This section reviews the most well-known current measures for the estimation of intellectual deterioration following injury or illness. The majority of the tests reviewed rely upon the measurement of verbal ability to estimate premorbid IQ. The rationale for using word-reading ability as a measure of premorbid IQ is that the ability to read irregular words has been shown to remain relatively unimpaired throughout the life span, even when faced with neurological damage or deterioration (Willshire, Kinsella, & Prior, 1991). There are those within the research community who have challenged the assumption that word-reading ability is resistant to cognitive deterioration due to illness or injury, and some of the research support-ing this challenge will also be discussed.

National Adult Reading Test

The National Adult Reading Test (NART) has been one of the most popular tests used to assess premorbid functioning postinjury/illness. The NART is a reading test, which consists of 50 irregularly spelled words. The subject is required to pronounce each word and only receives credit if his/her pronunciation is correct.

There are three main versions of the NART. The original test was developed and standardized in the United Kingdom in the early 1980s for use with the original Wechsler Adult Intelligence Scale (WAIS) (Nelson, 1982). Nelson and Willison (1991) published a second version of the NART (NART-2), which was standardized for use with the revised WAIS (WAIS-R). Blair and Spreen (1989) developed an alternate version of the test for use in the United States and Canada, which is known as the NAART or NART-R (North American Adult Reading Test). Other versions include the American modification of the National Adult Reading Test (AMNART) (Grober & Sliwinski, 1991) and the American National Adult Reading Test (ANART) (Schwartz & Saffran, 1987), which were developed solely for use within the United States.

The NAART, which was developed for use in the United States, has been shown to be both a valid and reliable measure of verbal intelligence (Uttl, 2002). The data show that NAART performance is not affected by gender, but that scores increase throughout adulthood and with level of education (Uttl, 2002). To investigate what exactly the NART correlates with in terms of performance on the WAIS, a factor analysis was conducted, and found that the NART only loads on verbal IQ as measured by the WAIS (Crawford, Stewart, Cochrane, Parker, & Besson, 1989).

Crawford et al. (1989) conducted a study on the construct validity of the NART by analyzing performance scores on the NART and the WAIS of 139 normal subjects. According to the results, the NART loaded highly on the WAIS measures of verbal intelligence, but not on factors of non-verbal intelligence, attention, and/or concentration. These results indicate that although the NART may provide an accurate estimate of verbal intelligence as measured by the WAIS, it does not provide a complete picture because the NART does not assess non-verbal intelli-gence. Additional research investigating the utility of the ANART demonstrates the weakness of the test in predicting performance on any non-verbal subtest measures in the WAIS-R (Gladsjo, Heaton, Palmer, Taylor, & Jeste, 1999).

Schretlen, Buffington, Meyer, and Pearlson (2005) administered an abbreviated form of a WAIS measure, as well as the NART-R and various other neuropsycholog-ical test measures, to 322 participants who ranged in age from 18 to 92. They reported that performance on the NART-R correlated highly with both Verbal and Full-Scale IQ scores in healthy adults. Performance on the NART-R did not corre-late significantly with any of the other 26 neuropsychological measures adminis-tered. Schretlen et al. (2005) concluded that these results indicate that the NART-R can be useful in providing information on premorbid IQ, but not in performance in the other areas examined.

Currently, there is some debate about the usefulness of the NART as a measure of premorbid intellectual functioning. O'Carroll (1995) reviewed the literature and reported various studies in which the efficacy of the NART was found to be compromised in certain neurological disorders. These include Alzheimer's disease, Korsakoff's syndrome, Huntington's disease, schizophrenia, and long-term survivors of glioma who have received whole-brain prophylactic irradiation.

In support of the research reviewed by O'Carroll (1995) as mentioned previously, more recent studies show that performance on the NART is sensitive to cognitive deterioration in Alzheimer's type dementia, and may not be the best estimate of premorbid intellectual functioning with this population (Paolo, Tröster, Ryan, & Koller, 1997; Taylor, 1999; McFarlane, Welch, & Rodgers, 2006). Performance on the NART has also been shown to be sensitive to those who have previously sustained a traumatic brain injury (TBI) (Morris, Wilson, Dunn, & Teasdale, 2005).

There is research indicating that performance on the NART is not compromised and may be an accurate reflection of premorbid intellectual ability. Sharpe and O'Carroll (1991) found that the ability to perform well on the NART is not susceptible to cognitive decline in a small sample study of elderly individuals diagnosed with dementia causing neurological disorders. The study analyzed group differences in performance on the NART and the WAIS-R in a Canadian sample of 20 elderly demented and 20 elderly control subjects. The two groups differed significantly on all measures except for the Verbal-Performance IQ discrepancy.

Smith, Bohac, Ivnik, and Malec (1997) assessed the usefulness of the AMNART (Grober & Sliwinski, 1991) in predicting verbal IQ in a sample of subjects diagnosed with early-stage dementia. Each subject had a previous measure of verbal IQ obtained approximately five years prior to the current study. Performance on the AMNART correlated strongly with the subject's previous verbal IQ measures, indicating use of the AMNART as a tool to measure premorbid verbal IQ in early-stage dementia populations.

Use of the NART in estimation of premorbid IQ with closed head-injury populations has been supported in research, which found the test resistant to the effects of neurological damage (Watt & O'Carroll, 1999).

Spot-the-Word

The Spot-the-Word test was developed by Baddeley, Emslie, and Nimmo-Smith (1993) as a measure to test premorbid ability via examination of performance on a lexical decision-making task. The measure involves presenting the test taker with one real word and one invented word. The individual is scored on his/her ability to recognize the real word within the set of words presented. Three studies were conducted to investigate the utility of the Spot-the-Word test. The first study investigated the use of the Spot-the-Word test with 50 subjects considered to have normal intellectual functioning, the second with elderly subjects, some of whom were determined to have intellectual decline, and the third using 224 subjects to assess test norms and test validity, via comparison of performance on both the Spot-the-Word and the NART. Subjects in each study were presented with two alternate versions of the test, each containing 60 word pairs. Performance on the Spot-the-Word test was found to correlate strongly with a measure that has been found to correlate highly with verbal intelligence such as the Mill Hill Vocabulary

Scale (1972) Both the intellectually intact and impaired subjects performed well on both the Spot-the-Word and Mill Hill Vocabulary Scale, indicating that verbal ability, as examined by these measures, may remain intact in the face of cognitive decline. The validity of the Spot-the-Word was assessed in the third study by calculating the correlation between performance on Spot-the-Word and the NART; there was a significant correlation between subjects' performances on both measures, which was stated to support the utility of the Spot-the-Word in predicting verbal intelligence (Baddeley et al., 1993).

McFarlane et al. (2006) assessed the resistance of three measures of premorbid intellectual functioning to the cognitive decline inherent in Alzheimer's disease. Sixty-six subjects with probable Alzheimer's disease and 32 cognitively intact age-matched controls were administered the NART, the Wechsler Test of Adult Reading (WTAR), the Cambridge Contextual Reading Test (CCRT), and Spot-the-Word. The Spot-the-Word was the only measure that did not find significant differences in performance between the two groups. These results indicate that Spot-the-Word estimation of premorbid IQ may provide a more accurate estimation of premorbid IQ in individuals with Alzheimer's disease than the other measures assessed.

Watt and O'Carroll (1999) found that performance on Spot-the-Word was sensitive to severity of head injury in a small sample of subjects who had sustained a closed head injury. In contrast to the results of the aforementioned study, in a large-scale study of almost 2,500 community-dwelling older adults, the Spot-the-Word Test was found to be resistant due to cognitive decline as a result of dementia (Mackinnon & Christensen, 2007). These results are also supported by the findings of Law and O'Carroll (1998).

Cambridge Contextual Reading Test

The CCRT, developed by Beardsall & Huppert (1994), was created by modifying the NART. The words used in the NART were placed into sentences to provide the test-taker with a contextual clue. In the original study (Beardsall & Huppert, 1994), 85 elderly British subjects (all over age 75) were assessed, and only 20 of the subjects were diagnosed with dementia. All subjects were administered the CCRT and the NART; regardless of cognitive functioning, all performed better on the CCRT. The subjects identified as having low reading ability gained the most from the CCRT approach of providing words within context, in comparison with their performance on the NART. Both the minimally and the mildly/moderately demented subjects increased in their ability to recognize and pronounce words when administered the CCRT, in comparison with their performance on the NART.

Additional research indicates significantly increased performance on the CCRT in comparison with the NART in British individuals diagnosed with dementia-causing conditions (Beardsall & Huppert, 1994; Conway & O'Carroll, 1997). The results may be interpreted to indicate that estimates of premorbid IQ based on performance on the CCRT are more valid than those obtained from the NART in the groups assessed. It is important to note that each of the studies cited used small group designs and lacked matched control groups.

The use of the CCRT in TBI patients has produced conflicting findings. According to Morris et al. (2005), the CCRT is sensitive to TBI-induced cognitive impairment. In contrast, Watt and O'Carroll (1999) reported that the CCRT is useful as a measure of premorbid IQ in TBI patients.

Beardsall (1998) developed an equation to convert CCRT errors to WAIS-R Verbal IQ scores based on a relatively small sample of healthy British individuals aged 70 years and older. The inclusion of the demographic information (education, gender) improved prediction. The CCRT has not yet been remodeled for use in North America.

Wechsler Test of Adult Reading

The 50-item WTAR was developed for use in the United States and the United Kingdom; the test was published in 2001. According to a review, it is unclear as to who shares authorship of the test, rather, it seems have been developed by a group of neuropsychologists interested in the estimation of premorbid IQ (Ginsberg, 2003). It has the advantage over other similar reading tests, as it was co-normed with the Wechsler Adult Intelligence Scale-III (WAIS-III) and the Wechsler Memory Scale-III (WMS-III). Co-norming the WTAR with the WAIS-III and the WMS-III allows for direct comparison between predicted and actual functioning with regard to general intellectual status and memory. The age norms developed for the WTAR span from adolescence to late adulthood (16–89 years). The WTAR appears to be an appropriate assessment for the estimation of IQ as measured by the WAIS-III (Strauss, Sherman, & Spreen, 2006).

Use of the WTAR has been shown to reliably estimate IQ in samples in the United Kingdom and the United States; however, recent research in an Australian sample (Mathias, Bowden, & Barrett-Woodbridge, 2007) has reported that the IQ estimates based upon the WTAR were significantly influenced by the phenomenon of regression to the mean. Specifically, the WTAR overestimated the intellectual functioning among those with lower IQ scores and underestimated the intellectual functioning of individuals with higher IQ scores. Furthermore, the WTAR may be sensitive to cognitive deterioration accompanying Alzheimer's disease (McFarlane, Welch, & Rodgers, 2006) and, therefore, may be of limited clinical utility.

The clinical utility of the WTAR among severe TBI patients has been demonstrated to be useful because their performance on WAIS-III subtests significantly improved from 2 to 5 months post-TBI (Green, Melo, Christensen, Ngo, Monette, & Bradbury 2008), although the performance of the patients on the WTAR remained *stable* across the assessments.

Spotting Books and Countries

The Spot-the-Book or Spot-the-Country tests (Scott, de Wit, & Deary, 2005) were developed as alternative techniques to word-reading-based measures for the assessment of premorbid intelligence. These alternative measures require subjects to discriminate between pairs of real and invented book titles, as well as the ability to view outlines of countries and correctly identify the country in question. To investigate the utility of the measures, Scott et al. (2005) administered the NART and Spot-the-Word, Spot-the-Book, and Spot-the-Country tests to over 100 healthy adults. Performance on the Spot-the-Book and Spot-the-Country tests correlated highly with performance on the NART and Spot-the-Word test. The results suggest that premorbid IQ may be estimated with measures that are not dependent strictly on reading ability.

Regression Equations

Some researchers propose that the results obtained with regression-based premorbid IQ equations are inherently flawed (Basso, Bornstein, Roper, & McCoy, 2000; Veiel & Koopman, 2001). Veiel and Koopman (2001) claim that the IQ scores estimated by a regression-based premorbid IQ equation will inevitably overestimate the IQ of an individual whose true IQ is below the population average, as well as underestimate the IQ of an individual whose true IQ score is above the population average. This occurs, in part, because the very essence of regression is to pull values closer to the mean. They propose statistical corrections, which will theoretically adjust for the bias. Yet the removal of the bias results in an increased standard error of estimate under certain circumstances. The authors state that in the case of the Barona index formula, it would only make sense to use their corrective measures when the correlation between the Barona index-estimated IQ and the current measured IQ is at 80 or above, thus creating a situation in which the corrective measures would correct the bias issue and not cause a significant increase in the standard error of estimate.

Basso et al. (2000) investigated the efficacy of regression-based formulas for the estimation of premorbid intelligence. The Barona Demographic Equations, Oklahoma Premorbid Intelligence Estimate (OPIE), and the BEST-3 approaches were included in the assessment. The WAIS-R was administered to 150 neurologically intact adults. The estimated Verbal IQ, Performance IQ, and Full-Scale IQ were estimated according to the procedures required by each of the above-mentioned regression-based assessment techniques. The results indicated that each of these regression-based formulas displayed a tendency of regression to the mean. This implies that all three techniques poorly predict premorbid Full-Scale IQ in subjects who fall on the outskirts of the normal range of Full-Scale IQ scores. Hence, an individual who would have obtained a very high or low Full-Scale IQ prior to injury would have an under- or overestimated Full-Scale IQ, respectively, as estimated by these techniques after intellectual deterioration. This issue is further elaborated on in Graves (2000).

Research has been published that supports the clinical utility of regression equations in predicting premorbid IQ. This research also supports the notion that regression to the mean may not be a significant issue in the use of regression formulas for predicting IQ scores (Vanderploeg & Schinka, 1995). Regression formulas for predicting WAIS-R performance were calculated using the original WAIS-R standardization sample. Thirty-three regression formulae were created by combining 1 of the 11 WAIS-R subtests with subject demographic variables. The predicted IQ scores calculated by the regression equations reportedly accounted for more variance in WAIS-R IQ scores than any other currently available methods (Vanderploeg & Schinka, 1995).

Barona Demographic Regression Equations

The Barona demographic regression approach was developed by Barona, Reynolds, and Chastain (1984). Barona demographic regression equations have been found to underestimate premorbid intelligence for persons with IQs less than 80 and overestimate intellectual ability for persons with IQs greater than 119, as measured by the WAIS-R. The Barona approach has also been found to overestimate the IQ scores of individuals with a validated brain dysfunction (Paolo, Ryan, Tröster, & Hilmer, 1996).

Powell, Brossart, and Reynolds (2003) investigated the use of the Barona demographic equation (Barona, Reynolds, & Chastain, 1984) and the OPIE equation (Krull, Scott, & Sherer, 1995). The study compared the accuracy of the two equations in estimating IQ in a cognitively intact sample and a brain-impaired sample. The Barona demographic equation was found to be the most accurate in estimating IQ scores as assessed by the WAIS-R. Axelrod, Vanderploeg, and Schinka (1999) found that estimates of IQ according to the Barona approach did not differ significantly from those calculated by the BEST-3, OPIE, OPIE-2, and OPIE-3 methods.

In contrast to the results found by Powell et al. (2003), Griffin, Mindt, Rankin, Ritchie, and Scott (2002) reported that premorbid IQ estimates calculated by the Barona demographic equation were inferior in terms of accuracy, in comparison with those computed with the OPIE method. The Barona method was susceptible to the phenomenon of regression to the mean in as much as the formula tended to systematically underestimate the intellectual functioning of individuals with higher level IQ scores and to overestimate the IQ scores of those who were lower functioning (Griffin et al., 2002).

Oklahoma Premorbid Intelligence Estimate-3

Scott, Krull, Williamson, Adams, and Iverson (1997) introduced the OPIE-3 in a study in which 215 subject files of individuals with a clinical diagnosis (e.g., epilepsy, dementia, TBI) from the University of Oklahoma Health Sciences Center were evaluated. Calculation of the OPIE-3 involves consideration of premorbid demographic variables of age, education, occupation, and race, as well as current scores obtained on WAIS-R/WAIS-III subtests. The results reported indicate that the OPIE-3, in comparison to the NART-R, Demographic, and Best Performance methods, was less susceptible to over- or under-predicting premorbid IQ.

A study conducted by Schoenberg, Duff, Scott, and Adams (2003) found that the OPIE-3 (2ST), OPIE-3V, and OPIE-3MR equations did not over- or underestimate premorbid IQ in subjects with brain injury or depression. The OPIE-3 (Best) procedure minimally overestimated Full-Scale IQ in the depressed group. These results indicate use of the OPIE-3 (2ST), OPIE-3V, or OPIE-3MR for use with clinical populations, and the OPIE-3 (Best) with patients who have suffered a mild-to-moderate brain trauma. Further research conducted supports the validity of the OPIE regression equations in predicting WAIS-III verbal, performance, and full-scale IQ scores via use of the WAIS-III standardization sample (Schoenberg, Duff, Dorfman, & Adams, 2004).

Research suggests that the OPIE-3 method for the estimation of premorbid IQ may not be subject to the skewed scores, which are obtained through many other methods, due to regression to the mean/range restriction of scores. In a study investigating the utility of the OPIE-3 for estimating premorbid IQ, Langeluddecke and Lucas (2004) evaluated a TBI group, which ranged in severity from moderate to extremely severe, and a cognitively intact control group. In contrast to the scores calculated using a purely demographic method, the IQ scores calculated with the OPIE-3 IQ method were not influenced by the phenomenon of regression to the mean. The results obtained by the OPIE-3 method were susceptible to neurological damage and resulted in lower-than-expected IQ scores. The outcomes support the use of the OPIE-3 in more severe TBI cases. The use of the OPIE-3 with patients who have sustained a mild to moderate TBI is questionable, as their Full-Scale IQ scores were overestimated by approximately one-third of a standard deviation.

Estimating Premorbid Functioning in Children

Schoenberg, Lange, Brickell, and Saklofske (2007) addressed the premorbid assessment of intellectual functioning in children through the creation of algorithms to predict prior IQ. The study used the standardization sample from the *Wechsler Intelligence Scale for Children-Fourth Edition* (WISC-IV). The sample of 2,172 children was randomly separated into two groups, one for validation, and the other for development. Twelve algorithms were created from the scores in the development group. The algorithms were found to accurately estimate performance on the WISC-IV. The outcome of this study is promising for the development of valid techniques to assess premorbid intellectual functioning in children.

Estimating Premorbid Functioning in Schizophrenia

Cognitive impairment is commonly associated with schizophrenia. Approximately 75–85% of individuals with schizophrenia exhibit abnormal intellectual functioning, memory impairments, and impaired attention and executive functioning skills (Reichenberg et al., 2006).

The diagnosis of schizophrenia and schizophrenia-related disorders is associated with low premorbid IQ scores relative to the general population. In a large-scale, longitudinal study investigating the association between premorbid IQ and risk for the development of psychiatric disorder, low premorbid IQ scores were associated with a higher risk of developing schizophrenia, as well as severe depression and other non-affective psychoses (Zammit et al., 2004). The presence of lower premorbid IQ associated with diagnosis of schizophrenia has also been demonstrated in comparison of IQ scores of individuals diagnosed with schizophrenia and their non-affected family members. Nonaffected family members were found to have average IQ scores, whereas the affected member was generally found to have a lower than average IQ (Toulopoulou, Quraishi, McDonald, & Murray, 2006).

Global intellectual functioning has been shown to remain stable across age groups in individuals diagnosed with schizophrenia, as assessed by subtests from the WAIS (Hijman, Hulshoff Pol, Sitskoorn, & Kahn, 2003), indicating that the lower intellectual ability associated with schizophrenia is present prior to the onset of the disorder. In related research, Reichenberg et al. (2006) investigated the association of premorbid IQ and future development of schizophrenia and schizophrenia spectrum disorders. Lower premorbid IQ assessed at 17 years of age in 54,000 male Israeli Army conscripts was significantly associated with the development of schizophrenia and schizophrenia spectrum disorders. There was no association found between IQ and age of onset of illness.

Russell and colleagues (2000) investigated the use of the NART in a population of British adults with schizophrenia. Only adults who had a childhood measure of IQ were included in the study. Actual IQ scores did not differ significantly from childhood to adulthood. However, the IQ scores estimated by the NART were significantly different from both of the IQ scores measured during the subject's child and adulthood. This was particularly evident when an IQ score deviated significantly from general population mean performance scores.

Discussion

Cognitive Reserve Hypothesis

The cognitive reserve hypothesis suggests that higher levels of educational and occupational achievement, as well as higher measures of general intelligence, serve as protective factors for cognitive ability in circumstances in which cognitive decline is expected (e.g., neurodegenerative disorders, TBI). Individuals who are categorized with higher levels of intelligence and achievement are theorized to "resist" presentation of symptoms of cognitive decline at the same stage in a disease or injury in which an average person would be displaying expected decline.

Several studies published over the past decade or so seem to support the concept of cognitive reserve. Roe, Xiong, Miller, and Morris (2007) conducted an archival analysis in which statistical methods were used to determine whether level of education was correlated with later-than-expected onset of dementia in three national registries of individuals diagnosed with Alzheimer's disease. Higher educational attainment was positively correlated with a "resistance" to the development of dementia in all three registry populations.

Ropacki and Elias (2003) assessed current IQ in a small group of patients who had all recently sustained a TBI. They found that individuals who had sustained a previous TBI obtained lower IQ scores than those subjects who had only experienced the recent injury. The results suggest that those who have sustained a previous TBI may have a decreased level of cognitive reserve in comparison to those with no prior history of injury.

The long-term consequences of experiencing a TBI were examined in a large-scale study of Vietnam veterans (Raymont, Greathouse, Reding, Lipsky, Salazar, & Grafman, 2008). The majority (92%) of the veterans suffered a penetrating head injury approximately 30 years prior to the study. The veterans who had a history of TBI experienced significantly greater decreases in measure intelligence in the long term, compared with veterans with no history of TBI.

Forensic Implications

The estimation of premorbid cognitive functioning has focused historically on intellectual functioning. The estimation of premorbid functioning in cognitive/

neuropsychological domains such as attention, concentration, learning, memory, and executive functioning have not been subjected to the same level of inquiry (Kaufman& Lichtenberger, 2006). This remains an area in need of further investigation. Although the estimation of an individual's premorbid level of intellectual functioning may occur as an issue before the trier of fact (court), the more pertinent issues tend to focus on alterations in other cognitive domains. At present, there is very little empirical data regarding the estimation of premorbid neuropsychological functioning per se, and the estimations of premorbid intellectual functioning are often associated with considerably large confidence intervals (cf. Strauss, Sherman, & Spreen, 2006) that render the accuracy of estimated premorbid IQ scores questionable.

References

Axelrod, B. N., Vanderploeg, R. D., & Schinka, J. A. (1999). Comparing methods for estimating premorbid intellectual functioning. *Archives of Clinical Neuropsychology, 14*(4), 341–346.

Babcock, H. (1930). An experiment in the measurement of mental deterioration. *Archives of Psychology, 18*, 1–105.

Babcock, H., & Levy, L. (1940). *Test and manual of directions: The revised examination for the measurement of efficiency of mental functioning*. Chicago: C. H. Stoelting.

Baddeley, A., Emslie, H., & Nimmo-Smith, I. (1993). The Spot-the-word test: A robust estimate of verbal intelligence based on lexical decision. *British Journal of Clinical Psychology, 32*(1), 55–65.

Barona, A., Reynolds, C., & Chastain, R. (1984). A demographically based index of premorbid intelligence for the WAIS-R. *Journal of Consulting and Clinical Psychology, 52*, 885–887.

Basso, M. R., Bornstein, R. A., Roper, B. L., & McCoy, V. L. (2000). Limited accuracy of premorbid intelligence estimators: A demonstration of regression to the mean. *Clinical Neuropsychologist, 14*(3), 325–340.

Beardsall, L. (1998). Development of the Cambridge contextual reading test for improving the estimation of premorbid verbal intelligence in older persons with dementia. *British Journal of Clinical Psychology, 37*(Pt. 2), 229–240.

Beardsall, L., & Huppert, F. A. (1994). Improvement in NART word reading in demented and normal older persons using the Cambridge contextual reading test. *Journal of Clinical and Experimental Neuropsychology, 16*(2), 232–242.

Blair, J. R., & Spreen, O. (1989). Predicting premorbid IQ: A revision of the national adult reading test. *Clinical Neuropsychologist, 3*, 129–136.

Cao, M., Ferrari, M., Patella, R., Marra, C., & Rasura, M. (2007). Neuropsychological findings in young-adult stroke patients. *Archives of Clinical Neuropsychology, 22*(2), 133–142.

Conway, S. C., & O'Carroll, R. E. (1997). An evaluation of the Cambridge contextual reading test (CCRT) in Alzheimer's disease. *British Journal of Clinical Psychology, 36*, 623–625.

Crawford, J. R., Millar, J., & Milne, A. B. (2001). Estimating premorbid IQ from demographic variables: A comparison of a regression equation vs. clinical judgment. *British Journal of Clinical Psychology, 40*(1), 97–105.

Crawford, J. R., Stewart, L. E., Cochrane, R. H. B., Parker, D. M., & Besson, J. A. O. (1989). Construct validity on the national adult reading test: A factor analytic study. *Personality & Individual Differences, 10*(5), 585–587.

Fleming, G. W. T. H. (1943). The Shipley-Hartford retreat scale for measuring intellectual impairment. *Journal of Mental Science, 89*, 64–68.

Ginsberg, J. P. (2003). Book and test reviews: Wechsler Test of Adult Reading, the Psychological Corporation, Harcourt Assessment Company, San Antonio, TX, 2001. *Applied Neuropsychology, 10*(3), 182–190.

Gladsjo, J. A., Heaton, R. K., Palmer, B. W., Taylor, M. J., & Jeste, D. V. (1999). Use of oral reading to estimate premorbid intellectual and neuropsychological functioning. *Journal of the International Neuropsychological Society, 5*(3), 247–254.

Graves, R. E. (2000). Accuracy of regression equation prediction across the range of estimated premorbid IQ. *Journal of Clinical and Experimental Neuropsychology, 22*(3), 316–324.

Green, R. E., Melo, B., Christensen, B., Ngo, L. A., Monette, G., & Bradbury, C. (2008). Measuring premorbid IQ in traumatic brain injury: An examination of the validity of the Wechsler test of adult reading (WTAR). *Journal of Clinical and Experimental Neuropsychology, 30*(2), 163–172.

Griffin, S. L., Mindt, M. R., Rankin, E. J., Ritchie, A. J., & Scott, J. G. (2002). Estimating premorbid intelligence: Comparison of traditional and contemporary methods across the intelligence continuum. *Archives of Clinical Neuropsychology, 17*(5), 497–507.

Grober, E., & Sliwinski, M. (1991). Development and validation of a model for estimating premorbid verbal intelligence in the elderly. *Journal of Clinical and Experimental Neuropsychology, 13*(6), 933–949.

Harvey, P. D., Friedman, C. B., Reichenberg, A., McGurk, S. R., Parrella, M., White, L., et al. (2006). Validity and stability of performance-based estimates of premorbid educational functioning in older patients with schizophrenia. *Journal of Clinical and Experimental Neuropsychology, 28*, 178–192.

Hijman, R., Hulshoff Pol, H. E., Sitskoorn, M. M., & Kahn, R. S. (2003). Global intellectual impairment does not accelerate with age in patients with schizophrenia: A cross-sectional analysis. *Schizophrenia Bulletin, 29*(3), 509–517.

Horner, M. D., Teichner, G., Kortte, K. B., & Harvey, R. T. (2002). Construct validity of the Babcock story recall test. *Applied Neuropsychology, 9*(2), 114–116.

Hothersall, D. (1995). *History of psychology.* New York: McGraw-Hill.

Karekan, D. A. (1997). Judgment pitfalls in estimating premorbid intellectual function. *Archives of Clinical Neuropsychology, 12*(8), 701–709.

Kaufman, A. S., & Lichtenberger, E. O. (2006). *Assessing adolescent and adult intelligence.* Hoboken, NJ: Wiley.

Krull, K., Scott, J., & Sherer, M. (1995). Estimation of premorbid intelligence from combined performance and demographic variables. *Clinical Neuropsychologist, 9*, 83–88.

Langeluddecke, P. M., & Lucas, S. K. (2004). Evaluation of two methods for estimating premorbid intelligence on the WAIS-III in a clinical sample. *Clinical Neuropsychology, 18*(3), 423–432.

Law, R., & O'Carroll, R. E. (1998). A comparison of three measures of estimating premorbid intellectual level in dementia of the Alzheimer's type. *International Journal of Geriatric Psychiatry, 13*(10), 727–730.

Lezak, M. D., Howieson, D. B., & Loring, D. W. (2004). *Neuropsychological assessment.* New York: Oxford University Press.

Lynch, J. K., & McCaffrey, R. J. (1997). Premorbid intellectual functioning and the determination of cognitive loss. In R. J. McCaffrey, A. D. Williams, J. M. Fisher, & L. C. Laing (Eds.), *The practice of forensic neuropsychology: Meeting challenges in the courtroom.* New York: Plenum Press.

Mackinnon, A., & Christensen, H. (2007). An investigation of the measurement properties of the spot-the-word test in a community sample. *Psychological Assessment, 19*(4), 459–468.

Mathias, J. L., Bowden, S. C., & Barrett-Woodbridge, M. (2007). Accuracy of the Wechsler Test of adult reading (WTAR) and national adult reading test (NART) when estimating IQ in a healthy Australian sample. *Australian Psychologist, 42*(1), 49–56.

McFarlane, J., Welch, J., & Rodgers, J. (2006). Severity of Alzheimer's disease and effect on premorbid measures of intelligence. *British Journal of Clinical Psychology, 45*(4), 453–463.

Morris, P. G., Wilson, J. T., Dunn, L. T., & Teasdale, G. M. (2005). Premorbid intelligence and brain injury. *British Journal of Clinical Psychology, 44*(2), 209–214.

Mortensen, E. L., Gade, A., & Reinisch, J. M. (1991). A critical note on Lezak's 'best performance method' in clinical neuropsychology. *Journal of Clinical and Experimental Neuropsychology, 13*(2), 361–371.

Nelson, H. E. (1982). *National adult reading test (NART).* Windsor, UK: NFER-Nelson Publishing.

Nelson, H. E., & Willison, J. (1991). *National adult reading test (NART): Test manual* (2nd ed.). Windsor, UK: NFER-Nelson Publishing.

O'Carroll, R. (1995). The assessment of premorbid ability: A critical review. *Neurocase, 1*(1), 83–89.

Paolo, A. M., Ryan, J. J., Tröster, A. I., & Hilmer, C. D. (1996). Utility of the Barona demographic equations to estimate premorbid intelligence: Information from the WAIS-R standardization sample. *Journal of Clinical Psychology, 52*(3), 335–343.

Paolo, A. M., Tröster, A. I., Ryan, J. J., & Koller, W. C. (1997). Comparison of NART and Barona demographic equation premorbid IQ estimates in Alzheimer's disease. *Journal of Clinical Psychology, 53*(7), 713–722.

Powell, B. D., Brossart, D. F., & Reynolds, C. R. (2003). Evaluation of the accuracy of two regression-based methods for estimating premorbid IQ. *Archives of Clinical Neuropsychology, 18*(3), 277–292.

Pressey, S. L., & Cole, L. W. (1918). Irregularity in a psychological examination as a measure of mental deterioration. *Journal of Abnormal and Social Psychology, 13*, 285–294.

Raven, J.C., Raven, J., & Court, J. H. (1972), *Mill Hill Vocabulary Scale*. Oxford, UK: Oxford Psychologists Press.

Raymont, V., Greathouse, A., Reding, K., Lipsky, R., Salazar, A., & Grafman, J. (2008). Demographic, structural and genetic predictors of late cognitive decline after penetrating head injury. *Brain, 131*, 543–558.

Reichenberg, A., Weiser, M., Caspi, A., Knobler, H. Y., Lubin, G., Harvey, P. D., et al. (2006). Premorbid intellectual functioning and risk of schizophrenia and spectrum disorders. *Journal of Clinical and Experimental Neuropsychology, 28*(2), 193–207.

Roe, C. M., Xiong, C., Miller, J. P., & Morris, J. C. (2007). Education and Alzheimer's disease without dementia: Support for the cognitive hypothesis. *Neurology, 68*(3), 223–238.

Ropaki, M. T., & Elias, J. W. (2003). Preliminary examination of cognitive reserve theory in closed head injury. *Archives of Clinical Neuropsychology, 18*(6), 643–654.

Russell, A. J., Munro, J., Jones, P. B., Hayward, P., Hemsley, D. R., & Murray, R. M. (2000). The national adult reading test as a measure of premorbid IQ in schizophrenia. *British Journal of Clinical Psychology, 39*(3), 297–305.

Schoenberg, M. R., Duff, K., Dorfman, K., & Adams R. L. (2004). Differential estimation of verbal intelligence and performance intelligence scores from combined performance and demographic variables: The OPIE-3 verbal and performance algorithms. *Clinical Neuropsychologist, 18*(2), 266–276.

Schoenberg, M. R., Duff, K., Scott, J. G., & Adams, R. L. (2003). An evaluation of the clinical utility of the OPIE-3 as an estimate of premorbid WAIS-III FSIQ. *Clinical Neuropsychologist, 17*(3), 308–321.

Schoenberg, M. R., Lange, R. T., Brickell, T. A., & Saklofske, D. H. (2007). Estimating premorbid general cognitive functioning for children and adolescents using the American Wechsler intelligence scale for children-fourth edition: Demographic and current performance approaches. *Journal of Child Neurology, 22*(4), 379–388.

Schretlen, D. J., Buffington, A. L., Meyer, S. M., & Pearlson, G. D. (2005). The use of word-reading to estimate "premorbid" ability in cognitive domains other than intelligence. *Journal of the International Neuropsychological Society, 11*(6), 784–787.

Schwartz, M., & Saffran, E. (1987). *The American-NART: Replication and extension of the British findings on the persistence of word pronunciation skills in patients with dementia*. Unpublished manuscript.

Scott, J. G., Krull, K. R., Williamson, D. J. G., Adams, R. L., & Iverson, G. L. (1997). Oklahoma premorbid intelligence estimation (OPIE): Utilization in clinical samples. *Clinical Neuropsychologist, 11*(2), 146–154.

Scott, K. M., de Wit, I., & Deary, I. J. (2005). Spotting books and countries: New approaches to estimating and conceptualizing prior intelligence. *Intelligence, 34*(5), 429–436.

Sharpe, K., & O'Carroll, R. (1991). Estimating premorbid intellectual level in dementia using the national adult reading test: A Canadian study. *British Journal of Clinical Psychology, 30*, 381–384.

Shipley, W. C. (1940). A self-administering scale for measuring intellectual impairment and deterioration. *Journal of Psychology, 9*, 371–377.

Smith, G. E., Bohac, D. L., Ivnik, R. J., & Malec, J. F. (1997). Using word recognition tests to estimate premorbid IQ in early dementia: Longitudinal data. *Journal of the International Neuropsychological Society, 3*, 528–533.

Strauss, E., Sherman, E. M. S., & Spreen, O. (2006). *A compendium of neuropsychological tests: Administration, norms, and commentary*. New York: Oxford University Press.

Taylor, R. (1999). National adult reading test performance in established dementia. *Archives of Gerontology and Geriatrics, 29*(3), 291–296.

Toulopoulou, T., Quraishi, S., McDonald, C., & Murray, R. M. (2006). The Maudsley family study: Premorbid and current general intellectual function levels in familial bipolar I disorder and schizophrenia. *Journal of Clinical and Experimental Neuropsychology, 28*, 243–259.

Uttl, B. (2002). North American adult reading test: Age norms, reliability, and validity. *Journal of Clinical and Experimental Neuropsychology, 24*(8), 1123–1137.

Vanderploeg, R. D., & Schinka, J. A. (1995). Predicting WAIS-R IQ premorbid ability: Combining subtest performance and demographic variable predictors. *Archives of Clinical Neuropsychology, 10*(3), 225–239.

Veiel, H. O., & Koopman, R. F. (2001). The bias in regression-based indices of premorbid IQ. *Psychological Assessment, 13*(3), 356–368.

Watt, K. J., & O'Carroll, R. E. (1999). Evaluating methods for estimating premorbid intellectual ability in closed head injury. *Journal of Neurology, Neurosurgery, and Psychiatry, 66*(4), 474–479.

Wechsler, D. (1958). *The measurement and appraisal of adult intelligence* (4th ed.). Baltimore: Williams & Wilkins.

Willshire, D., Kinsella, G., & Prior, M. (1991). Estimating WAIS-R IQ from the national adult reading test: A cross-validation. *Journal of Clinical and Experimental Neuropsychology, 13*(2), 204–216.

Yates, A. J. (1956). The use of vocabulary in the measurement of intellectual deterioration—A review. *Journal of Mental Science, 102*, 409–440.

Yerkes, R. M., Bridges, J. W., & Hardwick, R. S. (1915). *A point scale for measuring mental ability.* Baltimore, MD: Warwick & York.

Zammit, S., Allebeck, P., David, A. S., Dalman, C., Hemmingsson, T., Lundberg, I., et al. (2004). A longitudinal study of premorbid IQ Score and risk of developing schizophrenia, bipolar disorder, severe depression, and other nonaffective psychoses. *Archives of General Psychiatry, 61*(4), 354–360.

Ecological Validity Issues That Arise in Medi-Legal Cases When Neuropsychologists Are Asked to Assess Patients With Traumatic Brain Injuries

18

Robert J. Sbordone

Introduction

This chapter examines many of the critical issues that arise when neuropsychologists are asked to assess individuals who have sustained traumatic brain injuries (TBIs) in medi-legal cases. It focuses on the inadequacies of the widely used standardized neuropsychological tests and batteries that have been traditionally used to assess an individual's cognitive functioning following a TBI. It describes why neuropsychological tests were never designed to evaluate changes in a patient's neurobehavioral functioning following traumatic brain damage, and are quite poor at doing this. It examines whether neuropsychological test data should be used to make a diagnosis of brain damage in the absence of the patient's clinical history and medical records, absence of interviews with significant others, and observations of the patient's behavior in real-world settings.

In addition this chapter considers why many neuropsychologists have traditionally based their opinions in the courtroom about the patient's ability to function in real-world settings on his or her test performance in a controlled and highly structured environment that bears little resemblance to the real world, rather than observe how these patients function in real-world settings that are typically complex, noisy, unstructured, and at times even chaotic. It also explores why many neuropsychologists do not rely on the observations of collateral sources about how a brain-injured patient functions in real-world settings, even though they make no effort to observe how these patients function in such settings.

The chapter also examines why many of our widely used standardized neuropsychological tests are inadequate when they are used to assess the cognitive and neurobehavioral effects of damage to the frontal lobes of the brain. It considers why many neuropsychologists fail to recognize the neurobehavioral syndromes that patients frequently exhibit when specific areas of the frontal lobes of the brain are injured. It examines why strict reliance on the use of standardized neuropsychological tests can prevent neuropsychologists from determining whether a patient can live independently, work, return to school, or function effectively after a TBI. This chapter also discusses the importance and the significance of the ecological validity of neuropsychological test data in medi-legal cases.

It examines why many neuropsychologists have traditionally administered standardized neuropsychological tests (e.g., Halstead-Reitan Battery, Trail-Making test, etc.) to brain-injured patients to assess their executive functions, even though such tests were never designed to assess the executive functions of the brain, and may produce inaccurate information about a brain-injured patient's executive functions.

Development of the Halstead-Battery Neuropsychological Battery

Neuropsychological testing in the United States grew out of the American psychometric tradition that used intelligence tests in the 1930s to evaluate the intellectual and cognitive functioning of children and adults. Ward Halstead set up the first neuropsychological laboratory in the United States in 1935. He developed neuropsychological tests based on his observations of brain-damaged patients to evaluate the cognitive, perceptual, and sensory motor functions of individuals to determine whether they had brain damage (Halstead, 1950). With the assistance of his former graduate student, Ralph M. Reitan, he developed a battery of neuropsychological tests that became known as the Halstead-Reitan Neuropsychological Battery.

The Halstead-Reitan Battery consisted of 14 different tests that could be scored numerically (Halstead, 1947; Reitan, 1955). It was administered to a number of patients with documented focal and diffuse brain damage, as well as a group of hospitalized control patients, presumably free of brain disease. The scores obtained by the brain-damaged group were compared with the scores of the controls to identify individuals with brain damage. Reitan developed an index of brain damage (e.g., Halstead Impairment Index) based on the patient's scores and performance patterns (Reitan, 1955) that allowed him to localize areas of the brain that had been damaged, as well as to infer the cause of the patient's neurological injury (e.g., a brain tumor, stroke, or TBI) (Wheeler, Burke, & Reitan, 1963; Wheeler & Reitan, 1962, 1963).

The primary focus of the Halstead-Reitan battery was to assess brain–behavior relationships through a careful analysis of the patient's quantitative test scores. Although the battery was helpful in identifying the location of brain tumors and vascular abnormalities prior to surgery, the success of this battery may have also reflected the lack of sophisticated neurodiagnostic tests (e.g., pneumoencephalogram and electroencephalograph [EEG]) available at that time to identify and localize brain abnormalities or dysfunction.

Problems With the Original Halstead-Reitan Norms

Many neuropsychologists continue to use Reitan's original norms, that were based on a total of only 50 patients ranging in age from 14 to 50 years, with the mean age of 28.3. As a consequence, when these norms are applied to older patients after they have been administered this battery, they may be misclassified as brain damaged. For example, Reitan (1955) reported that after age 45, normal test subjects often scored in the impaired range. Thus, an "average" performance of an older or elderly patient may be interpreted as abnormal or brain damaged. When these norms were used to classify healthy volunteers between ages of 55 and 67, the majority of these individuals were inaccurately classified as brain damaged based on their score on the Halstead impairment index (Elias, Podraza, Pierce, & Robbins, 1990).

Reitan's original norms have been severely criticized by Lezak, Howieson, and Loring (2004) For example, 10 of the 28 control subjects had been receiving care for psychiatric disturbances, some of whom had military combat experience. One control subject was a military prisoner facing imminent life or death imprisonment or execution. Three other control subjects were awaiting frontal lobotomies because of severe behavioral problems (two of which were described as having homicidal tendencies; one had suicidal impulses and was described as having strong homosexual tendencies).

Because Reitan and his associates made no attempt to use demographic corrections for the patient's age, education, or gender, some neuropsychologists (e.g., Heaton et al., 1986, 1996) raised serious concerns about the applicability of Reitan's original norms to individuals whose age, educational background, and gender fell outside the clinical sample used by Reitan. This resulted in the development of demographic normative corrections to interpret the significance of an individual's test scores (e.g., Heaton et al., 1991). Reitan and Wolfson (1986, 1995, 2005) criticized the use of such norms by arguing that the presence of brain damage obviated the need for any demographic corrections. Moses et al. (1999) compared the validity of Reitan's original norms to the Heaton et al. (1991) norms, and found that the Heaton et al. (1991) norms were clearly superior to Reitan's original norms in minimizing the confounding effects of age and education in the interpretation of the test scores. Golden and van den Broek (1998), however, found value in using both sets of norms. Sweeney(1999) on the other hand, identified problems using the Heaton et al. (1991) norms in a brain-injured sample. Horton (1999) and Yantz, Gavett, Lynch, and McCaffrey (2006) also noted problems in using the Heaton et al. norms in a brain-injured sample.

The Limitations of the Halstead-Reitan Battery

The Halstead-Reitan Battery was designed to identify the presence of brain damage; it was *never* designed to identify neurobehavioral problems such as irritability, diminished frustration tolerance, circumstantial and tangential thinking, egocentricity, rapid mood swings, or viscosity following brain damage, neurobehavioral syndromes caused by damage to specific areas of the brain (e.g., orbital frontal lobe syndrome) (Reitan, 1964); or predict how the patients who were identified as brain damaged would function at work, school, home, in the community, or could live independently.

Reitan and his associates have been misunderstood regarding their research approach to interpretation. This misunderstanding when interpreting the patient's test data may have inadvertently handicapped neuropsychologists who mistook a research study procedure for recommendations for clinical practice. For example, when doing the initial research which was supported largely by federal government research grants, Reitan would not consider factors such as the patient's current medical problems, medications, neurobehavioral symptoms, and preexisting psychiatric and neurological problems, as well as information from collateral sources such as the patient's spouse, parents, siblings, friends, and coworkers in analyzing test data because the research design required the interpretation to be based on the patients' test scores alone (Reitan, 1974). The research procedure was needed because the contention by neurologists and neurosurgeons at that time was that extra-test information was the basis for a neuropsychologist's findings rather then the actual test data (Reitan, 1974). In terms of clinical practice, the extra-test information would be integrated with the test interpretation information prior to reaching final conclusions and making recommendations (Reitan & Wolfson, 1986).

Because of this misunderstanding, many neuropsychologists make no effort to observe and record the patient's neurobehavioral symptoms during the examination or observe how brain-damaged patients functioned in unstructured, noisy, complex, and unpredictable real-world settings instead of the controlled, quiet, predictable, and highly structured environment in which they had been tested.

This misunderstood methodology can ignore factors such as a patient's effort, motivation, or fatigue during testing, even though 8–10 hours were required to administer the entire battery. As a consequence, many patient populations (e.g., elderly patients, patients in the acute stages of recovery following a brain injury, patients with serious medical problems, patients with a prior history of neurological disorder or brain damage, or patients who were in pain at the time of testing as a result of arthritis or orthopedic injuries) were often unable to complete the battery or performed poorly.

Reitan (Reitan & Wolfson, 1986) advocates using the battery as a whole when possible but has supplemented the Halstead-Reitan battery, with other tests based on clinical needs. There are concerns that tests in the Halstead-Reitan battery do not adequately assess a patient's verbal and visual learning and memory (Jarvis & Barth, 1994) or frontal lobe functioning (Reitan, 1964) and that use of additional tests is needed based on the clinical needs of patients to be assessed.

Other Approaches to Neuropsychological Assessment

Alexander Luria was initially trained as a cognitive psychologist, and later as a physician and neurologist in Russia. He spent over 40 years studying the cognitive functioning, behavior, and psychological impairments of over 57,000 head-injured war victims and neurosurgical patients. He developed relatively simple neuropsychological tasks that could be administered at the patient's bedside based on his extensive clinical experience and theoretical model of brain–behavior relationships. Luria focused on how patients with damage to specific areas of their brain went about performing these tasks. This methodology allowed him to understand how the brain is organized, functions, and compensates following an injury. Unlike Reitan's approach, Luria's approach relied heavily on the background, competence, and training of the examiner to understand how damage to specific regions of the brain resulted in a disruption of the patient's complex cognitive functions. His approach allowed clinicians to determine whether brain dysfunction was present and, if present, the specific nature of the dysfunction (Luria, 1966).

Luria briefly tried using the tests developed by Halstead, but did not find them helpful because they did not allow him to identify neurobehavioral syndromes caused by damage to specific regions of the brain (Luria, 1966).

American neuropsychologists who had been trained in the use of the Halstead-Reitan battery perceived Luria's nonquantitative approach as lacking in scientific objectivity because it relied heavily on the clinician's expertise, rather than the patient's quantitative test data. Three American neuropsychologists (Charles Golden, Thomas Hammeke, and Arnold Purisch) tried to rectify this by administering several hundred test items contained in Luria's neuropsychological investigation that had earlier been developed by Anne-Lise Christensen (Christensen, 1979), one of Luria's former students, to normal controls, and later to neurological patients. They used discriminant function statistical analysis techniques to determine which test items were sensitive to the presence of brain damage. Their research (Golden, Hammeke, & Purisch, 1978) resulted in a battery of 269 items that was named the Luria-Nebraska Neuropsychological Battery and was first introduced in 1978. Unfortunately, Reitan and many of his students strongly criticized the use and validity of this battery and Luria's approach, which significantly diminished its popularity and use.

Commonly Used Neuropsychological Tests in Medi-Legal Cases

Most neuropsychologists in medi-legal cases are asked to determine whether a patient sustained brain damage when the neurological examination and neurodiagnostic tests (e.g., computed tomography [CT], magnetic resonance imaging [MRI], and EEG studies) are normal. The overwhelming majority of neuropsychologists practicing today in the United States and Canada have either relied on the Halstead-Reitan Neuropsychological Battery or use what has been termed a "flexible neuropsychological battery," which often includes some of the tests found in the Halstead-Reitan battery to evaluate patients with suspected or known brain damage. The choice of tests that are administered by neuropsychologists who use a flexible battery approach often depends on the patient's age, ethnic and linguistic background, physical limitations, type of brain damage, the background, education, and training of the psychologist, and the particular neuropsychological tests favored by the psychologist.

Many neuropsychologists naively assume that the patient's neuropsychological test data can be used to make a diagnosis of brain damage in the absence of the patient's clinical history, medical records, interviews with significant others, and observations of the patient's behavior in real-world settings. In other words, poor performance on a set of neuropsychological tests is often seen as prima facie evidence of brain damage, even if the patient's clinical history or medical records do not show evidence of brain damage (Sbordone & Purisch, 1996).

This mistaken assumption is often made without any appreciation of the complex factors that can influence a patient's performance on these tests (Sbordone & Purisch, 1996) and the patient's ability to function in real-world settings. The patient's neuropsychological test data are often seen as objective, and at times even reified, to possess the same diagnostic certainty of blood gas values or x-rays. As a consequence, many neuropsychologists have offered opinions in medi-legal or forensic cases about the presence and severity of a patient's "brain damage" that are not only inaccurate, but often are absurd.

Problems Related to Inadequate Training in Neuropsychology

Psychologists who have only learned in workshops how to administer, score, and interpret the quantitative test data of patients are likely to be inadequately trained. Workshops typically do not allow the student to administer any tests to patients because they typically do not include any patients. After completing workshops, psychologists often receive little or no supervision by experienced neuropsychologists on how to correctly interpret the test data produced. As a consequence, psychologists trained only in workshops are prone to making repeated errors in their interpretation of the test data.

Because many psychologists may only administer a neuropsychological test battery once a month or even less after completing workshop training, this limited experience does not permit them the opportunity to develop sufficient expertise in its use. As a result, they are likely to overlook the influence of confounding factors such as prior physical injuries or neurological insults, pain and discomfort at the time of testing, headaches, poor vision, impaired hearing, cultural and linguistic factors, the effects of medications and medical diseases (e.g., hypothyroidism, diabetes, and endocrine disorders), psychotic thinking, depression, anxiety, histrionic behavior, or poor motivation to perform to the best of one's ability on the administered tests, when interpreting the patient's test data (Sbordone & Purisch, 1996), even though such factors can cause individuals to perform poorly on neuropsychological tests without ever having sustained a brain injury (Sbordone, Saul, & Purisch, 2007).

Case Example

A neuropsychologist concluded that the patient he examined had sustained a severe TBI as a result of an automobile accident that occurred 3 years ago based on his poor neuropsychological test scores, particularly on tests that assessed his recent memory and problem-solving skills. In doing so, the psychologist ignored the following information: this patient's medical records that made no mention of any head trauma or alteration or loss of consciousness; the patient's clinical history that indicated the patient was not seen or taken to the emergency room after the accident, and was able to safely drive 40 miles home in heavy traffic from the scene of the accident; the patient's vocational history that indicated that the patient had received a promotion, excellent job evaluations, and two pay raises at work after he returned to work two days after the accident. The neuropsychologist also ignored the fact that when this patient arrived at his office, the patient was able to recall the date and time of the appointment, indicated that he had driven over 80 miles to the appointment, arrived on time and was neatly dressed, was able to provide a detailed clinical history that included the names of all of the doctors he had seen and locations of their offices, and the names of the various diagnostic tests he had undergone since the accident; returned from lunch promptly after an hour, and recalled where he had gone to lunch and what he ate; and accurately described the sports and news events that took place during the past week.

Analysis

This case illustrates the danger of basing your opinion of whether a patient has sustained brain damage solely on the patient's test scores. Although a patient may perform poorly on tests that assess his or her memory and problem-solving skills, this does not mean they have cognitive difficulties or have sustained a brain injury. Unfortunately, this neuropsychologist failed to recognize the discrepancies between this patient's test data and his ability to function in a manner that was inconsistent with an individual with severe brain damage. Had he reviewed the patient's medical records and taken a careful clinical history, he would have realized that the patient's test scores had virtually no ecological validity and most likely reflected motivational factors.

The real issue is what should the neuropsychologist be focusing on during the examination: the neuropsychological test scores or the patient's behavior in real-world settings. Some neuropsychologists have difficulty dealing with this ambiguity, and tend to ignore inconsistencies, when they occur. They rely instead on the neuropsychological test data because they believe it to be more "scientific" than the patient's real-world behavior, even though they are usually asked to opine in medi-legal cases about the patient's ability to function in a variety of real-world settings. The issue that often gets overlooked is how the patient's neuropsychological test data can be considered "scientific" if it is not supported by the patient's medical records and ability to function in real-world situations. This predicament is similar to an engineer, who has never seen a hummingbird fly, testify in court that based on his research, it is scientifically impossible for a hummingbird to fly.

The Generalizability of the Normative Test Data

The normative test data used by neuropsychologists to determine whether a particular individual is cognitively impaired or brain damaged is typically obtained in quiet environments that are usually free of any distractions. The furniture and temperature in the room in which the tests were administered are usually quite comfortable. The examiners who administer these tests are usually polite, kind, and professional. They usually speak to the test subjects in a calm manner, provide clear instructions, and whenever necessary provide examples to help the patient complete the tests they are administered. Unfortunately, the normative test data obtained in this highly structured and professional setting to determine whether a patient is brain damaged is most likely not applicable when neuropsychological tests are administered to patients in settings that are dramatically different from the setting in which the normative data were collected.

For example, when individuals are tested in jails or prisons after being arrested for major crimes, many of these settings require the examinee to sit in a small booth behind the thick wire mesh screen, as the examiner and examinees are located in different booths that are electronically linked. The examiner frequently has no control of the lighting (that is often poor), the temperature of the room (that is often too cold or hot), or the background ambient noise (that is often considerable).

The examiner and examinee are often required to sit on small uncomfortable round metal stools that are attached to the floor. Guards who stand several feet away often talk loudly to each other and frequently yell at the prisoners. Testing is often interrupted by loud announcements that are broadcast over the PA system. The guards frequently stare at the examiner and examinee during the examination. Other prisoners who are nearby can often overhear the patient, which eliminates any confidentiality or privacy. If the examinee normally wears glasses or a hearing aid, these devices may not be brought to the examination. If the examinee needs to retrieve them, he or she must notify a guard who must take him or her back to his/her cell. This process not uncommonly takes one or two hours. If the examination is tested around the inmates' feeding and counting schedules, the examinee often must leave the room in the middle of the test they are being administered and may not return until the following day.

Because the neuropsychological tests that are administered to the examinee must be small enough to fit under the wire mesh screen, many neuropsychological tests do not fit under the wire mesh screen and cannot be administered. The background noise (that is often quite distracting) in this setting often compromises the patient's performance on tests that assess their attention, concentration, and memory. Tests that assess the examinee's visual perceptual skills and visual memory often must be viewed through a thick wire mesh screen in a dimly lit room. Finally, the examinee may be forced to wear uncomfortable metal restraining devices on his or her arms and legs throughout the entire examination, which restrict his/her movements.

Testing an individual in this environment is dramatically different from the standard clinical environment in which the test norms were obtained. Because there are no norms available for individuals who are being tested in such environments (Sbordone, Seyranian, & Ruff, 2000), the use of standardized clinical norms for any neuropsychological tests that are administered under these circumstances is likely to lead to a high rate of false positive errors (e.g., determining that the individual is cognitively impaired or brain damaged on the basis of the test data when he or she is not).

It is also very difficult to determine whether there has been any change in the examinee's cognitive functioning if he or she was previously tested in a standard clinical environment or had been previously tested in another jail, or even in the same jail or prison, because the conditions under which he or she had been previously tested may have been quite different.

Use of Symptom Questionnaires to Identify Cognitive Problems and Neurobehavioral Symptoms

Many neuropsychologists use symptom questionnaires and rating scales that are usually completed by patients as they are seated in the waiting room to identify their cognitive and neurobehavioral symptoms, rather than directly interview them. This is commonly done to save time and reduce the cost of the examination. This policy unfortunately ignores the fact that many brain-damaged patients have a poor or limited awareness of their neurobehavioral and cognitive problems, and are often unable to recognize such problems even when they are pointed out to them (Sbordone, Seyranian, & Ruff, 1998).

Rather than giving symptom questionnaires and rating scales to brain-damaged patients to identify their cognitive and neurobehavioral symptoms, these materials should be given to the patient's spouse and/or parents to complete. They are usually able to recognize subtle changes in the patient's cognitive and neurobehavioral functions following a brain injury and the patient's ability to function in real-world settings, as a result of their familiarity with the patient prior to the brain injury and their observations of the patient's behavior since his/her brain injury. Sadly, this is infrequently done by neuropsychologists, because such information is often assumed to lack objectivity and hence compromise the interpretation of the test data.

This makes little sense in light of the fact that if you were applying for a top-secret security clearance to work on highly classified military projects, the evaluators would not solely rely on the results of the psychological tests you were administered. They would carefully interview your spouse, family, friends, teachers, and virtually everyone who ever knew you to assess your ability to adequately perform your duties in a diligent manner, work effectively with others, and handle classified information. This would include a careful background check including your previous job history, marriage, finances, political and religious beliefs, family background, friends, memberships, medical and psychiatric history, history of alcohol or drug use, criminal behavior, loyalty, character, and integrity. If any discrepancies were found between your psychological test scores and the information obtained by them, they would probably ignore the results of the psychological tests you were administered and rely on how you have behaved in the past.

Within the past decade, questionnaires and rating scales have been developed to assess changes in a brain-damaged patient's cognitive, executive, and neurobehavioral functions. These questionnaires and rating scales can be completed by brain-damaged patients and/or their significant others.

The Frontal Systems Behavior Scale (FrSBe), formerly the Frontal Lobe Personality Scale (FLOPS) (Grace, Stout, & Malloy, 1999), is a rating scale that has been designed to measure behaviors associated with damage to the frontal lobes and frontal systems of the brain. Because research has shown that many individuals with frontal lobe dysfunction are capable of normal performance on traditional neuropsychological tests and measures, their behavior in real-world settings can be disordered, which produces an impairment of a person's occupational and social functioning (Sbordone & Purisch, 1996).

The FrSBe was based on the research of Cummings and colleagues (1994) that linked three clinical observable frontal neurobehavioral syndromes to three frontal-striato-thalamic circuits that play a major role in the executive functions of the brain: the dorsolateral prefrontal circuit has been associated with executive dysfunction; the orbital prefrontal circuit has been associated with disorders of emotional and behavioral self-regulation; and the anterior cingulate circuit has been associated with disorders of activation, spontaneous behavior, and motivation, resulting in syndromes of apathy or frontal abulia.

The FrSBe was specifically designed to identify and quantify a brain-damaged patient's neurobehavioral problems and assess changes in his/her behavior since his/her brain injury, by comparing the patient's present neurobehavioral functioning to his/her premorbid state. This also allows the clinician to keep track of any changes in a brain-damaged patient's cognitive and neurobehavioral functioning over time.

The FrSBe can be completed by the patient's significant others and allows input from multiple observers. The manual provides information about the FrSBe materials, administration, scoring procedures, interpretation, and psychometric properties, and contains normative data based on a community-based sample of 436 adults (men and women). The manual also summarizes the research that establishes its reliability and validity.

The Behavior Rating Inventory of Executive Function (BRIEF) is a psychometrically sound questionnaire with large-scale norms. It was designed for parents and teachers of children ranging in age from 5 to 18 years of age (Gioia, Isquith, Guy, & Kenworthy, 2000). The Parent and Teacher questionnaires both consist of 86 items that produce eight theoretically and empirically derived clinical scales that measure different aspects of executive functioning: inhibit, shift, emotional control, initiate, working memory, plan/organize, organization of materials, and monitor. It contains two validity scales (inconsistency and negativity). The clinical scales form two broader indexes: behavioral regulation and metacognition, and an overall score, the Global Executive Composite.

The BRIEF-Adult Version (BRIEF-A) has been designed for patients who are over 18 years of age (Roth, Isquith, & Gioia, 2005). It can be completed by patients and/or their informants. The patient and informant questionnaires both contain 75 items. One of the primary advantages of the adult version is that comparisons can be made between the clinical profiles of brain-damaged patients and their informants to shed light on the patient's awareness of his or her executive functioning. The BRIEF-A can be given repeatedly to assess any changes in the patient's executive functions and his/her awareness of his/her executive dysfunction. The BRIEF-A contains the same clinical scales and index scores as the BRIEF. The BRIEF and BRIEF-A test item scores can be evaluated by computer software programs that can be purchased from Psychological Assessment Resources, Inc. (PAR). Both programs produce detailed statistical analyses and narrative descriptions of the clinical scales and index scores.

Interviewing Brain-Damaged Patients

When brain-damaged patients are interviewed in a highly structured setting, such as a psychologist's or physician's office or by an attorney during a deposition, they may not exhibit neurobehavioral symptoms if they are asked simple, straight-forward questions that can be answered by a simple yes or no response. They are more likely to exhibit cognitive and neurobehavioral deficits when they are asked broad open-ended questions that challenge their frontal lobes and the executive functions of their brains. Under such circumstances, these patients may exhibit circumstantial and tangential thinking, confusion, memory difficulties (e.g., being unable to recall the question), a loss of their train of thought, word-finding difficulties, or confabulation, particularly when they become fatigued, even though they did not indicate that they were having such problems during the clinical interview or on the symptom questionnaires they had completed.

The Validity of the Brain-Injured Patient's Subjective Complaints

Neuropsychologists often fallaciously assume that the patient's neuropsychologi-cal test performance should be consistent with his/her subjective complaints of cognitive difficulties (e.g., the patient complains of severe memory difficulties and performs poorly on memory tests). Unfortunately, nothing could be further from the truth, because the neuropsychological test performance of a brain-dam-aged patient is typically *inconsistent* with his/her subjective complaints (e.g., he/she typically complains of relatively few cognitive symptoms, in contrast to his/her neuropsychological test data that demonstrate significant cognitive deficits).

His/her neuropsychological test performance is more likely to be consistent with the observations of the patient's cognitive and neurobehavioral functioning as obtained by the patient's significant others (providing they are not in denial and accurately reporting the patient's problems) and medical records. When a brain-injured patient's subjective complaints are consistent with his/her neuropsy-chological test performance or are of greater severity than reported by his/her significant others, malingering should be suspected unless the significant others are in denial (Sbordone et al., 2000).

Necessity of Interviewing Collateral Sources or the Patient's Significant Others

Because many neuropsychologists do not interview family members or the patient's significant others (e.g., coworkers, teachers, friends, employers), they are forced to rely almost entirely on their observations of the patient in a highly structured clinical setting and the patient's quantitative test data to determine whether the patient has any cognitive and neurobehavioral problems, even though brain-damaged patients frequently do not exhibit such problems in this environ-ment, and the standardized tests that are traditionally used to evaluate them are often insensitive to their cognitive problems and neurobehavioral symptoms.

Interviewing family members and significant others can often improve the ecological validity of the psychologist's opinions about whether the patient can return to school, work, live independently, or function effectively in the community.

Testing Brain-Damaged Patients in Controlled Artificial Settings Can Mask Their Cognitive and Neurobehavioral Problems

Testing brain-damaged patients in quiet, highly structured settings, combined with the gentle and calm manner of the examiner, not to mention the examiner's patience and concerted efforts to prevent the patient from becoming fatigued or emotionally upset, frequently mask many of the patient's neurobehavioral and cognitive problems that may only be seen when the patient is seen in an unstructured, complex, noisy, stressful, or cognitively demanding situation, particularly when they are fatigued.

Under such conditions, a patient's cognitive and behavioral functioning is often quite discrepant from how they appeared in the quiet, highly structured, and controlled environment in which they had been tested. As a consequence, predictions of how they are expected to function in real-world settings (e.g., work, school, home, community) based on the quantitative test data obtained in this setting are often inaccurate.

Case Example

A 27-year-old female was referred for neuropsychological testing after she sustained a severe closed-head injury during a bicycle versus motor vehicle accident. She had been rendered comatose for 2 weeks. CT and MRI studies revealed bilateral contusions to her frontal and temporal lobes. Prior to the accident, she had worked as a TV news broadcaster, spoke several languages, and had earned a master's degree in economics. During her examination, she appeared articulate, demure, and cooperative. Testing revealed a Wechsler full-scale IQ of 138, which placed her in the 99th percentile, which was consistent with her academic and vocational achievements.

With the exception of some mild cognitive difficulties on tests that assessed her divided attentional skills, her performance on the standardized neuropsychological tests that were administered to her was essentially intact. Her performance on standardized neuropsychological tests that assessed her intellectual functioning, memory, language, perception, judgment, executive functions, motor skills, problem solving, and speed of cognitive processing was intact.

To assess how this patient functioned in a highly unstructured, complex, and noisy environment with numerous distracting stimuli, she was taken to a large, crowded mall on a Saturday afternoon. Before being taken to the mall, she was given a total of $100 by her husband who instructed her to purchase five specific items at the mall.

Her behavior in this setting was covertly videotaped by a professional investigator. Another investigator (a strikingly attractive woman in her late 20s) stood next to her the entire time and covertly recorded whatever she said. Both observers were never introduced to her, but remained at her side throughout the entire 4 hours that she spent at the mall. At no time was either investigator more than 3 feet away from her. Despite this, she never recognized their presence or asked why they were constantly at her side as she walked through the mall. Other shoppers and a security guard noted their presence and came over and asked what was going on.

Shortly after she entered the mall, she walked up to a large posted mall directory trying to locate the kitchen utensils that her husband had asked her to purchase. Although the directory listed where the household items were located, she indicated that she could not find where the kitchen utensils were located. She then walked aimlessly throughout the mall without any apparent goal or plan, even though her husband had written down on a sheet of paper the items that he had wished her to purchase. At no time did she ever pull out this list from her purse to examine its contents or check to see whether any of the items she had purchased were on the list.

She walked through the mall with little or no regard to other shoppers, which resulted in her walking into three shoppers. At no time did she apologize or seem the least bit concerned about what had occurred. On several occasions, she walked to the front of a long line of shoppers and demanded the immediate attention of the salesperson. When she was told by the salesperson that she was waiting on another shopper and to please stand in line, she began cursing very loudly. Thus, she appeared to have little or no regard for the rights or welfare of other shoppers.

When she went into a department store, she walked around on one of the floors several times without realizing that she had done this. She would often pick up items and walk away with them rather than take them to the checkout stand.

She was taken to a restaurant at the mall for lunch, where she was seated only a few feet away from several young children. When the waitress did not immediately wait on her, she began cursing in a very loud manner, which created a scene at the restaurant that resulted in her being asked to leave the restaurant by the manager. Although she had spent the $100 that had been given to her by her husband, she did not purchase any of the items that he had requested.

Analysis

This case demonstrates the discrepancies that can occur between a PUT BACK brain-damaged patient's test results on standardized neuropsychological tests in a quiet and highly structured artificial setting, and how he or she behaves in an unstructured, complex, novel, noisy, and crowded setting. This patient's behavior in this latter setting would not have been remotely predicted by observing her in the quiet and highly structured artificial test setting or by a review of her quantitative test data.

The Ecological Validity of the Neuropsychological Test Data

Ecological validity in the area of neuropsychological testing refers to the functional and predictive relationship between a patient's performance on a particular neuropsychological test, set of tests, or battery, and his/her behavior at home, work, school, or in the community (Sbordone, 1996; Sbordone & Guilmette, 1999; Sbordone, 2007).

Neuropsychologists have traditionally used two major approaches to enhance the ecological validity of their neuropsychological test data. The first approach involves using tests that mimic the demands of the patient's everyday functioning. The second approach involves using neuropsychological tests that have been empirically shown to be correlated or can be used to predict the patient's everyday functioning.

The first approach is known as *verisimilitude*, and refers to the degree to which the tests and measures used mimic the cognitive demands of the patient's environment (Franzen & Wilhelm, 1996). This definition assumes that the neuropsychologist's choice of tests should be determined by the cognitive demands in the settings the patient currently functions within or will function within in the future. Several tests have been developed for this purpose. For example, the Rivermead Behavioral Memory Test (Wilson, Cockburn, & Baddeley, 1985) tries to mimic the demands that are made on a patient's memory in everyday situations.

The primary focus of this approach is to avoid using tests that were primarily designed to identify brain damage, but rather use tests that simulate the cognitive demands of the patient's everyday environment. This approach, however, often overlooks whether the data obtained from such tests, often under highly artificial conditions (e.g., the quiet highly structured environment in which he or she is tested) irrespective of his/her empirical verisimilitude, accurately reflect the demands of the patient's environment.

Sadly, neuropsychologists frequently ignore this issue and use tests that were primarily designed to detect brain damage rather than mimic the demands of the patient's environment. In addition, neuropsychologists often do not interview significant others who are familiar with the demands of these environments, and routinely observe how the patient functions in these environments. In other words, neuropsychologists, as a rule, rarely leave their laboratories or offices to determine whether the tests and the environment in which the tests were administered accurately represent the demands of the patient's environment, and whether the test data obtained under such conditions corroborates the observations of the patient's significant others.

The second approach refers to the degree to which the administered neuropsychological tests are empirically related to measures of everyday functioning (Franzen & Wilhelm, 1996). This approach has been labeled *veridicality*, and typically involves the use of statistical techniques to relate a patient's performance on traditional neuropsychological tests to measures of real-world functioning, such as work performance evaluations, questionnaires completed by significant others, or clinician ratings.

One issue that confounds the validity of this approach is whether the chosen outcome measure accurately reflects the patient's real-world functioning, because the use of inappropriate outcome measures can lead to inaccurate predications of the ecological validity of a particular neuropsychological test or battery. For example, Chaytor and Schmitter-Edgecombe (2003) found after carefully reviewing 17 empirical studies of the ecological validity of neuropsychological tests and outcome measures of everyday functioning that there was considerable variability in the choices of neuropsychological tests and outcome measures that were used, even within the same cognitive domain. For example, they found that these studies frequently ignored the issue of specificity between the tests and the outcome measures that were used. They also found that many of these studies did not specify a priori which neuropsychological tests would be expected to be related to specific measures of everyday functioning and which should not.

Irrespective of these methodological issues, they found that tests of memory had the best ecological validity, whereas tests that purported to assess the executive functions of the brain had the poorest ecological validity. They also noted in their review of these studies that many clinicians seemed perplexed that patients, whose test scores on standardized neuropsychological tests were within normal limits, had impaired executive functions on measures of everyday functioning.

Although the vast majority of widely used neuropsychological tests were never specifically designed to assess a patient's functioning in real-world or everyday settings, within the past decade, some effort has been made to determine whether many of our widely used neuropsychological tests and measures possessed ecological validity in predicting real-world functions such as job performance, activities of daily living, academic performance, work behavior, shopping, everyday life problems, executive functions, adaptive decision making, functional status, driving, and work-related skills (Chaytor & Schmitter-Edgecombe, 2003; Sbordone,1996, 1997, 2007).

The major problem inherent in such studies is that the environments in which these patients were administered neuropsychological tests had little or no resemblance to real-world settings. For example, individuals who were administered neuropsychological tests are usually tested in a quiet and highly structured setting that is relatively free of extraneous or distracting stimuli to optimize their test performance. This type of environment has been a standard in the field for the expressed purpose of reducing extraneous negative influences during the evaluation process, and allows different psychologists to compare the patient's quantitative test data (Sbordone & Purisch, 1996).

Unfortunately, although these particular conditions may optimize the patient's test performance, particularly when they are given tasks that require a high level of attention and concentration, the real issue is whether the test results obtained under such highly artificial conditions can generalize to the patient's environment, which is often unstructured, chaotic, noisy, contains numerous and distracting stimuli, and is highly dissimilar to the conditions under which the quantitative test data were obtained (Sbordone, 2007).

The Use of Significant Others to Improve the Ecological Validity of Neuropsychological Test Data

The presence of family members and/or significant others during clinical interviews can shed considerable light on a patient's neurobehavioral symptoms, and improve the ecological validity of the neuropsychologist's opinions about the patient's ability to return to school or work, live independently, or function in the community. When neuropsychologists rely solely on the brain-injured patient's assessment of his/her ability to function at work, they are often likely to make predictions about the patient's ability to return to work or school that are frequently inaccurate, and potentially harmful to the patient's economic and psychological welfare.

Case Example

A 37-year-old male laborer had fallen 12 feet from a ladder at work and struck his head against the asphalt. He was unconscious for less than a minute, according to his medical records. A CT scan failed to identify any intracranial abnormalities. He was placed on medical leave for 2 weeks and was referred by his physician for neuropsychological testing to determine whether he could return to work. When the patient was seen by the neuropsychologist, he denied any behavioral or cognitive deficits and tested within the normal range on all of the neuropsychological tests that were administered to him. When the psychologist asked him if he felt he was ready to return to work, the patient said he did not see any reason why he could not return to work. Based on this information, this neuropsychologist recommended that this patient was able to return to work. Shortly after the patient returned to work, his coworkers and supervisor observed that he frequently used crude and coarse language, became easily fatigued, often cursed at them, and made serious errors of judgment that jeopardized their safety. As a consequence, he was terminated and had considerable difficulty finding a similar job.

Conditionality

In his dialogue, Meno, Plato demonstrated how Socrates was able to convince Meno that a simple slave boy knew all the principles of geometry by asking him leading questions to prove that all knowledge was innate (Plato, 1952). This phenomenon with respect to the ecological validity of our test data has been termed *conditionality* (Sbordone, 1996, 1997, 2007; Sbordone & Guilmette, 1999).

Conditionality refers to specific modifications of the test protocol or instructions during testing and/or the use of compensatory techniques during testing that allow the patient to ignore extraneous or distracting stimuli, attend to the examiner and task, comprehend and recall the test instructions, perform according to the test requirements, use cues and prompts to minimize problems of initiation and organization, and foster a positive emotional and/or psychological state and attitude during the examination to compensate for the patient's cognitive and neurobehavioral deficits, to allow the patient to perform at an optimal level of cognitive efficiency throughout the entire test or battery.

If most people were asked whether they could fly a 747 jet, they would probably state that they could not do this. The truth, however, is that most people are capable of flying a 747 without even going to flight school, if the pilot were sitting next to them in the cockpit as they were flying at altitude instructing them what to do in a gentle, simple, and reassuring manner. However, if the pilot suddenly passed out or died, the individual who had been following the instructions of the pilot would most likely be unable to continue flying the aircraft. In other words, under the right set of conditions, many individuals would be capable of flying an aircraft without ever attending flight school. However, if these conditions changed, then this individual would be unable to fly and land the aircraft.

In reality, many neuropsychologists consciously or unconsciously modify standard test instructions or procedures when they are evaluating patients with brain damage. For example, the examiner may repeat the test instructions or permit the patient to spend more time warming up prior to administering a test to them. The examiner may provide frequent cues and prompts throughout testing to minimize the patient's problems of initiation and the effects of fatigue, redirect the patient back to the task, and keep the patient as motivated as possible to facilitate his/her test performance (e.g., using praise or rewards).

Unfortunately, these modifications are usually not recorded by neuropsychologists, because the traditional focus of testing has been placed on the patient's quantitative test performance rather than his/her behavior during testing.

If the examiner follows strict test guidelines that specify precisely what can be said or done with a patient during the administration of a test and does not provide any cues, prompts, or any more rehearsal or practice time than is specified by the test manual, the patient's test scores will most likely be significantly impaired. This will often cause the neuropsychologist to report that the patient has significant cognitive deficits that render him or her incapable of competitive employment or returning to the job he/she held at the time of his/her brain injury.

If brain-damaged patients are placed in a highly structured and familiar work setting that provides them with frequent cues, prompts, and contains caring and patient individuals who compensate for the patient's cognitive and neurobehavioral deficits, a surprising number of brain-damaged patients can function reasonably well at their jobs even though their cognitive functioning is impaired.

Case Example

A 40-year-old attorney who sustained a severe TBI in a motor vehicle accident was referred for neuropsychological testing 2 years postinjury. Review of his medical records revealed that he had sustained bilateral contusions to the anterior frontal and temporal lobes, a subdural hematoma, and a subarachnoid hemorrhage. The damage to his right temporal lobe was so severe that the anterior 6 cm had to be surgically removed.

The neuropsychologist who had tested this patient at the 1-year post-injury mark strongly felt that this patient was incapable of ever practicing law based on his poor test scores. When another neuropsychologist later saw him after he had gone back to work, the patient indicated that he was doing well at his job and as a husband and father at home.

When the latter neuropsychologist interviewed the staff at his law firm, they admitted that they had felt sorry for him when he returned to work, and had provided him with a great deal of organization, structure, cues, frequent prompts, and reminders to help him function more effectively at work. For example, although the other attorneys in the firm had shared a secretary with one or two other attorneys, this patient needed three full-time secretaries and two legal assistants to help him perform his job, even though he was billing considerably less than any other attorney in the firm.

The patient compensated for his cognitive impairments by putting in long hours each day (usually 11–12 hours a day) and working weekends, in comparison with only working 6 or 7 hours a day 4 days a week prior to his accident. At home, his wife, who was no longer practicing law after she had decided to become a full-time homemaker to care for their two young children, admitted that since her husband's accident she had been making all of the family decisions at home, which her husband had made prior to his accident. She also indicated that she had taken over all of the household duties and responsibilities that had been previously performed by her husband, and would often assist her husband with his legal work at night.

Analysis

This case illustrates that when a severely brain-injured patient is placed in a highly structured environment that contains individuals who serve as his/her "ancillary frontal lobes" by providing him or her with frequent reminders, cues, prompts, guidance, structure, feedback, organization, and take over many of his/her responsibilities to compensate for his/her cognitive impairments, he or she often can return to work and create the superficial appearance that he or she has made an excellent recovery. Neuropsychologists should recognize the issue of conditionality when they are asked to predict whether a patient can return to work and maintain his/her job. Unfortunately, many neuropsychologists fail to interview the patient's family, coworkers, employers, friends, or spouses to determine how the patient is performing at work and under what conditions the patient is able to perform his job duties and responsibilities.

Widely Held Assumptions by Neuropsychologists

Neuropsychologists as a result of their educational background, training, and experience often hold assumptions about how neuropsychological testing should be performed that may actually handicap them in dealing with the issue of the ecological validity of their test data. For example, many neuropsychologists take workshops in which they are not told that it is necessary to take a detailed clinical history or interview collateral sources,. These workshops may emphasize that neuropsychologists should rely on a patient's quantitative neuropsychological test data and not emphasize that having knowledge of the patient's medical records is necessary to arrive at accurate opinions about the patient's brain–behavior relationships and/or localization of brain dysfunction.

Neuropsychologists may be taught in these workshops that it is essential that standardized tests and/or batteries be used to arrive at any meaningful opinions about the presence or absence of cognitive dysfunction and/or brain damage. They are taught that any changes in the patient's cognitive functioning over time can best be determined by a careful examination of the patient's serial test data. They are also taught that the neuropsychologist's (or technician who administers the tests) primary responsibility is to record and score the patient's quantitative responses to specific test stimuli during testing.

As result of taking these workshops, many neuropsychologists assume that it is not necessary to record the amount and type of practice or the various cues, prompts, or strategies that are given to the patient or are used by the patient during testing, because a review of the patient's raw test data is sufficient to determine the patient's cognitive impairments (Sbordone, 1996, 1997, 2007).

Many neuropsychologists assume incorrectly that the neuropsychological test data can be best interpreted in the absence of information from other sources (e.g., historical information, medical records, academic records, interviews with significant others, etc.). Observations of the patient's behavior outside of the testing environment or in real-world settings is often seen as irrelevant and misleading, and in some cases, even unethical, because they often assume that careful interpretation of the test data is sufficient to predict how a patient is likely to function in real-world settings (e.g., return to work or school, or live independently), even though the tests they are relying on were never designed to do this and usually have little ecological validity.

Many neuropsychologists assume that intact performance on standardized neuropsychological tests or batteries can determine whether the patient has cognitive deficits and/or has a brain injury. They often assume that it is not necessary to review the patient's medical chart if they are trying to determine whether the patient has sustained a brain injury, because this can best be determined by careful examination of the quantitative test data.

Irrespective of whether such assumptions are faulty or have any merit, neuropsychologists who hold such assumptions are likely to find it difficult to deal with the issue of the ecological validity of their neuropsychological test data (Reitan, 1964). For example, if you fail to observe the patient's ability to function outside of the highly structured and artificial environment in which they were administered neuropsychological tests, and do not interview significant others to obtain information about how the patient functions at home or in the community, both prior and following his/her brain injury, it is nearly impossible to determine whether the test data has any ecological validity (Sbordone & Purisch, 1996).

Some neuropsychologists believe that using standardized neuropsychological tests and their careful interpretation of the test data is more scientific than observing the patient functioning in real-world settings, and that any information obtained from significant others is unscientific. In other words, they assume that any digression from the standard test protocol would not yield valid or reliable data (Sbordone & Purisch, 1996).

Neuropsychological Tests Were Never Designed to Assess Neurobehavioral Problems

Neuropsychologists frequently assume that a patient's neurobehavioral problems can be detected by standardized neuropsychological tests, even though such tests were never designed to indentify these problems, and are actually quite poor at this (Reitan, 1964). For example, standardized neuropsychological tests are essentially unable to detect neurobehavioral problems following a brain injury, such as irritability, rapid mood swings, poor safety judgment, problems with emotional and behavioral regulation, loss of curiosity, impulsivity, uninhibited speech or behavior, use of crude or coarse language, circumstantial and tangential thinking, poor frustration tolerance, inability to feel compassionate or show affection toward others, loss of libido, uninhibited social behavior, rapid fatigue, viscosity, emotional lability, apathy, inappropriate social behavior, egocentricity, poor judgment, anhedonia, inability to plan for future events, reduced responsiveness to environmental cues, hyperverbosity, or hypersomnia, even though such problems have been commonly reported by their significant others.

Because neuropsychological tests were not specifically designed to identify a patient's neurobehavioral problems (Reitan, 1964), these problems must be recognized by the neuropsychologist during the examination when and if they occur. Unfortunately, the training of many neuropsychologists is usually focused on how to administer, score, and interpret standardized quantitative tests, rather than observe the patient's neurobehavioral functioning during the examination (Sbordone & Purisch, 1996).

Because most neuropsychologists rely on the use of questionnaires to gather information about the patient's symptoms and background, and use technicians to administer and score the neuropsychological tests that are administered to patients who have sustained brain injuries, they may spend only 15–20 minutes with patients, even though the entire examination may last for 8–10 hours. This dramatically limits the amount of time available to observe and identify a patient's neurobehavioral problems when they occur (Sbordone & Purisch, 1996).

The patient's significant others, when they are interviewed for a lengthy period of time, will frequently report observing significant changes in the patient's neurobehavioral functioning without recognizing their relationship to the patient's TBI. When they are asked to describe any changes they have observed in the patient's behavior and cognitive functioning since the patient's accident, they will often report observing a dramatic change in the patient's personality since the accident that includes poor frustration tolerance, increased irritability, marked egocentricity, an inability to express affection toward others, a negative change in the patient's personal hygiene and grooming, loss of libido, circumstantial and tangential thinking, word-finding difficulties, apathy, poor judgment, confusion, difficulty initiating and following through on tasks, and rapid mood swing. They often admit that they are puzzled by the patient's poor awareness of these problems, and how the patient believes that he or she is fine and can return to work or school without any difficulty.

Standardized Neuropsychological Tests Were Never Designed to Assess the Frontal Lobes of the Brain

Stuss and Benson (1986) stressed that neuropsychological tests were not specifically designed to evaluate the frontal lobes of the brain. They emphasized that identification of the neurobehavioral and cognitive symptoms of frontal lobe pathology depended to a large degree on the *competence and experience of the neuropsychologist*. They stressed that a patient's neuropsychological test data needed to be supplemented by interviews with significant others, observations of the patient's behavior in real-world settings, and a review of the patient's medical records to determine how the patient was functioning while he or she was receiving treatment following his/her brain injury, and after he or she returned home and to his/her community.

A number of prominent neuropsychologists and behavioral neurologists has pointed out how inadequate neuropsychological tests are to assess damage to the frontal lobes and the regions connected to the frontal lobes of the brain. For example, Reitan (1964) documented difficulties in assessing the frontal lobes with the Halstead-Reitan Battery. In addition,, Bigler (1988) stressed that traditional neuropsychological tests and measures were generally insensitive to alterations in the patient's behavior caused by frontal lobe damage. He stressed that the patients themselves lacked awareness that such alterations had occurred. He strongly emphasized the importance of careful observations of the patient's behavior and detailed interviews of the family members and significant others who have observed the patient to assess any alterations in the patient's executive functions.

Although standardized neuropsychological tests are widely used to assess patients who have sustained frontal lobe injuries, Damasio (1985) reported that patients who had most of their prefrontal lobes surgically removed often tested in the normal range on IQ tests and other standardized neuropsychological tests. He found, however, that in real-world settings, these patients frequently exhibited the following neurobehavioral symptoms: loss of initiative, curiosity, exploratory behavior, motivation, creativity, and libido; an inability to regulate their behavior and emotions; an inability to organize their thoughts, plan, remain on task, monitor their actions, problem solve, recognize their mistakes, or rectify them when they were made aware of them by others; impaired social behavior, inflexible thinking, poor judgment, impulsivity, egocentricity, an inability to show affection or feel compassion toward others; crude or coarse language; lack of plans or concern for future events; an inability to profit from experience; and a tendency to confabulate when they were asked to recall information .

Mesulam (1986) felt that the behavioral changes associated with frontal lobe damage were almost impossible to quantify through traditional neuropsychological tests and batteries. He felt that our traditional methods of testing the frontal lobes were often overly simplistic. For example, some neuropsychologists have naively assumed that a patient's performance on the Trail-Making Test can assess his/her frontal lobes or executive functions. Zangwill (1966) has also pointed out that patients with frontal lobe injuries will often perform in the normal range on standardized neuropsychological tests. As a consequence, he felt that the standardized neuropsychological tests were inadequate to assess the cognitive deficits caused by frontal lobe injuries.

Despite this evidence, many neuropsychologists continue to use and rely on standardized neuropsychological tests to determine whether a patient has sustained frontal lobe damage. Many neuropsychologists continue to assume that, if a patient's test scores on standardized neuropsychological tests (that they believe assess the frontal lobes) fall in the average or expected range, the patient's frontal lobes are intact, even though the patient is observed by his/her significant others to exhibit neurobehavioral problems consistent with frontal lobe damage or dysfunction.

Many neuropsychologists assume a patient's performance on the Wisconsin Card Sorting Test, which has been frequently used to assess the integrity of the frontal lobes, can determine whether a patient has sustained damage to his/her frontal lobes, even though it is generally well known that individuals who sustain damage to their orbital frontal lobes typically perform well on this test (Stuss & Benson, 1986).

Luria and Tsvetkova (1990) observed that although many patients with frontal lobe lesions typically did fairly well on neuropsychological tests, they exhibited qualitative changes in cognitive functioning when they were asked to solve problems. They observed that they approached the problem-solving task quite differently, and were generally unable to formulate a plan that was needed to solve the problem when the task required a preliminary analysis of the problem itself.

Sadly, many neuropsychologists do not understand the effects of damage to the frontal lobes. For example, patients who are involved in motor vehicle accidents frequently sustain damage to their lateral orbital frontal lobes when they are struck by a motor vehicle. Although these patients will usually deny any behavioral or cognitive symptoms and typically perform in the normal range on standardized neuropsychological tests, they frequently exhibit neurobehavioral problems such as a dramatic change in their personalities, which is observed by their families and significant others but not by the patients. They are unable to control their behavior or regulate their emotions. They exhibit a loss of social tact, poor impulse control, an inability to empathize with others, marked egocentricity, frequently use crude and coarse language at home, exhibit inappropriate social behavior, poor frustration tolerance, rapid mood swings, poor judgment, and have little or no awareness of how their neurobehavioral problems affect others, which prevent them from maintaining employment and alienate their families, friends, and coworkers. These patients often have problems with law enforcement authorities because of their poor judgment, impulsivity, and inability to regulate their emotions and behavior.

Most neuropsychologists do not understand the neurobehavioral sequelae of damage to the medial orbital frontal lobes, even though this area of the brain is commonly injured during high-speed motor vehicle accidents. Although individuals with such injuries will usually perform in the normal range on standardized neuropsychological tests, they typically exhibit the following neurobehavioral problems: a loss of motivation, loss of energy and drive, loss of pleasure from the environment, pseudodepression, psychomotor retardation, a change in their eating habits, loss of sex drive, loss of curiosity, and obsessive-compulsive behavior that typically does not respond to psychiatric treatment (Sbordone & Purisch, 1996).

Why Do the Neurobehavioral Symptoms of Patients With Frontal Lobe Injuries Go Unrecognized?

This commonly occurs when the neuropsychologist fails to interview the patient's significant others and bases his or her opinions on the patient's performance on standardized neuropsychological tests, which are often administered by a technician or someone in training, often without the neuropsychologist being present. It can also occur when the neuropsychologist has a poor understanding of the neurobehavioral symptoms of orbital frontal lobe pathology, takes an inadequate history, fails to review the patient's medical and/or rehabilitation records, and naively assumes that poor performance on neuropsychological tests indicates brain damage and relatively normal performance indicates no brain damage. It can also occur when the neuropsychologist does not spend any time observing how the patient functions in unstructured, noisy, complex, and novel settings (Sbordone & Purisch, 1996).

Some neuropsychologists stress the importance of interpretation of the patient's test data and do not adequately review the patient's clinical history and medical records. This practice can result in the neuropsychologist forming opinions based primarily on neuropsychological tests that are often insensitive to the neurobehavioral symptoms caused by orbital frontal lobe damage. This increases the likelihood that the neuropsychologist's predictions about the patient's ability to function in real-world settings will be inaccurate and misleading, and has the potential of arriving at opinions that may be harmful to the patient's welfare and/or the patient's significant others (Sbordone & Purisch, 1996).

Case Example

A 27-year-old male sustained a blunt head injury as a result from falling from a ladder and striking his head on the ground. He sustained a brief loss of consciousness and was observed to be combative at the scene of the accident. He had a Glasgow Coma Scale rating of 14 when the paramedics arrived. He was taken into the emergency room and was released later that day after his x-rays and a CT scan of his head were normal. Within a few weeks, his wife observed a dramatic change in her husband's personality. Specifically, she observed that her husband had a great deal of difficulty controlling his emotions and temper, and would often hit her and throw things with little or no provocation. She denied that he had ever acted this way prior to the accident. She contacted her family physician, who referred her husband to a psychologist for neuropsychological testing. When he was seen, he denied any cognitive difficulties or problems controlling his emotions.

Because his test scores on each of the neuropsychological tests that were administered to him fell into the normal range, the psychologist contacted the referring physician and informed him that the patient showed no evidence of brain damage or cognitive deficits. Unfortunately, 3 weeks later, the patient struck his wife with a heavy metal crowbar during an argument and killed her.

Analysis

The psychologist based his opinions on the patient's intact performance on the neuropsychological tests that he administered to the patient. The psychologist had never interviewed the patient's spouse or had ever observed how this patient functioned outside of his office or in stressful situations. The psychologist was apparently unfamiliar with the neurobehavioral symptoms of an orbital frontal lobe contusion and the insensitivity of standardized neuropsychological tests to assess damage to this region of the brain.

Neuropsychological Tests Were Never Designed to Assess the Executive Functions of the Brain

The executive functions of the brain are a complex process of integrated cognitive activities. For example, Sbordone (2000) has described it as a complex process by which an individual goes about performing a novel problem-solving task from its inception to completion. This process includes an awareness that a particular problem or need exists, an evaluation of the particular problem or need, an analysis of the conditions of the problem, formulation of specific goals necessary to solve this problem, development of a set of plans to determine which actions are needed to solve this problem, an evaluation of the potential effectiveness of these plans, the selection and initiation of a particular plan to solve the problem, evaluation of any progress made toward solving the problem or need, modification of the plan if it is not effective, disregarding ineffective plans and replacing them with more effective plans, comparing the results achieved by the new plan with the conditions of the problem, terminating the plan when the conditions of the problem have been satisfied, storing the plan, and retrieving it later if the same or similar problem appears.

Although neuropsychological tests were primarily designed to assess whether a person has brain damage, they were never designed to assess the executive functions of the brain. Much like the man crawling on his hands and knees along the street at night trying to find his keys on the street in front of his house that he lost two blocks away, because the light is better at this location, neuropsychologists frequently rely on neuropsychological tests that are believed to be sensitive to the frontal lobe damage to assess the executive functions of the brain, because they assume that the executive functions are located in the frontal lobes. This assumption, however, is faulty, because injuries to subcortical and other non-frontal brain structures that have connections to the frontal lobes can produce executive dysfunction, even though the patient's frontal lobes are intact (Cummings, 1995). For example, subcortical disorders such as Parkinson disease, progressive super nuclear palsy, Huntington's disease, Korsakoff's syndrome, and dementia caused by carbon monoxide exposure and inhalation of organic solvents are well known to produce executive dysfunction (Sbordone, 2000).

Many neuropsychologists assume that the best way to assess the executive functions of the brain is to administer standardized neuropsychological tests. However, a patient's performance on these tests may not provide accurate information about his/her executive functions, because they may only assess a few, but not all, of the complex steps that involve the executive functions of the brain (Cripe, 1996; Sbordone, 2000, 2007). By analogy, using these tests to assess a patient's executive functions is comparable to being asked to write a review of the movie *Titanic* after watching only 10 minutes of the film. This would not provide sufficient time to comprehend the complexity, richness, and drama of this movie. The only way to fully appreciate the movie and write a meaningful review would be to watch the entire movie from start to finish. Unfortunately, the manner in which neuropsychologists currently practice today (e.g., administering tests rather than observing the patient function in real-world settings) is the primary reason why we do not understand the executive functions of the brain or how to adequately assess them.

Whereas a patient's score on a particular neuropsychological test or measure may not adequately assess a patient's executive functions, or have any bearing on a patient's ability to function effectively in real-world settings (e.g., home, work, school, community), some relatively non-standardized tests have shown some promise in predicting the efficacy of a brain-damaged patient's executive functions in a variety of everyday settings. For example, tests such as the Behavioral Assessment of the Dysexecutive Syndrome (BADS) (Wilson, 1993; Wilson, Alderman, Brugess, Emslie, & Evans, 1996), Tinker Toy (Lezak, 1987, 1995), and the Behavioral Assessment of Vocational Skills (BAVS) (Butler, Anderson, Furst, & Namerow, 1989; Butler, Rorsaman, Hills, & Tumama, 1993), may be helpful in identifying subtle executive dysfunction in a patient's everyday behaviors that is not identified by standardized neuropsychological tests (Sbordone & Guilmette, 1999).

How to Best Determine the Ecological Validity of the Test Data

Sbordone, 1997 and 2007; Sbordone and Guilmette, 1999; and Sbordone and Purisch (1996) have recommended that neuropsychologists use what has been termed a "vector analysis approach" to evaluate the ecological validity of a patient's neuropsychological test data. Sbordone and his associates have stressed that if the information obtained about the patient's neurobehavioral functioning from different sources such as the significant others, medical, academic, and vocational records is consistent with the patient's neuropsychological test data, there is a high probability that the test data is ecologically valid. On the other hand, if the test data is inconsistent with this information (e.g., the test data indicates that the patient is severely impaired three years postmotor vehicle accident in the face of medical records indicating no loss of consciousness, amnesia, disorientation, or brain or head trauma combined with academic and vocational records, which document appreciable educational and vocational attainment subsequent to the accident), there is a high probability that the ecological validity of the test data is poor. When the latter occurs, neuropsychologists should explore alternative explanations of the test data to avoid at arriving at premature diagnoses, opinions, or predictions about the patient's functioning in real-world situations.

The Importance of Considering the Ecological Validity of the Test Data in Medi-Legal Cases

Because many psychologists often perceive their role in medi-legal cases as determining whether a person has sustained a brain injury and its severity, they often have ignored the issue of the ecological validity of their test data. Unfortunately, the courts today are interested in knowing whether a plaintiff can engage in competitive employment, return to the job he or she held at the time of his/her accident, successfully return to school, complete his/her educational requirements to obtain a diploma or degree, manage his/her finances, operate an automobile or machinery, return to his/her household duties and responsibilities, safely raise his/her children, and/or live independently. Determining that a patient has brain damage does not automatically permit a neuropsychologist to predict how this patient will function in real-world settings and/or cope with the demands of his or her environment unless the brain injury is catastrophic.

The importance of the ecological validity of the test data cannot be overemphasized, because this issue can significantly affect a neuropsychologist's credibility in the courtroom. For example, if the test findings are consistent with the observations of the patient's significant others and the medical records, then the test results are likely to be seen by the court as accurately reflecting the patient's cognitive deficits. Any opinions offered by the neuropsychologist at time of trial will most likely be given more weight by the court. On the other hand, if the neuropsychologist's opinions based on the test data are seen as discrepant from the patient's functioning in real-world settings, the opinions of the neuropsychologist will most likely be given little weight by the court.

Acknowledgment

Part of this chapter was presented at a Conference on Medical and Legal Issues on Brain Injury in Vancouver, BC, Canada, on March 28–29, 2008.

References

Bigler, E. D. (1988). Frontal lobe damage and neuropsychological assessment. *Archives of Clinical Neuropsychology, 3,* 279–297.

Butler, R. W., Anderson, L., Furst, C. J., & Namerow, N. S. (1989). Behavioral assessment in neuropsychological rehabilitation: A method for measuring vocational related skills. *Clinical Neuropsychologist, 3,* 235–243.

Butler, R. W., Rorsaman, I., Hills, J. M., & Tumama, R. (1993). The effects of frontal brain impairment on fluency: Simple and complex paradigms. *Neuropsychology, 7,* 519–529.

Chaytor, N., & Schmitter-Edgecombe, M. (2003). The ecological validity of neuropsychological tests: A review of the literature on everyday cognitive skills. *Neuropsychological Review, 13*(4), 181–197.

Christensen, A. L. (1979). *Luria's neuropsychological investigation* (2nd ed.). Copenhagen, Denmark: Munksgaard.

Cripe, L. I. (1996). The ecological validity of executive function testing. In R. J. Sbordone & C. Long (Eds.), *Ecological validity of neuropsychological testing* (pp. 129–146). Delray Beach, FL: GR/St. Lucie Press.

Cummings, J. L. (1993). Frontal-subcortical circuits and human behavior. *Archives of Neurology, 50*(8), 873–880.

Cummings J. L. (1995). Anatomic and behavioral aspects of frontal-subcortical circuits. In J. Grafman, K. J. Holyoak, & F. Boller (Eds.), *Structure and function of the human pre-frontal cortex: Vol. 769: Annals of the New York Academy of Sciences* (pp. 1–13). New York: Academy of Sciences.

Cummings, J. L., Mega, M., Gray, K., Rosenberg-Thompson, J. Carusi, D. A., & Gornbein, J. (1994). The neuropsychiatric inventory: Comprehensive assessment of psychopathology in dementia. *Neurology, 44*(12), 2308–2314.

Damasio, A. R. (1985). The frontal lobes. In K. M. Heilman & E. Valenstein (Eds.), *Clinical neuropsychology* (2nd ed., pp 409–460). New York: Oxford Press.

Elias, M. F., Podraza, A. M., Pierce, T. W., & Robbins, M. A. (1990). Determining neuropsychological cut scores for older healthy adults. *Experimental Aging Research, 16*, 209–220.

Franzen, M. D., & Wilhelm, K. L. (1996). Conceptual foundations of ecological validity in neuropsychology. In R. J. Sbordone & C. J. Long (Eds.), *The ecological validity of neuropsychological testing* (pp. 51–69). Orlando, FL: GR/St. Lucie Press.

Gioia, G. A., Isquith, P. K., Guy, S. C., & Kenworthy, L. (2000). *Brief rating inventory of executive function.* Lutz, FL: Psychological Assessment Resources.

Golden, C. J., Hammeke, T. A., & Purisch, A. D. (1978). Diagnostic validity of a standardized neuropsychological battery derived from Luria's neuropsychological tests. *Journal of Consulting and Clinical Psychology, 5*, 221–238.

Golden, C. J., & van den Broek, A. (1998). Potential impact of age and education scores on HRNB score patterns in participants with local brain injury. *Archives of Clinical Neuropsychology, 13*(8), 683–694.

Grace, J., Stout, K., & Malloy, P. F. (1999). *Frontal systems behavioral scale.* Lutz, FL: Psychological Assessment Resources.

Halstead, W. C. (1947). *Brain and intelligence: A quantitative study of the frontal lobes.* Chicago: University of Chicago.

Halstead, W. C. (1950). Frontal lobe functions and intelligence. *Bulletin of the Los Angeles Neurological Society, 15*, 205–212.

Heaton, R. K., Grant, I., & Matthews, C. G. (1986). Differences in neuropsychological test performance associated with age, education and sex. In I. Grant & K. Adams (Eds.), *Neuropsychological assessment of neuropsychiatric disorders* (pp. 100–120). New York: Oxford.

Heaton, R. K., Grant, I., & Matthews, C. G. (1991). *Comprehensive norms for an expanded Halstead-Reitan Battery.* Odessa, FL: Psychological Assessment Resources.

Heaton, R. K., Miller, S. W., Taylor, M. J. & Grant, I. (2004). *Revised comprehensive norms for an expanded Halstead-Reitan Battery.* Odessa, FL: Psychological Assessment Resources.

Heaton, R. K., & Pendleton, M. G. (1981). Use of neuropsychological tests to predict adult patients every day functioning. *Journal of Consulting and Clinical Psychology, 49*, 807–821.

Horton, A. M., Jr. (1999). Prediction of brain damage severity: Demographic corrections. *International Journal of Neuroscience, 97*, 179–183.

Jarvis, P. E., & Barth, J. T. (1994). *Halstead-Reitan test battery: An interpretive guide* (2nd ed.). Odessa, FL: Psychological Assessment Resources.

Lezak, M. D. (1987). Relationships between personality disorders, social disturbances, and physical disability following traumatic brain injury. *Journal of Head Trauma Rehabilitation, 2*, 57–69.

Lezak, M. D. (1995). *Neuropsychological assessment* (3rd ed.). New York: Oxford University Press.

Lezak, M. D., Howieson, D. B., & Loring, D. W. (2004). *Neuropsychological assessment* (4th ed.). New York: Oxford University Press.

Luria, A. R. (1966). *Human brain and psychological processes.* New York: Harper and Row.

Luria, A. R., & Tsvetkova, L. S. (1990). *Neuropsychological analysis of problem solving.* Delray Beach, FL: GR/St. Lucie Press.

Mesulam, M. M. (1986). Frontal cortex and behavior: Editorial. *Annals of Neurology, 19*, 320–325.

Plato. (1952). The dialogues of Plato (B. Jowett, Trans.). In R. M. Hutchins (Ed.), *Great books of the western world* (Vol. 7). Chicago: Encyclopedia Britannica.

Reitan, R. M. (1955). The distribution according to age of a psychological measure dependent upon organic brain functions. *Journal of Gerontology, 10*, 338–340.

Reitan, R. M. (1964). Psychological deficits resulting from cerebral lesions in man. In J. M. Warren & K. A. Akart (Eds.), *The frontal granular cortex and behavior* (pp. 23–34). New York: McGraw-Hill.

Reitan, R. M. (1974). Methodological problems in clinical neuropsychology. In R. M. Reitan & L. A. Davison (Eds.), *Clinical neuropsychology: Current status and application* (pp. 19–46). New York: Wiley.

Reitan, R. M., & Wolfson, D. (1986). The Halstead-Reitan neuropsychological test battery. In D. Wedding, A. M. Horton, Jr., & J. S. Webster (Eds.), *The neuropsychology handbook* (pp. 134–160). New York: Springer Publishing Company.

Reitan, R. M., & Wolfson, D. (1995) Influence of age and education on neuropsychological test results. *Clinical Neuropsychologist, 9*, 151–158.

Reitan, R. M., & Wolfson, D. (2005). The effect of age and education transformations on neuropsychological test scores of persons with diffuse or bilateral brain damage. *Applied Neuropsychology, 12* (4), 181–189.

Reitan, R. M., & Wolfson, D. (1993). Validity of the trail-making test as an indicator of organic brain damage. *Perceptual and Motor Skills, 8,* 271–276.

Roth, R. M., Isquith, P. K., & Gioia, G. A. (2005). *Brief rating inventory of executive function—Adult version.* Lutz, FL: Psychological Assessment Resources.

Sbordone, R. J. (1996). Ecological validity: Some critical issues for the neuropsychologist. In R. J. Sbordone & C. J. Long (Eds.), *The ecological validity of neuropsychological testing* (pp. 15–41). Orlando, FL: GR/St. Lucie Press.

Sbordone, R. J. (1997). The ecological validity of neuropsychological testing. In A. M. Horton, D. Wedding, & J. Webster (Eds.), *The neuropsychology handbook, Vol. 1: Foundations and assessment* (2nd ed., pp. 365–392). New York: Springer Publishing Company.

Sbordone, R. J. (2000). The executive functions of the brain. In G. Groth-Marnat (Ed.), *Neuropsychological assessment in clinical practice: A guide to test interpretation and integration* (pp. 437–456). New York: Wiley.

Sbordone, R. J. (2007). The ecological validity of neuropsychological testing: Critical issues. In *Neuropsychologist's handbook.* New York: Springer Publishing Company.

Sbordone, R. J., & Guilmette, T. J. (1999). Ecological validity: Prediction of everyday and vocational functioning from neuropsychological test data. In J. J. Sweet (Ed.), *Forensic neuropsychology* (pp. 227–254). Lisse, The Netherlands: Swets and Zeitlinger.

Sbordone, R. J., & Purisch, A. D. (1996). Hazards of blind analysis of neuropsychological data in assessing cognitive disability. *Neurorehabilitation, 7,* 15–26.

Sbordone, R. J., Saul, R. E., & Purisch, A. D. (2007). *Neuropsychology for psychologists, health care professionals, and attorneys* (3rd ed.). Boca Raton, FL: CRC Press.

Sbordone, R. J., Seyranian, G. D., & Ruff, R. M. (1998). Are the subjective complaints of brain-injured patients reliable? *Brain Injury, 12*(6), 505–515.

Sbordone, R. J., Seyranian, G. D., & Ruff, R. M. (2000). The use of significant others to enhance the detection of malingers from traumatic brain-injured patients. *Archives of Clinical Neuropsychology, 15,* 465–477.

Stuss, D. T., & Benson, D. F. (1986). *The frontal lobes.* New York: Raven Press.

Sweeney, J. E. (1999). Raw, demographically altered and composite Halstead-Reitan Battery data in the evaluation of adult victims of nonimpact acceleration forces in motor vehicle accidents. *Applied Neuropsychology, 6*(2), 79–87.

Wheeler, L., Burke, C. J., & Reitan, R. M. (1963). An application of discriminant functions to the problem of predicting brain damage using behavioral variables. *Perceptual and Motor Skills, 16,* 417–440.

Wheeler, L., & Reitan, R. M. (1962). The presence and laterality of brain damage predicted from responses to a short Aphasia Screening test. *Perceptual and Motor Skills, 15,* 789–799.

Wheeler, L., & Reitan, R. M. (1963). Discriminant functions applied to the problem of predicting cerebral damage from behavior tests: A cross validation study. *Perceptual and Motor Skills, 16,* 681–701.

Wilson, B. A. (1993). Ecological validity of neuropsychological assessment. Do neuropsychological indexes predict performance in everyday activities? *Applied and Preventive Psychology, 2,* 209–215.

Wilson, B. A., Alderman, N., Brugess, P. W., Emslie, H., & Evans, J. J. (1996). *Behavioral assessment of the dysexecutive syndrome.* Bury St. Edmunds, UK: Thames Valley Test Company.

Wilson, B. A., Cockburn, J., & Baddeley, A. D. (1985). *The Rivermead behavioural test manual.* Bury St. Edmunds, U.K.: Thames Valley Test Company.

Yantz, C. L., Gavett, B. E., Lynch, J. K., & McCaffrey, R. J. (2006). Potential for litigation disparities of Halstead-Reitan neuropsychological battery performance in a litigating sample. *Archives of Clinical Neuropsychology, 21*(8), 809–817.

Zangwill, O. L. (1966). Psychological deficits associated with frontal lobe lesions. *International Journal of Neurology, 5,* 395–402.

Part IV

Special Areas and Populations in Neuropsychology

The Admissibility of Neuropsychological Evidence: A Primer

19

Larry Cohen

Introduction

Neuropsychologists, like health care witnesses generally, are familiar with the idea that courts impose restrictions on the substance of the testimony "expert witnesses" are allowed to present in formal legal proceedings. The scope of that familiarity is rather limited, though. Most practitioners have heard of the so-called "Frye" and "Daubert" standards for the admissibility of expert testimony. However, few are familiar enough with the details of these standards to know how application of one or the other will bear on their ability to present their opinions in formal legal proceedings. Even fewer are familiar enough with the other evidentiary and procedural restrictions on the admissibility of evidence to understand the limitations that may be placed on the content and scope of their proposed testimony or consideration of their records and reports.

Practitioners might respond to this lack of familiarity with evidentiary and procedural rules by observing that these are concerns best left to the lawyers who are responsible on behalf of their respective clients to get evidence admitted or keep it excluded. It is sufficient in this view for the practitioner to be guided by the lawyer in what and how to present at the various stages of formal proceedings. Although there is some wisdom to this response, it puts the neuropsychologist at considerable risk, both of failing to accomplish the practitioner's goals in delivering information about a case, and of appearing inadequate, and perhaps even incompetent, in the work the neuropsychologist has performed.

There are many reasons why the neuropsychologist may be exposed to such risks. One is that neuropsychologists and lawyers have different goals, the former being concerned primarily with accuracy and the latter being concerned primarily with advocacy. The likelihood of those goals diverging is significant when dealing with a subject matter, brain–behavior relationships, about which there is so much controversy in description, assessment, and explanation.

Another reason neuropsychologists may be at risk is that there is considerable variability in the quality of practice among attorneys. Most lawyers do not know enough about the practice of neuropsychology to appreciate the foundation that has to be laid to ensure proposed testimony and documents will be permitted in formal proceedings. Even those lawyers who make an effort to be familiar with the field may not be aware of developments bearing on the admissibility of proposed opinions.

Lawyers may fail, in a given case, to meet certain impending evidentiary or procedural deadlines. As a result, part or all of proposed testimony, records, or reports may be excluded, because necessary requests may not have been timely presented to the court or disclosures may not have been timely made to the opposing party.

Still another reason neuropsychologists may be at risk in presenting what they want to submit through oral testimony or documents is that there may be financial limitations on the attorneys with whom they are dealing. Collateral information may not be collected or passed along. The scope of the assessment authorized by the attorney may be limited. In either event, the neuropsychologist may be unable to meet applicable evidentiary standards.

Finally, there are many circumstances in which practitioners confront the legal system on their own, without the benefit of whatever assistance lawyers may provide. As treating providers, they may not be so aligned with either side that the attorneys involved believe it in their respective client's interests to spend time or resources interacting with them before a formal proceeding. Neuropsychologists may become involved at the request of the court or pursuant to some law or regulation, rather than through the actions of an attorney.

The solution proposed by the discussion that follows is not to make neuropsychologists into lawyers. It is not to suggest that neuropsychologists devote a substantial amount of time learning the laws of evidence and procedure, either. The point of this discussion is to so inform neuropsychologists about how the legal system functions, with respect to the admissibility of the kind of testimony, records, and reports neuropsychologists offer, that they can ask appropriate questions of the attorneys with whom they interact and be better consumers of what they are told. They will have some idea about when lawyers with whom they are dealing are failing to take actions the neuropsychologist understands are needed to permit them to testify effectively and completely on the issues they are addressing with the court. Finally, it will help practitioners to appreciate when they need to be proactive on their own behalf to meet the necessary evidentiary and procedural criteria, so their proposed opinions will not be compromised or precluded.

Multiple Decision-Making Systems

There are a number of different fora in which disputes are resolved and decisions are made. The admissibility standards vary to a greater or lesser extent across these different fora.

Starting with courts, there are two separate court systems, the federal system and the state system.[1] Although many of the formalities of the respective court systems are the same, the evidentiary and procedural rules differ in some very important ways across these systems.

Further, federal judges collectively have the reputation of being stricter in the application of procedural rules than state court judges collectively. There is, of course, variability among the judges within the respective court systems. As a general proposition, though, practitioners can expect federal judges to be stricter than state judges in their adherence to the procedural rules.

Focusing next on courts across the various states, there is variability both in letter of the evidentiary and procedural rules, and in how strictly or how liberally they are applied. Neuropsychologists who testify or are invited to testify in multiple states need to inquire as they move from state to state about the applicable rules of the courts in the state where the practitioner will be appearing. They should inquire, as well, about how the judge in any particular court within a state is likely to apply the rules.

Within court systems, cases may be tried to a jury or to the judge (also referred to as "to the bench" or "to the court").[2] Judges sometimes will seemingly relax evidentiary standards in cases tried to the court, on the theory that they, as judges, will not be influenced as members of a jury might be by prejudice, bias, credibility, or integrity issues with purported evidence.

In addition to these judicial court proceedings, there are also administrative court proceedings. The latter are courts created to deal with disputes arising in the context of an administrative agency. In some states, for example, the worker's compensation cases are tried by specially created administrative courts, presided over by administrative law judges. Cases in administrative courts usually are tried only to the court. These administrative courts have their own procedural rules, and the rules of evidence usually are relaxed to a greater or lesser extent.

Finally, parties sometimes choose to resolve their disputes through private proceedings. Although these proceedings may be referred to as courts, they are more typically referred to as arbitrations. Once more, there are usually some procedural formalities and some adherence to evidentiary rules. The precise nature and application of these formalities and rules are determined by the parties, and so will vary greatly from case to case.

The point for neuropsychologists is to inquire about the forum in which the matter in issue is being processed, including the formalities and rules that will be applied and the judicial officer or other presiding person who will be governing the proceeding. Only in this way will the neuropsychologist know what standards will be applied and what procedures must be followed to accomplish the presentation of the evidence the neuropsychologist proposes to present in the case.

Procedural Rules

Principles of Procedure

Procedural rules govern the method and manner of processing a case from inception to conclusion. The purpose of procedural rules in legal proceedings is to ensure each side has a reasonable and substantially equivalent opportunity to present and defend their respective positions.[3] The rules function as guidelines for the acquisition and distribution of information in any given case.

There are two sources of procedural rules. The first are rules established for processing cases submitted to the trial courts within the federal trial court system or the trial courts of any particular state. The federal trial courts have their procedural rules for civil and criminal proceedings, just as do the trial courts in each of the respective states.[4] Although many of these procedural rules are identical across the federal and state systems, or at least substantially similar, there are differences as well that may quite important for the processing of a given case.

These rules may be or may appear to be clear as written. Questions nonetheless arise about how they should be applied generally or in the context of a particular set of circumstances. Trial judges may be guided in applying the rules by the comments of those who drafted the original rules or subsequent amendments to the rules. More typically, though, trial court judges look to how appellate courts have interpreted them. The federal trial courts across the country are assembled into circuits, and federal trial court judges are obliged to look to the appellate courts within their respective circuits for guidance in applying these procedural rules. State trial court judges likewise are obliged to look to the appellate courts within their respective states for guidance. Where the body of judicial decisions, or case law, within their own respective appellate courts do not provide definitive guidance, trial court judges may then look to the appellate courts of other jurisdictions, federal or state, for suggestions about how to apply the procedural rules.

These forum rules usually are supplemented by rules for the individual case established by the judicial officer responsible for that case. These rules almost always are set forth in writing, in the form of orders presented to the parties. They may be rules the judge uses in every like case in that judge's court, or they may be rules put in place because of the special circumstances of that case. In any event, they have the same force and effect as the published forum rules, and may not be ignored.

The most important point for neuropsychologists to appreciate about the procedural rules is that they establish deadlines by which actions must be taken. A party who fails to complete an information or acquisition task within a procedural deadline risks being unable to collect or disseminate the information before trial, or being able to use or challenge the information at trial. This may have an impact on the admissibility of proposed evidence, including opinion testimony generally, or a part of the proposed testimony. The resulting exclusion has nothing to do with the relevance, integrity, or credibility of the excluded information, but rather is simply a consequence of failing to abide by a procedural deadline. Neuropsychologists thus need to be aware of deadlines bearing on the evidence they will submit in a case to ensure that the scope and substance of their testimony is not restricted or limited because of a lawyer's failure to meet a procedural deadline.

Key Procedural Rules for the Neuropsychologist[5]

Neuropsychologists are mostly interested in procedural rules as they bear on the exchange of information. In the federal court system, and in an increasing number of state court systems, there are two means of exchanging information. The first means, familiar to most people experienced with the legal system, are discovery rules. Under these rules, one party seeks information from another, identifying the matters about which information is sought generally, and detailing the information sought specifically. The second means, provided for in the federal system and in an increasing number of state systems, are disclosure rules. Parties are required by these rules affirmatively to provide information on specified subjects to the other side. It bears emphasizing again that the failure to provide information within the time required may result in the exclusion of evidence relating to that information.

Rule 26(a)(2), Federal Rules of Civil Procedure (FRCP)[6]

This is the federal rule dealing with the disclosure of expert testimony. It is among the most demanding of the expert witness disclosure rules. Most states have disclosure counterparts, or leave it to the parties to ask through written questions (interrogatories) for information about expert witnesses. As a practical matter, most attorneys seek through disclosure or written questions the level of detail requested in this rule.

The federal rule requires the expert to provide by a specified date a written report stating all opinions the expert will present, plus the bases for each opinion. The expert must also provide the data or information on which the opinion is based. Finally, the expert must identify the exhibits that will be used in support of the opinions to be presented. Information not included with the report may be excluded at trial, unless a good reason is given why the information was not provided with the original report.

Additionally, the expert must state his or her qualifications to give the opinions to be presented. Further, the expert must report all publications within the preceding 10 years, all cases in which the expert has testified at deposition or trial within the preceding 4 years, and the compensation the expert is being paid. Failure to affirmatively disclose this information may result in the expert being restricted in what he or she may say at trial or excluded altogether.

Rule 26(b)(1), FRCP

This rule defines the scope of discovery very broadly:

> Parties may obtain discovery regarding any matter, not privileged, that is relevant to the claim or defense of any party....Relevant information need not be admissible at trial if the discovery appears reasonably calculated to lead to the discovery of admissible evidence.

Courts tend to interpret this rule in a way that allows lawyers to pursue almost any subject in great detail. There are limits, however, and objections to information entirely unrelated to the case or very personal in nature may be sustained. Finally, every state has a similar rule and interprets its rule similarly.

Rule 26(b)(4), FRCP

This rule deals with the discovery by a party of information about the opposing party's experts. It draws an important distinction between experts who will testify and experts who are only used as consultants.

As a general proposition, the opposing party can inquire into all aspects of the opinions of and underlying work performed by a testifying expert. This includes all communications between the attorney who retained the expert and the expert.

By contrast, except under very unusual circumstances, the opposing party may not learn anything about a consultant. This extends even to the name of the consultant and the fact that an attorney has a consultant.

The law on discovery and disclosure becomes somewhat complicated when a person wants to switch an expert between testifying and consulting roles. Neuropsychologists should avoid such situations, because communications that were freely exchanged between an attorney and consultant when they expected it would remain private could be used at deposition or trial, even if unfairly, to challenge the credibility and integrity of the neuropsychologist.

This federal rule requires payment of the expert in advance for participating in discovery by the party seeking discovery. Many states do not have such an express requirement, leaving the expert to resort to the court for assistance when the party seeking discovery fails to pay.

Rule 26(c), FRCP

This is the rule through which one may ask the court for a protective order, limiting the extent of discovery, or what may be done with information received through discovery. A neuropsychologist would resort to this rule to try to stop lawyers from getting their raw data or protocols, or to restrict the use and retention of raw data or protocols if they are produced.

Rule 30, FRCP

The method and manner of taking depositions is governed by this rule. In the federal system and in many states, the presumptive length of depositions is limited by this rule. In the federal system, for example, depositions are presumptively limited to 7 hours. In Arizona, they are limited to 4 hours.

Rules 33, 34 FRCP

These rules provide for written questions (interrogatories) and requests for documents (requests for production) to be submitted to the opposing party. Such requests may be important to the neuropsychologist to the extent that they include information about treating providers and expert witnesses. When requested information and documents are not timely produced, the treating provider or expert may be restricted in what the expert may testify about, or be precluded altogether.

Rule 35, FRCP

The defendant in a civil injury proceeding may seek a neuropsychological assessment of the plaintiff through this rule. The examiner is required by this rule to provide a written report of the examination, including, among other things, "results of all tests made." The rule does not specifically require production of raw test data or protocols, but may be used as a means to try to get that kind of information. Finally, the examiner who fails to provide the report required by this rule may be precluded from testifying at trial.

In many states, provisions have been incorporated into this rule that may bear on how the neuropsychologist conducts a requested examination of a plaintiff. For example, some states permit the party being examined to have a person be present during the examination, or to record by audio or video the course of the examination. Some attorneys will argue that this rule permits inquiry before the examination about what the neuropsychologist will do in the course of the examination, including what tests will be performed. The neuropsychologist who objects to such invasion into the examination process will need to provide the court with principled reasons why the proposed activities would compromise the examination process, supported if available by research in the field. The first step in raising such an objection, though, is to know what exactly the rule permits and what limitations, if any, the applicable appellate courts have imposed on efforts to use the rule in this way.[7]

Jury Questions

In some jurisdictions, jurors are permitted to ask questions of witnesses during the trial of the case.[8] The idea is to permit jurors to focus on issues they consider important to their deliberations. Neuropsychologists should inquire before trial about whether this procedure is permitted in the jurisdiction in which they will be testifying, so they can be prepared for such inquiries, should they take place. For example, the unprepared neuropsychologist may not respond in a way that the juror considers responsive or respectful, and so be held in less regard by the inquiring juror and perhaps the entire jury. Although not a formal restriction on or exclusion of opinion testimony, the practical result will be the same, in that the juror or jury may reject the opinions the neuropsychologist is trying to provide in the matter at issue.

Evidentiary Rules

Principles of Evidence

Evidence law deals with the kind of information that may be used by a decision maker to determine the facts dealing with an issue. Evidence is considered relevant when "it has the tendency to make the existence of a fact that is of consequence to the determination of an issue more or less probable than it would be without the evidence."[9]

Generally speaking, there are two kinds of evidence. Direct evidence is evidence that proves a proposition directly, in one step and without inference from other information. Circumstantial evidence is evidence that proves a proposition through an inference based on one or more pieces of information. For example, if a parent sees a child placing a cookie into the child's mouth, the parent has direct evidence that the child is eating a cookie. If a parent does not see the child eating the cookie, but sees cookie crumbs around the child's mouth, the parent has circumstantial evidence that the child ate a cookie.

Evidence is presented through several means. Testimonial evidence is oral testimony presented under oath and in court. Tangible evidence may be real, that is to say, the thing itself, as in a preserved portion of a deceased client's brain. Tangible evidence may also be demonstrative, as in a physical aid designed to help the decision maker understand the evidence, as in a model of the brain. Finally, there may be hybrids of real and tangible evidence, as in a deposition transcription that is read to the jury or the written report of an expert.

As a general proposition, relevant evidence is admissible for the purpose of deciding some issue. However, relevant evidence may be excluded for a number of reasons, including questions about the integrity of the information, for example, credibility, trustworthiness, accuracy, or bias.[10] Relevant evidence may also be excluded because its prejudicial effect on the decision maker is believed to outweigh whatever probative value it may have. Finally, relevant evidence may be excluded because admission may be considered unfair to one party or another or as a matter of public policy.

Key Evidentiary Rules for the Neuropsychologist

The rules of evidence are very similar across the various court systems. Indeed, the most significant differences in the rules, for the purposes of this discussion, are the rules dealing with expert witnesses.

Unlike the procedural rules, which differ in civil and criminal proceedings, the evidence rules apply across different types of cases. Constitutional and public policy issues may affect how the evidence rules are applied to civil and criminal litigants, but for the most part, the rules are the same in all types of cases.

Like the procedural rules, there is a substantial body of case law interpreting the evidence rules. Once more, courts within their respective federal and state jurisdictions look to their respective appellate courts for direction in how to apply the rules in any given circumstances. Where there remains uncertainty, either because the issue presented has not been addressed as yet by respective appellate courts, or because the available case decisions are not entirely clear, trial courts will consider decisions from appellate courts in other jurisdictions for guidance on the issue.

Nowhere are the rules of evidence more subject to interpretation than in the area of opinion testimony. For that reason, it is always prudent for the neuropsychologist to inquire of the attorneys with whom they are working in a case, or of other attorneys from the jurisdiction, where available, about the prevailing law on the admissibility of opinion testimony. Neuropsychologists will encounter some variability, but much consistency, across federal courts in different geographic locations. Neuropsychologists will encounter considerable variability, though, as they move from one state to another.

Neuropsychologists should also be prepared for variability in the application of evidence rules as they move from courtroom to courtroom within their own geographic location, both in federal and state courts. Stated simply, different judges will interpret and apply the rules differently, even in light of the same prevailing evidence case law. For a variety of reasons, the consideration of which is beyond the scope of this discussion, individual trial judges may interpret and apply evidence rules differently. This variability is tolerated by appellate courts to the extent they review trial judge decisions on evidence issues by what is called an "abuse of discretion" standard, meaning that instead of reviewing for themselves whether the evidentiary decision was the one they would have made,[11] appellate courts review evidence decisions to determine whether the trial judge acted within the range of his/her discretion in applying the respective rule to the facts of the case.

The fact of this variability across jurisdictions and across courtrooms makes it important for neuropsychologists to consult with attorneys familiar with the rules of evidence, generally within the applicable jurisdiction, and with the specific judge who will be hearing the case. This will help the neuropsychologist confronting a challenge to the admissibility of opinion testimony generally, or some part of the foundation or basis for the testimony, to be fully prepared to make the best possible case for acceptance of the proposed evidence. Uninformed neuropsychologists risk speaking past the judge in failing to address the issue in a way the judge will find persuasive or compelling.

Rule 104(a), Federal Rules of Evidence

Challenges to the qualifications of an expert witness to testify and the admissibility of evidence, including proposed expert opinion testimony, are pursued through this rule.

Preliminary questions concerning the qualification of person to be a witness, the existence of a privilege, or the admissibility of evidence, shall be determined by the court.

The most important provision in this rule deals with the evidence the court may consider in making its decision about the qualifications of the witness or the admissibility of proposed evidence.

In making its determination [the court] is not bound by the rules of evidence except those with respect to privileges (Federal Rules of Evidence, p. 1)

This means the neuropsychologist can rely on virtually anything, including especially hearsay information, to support his/her own qualifications or to establish the credibility and integrity of the opinion testimony they propose to offer at trial. They should take advantage of this in trying to persuade the judge to overrule pretrial admissibility objections.

Rule 602, FRE

Though simple and seemingly innocuous on its face, this rule is quite important for neuropsychologists. It provides that the only witnesses competent to testify are those with first-hand knowledge.

> *A witness may not testify to a matter unless evidence is introduced sufficient to support a finding that the witness has personal knowledge of the matter.*

A neuropsychologist specially retained to express opinions in a case relies entirely or, at best, to a great extent on information supplied by the attorney or some other like source. As such, the neuropsychologist as retained expert would not be testifying from first-hand knowledge, and so ordinarily would not be permitted to testify in the proceeding. There must be some other basis in the rules that permits the neuropsychologist to testify, and that basis is the opinion rules for expert witnesses.

There are circumstances, though, in which the neuropsychologist does testify based on first-hand knowledge. This is where the neuropsychologist is a treating provider, reporting as a matter of fact the observations the neuropsychologist made, the opinions reached, and the work performed in the course of treating a patient in the course of neuropsychological practice. There is an argument to be made here that the neuropsychologist is not limited by or subject to the opinion rules for expert witnesses, but rather is a competent witness in the neuropsychologist's own right, consistent with Rule 602. This is certainly true to the extent of the observations the neuropsychologist has made in the course of clinical work. The argument could be made that opinions are reported as an historical fact in describing the clinical work, and so should not be subjected to the scrutiny that may be applied to opinion testimony generally. Alternatively, at the very least, such scrutiny should be limited to those opinions, and not be a basis for restricting or excluding the clinical observations made and treatment provided by the neuropsychologist.

Rules 607, 608, and 609, FRE

These three rules provide the means through which the integrity of a witness can be challenged on the basis of the witness' credibility. The focus here is on the truthfulness of the witness, including the witness' character or prior acts that raise questions about the likely truthfulness of the witness.

Rule 611, FRE

Judges control the mode and order of the presentation of the evidence through this rule. It is the means through which a neuropsychologist may seek help for problems with scheduling. The judge relies on the power conferred by this rule, for example, to permit a witness to testify out of order to accommodate that witness' availability. The central concern for the court in every case is to keep the case moving along and help make the evidence accessible to the decision maker, whether that is the jury or the court. A neuropsychologist seeking assistance from the court for scheduling would be well advised to reference these considerations, along with whatever the reason is for the scheduling accommodation.

The rule is also a vehicle through which the court may ask questions of a witness during the trial of a case. The underlying reasoning is that the court may, through appropriate questions, focus the witness on matters that will help the jury or the judge, if the case is being tried to the court, to resolve issues. It would be helpful for the neuropsychologist to know in advance of the trial whether the judge is someone with a reputation for asking questions. In this way, the neuropsychologist will be prepared to address any questions if and when they are presented.

Rule 615, FRE

This so-called "rule of exclusion" permits a party to exclude any person from trial proceedings in which that person is going to be called as a witness for that trial. The reasoning is that the witness should not be influenced in what he or she has to say by what others have said before that witness.

There is an important exception to this rule that permits a person to be present, "who is shown by a party to be essential to the presentation of the party's cause." That exception could be used to argue that an expert witness should be allowed to observe the testimony of other witnesses, and particularly of the plaintiff and of "collaterals," where the expert will be relying on what those persons have to say in expressing opinions about matters at issue in the case. The opposing argument, particularly compelling in jurisdictions where there is a disclosure requirement, is that each party is entitled to know in advance of trial the bases for the expert's opinions, and should not have to deal with opinions newly formed based on information obtained at the time of trial, especially where that information was available before the trial.

Most attorneys will try to use this rule to exclude the expert from depositions, as well as for trial. The reasoning is that the deposition is a formal proceeding in which the same concerns about the integrity of the witness' testimony apply. The opposing view is that experts will have access to the same information they would hear during a deposition by reading the transcript of the deposition. Further, the expert can be very helpful during the deposition in guiding the attorney in the exploration of matters that will be helpful to the neuropsychologist in formulating opinions for the case.

Rules 801-805, FRE

These are the hearsay rules. Hearsay is any statement made outside of trial or other hearing, offered as evidence of the truth of the matter at issue.[12] Hearsay "statements" may be oral statements, written statements, or even actions.

The reason hearsay generally is excluded is because there is no opportunity for a party who may want to challenge the statement to explore the trustworthiness of the statement. Absent that opportunity, it is unfair to subject that party to whatever impact the statement may have on the judge, jury, or whomever is determining the facts and deciding disputed issues in the case.

There are many exceptions to the hearsay rule.[13] In each instance, these are circumstances in which there is some reason to believe the out-of-court statement is sufficiently trustworthy that it may be considered as evidence by the factfinder. The following exceptions should be of particular interest to the neuropsychologist.

Rule 803(4), FRE

Statements made for medical diagnosis or treatment are not excluded by the hearsay rule. The reasoning is that when persons present themselves for health care, it is assumed that they are truthful about what they say because they are intent on getting an accurate diagnosis and appropriate treatment. Likewise, statements made by the health care provider are assumed to be focused on the health care needs of the patient and not other matters.

It is important to appreciate that this exception for treatment records does not extend to a report prepared by an expert specially retained in a legal proceeding to evaluate a party to that proceeding. In that case, none of the reasoning applicable to the medical exception rule applies. The subject of the examination is not seeking help with a health care problem, and so cannot be trusted implicitly to make accurate statements. Likewise, the health care provider's agenda is focused on matters other than assessment and treatment for the clinical benefit of a patient.

Rule 803(18), FRE

A neuropsychologist may want to refer during trial to an authoritative source that supports the opinion or methodology testimony. Such sources are hearsay, of course, because they are statements made out of court. However, there is an exception for so-called "learned treatises" when they are established as "reliable authorities" on the issue. This can be accomplished, for example, by the neuropsychologist testifying that it is a reliable authority in the field. When that condition or foundation is established, the neuropsychologist may reference the source, including reading directly from it. However, the source itself may not be admitted in evidence as a document that the jury or other trier of fact can review and consider during deliberations on the issues presented.

Attorneys often press experts in the course of discovery, and particularly during depositions, to identify sources the expert considers authoritative on an issue, or authoritative in the field generally. The attorney's usual purpose is to develop information through which the expert can then be challenged with some author's opposing view or position on a matter at issue. Experienced experts, knowing this likely purpose, tend to be reluctant to concede that an identified publication is authoritative, at least not until the expert is certain about what information is contained in the "authority" and has considered how it may be used to challenge the expert in some way.

Rules 702–706, FRE

These are the expert opinion rules. They deal first with the circumstances under which expert opinion testimony is permitted, then with the bases for opinion testimony, next with certain kinds of opinions that are permitted and excluded, and finally, with disclosure of the facts or data underlying expert opinions. There is also a special rule permitting the court to select an expert where the court believes opinion testimony would be helpful on an issue.

The case authority interpreting these rules is substantial indeed, both in the federal and the state courts. The overwhelming principle expressed in those cases is that courts need to serve as gatekeepers to ensure that there is a least a minimum level of integrity to the opinions proposed to be presented the jury. The concern is that without such oversight by the courts, there is a great risk that triers of fact, and particularly jurors, will be led to believe baseline opinions because they have been presented by someone who has, or claims to have, the appearance of expertise in the field. The ensuing debate within the courts has been how that gatekeeping function should be exercised generally, and what should be the standards for admissibility. Neuropsychologists' intent on overcoming a challenge to the admissibility of proposed opinion testimony should consider this underlying purpose as they prepare the substantive response to the challenge. In other words, the goal should be to demonstrate the integrity of the proposed testimony in light of whatever factors will be considered by the court in the applicable jurisdiction.

Another approach, presently in the distinct and small minority, starts with the proposition that cross examination is well established as an effective means of challenging proposed witnesses' testimony toward the end of ferreting out the integrity of the proposed evidence.[14] On this view, there is no need for special standards to protect jurors from receiving information from witnesses, at the expense of excluding what otherwise would be conceded as relevant information. Jurors should be trusted to understand the information presented and to see, through observing cross examination, the strengths and weaknesses of proposed opinion testimony.

The result of the battles in the appellate courts over the admissibility of expert testimony is the development of the so-called "Frye" and "Daubert" standards, and to the evolution of these standards as they have been applied in the various federal and state proceedings. Before addressing how these standards bear on the admissibility of neuropsychological opinion testimony in particular, we should look at the evidence rules to which these standards apply.

Rule 702, FRE

This rule provides the justification for expert opinion testimony in the first instance. Such opinion testimony is permitted when it will assist the trier of fact either to understand the evidence or to determine a fact at issue. If the jury does not need such help, as, for example, in deciding whether a person is credible, or if the opinion will not provide such help, then the expert opinion testimony is not permitted.

It may be argued, for example, that expert opinion as to whether a person is "malingering" is outside the scope of what is permitted by this rule. The argument would be that insofar as the concept of malingering includes a component dealing with whether a person is being dishonest, the trier of fact is quite capable of making that determination on its own, without the assistance of an expert. Opinion testimony may still be helpful in addressing the other component of the concept of malingering, whether a person is performing at a level of functioning that would be expected of someone with that person's functional capacity. The trier of fact would not be in a position to make that determination without expert assistance. Questions as to the person's credibility, and so the ultimate determination of whether the person is, in fact, malingering, as opposed to failing to perform at the predicted level for some other reason, is within the scope of the trier of fact's own understanding and no expert opinion is needed on the issue.

This rule also addresses the kind of knowledge an expert must have to qualify as an expert witness. The rule directs courts to look for scientific, technical, or other specialized knowledge. At various times, other requirements have been suggested. For example, courts have been urged to require that neuropsychologists be board-certified to qualify as trial experts.[15] Such proposals have been rejected because they impose a level of credentialing not required by the rule. Any person with the requisite knowledge who can help the jury should be permitted to express the opinion. It is then up to the party challenging the opinion to try to persuade the trier of fact not to consider or to give little weight to the opinion, because the purported expert lacks the necessary qualifications to speak on the subject.

The "Frye" standard, the "Daubert" standard, and the various hybrids of these standards are all consistent with these elements of Rule 702. The federal courts and some state courts have gone further, however, and imposed certain additional requirements as part of the rule itself. These further requirements are grounded in the reasoning of the Supreme Court in the Daubert line of cases.[16] In these courts, the expert opinion is permitted only where

> (1) the testimony is based upon sufficient facts or data, (2) the testimony is the product of reliable principles and methods and (3) the witness has applied the principles and methods reliably to the facts of the case.

Most state courts do not impose these further requirements within the scope of the rule itself. However, state courts that have adopted the Daubert standard as part of their case law through appellate court decisions still impose these requirements.

Briefly, the "Frye" standard, or general acceptance standard, requires only a showing that opinion is based on theories or principles that are "generally accepted" within the applicable field.[17]

> [T]he thing from which the deduction is made must be sufficiently established to have gained general acceptance in the particular field in which it belongs.

The court in *Frye v. U.S.* developed this standard in light of its recognition that it is not always clear when an idea has moved from the exploratory to the established side of scientific understanding:

> Just when a scientific principle or discovery crosses the line between the experimental and the demonstrable stages is difficult to define. Somewhere in this twilight zone the evidential force must be recognized.

The court in that case decided that "general acceptance" in the field would be that dividing point.

Neuropsychologists intent on meeting this standard should understand that the court is looking for indications of general acceptance. As we discussed previously, information providing those indications is not limited to what is admissible under the rules of evidence. Accordingly, the neuropsychologist trying to meet this standard should present the court with evidence from all manner of sources that will demonstrate such acceptance. This might include, for example, presidential addresses at professional meetings, research grants made by government agencies, symposia at professional conferences, exchanges of written or electronic communications among respected persons within the field, and, of course, publications, particularly in peer-reviewed journals. The point is to understand what kind of information the court is seeking when considering an admissibility challenge under this standard, and to provide information that is responsive to what the court is seeking.

The Daubert standard focuses on four factors suggested by the United States Supreme Court in the Daubert case that the Court thought would be indicative of "reliable" scientific activity:[18]

1. Whether it can be falsified through testing;
2. Whether it has been subjected to peer review and publication;
3. With respect to an assessment technique, whether there is a known rate of error;
4. Whether it has been generally accepted in the field.

Whereas the Court in the *Daubert* decision was clear that these four factors were not intended to be exclusive or exhaustive of how the reliability of a proposed opinion might be established, as a practical matter, these four factors have become established as the "Daubert" factors. State court decisions have, in some instances, identified other factors, and some federal courts have been willing to consider other factors as well to establish the necessary reliability. For the most part, though, the Daubert factors remain, for the most part, those four referenced by the United States Supreme Court in its original decision.

Neuropsychologists confronted with challenges to the admissibility of proposed testimony would be well served to present information satisfying all, or as many of the Daubert factors as possible. As the law of scientific evidence continues to evolve, it is more likely than not that courts will move away from the Frye standard and toward the Daubert standard, or something like it. Meeting all of these criteria thus minimizes the risk of a change in the law that would find that the information provided by the neuropsychologist in any given case is insufficient. Moreover, because "general acceptance" is one factor among the four Daubert factors, the neuropsychologist who tries to address all the Daubert factors will necessarily address the Frye factor, as well.

Rule 703, FRE

This is a crucial rule for expert witnesses, because it allows them to testify based on something other than personal knowledge. As we noted previously, Rule 602 limits witnesses to testifying based on personal knowledge. Without a rule permitting testimony based on other information, expert witnesses would not be able to express opinions on anything they did not observe directly.

The facts or data in the particular case upon which an expert bases an opinion or inference must be those perceived by or made known to the expert at[19] or before the hearing.

As we have seen, though, information made known to a person is hearsay, raising an admissibility problem on that basis. The rule solves that problem as well, though, by providing for circumstances in which the facts or data on which the expert relies need not be admissible in evidence:

If of a type reasonably relied upon by experts in the particular field in forming opinions or inferences upon the subject, the fact or data need not be admissible in evidence in order for the opinion or inference to be admitted.

However, the rule ordinarily does not permit those inadmissible facts or data to be disclosed to the jury, thus ensuring that they will not be given too much weight by the jury under circumstances in which the opposing party is not in a position to challenge them effectively. [20]

Considering the broad scope of this rule, the neuropsychologist should be expansive in seeking information that will be helpful in forming and supporting an opinion on the matters at issue. However, in doing so, the neuropsychologist must be prepared to demonstrate that the information is of the kind neuropsychologists performing similar work would rely upon in clinical work or research, outside of what takes place in forensic settings. Information developed exclusively for the litigation, such as the report of another forensic expert, might be excluded because it is not of the kind relied upon by experts in the field.

Rule 704, FRE

This rule permits experts to testify broadly as to matters at issue in a case. Specifically, the rule provides that an opinion otherwise admissible is not objectionable, "because it embraces an ultimate issue to be decided by the trier of fact." Courts usually will not allow experts to express opinions that fully cover the ultimate issues that must be decided by the trier of fact, but will allow opinions that bear on those ultimate issues. Thus, a neuropsychologist may be permitted to testify that a person's brain injury was caused by a particular event, and may be permitted to describe how the defendant's conduct contributed to that result, but would not be permitted to testify that the defendant acted unreasonably, or that the defendant caused the outcome.

Rule 705, FRE

An expert is permitted to express opinions without revealing the underlying facts or data. This can be extremely helpful when the neuropsychologist testifies early in the direct examination, when the jurors are most likely to be attentive. The alternative is to spend a considerable amount of time introducing the neuropsychologist, reviewing background and credentials, and then describing in detail the work performed before reporting any opinions. By that time, it may be questionable whether jurors remain sufficiently attentive to fully receive and appreciate the opinions being offered.

However, the court has the power under this rule to require the expert to disclose the underlying facts or data first. This may happen, for example, when there is a challenge to the adequacy of the factual basis for the expert's opinion. The opposing party may insist that these facts be disclosed as part of an effort to try to convince the court not to allow the expert to testify about some or all of the proposed opinions. In that case, the neuropsychologist will have to report the facts before expressing any opinions.

Additionally, the opposing counsel may require the expert to disclose the opinions during cross examination. This is likely to occur when the opposing party has been unsuccessful or believes it will be unsuccessful in persuading the court to exclude some or all of the opinions. Lacking that option, the opposing party may want to have the neuropsychologist testify about the underlying facts and data toward the goal of trying to persuade the trier of fact that the information on which the neuropsychologist is relying is incomplete or inadequate in some way.

Regardless of why the neuropsychologist may be required to disclose the underlying facts or data, it would be prudent to be prepared to do so in an organized and clear way. This will maximize the opportunity for the court to find the underlying facts and data to be sufficient, and will help make the information accessible to the jury so it can see how and why the information on which the neuropsychologist depended was appropriate and sufficient to support the opinions rendered.

Rule 706, FRE

There are times when the court determines on its own that an expert is needed, or when the parties agree that an expert is needed and prefer to have one appointed by the court rather than either of the parties. This rule deals with that situation. Neuropsychologists appointed through this Rule enjoy greater credibility in the eyes of the trier of fact. They remain at risk to be challenged, though, because the Rule still permits either party to employ their own expert witness on the matters at issue, and to cross-examine the court-appointed expert to whatever extent they deem appropriate.

Notes

1. Individual courts are generally referred to as jurisdictions. The term *system* is used here to refer to collections of courts, as in the federal system of courts and the state system of courts.
2. The person or group of persons to whom the matter is tried, for purposes of deciding what the facts are and how to apply the law to those facts in deciding matters at issue, is the "trier of fact." The trial judge, in making decisions based on the applicable law, is the "trier of law." In jury trials, the jury is the trier of fact. In trials conducted without juries, the judge is the trier of fact and the trier of law. In arbitrations, the arbitrator or the arbitration panel is the trier of fact and the trier of law.

3. See Rule 1, Federal Rules of Civil Procedure, and, generally speaking, the corresponding first rule of civil procedure is in the respective of the court.

4. In addition to forum rules applicable to the federal trial courts generally, and the trial courts within any particular state, there may be so-called "local rules" developed by courts within a geographic area, such as a state within the federal system or a county within a state, to deal with circumstances considered special or unique to that setting.

5. This discussion will focus on the federal rules for simplicity and because of space limitations. Unless otherwise indicated, there are counterparts to the concepts discussed here in the state systems, though the specific details of these concepts may differ, and sometimes significantly so, in the various states.

6. This discussion focuses on rules of civil procedure. Criminal rules are generally similar in principle, but often very different in substance.

7. For example, the court in *Raage v. MCA/Universal Studios, 165 F.R.D. 605 (C.D. Cal. 1995)* refused the plaintiff's request for a list of tests to be performed, on the grounds that it would compromise the integrity of the neuropsychologist's proposed examination.

8. In Arizona, for example, Rule 39(b), Arizona Rules of Civil Procedure, provides a mechanism through which jurors can seek information from witnesses.

9. This principle is stated in Rule 402, Federal Rules of Evidence, and likewise is to be found in the rules of evidence of the respective state courts.

10. These issues are addressed throughout the rules of evidence, including especially rules dealing with relevance (the 400 series in the federal and most state rules), competency (the 600 series), opinions (the 700 series), hearsay (the 800 series), and the authenticity of documents (the 900 series).

11. Such review is called "de novo," meaning that the reviewing court makes its own determination of how the rule should be applied in light of the applicable facts and circumstances.

12. For the neuropsychologist's purposes, it is simpler to think of hearsay as any statement made out of court.

13. There are 23 exceptions in the federal rules, and more in most state rules, where the person who made the hearsay statement is available to testify at the proceeding. There are another five exceptions when the declarant is not available. There is also a so-called "residual exception," when "justice" would be served by admitting the out-of-court statement into evidence. Finally, there are two circumstances in which a prior statement by a party or a witness is defined as other than hearsay.

14. See, for example, *Logerwuist v. McVey, 196 Ariz. 470, 1 P.3d 113 (2000),* in which the Arizona Supreme Court wrestled with the admissibility of testimony by a psychologist dealing with repressed memory syndrome.

15. The Iowa Supreme Court rejected this proposal in *Hutchinson v. American Family Mutual Insurance, 514 N.W.2d 882 (Iowa 1990),* reasoning that a person who can show the required scientific, technical, or other specialized knowledge on a subject may express opinions. The strength or weakness of the expert's credentials may then be challenged through cross examination in an effort to persuade the trier of fact to give more or less weight to the opinion testimony.

16. The so-called Daubert trilogy includes *Daubert v. Merrell Dow Pharmaceuticals, 509 U.S. 579, 113 S.Ct. 2786, 125 L.Ed.2d 469 (1993), General Electric Co. v. Joinder,*

522 U.S. 136, 118 S.Ct. 512, 139 L.Ed.2d 508 (1997), and *Kumho Tire Co. Ltd v. Carmichael, 526 U.S. 137, 119 S.Ct. 1167, 143, L.Ed.2d 238 (1999).*

17. The Frye standard was announced by the Court of Appeals for the District of Columbia in *Frye v. United States, 293 F. 1013 (D.C. Cir. 1923).* The matter at issue was the admissibility of testimony based on research performed with a version of a lie detector test. The Court refused to allow the proposed testimony because lie detectors were not a generally accepted means of determining a person's truthfulness.

18. It should be noted that what the court means by the term "reliable" is not the same as what behavioral and social scientists mean by the term. The court's use of the term combines what is generally referred to as "validity," meaning that the thing measures what it purports to measure, and "reliability," meaning that whatever is being measured is being measured consistently. One might go further and suggest that the court's use of the term "reliable" also incorporates further indications of precision in assessment, as would be the case when the "sensitivity" and "specificity" of a measure is known as well. All together, the idea is that the enterprise at issue has a determinable measure of scientific integrity.

19. This provision that opinion testimony may be based on information made known to the expert "at" the hearing is intended to deal with hypotheticals presented to the expert while testifying. An argument could be made, though, that this rule supersedes the exclusion provision in Rule 615, and so provides a basis for permitting expert witnesses to be present during the trial, even when other witnesses are excluded because of the invocation of Rule 615.

20. There is an exception to this rule of exclusion, though, in which the court determines that the probative value of these facts and data in assisting the jury in evaluating the expert's opinion substantially outweighs their prejudicial effect. Usually, what will happen is that the party opposing the expert's opinion will ask the court to admit the facts or data as part of a challenge to the credibility or integrity of the expert's opinion.

References

Arizona Rules of Civil Procedure. (2009).
Arizona Rules of Evidence. (2009).
Daubert v. Merrell Dow Pharmaceuticals, 509 U.S. 579, 113 S.Ct. 2786, 125 L.Ed.2d 469 (1993).
Federal Rules of Civil Procedure. (2009).
Federal Rules of Evidence. (2009)
Frye v. United States, 293 F. 1013 (D.C. Cir. 1923).
General Electric Co. v. Joinder, 522 U.S. 136, 118 S.Ct. 512, 139 L.Ed.2d 508 (1997).
Hutchinson v. American Family Mutual Insurance, 514 N.W.2d 882 (Iowa 1990).
Kumho Tire Co. Ltd v. Carmichael, 526 U.S. 137, 119 S. Ct. 1167, 143, L.Ed.2d 238 (1999).
Logerquist v. McVey, 196 Ariz. 470, 1 P.3d 113 (2000).
Raage v. MCA/Universal Studios, 165 F.R.D. 605 (C.D. Cal. 1995).

Neuropsychological Assessment in Disability Determination, Fitness-for-Duty Evaluations, and Rehabilitation Planning

20

Thomas L. Bennett
Michael J. Raymond

Introduction

In forensic neuropsychology, not only is the neuropsychologist expected to determine the presence versus absence of brain injury, but also she or he needs to relate the neuropsychological test data to disability. This, in turn, relates to the ever-present issue of the significance of specific test scores, and patterns of performance of these scores. For example, what does it mean if a person is mildly impaired on a test of attention, moderately impaired on a memory test, or severely impaired on a test of problem solving? Furthermore, what does the pattern of performance on these measures mean? Answering this question in a forensic context requires an understanding of the significance of test performances not just from a statistical framework, but also from a functional performance perspective. That is, what are the implications of a test score, or pattern of scores, for predicting a person's ability to successfully engage in normal life activities? Two issues that are germane to this question include the nature of disability and the ecological validity of neuropsychological tests.

Impairments, Disabilities, and Handicaps: Overview of Concepts

Barbara Wilson (1997) has observed that, using The World Health Organization's (1980) conceptual framework, one can classify the sequelae of brain injury (resulting from any neurological condition or injury) into three categories: *impairments, disabilities, and handicaps*. Impairments refer to physical damage (e.g., frontal lobe damage) or deficits on neuropsychological tests as reflected by test scores (e.g., a mild impairment on a test of attention). Impairments have the potential to produce disability. A person who has impairment but is able to meet normal life demands is not considered disabled.

Disabilities refer to the functional consequences of the impairment. For example, a mother may forget to pick up her child after school secondary to a memory deficit associated with temporal lobe damage. Disability is defined in the American Medical Association's *Guides to the Evaluation of Permanent Impairment, Fourth Edition* (1993) as "an alteration of an individual's capacity to meet personal, social, or occupational demands, or statutory or regulatory requirements because of impairment" (p. 3). Scores on neuropsychological tests (impairments) may overestimate or underestimate disabilities.

Handicaps can be conceptualized as problems imposed by the environment on an individual because of his or her disability. As Wilson noted, a person who is not handicapped in buildings that are wheelchair accessible may be handicapped in buildings that are not wheelchair accessible. As noted in the AMA Guides, "an impaired person is handicapped if there are obstacles to accomplishing life's basic activities that can be overcome only by compensating in some way for the effects of the impairment" (p. 5). However, "if an impaired individual is not able to accomplish a specific task or activity despite accommodations, or if no accommodation exists that will enable completion of the task, then that individual is both handicapped and disabled" (p. 5). Finally, an impaired individual who is able to accomplish a specific task is "neither handicapped nor disabled with regard to that task" (p. 5).

In a forensic context, impairments on test scores are important to the extent that they predict disability in the real world (have ecological validity; see Sbordone & Long, 1996). Not all deficits predict disability. A well-known example of this is seen on the Finger Tapping Test. This test was developed for and has the most power when used to make decisions about lateralization of a brain injury. The fact that a person is mildly slow on finger tapping, or does not show the typical 10% advantage in dominant hand speed over non-dominant hand speed, does not reliably predict disability in one's everyday activities. In contrast, if a person has developed a left upper-extremity paresis after brain injury, and cannot perform the Finger Tapping Test, that might be considered clinically significant. However, the examiner would know that without even attempting the test!

On the other hand, performance within normal limits does not necessarily indicate lack of disability. The first author of this chapter (Bennett) re-evaluated a woman who had a persisting memory disorder due to carbon monoxide overexposure. She successfully completed the Wisconsin Card Sorting Test (WCST). However, throughout the testing, she kept overtly repeating the appropriate sorting principle to stay on task. Overt verbal rehearsal was a compensatory strategy she had learned in occupational therapy to help her successfully stay on task when completing her daily activities. Did her normal performance indicate that her cerebral functions on which this task depends were normal? Certainly, it did not. Is she disabled, despite a lack of impairment on a test score? Probably, but certainly, her disability is reduced by her effective use of a specific compensatory strategy.

If the deficits do indicate that there is a probable disability, or a potential handicap, then the forensic neuropsychologist should be a resource for determining ways to reduce the impact of these deficits. If the forensic neuropsychologist can develop a plan of treatment to reduce a person's disability or if the environment can be changed to reduce a handicap, then the person will have a better chance of returning to productive activity and the damages would accordingly be reduced.

Americans with Disabilities Act

Individuals who experience residual neurological, cognitive, and/or behavioral alterations following acute or chronic injury, illnesses, or diseases are often forced to make changes to adapt to their environment. Unfortunately, this is often a difficult task, and one that has been hindered by societal views and structural or environmental barriers.

With the advent of federal legislation, namely Section 504 of the Rehabilitation Act of 1973 (United States Department of Health, Education, and Welfare, 1977) and the Americans with Disabilities Act (ADA) of 1990 (P.L. 101-336), a requirement of nondiscrimination toward individuals with disabilities was enacted. Specifically, Section 504 addressed basic civil rights, indicating that an individual with a disability, who was deemed qualified, could not be excluded from any activity, program, or other benefit that was federally funded. The ADA expanded the rights addressed in Section 504, and included all employers, industries, and private organizations. The ADA also expanded the definition of disability and eligibility requirements. Overall, it protected the civil rights of individuals with disabilities by mandating equal rights and opportunities in the following areas:

- Employment (Title I)
- State and local government services (Title II)
- Public accommodations (Title III)

Title I: Employment

Title I of the ADA promotes the practice of nondiscrimination against qualified individuals with disabilities. This addresses all phases of employment including recruitment, completion of the application, hiring, education and training, promotion, compensation, and all other privileges or conditions of employment. For example, if an individual demonstrates the ability to perform essential tasks of a designated position (job), then the employer may not discriminate against the individual. However, the employer is not required to give preference to individuals with disabilities in the aforementioned areas of hiring, promoting, compensating, or retaining, as the ADA is not considered an affirmative action law.

Title II: State and Local Government Services

In Title II of the ADA, state and local governments are prohibited from discriminating against individuals with disabilities by refusing them the opportunities of their services, programs, or activities. Provisions under Title II are regulated by the United States Department of Justice, especially with regard to accessibility. Specifically, all public agencies, at the time of enactment of this act, were required to submit, in writing, a formal plan to enable program accessibility through structural changes (e.g., barrier removal).

Title III: Public Accommodations

Included in Title III of the ADA is the requirement that all public agencies be accessible to all individuals with disabilities. All businesses that provide public accommodations must not discriminate against those individuals seeking services, procedures, and other associated accommodations. Alterations to public facilities in order to abide by these requirements had to be completed in an expedient manner, in addition to minimizing costs. New construction would be free of barriers, whereas reconstruction would ensure public accessibility. Adherence to these requirements is reviewed and controlled by the United States Department of Justice.

In essence, the ADA contends that the problems faced by individuals with disabilities are not disability, but merely a societal misperception and negative response. Dart and West (1995) indicated that, "the ADA affirms that disability is a natural fact of the human experience. It rejects the notion that disability is somehow an experience separate and different from the experience of being human" (p. 7).

Ecological Validity of Neuropsychological Tests

If neuropsychological test scores are to be used in disability determination, they must have ecological validity. This means that the tests are actually reflective of real-life processes. A memory test is useless in a forensic setting if a person does poorly on it (is impaired) but has no functional memory difficulties at home or at work. Similarly, the test would not have ecological validity if the person did very well on the test, but could not remember to take medicine, turn off stove burners, or remember important phone messages.

One must remember, as Sbordone (1996) has emphasized, that the assessment environment is not the real world. The conditions of testing are set up in such a way as to optimize performance. The assessment environment is typically free from distractions. The environment and the tests are structured, and the examiner is directing the patient regarding what to do and not to do. Feedback is typically clear, immediate, and unambiguous. Time demands are minimized. Instructions are repeated and/or clarified to optimize performance, and prompts are given to facilitate success. The testing environment minimizes the impact of one's emotional state, and because of the structure of the testing environment, problems with task initiation, organization, and follow-through are minimized. How different this is from the noise and distractions, time demands, lack of structure, and lack of direction and supervision that we typically experience in our homes, schools, workplaces, and communities! Indeed, these observations would suggest that neuropsychological testing data could potentially underestimate cognitive disability.

In evaluating disability, neuropsychologists often place too much emphasis on test scores, a potential error that the use of demographic norms has unfortunately reinforced. This can lead to behavioral observations made during testing, which may provide very important information about disability, being minimized. The importance of behavioral observations, that is, how an individual with a brain injury arrives at a solution or approaches a problem, was stressed early in the development of neuropsychology as a discipline.

Goldstein's (1942) work strongly argued that *only* qualitative evaluations were valid. He stated that quantitative assessments, with their focus on test scores, would confuse the issues, because a normal and a brain-injured individual might obtain the same score but arrive at the score quite differently. Goldstein's focus on the importance of behavioral observations is still important today.

The present authors believe that test scores and behavioral observations are both critically important. In their assessments, neuropsychologists need to obtain not only test scores, but also observe how the patient approaches and performs each task that contributes to the specific test score. If a person obtains a normal score but achieves this score in a manner that would never be successful in her or his daily activities, then the person is still disabled with respect to the cognitive ability being assessed.

It is essential, with regard to this latter point, to consider a person's test performance as well as behavioral observations after completion of rehabilitation. After neurorehabilitation, the individual who sustained a brain injury may achieve normal scores on tests in the supportive testing environment, but still report mild difficulties in attention, memory, and organization during everyday activities, especially when in an environment with various external distractions. Is such an individual perfectly normal and not disabled? We do not believe that such a person is without disability, but rather believe the improvements that have occurred during rehabilitation help such an individual compensate to the point at which her or his disability is significantly reduced. Improvements in test scores in all likelihood reflect, to a great extent, compensatory strategies gained during rehabilitation.

What application, then, do neuropsychological test results have for predicting disability? To answer this question, a distinction needs to be made between activities of daily living (ADL) versus instrumental activities of daily living (IADL). ADL are activities oriented toward one's own personal care. ADL include bathing and showering, dressing, getting in and out of bed or a chair, using the toilet, and eating. They enable basic survival and well-being. Generally speaking, neuropsychological testing does not provide critical information for determining a person's ability to successfully complete ADL; this is best done in a structured setting and/or in the patient's home by an occupational therapist.

IADL, on the other hand, are activities to support daily life within the home and community that typically require more complex interactions than self-care used in ADL. IADL enable a person to function independently within a community. Examples of IADL include care of others (including selecting and supervision of caregivers), care of pets, child rearing, communication management, community mobility, financial management, health management and maintenance, home management, meal preparation and cleanup, safety and emergency maintenance, transportation/driving, and shopping. Neuropsychological testing can provide an important source of information that is directly applicable to one's ability to successfully engage in IADL. Neuropsychological testing also can provide valuable information regarding possible impact of cognitive impairments on educational and vocational tasks. The use of neuropsychological assessment in fitness-for-duty evaluations will be discussed later in this chapter.

Improving the Ecological Validity of Neuropsychological Assessment by Interfacing With Allied Rehabilitation Professionals

Neuropsychologists can improve the ecological validity of their assessments, and thereby improve their ability to evaluate, predict the significance of, and rehabilitate disability, by combining their assessment procedures with those of allied health professionals. An example of this is found in the multi- or interdisciplinary rehabilitation settings of both authors. At these settings, neurocognitive assessment and the effects of cognitive impairments on performance of IADL are investigated and treated by a team approach that includes, but may not be limited to, neuropsychology, speech and language therapy, and occupational therapy. The general rehabilitation procedure, which is used across disciplines to reduce disability and handicap, includes the redevelopment of previous skills (remedial training), metacognitive awareness training, and instructing the patient to develop new skills to compensate for his or her cognitive deficits. Following the learning of new strategies, the patient has the opportunity to incorporate them into simulated or real-life environments (home, work, or community).

For the person with severe deficits, therapy services are initially provided in an inpatient hospital-based rehabilitation program, followed by home and community-based therapy to ensure direct generalization as much as possible. For the mild to moderately impaired patient, therapy is initially provided in outpatient clinic and home settings, and again as therapy progresses, the focus therapy is more community-based. For patients with mild brain injuries, who are still able to work to some extent, services will be provided in the workplace, and may include employer/coworker education and job coaching, with the focus often being on removing sources of handicap.

Resulting benefits for the neuropsychologist's assessment process in such a program include the ability to validate hypotheses generated in testing by evaluating their ecological validity as the patient meets typical challenges in his or her IADL. Both the assessment and treatment phases of this program are well integrated, and therefore, the neuropsychologist can increase the breadth and ecological validity of the neuropsychological assessment process by including testing results and behavioral observations obtained by allied professionals, such as an occupational therapist and speech and language pathologist. Evaluations by professionals in these latter two disciplines are different from basic neuropsychological assessments, in that they combine subjective and behavioral assessments of IADL with standardized assessment procedures (tests). They enable the evaluator to more directly assess disability and handicap by using assessment procedures that more closely reflect normal IADL than do neuropsychological tests.

Occupational Therapy

Occupational therapy assessment and treatment is "occupational" in nature, because it addresses difficulties in activities that "occupy" a patient's time and activity. Occupational therapy, by emphasizing task analysis of functional skills, can evaluate the impact of cognitive difficulties (impairments) on IADL (disabilities). A variety of behavior checklists, interviews, structured and unstructured behavior observations, as well as formal testing procedures to evaluate sensory, motor, sensory-motor integration, balance, and visual–perceptual and visual–motor problems, are used to determine the impact of brain injury on a person's IADL. Major areas that are evaluated, in addition to sensory and motor difficulties, include the following.

Occupational therapy's assessment of one's ability to re-engage in IADL uses interview and/or observations of such activities as personal care, driving or transportation, community interactive skills, cooking, house cleaning, grocery shopping, organization and decision making in the home, and ability to maintain, and engage in, leisure activities. Assessments are completed at the clinic, in a person's home, and in the community. Return-to-work assessment includes an evaluation of work readiness, a work-site analysis, and a determination of environmental modifications needed to enable a person to return to productive employment and to maintain his or her productivity. Thus, these procedures directly evaluate disability and handicap.

Functional cognitive assessment will evaluate how a person's cognitive deficits are impacting IADL, and determine the types of compensatory strategies that need to be developed and implemented to reduce the impact. Functional cognitive assessment can be completed in the clinic, in the person's home, at work, or in the community. What better way could there be to assess the impact of attention deficits on functional skills than to *directly observe how* attention/concentration problems are affecting the person when she or he tries to purchase food at a grocery store, find and purchase a shirt at a department store, or stay on task and be productive at work? This information can then be used to validate (or reject) predictions based on the neuropsychological testing.

The neuropsychologist can thereby develop confidence in the predictive validity of her or his data with respect to meaningful, functional abilities. Information from the occupational therapy evaluation can also aid us in determining how such factors as fatigue, balance problems, motor deficits, and visual–motor and visual perceptual difficulties are interacting with brain-injury-related cognitive impairments to influence our patients' functional abilities.

Speech and Language Pathology

A speech and language pathology assessment is completed to address several areas of functional communication that are typically not directly addressed through a neuropsychological evaluation. In addition, and from a functional evaluation standpoint, specific cognitive difficulties (e.g., speed of processing, attention and concentration, learning and memory, sequencing, and problem solving) may be directly observed through reduced functional communication skills. The communication skills, which we assess through a speech and language assessment, include auditory comprehension, reading comprehension, verbal expression, written language, and math.

As with the occupational therapy evaluation, the speech and language assessment uses standardized testing procedures along with subjective assessment (e.g., interview and observational data). Take the case of auditory comprehension as an example. Auditory comprehension translates into how well we can understand what others tell us. Auditory comprehension skills can be evaluated by standardized measures to identify possible problems in the areas of understanding and recalling vocabulary concepts, main ideas, details, and sequential information. A more subjective assessment is conducted via interview to assess a person's understanding and memory of these parameters during interpersonal communication (e.g., conversation, classroom lectures, understanding information communicated over the phone, and understanding information presented in group conversation).

Other aspects of auditory comprehension are addressed during the assessment, such as the patient's ability to understand and remember language if there is background noise present, if there are distractions present, or if a person can stay on track and listen while doing another activity. Taken together, the results of standardized testing and the subjective interview can be used to describe one's functional auditory comprehension skills.

Similar procedures can be used to evaluate other functional communication skills. Care must be taken, in formulating a rehabilitation program, to determine what a patient's functional communication skills were like before the brain injury and the level of ability that is required for his or her normal activities. A lawyer, for example, must have a much higher level of verbal expression skills than an over-the-road truck driver.

Deficits observed by the speech and language pathologist thus not only provide information regarding specific communication difficulties (e.g., aphasia, dysarthria), but they also provide greater insight into how these communication deficits are affecting our patients' ADL, thereby providing additional direct observation of disability and handicap. In addition, they can demonstrate how brain-injury-produced cognitive impairments are affecting one of our most important functional skills, the ability to communicate with others.

Like the occupational therapy evaluation, the speech and language pathology evaluation can be an extension of the neuropsychological assessment. Of greatest benefit is the fact that these evaluations by allied rehabilitation professionals can extend the ecological validity of our own investigations, and thereby improve our ability to estimate disability based on a person's neuropsychological testing performance.

Based on our own observations of correlations between neuropsychological test scores and disability, as well as those made by others, it does appear probable that patterns of cognitive strengths and weaknesses, as reflected by test scores obtained in a neuropsychological evaluation, can help us predict the types of problems (disability and potential sources of handicap) a person might have in her or his ADL. The relationship between impairments in neuropsychological test performance and disability in one's ADL has been discussed by Bennett (1988), Heaton & Pendleton (1981), Prigatano (1986), and others.

Implications of Neuropsychological Test Impairments for Functional Activities of Daily Living

In discussing the implications of neuropsychological test impairments for one's ability to function normally and meet the typical familial, social, educational, and vocational demands, our observations are based on results obtained using the expanded Halstead-Reitan Neuropsychological Test Battery (Reitan & Wolfson, 1993); the same was true for observations made by Heaton and Pendleton (1981), and by Prigatano (1986). Examples will be provided, but, of course, there are many combinations and permutations when analyzing test score profiles, and it is critical that one integrate test scores across and between cognitive abilities in arriving at conclusions regarding a patient's neuropsychological impairments, strengths, and capabilities. The discussion focuses on acquired cognitive impairments arising from traumatic brain injury (TBI). Additional information regarding the neuropsychology of mild brain injury is provided by Raymond, Bennett, Hartlage, and Cullum (1999), and regarding general TBI, by Bennett and Raymond (2008).

Impairments of Sensory and Motor Skills

In general, with the exception of visual field deficits or significantly reduced visual or auditory acuity, deficits on the Sensory-Perceptual Exam (unless severe) are not likely to significantly influence one's everyday functioning.

The same can be said for fine motor speed, as measured by the Finger Tapping Test. The Sensory-Perceptual Exam, along with finger tapping, is more diagnostic of lesion lateralization than functional ability. The exception would be in the case of jobs that require high levels of manual dexterity and sensory–motor integration.

Impairments in sensory abilities that may significantly affect ADL and IADL include balance or vestibular problems and visual tracking, visual accommodation, and visual processing problems secondary to, or associated with, TBI (Raymond, Bennett, Malia, & Bewick, 1996). Neuropsychological assessment, at best, only indirectly evaluates these problems. In our programs, these complaints are screened by occupational therapy or physical therapy, with subsequent referrals to specialists for further evaluation, as deemed appropriate (e.g., behavioral or neuro-optometrists).

Impairments on Tests of Attention and Concentration

Attention and concentration are critical for higher level neuropsychological functioning, and impairments in these domains are often the basis for reported disabilities among patients with brain injuries in learning and memory, communication, reading and writing, and executive functions (Bennett, Raymond, Malia, Bewick, & Linton, 1998). Basic attention skills can be evaluated with the Speech Sounds Perception Test and the Seashore Rhythm Test, sustained attention by Digit Vigilance, alternating attention by Trails B, and sustained attention in the face of interference by failures to maintain a correct set on the WCST.

Individuals who perform normally on the Speech Sounds Perception Test, but poorly on the Seashore Rhythm Test, can typically stay on task or track a conversation if the pace is slow, but they lose track of what is going on if the pace increases. People who make most of their errors on page 2 of Digit Vigilance have trouble processing information for more than a few minutes; they need information presented in small chunks. People whose basic attention skills are intact but have trouble maintaining a correct sorting principle on the WCST are particularly sensitive to outside interference as they go about their IADL. They need to work in a quiet, non-distracting environment. People who perform normally on Trails A but are impaired on Trails B have trouble alternating attention between simultaneous tasks; they need to do one task until it is completed before moving on to another activity.

Impairments on Tests of Learning and Memory

Disabilities with respect to "remembering" are the most common symptoms reported among neurological patients with cognitive complaints (Malia, Raymond, Bewick, & Bennett, 1996). Most individuals will report intact memory for premorbid events, but they report difficulties with remembering events that have happened recently. Aside from the Tactual Performance Test and Subtest 7 of the Category Test, the Halstead-Reitan Battery does not directly evaluate memory impairments. Fortunately, there are instruments now available to evaluate learning and memory abilities that also have predictive ecological validity. Some of these include the Memory Assessment Scales, the California Verbal Learning Test (CVLT), and the Rivermead Behavioral Memory Test (RBMT).

The RBMT is especially helpful in making predictions regarding one's functional memory skills, according to data published by Wilson, Cockburn, Baddeley, and Hiorns (1989). This is because the test items and conditions of learning are not highly structured, and because the actual subtests are designed to be analogs of the types of memory challenges we face in our normal endeavors. Significant impairments on memory batteries that have ecological validity are good predictors as to whether or not a person will have functional memory disabilities.

A strength of the CVLT is its ability to clarify the basis for an individual's memory deficits, and thereby provide helpful information regarding functional memory skills. By assessing memory skills, and by defining the contribution of attention, consolidation, and/or recall deficits to a person's functional memory, one can make recommendations regarding strategies to be used to remediate or compensate for the deficit, make predictions regarding the likely permanence of the memory deficit, and predict how a person will do with respect to functional skills. Some examples are as follows.

Some individuals have memory disabilities that are solely related to attention problems. If attention is improved and impairments are compensated for, and if distractions can be kept to a minimum, they will be able to consolidate information at a normal rate (and therefore not be disabled). On a long-term basis, such individuals rarely need more than a memory book compensatory system to demonstrate normal functional memory skills.

Some individuals, after brain injury, will learn information more slowly, but retention is normal following acquisition. Such individuals should be able to engage in regular educational or training programs, with a reduced course load. They will have to study more or have information repeated more often than will their fellow students or coworkers. Often, these individuals will benefit from academic accommodations. These patients do not report as many problems in everyday forgetfulness as do individuals with acquired retention deficits.

Some patients demonstrate reasonably normal acquisition, but retention is impaired. Such individuals have significant problems with everyday forgetfulness, as demonstrated by frequently forgetting where things have been placed, what they have been told by others, and what they need to do in the future. In patients with good attention, this disability is most effectively reduced by teaching them compensatory memory strategies that are routine and regimented.

Patients with both significant acquisition and retention deficits, such as those with a hypoxic brain injury, cannot retain new information after their attention has been diverted elsewhere. If attention and executive functions testing results are normal in such individuals, some such patients can be taught, with a great deal of effort and support, memory compensatory strategies that enable them to function independently in a highly structured and routine environment (e.g., Bennett & Moore, 1997). If not compensated for, such deficits render a person unable to work or live independently or to manage his or her own affairs.

In essence, these suggestions point to the wealth of information regarding a neurological patient's capabilities that may accrue following a comprehensive evaluation of learning and memory abilities.

Impairments on Tests of Language and Communication

Some neuropsychologists comprehensively evaluate communication skills, but for the most part, their evaluation is cursory. The Aphasia Screening Test from the Halstead-Reitan Battery is just a screening test, and one should not attempt to make significant conclusions based on it. It is designed to elicit pathognomonic signs of left versus right hemisphere damage. The power of this test is in diagnosing the likelihood of brain injury and determining evidence of lateralization of brain injury, not in evaluating a person's communication skills. Adding a test of verbal fluency or a test of naming objects does not add significantly to the Aphasia Screening Test. If a neuropsychologist suspects communication impairments, then a referral should be made to a speech and language pathologist for evaluation of verbal and written expression, verbal and reading comprehension, fluency, articulation, word finding, and so on.

Impairments on Tests of Executive Functions

Executive cognitive functions include problem solving, sequencing, thinking prospectively, cognitive flexibility, making a plan, starting an activity, self-monitoring and self-correcting, and completing a task (Bewick, Raymond, Malia, & Bennett, 1995). Executive functions depend on the integrity of the frontal lobes, but the frontal lobes cannot self-monitor and plan unless information arriving from the posterior association areas has been properly analyzed and transmitted forward. This is why damage to any quadrant of the brain will disrupt performance on the Category Test.

One can make some general statements regarding impairment on tests of executive functions and one's functional capabilities, but it must always be remembered that it is a long way from the testing room to real life, and some individuals who do very well in the structured testing environment will have very significant impairment of executive functions in their ADL. Indeed, such a disparity is pathognomonic for frontal lobe dysfunction.

Because of its dependency on alternating attention, brain-injured individuals who are impaired on Trails B (but do relatively better on Trails A) often have trouble "thinking on their feet." They have difficulty ordering and sequencing information and successfully engaging in activities that require sequential responding.

Performance on the Category Test can reflect, in a general way, a person's ability to cope with the complexities of a normal environment. Patients who are only mildly impaired on the Category Test can usually perform adequately in routine daily activities. These same individuals would, however, have difficulty understanding abstract information they would have understood prior to their brain injury, and thus, they would experience difficulty making decisions about matters that were complicated or out of the ordinary. Students who have even mild deficits on the Category Test often report problems with synthesizing and analyzing new information presented in the classroom or in textbooks. Patients who are severely impaired on the Category Test typically should not be making decisions on their own behalf nor live alone. Even routine decisions cannot be made in a reliable fashion by such individuals.

Perseverative responding, as reflected by poor performance on the WCST, can further reduce the adaptive ability of patients with deficits in sequential thinking, logical analysis, and problem-solving ability. Patients with high perseverative response scores on the WCST are, in general, inflexible in their thinking. If they start out with an ineffective approach to a new problem or situation, they will continue with that approach long after most people would try alternative strategies. They have trouble inhibiting an action before it is needed or after it should be stopped. They have trouble learning from mistakes as well as from successes.

As discussed earlier in this chapter, the neuropsychological assessment environment is not the real world, and in our assessment procedures, we typically do not create real-world situations. Although neuropsychological assessment has been criticized for being too sensitive, in reality, it is often not sensitive enough to detect deficits that follow brain injury. This is particularly true for executive functions that are assessed with highly structured tests such as Trails B, the Category Test, and the WCST, although the WCST is less structured and probably more sensitive to frontal lobe dysfunction than the other two.

The use of such highly structured tests may render it difficult for our assessments to adequately evaluate the integrity of the executive control system, because the very process of formally testing executive functions may mask an existing impairment (Sbordone, 1996; Ylvisaker & Szekeres, 1989). This is because the structure provided by the testing environment and the guidance provided by the examiner can serve as a prosthesis for deficits the individual with a brain injury normally has with respect to task planning, initiation, maintenance, and completion. The examiner typically tells the patient what to do, when to begin, and how to be successful; once the test begins, the examiner keeps the patient on task until it is completed. Formal testing can thus reduce or eliminate deficits in executive functioning that the patient normally experiences. In essence, a well-standardized and validated assessment, in conjunction with behavioral observations, should yield beneficial and meaningful information with regard to the assessment of executive functions.

A test battery with potentially improved ecological validity for predicting executive functions, Behavioral Assessment of the Dysexecutive Syndrome, has been published (Wilson, Alderman, Burgess, Emslie, & Evans, 1996). This test should add to our ability to accurately assess executive cognitive functions typically ascribed to the frontal lobes. In addition to using less structured assessment protocols, executive functions also should be evaluated through observations of the patient in his or her normal activities (Bewick, Raymond, Malia, & Bennett, 1995; Kay & Silver, 1989; Sbordone, 1996).

Effort and Symptom Validity Assessment

In all cases involving neuropsychological consultation, the primary role of the clinical neuropsychologist is to correctly administer, score, and interpret test results in order to render a professional opinion with a reasonable degree of neuropsychological certainty. This must be based on scientifically validated neuropsychological findings that yield valid and reliable data. Without valid information, the test results, in most instances, are uninterpretable and essentially meaningless. To ensure valid test results, measures of effort and symptom validity must be included in a standardized neuropsychological assessment.

The assessment of effort and symptom validity, to either rule in or rule out marginal effort, symptom exaggeration, or invalid test scores, has become a viable part of clinical and forensic neuropsychological assessment. This has become most evident over the past few years through an increase in clinical research and publications addressing this issue. Whereas the assessment of these areas may vary upon specific training and ideology of the neuropsychologist, referral question, and potential diagnoses, the assessment must occur and be part of a neuropsychological evaluation. The importance of assessing for effort and symptom validity was reviewed by a group of esteemed neuropsychologists who are all members of the National Academy of Neuropsychology (NAN). They developed a NAN position paper that was eventually published in 2005 (Bush et al., 2005). The primary purpose of the position paper and article was to summarize symptom validity testing and procedures, make specific recommendations regarding these procedures, and to provide an educational overview regarding the need for symptom validity testing. The terms "symptom validity," "response bias," "effort," "malingering," and "dissimilation" were all discussed and defined within the article. These are common terms that are generally associated with various procedures and measures used to assess effort and validity.

An overview of specific tests and procedures to assess effort and validity is included in a separate chapter of this text. Furthermore, please review the current literature regarding the development and clinical utility of each assessment procedure. For brevity purposes, the following is a partial list of commonly used tests and procedures to assess effort and symptom validity:

Portland Digit Recognition Test (PDRT)
(Binder, 1993)

Computerized Assessment of Response Bias (CARB)
(Allen, Conder, Green, & Cox, 1997)

Victoria Symptom Validity Test (VSVT)
(Slick, Hopp, Strauss, & Thompson, 1997)

Word Memory Test (WMT)
(Green, Allen, & Astner, 1996)

Test of Memory Malingering (TOMM)
(Tombaugh, 1996)

The use of effort testing is imperative in obtaining valid and interpretable test results that will be used in the determination of clinical syndromes, causality, and the neurocognitive and behavioral status of the individual assessed. Obviously, this information will prove beneficial in all clinical and forensic cases involved in disability determination, fitness-for-duty, and rehabilitation planning.

Neuropsychological Assessment and Fitness-for-Duty Examinations

Most neuropsychologists would agree that, in addition to providing important information regarding presence versus absence of brain injury and diagnostic information regarding different neurobehavioral syndromes, neuropsychological assessment can provide important information regarding impairments of cognition secondary to brain dysfunction, and the implications of these deficits for a person's ability to function and meet everyday challenges. Consequently, neuropsychological assessment is increasingly called on to evaluate the implications of possible cognitive impairments for employment following such neurological events as TBI or stroke. Such objective assessments can help to determine whether the examinee can do the job and to ensure that he/she is not a danger to himself/herself or others. Guidelines for such fitness-for-duty evaluations are available for several career categories, including physicians and police officers.

Fitness-for-duty neuropsychological evaluations can occur in several settings including return to work, continuing in one's occupation, or obtaining a new job, transfer, or promotion. The questions regarding fitness for duty can also arise because of possible problems in meeting the expectations of one's career secondary to other neurological conditions (e.g., epilepsy) or neurodegenerative disorders with cognitive components (e.g., multiple sclerosis, dementia, Parkinson's disease). This section of the chapter will provide some general guidelines and will discuss the utility of neuropsychological assessment in fitness-for-duty evaluations.

These evaluations must be consistent with human-rights legislation. With respect to prospective employees, a fitness-for-duty examination may only be given **after** a job offer has been made. It is strictly prohibited to ask a prospective employee in the preoffer stage to submit to a fitness for duty examination. However, a prospective employer can make pre-employment inquiries into the ability of the prospective employee to perform job-related functions. An employer is, on the other hand, allowed to make a job offer conditioned on successful completion of a fitness-for-duty examination, providing this is required of all entering employees in the same category. The outcome of such an exam would be to indicate that the employee would be able to perform the job and would not be a hazard to self or others, when working in that job. Similar conditions apply to situations when an employee applies for a job transfer or a promotion; the employee may only be given a fitness-for duty-evaluation after a job offer had been made. The job offer may be conditioned on passing the exam.

Under the ADA, employers may require a fitness-for-duty evaluation for those returning to work after a medical leave if the employer has reasonable belief that the employee's present ability to perform essential job functions will be impaired, or that the employee poses a direct threat to self or others because of the medical condition. Under the ADA, the examination must be limited in scope to information needed to assess the employee's ability to work, and the examination must be directed toward an assessment of the actual medical condition that caused the absence. Neuropsychological fitness-for-duty evaluations meet these requirements by focusing on the impact that one's neurological condition has on cognitive abilities, and how possible resulting impairments affect the ability of the employee to meet specific cognitive demands required by his/her job, including the ability to perform the job safely.

The primary referral questions for the neuropsychologist in fitness-for-duty evaluations are whether a possibly impaired individual can either return to work or maintain employment in a particular job. The evaluation requires informed consent from the examinee to participate in the examination. The informed consent must include a description of the nature and scope of the assessment; the limits of confidentiality, including any information that may be disclosed to the employer without the employee's specific authorization; the potential outcomes and use of the assessment findings; and other legal and ethical standards applicable to mental health assessments conducted at the request of third parties. The client in the fitness-for-duty evaluation is the employer, not the employee being evaluated, and this must be communicated to all involved parties prior to the beginning of the formal evaluation. The neuropsychologist, of course, owes an ethical duty to both parties to be fair and impartial, and to honor their interests and legal rights. In addition to obtaining informed consent, the examiner must obtain written authorization from the examinee to release the examiner's findings and opinions to the employer.

Prior to formal neuropsychological testing, the evaluator must often exert considerable effort to obtain and review all relevant medical and personnel records, as well as possible incident reports or memos. After the testing, additional information may be sought, if deemed necessary, from relevant third parties. In addition to medical records, pertinent information may be obtained from the examinee's significant others, the referral source, supervisors, and from anyone involved in monitoring the individual. The employer can provide a detailed job analysis, with the actual and anticipated essential requirements of the job and a review of the work environment, including the potential of situations that might aggravate any impairments that are discovered (e.g., significant distractions, need to multitask, need to make quick decisions, requirements of sustained attention, memory, and response speed/dexterity demands). It may be necessary to make a referral to, and consultation with, a specialist, if deemed necessary by the examiner.

There are no empirically derived guidelines for determining whether an impaired worker is fit to return to work, and to make a recommendation with a reasonable degree of neuropsychological confidence, one must be very familiar with the specific demands of a person's job. This may require a visit to a job site or shadowing a person doing the same job that the examinee did in the past. Knowledge of the applicability of test scores to everyday demands is also crucial. For example, a physician with Parkinson's disease may be found to be perfectly normal in our assessment from a cognitive perspective, but at the same time, be unable to complete certain motor dexterity tasks within the normal range. We would not want that physician to practice surgery, but a physician practicing as a psychiatrist would not be affected by this condition.

There has been significant interest in fitness-for duty evaluations in physicians because of the obvious implications that would arise if errors in practice were made. General guidelines for psychiatric fitness-for duty evaluations have been published (Anfang, Faulkner, Fromson, & Gendel, 2005; Wettstein, 2005), and neuropsychological testing of physicians has been discussed in an article by Rentz (2006). Rentz emphasizes the difficulty of evaluating physicians. This group is high-functioning, and by virtue of their intellectual abilities and extensive education, physicians typically perform very well on cognitive tests. Because people who have always been high-functioning cognitively are more adept at finding alternative strategies in response to task demands, Rentz noted that an impaired physician might perform within the normal range on neuropsychological tests because of the ability to compensate for brain damage or a progressive cognitive impairment. Therefore, Rentz concluded that the neuropsychologist needs to consider whether the test scores are consistent with the physician's estimated ability level and estimated demands of his/her career, rather than simply evaluating the physician against a normative standard (even demographically adjusted norms, we would add).

Based on the findings of the fitness-for-duty evaluation, there are three possible outcomes.

Fit: This conclusion means that the employee can meet all of the cognitive demands of the job and is able to perform the job without danger to self or others, without reservation. The subcategory "temporarily" can be used for any of these major conclusions. "Permanently," on the other hand, should never be used with a judgment of "fit" because the evaluator cannot see into the future.

Fit subject to work modifications: A statement in this category indicates that the person cannot successfully complete the normal job requirements, or might be a danger to self or others if required to do so. However, the person could be successful and safely meet job expectations if current working conditions were modified. This could include changes in the work environment or changes in the way the work is performed. Suggested modifications must be clearly described in the conclusions/recommendations section of the report. However, the determination as to whether or not a recommended restriction or accommodation is reasonable for the specific employee and job is a determination to be made by the employer, not the examiner.

If the modifications can be accommodated, the employee is considered fit for the modified job. If the modifications cannot be reasonably accommodated, the employee is deemed temporarily or permanently unfit. "Temporarily" means that as the employee's condition improves with time or further rehabilitation, the requirements for work modifications may be lifted. "Permanently" means that the employee will never be fit for the job without the modifications.

Unfit: This category describes the employee who is unable to meet cognitive demands of the job and/or is not able to safely perform the job, even if reasonable and necessary work modifications were in place. This category could be either "temporary" or "permanent," depending on whether the examiner believes that the employee's condition may improve with time or further rehabilitation interventions. Thus, "temporarily unfit" means that the employee may experience improvements over time, and may be able in the future to return to normal or modified work, or transfer to some other job. "Permanently unfit" usually implies that the employee will never be fit for the job, and neither rehabilitation interventions nor job modifications could reasonably be expected to change this situation. If "permanently" means that the employee is unable to do any available job, with or without work modifications, this conclusion should be stated in the results/conclusions section of the report.

When a fitness-for-duty evaluation is completed, the examiner's findings, conclusions, and opinions are based on all data and information available at the time of the assessment. If additional relevant information is obtained after completion of the evaluation, or if it was determined that the original evaluation was based on inaccurate information, the employer may request that the examiner reconsider his or her conclusions based on the additional information. Reconsideration or re-evaluation may also be appropriate in situations in which an employee, previously deemed unfit for work, subsequently provides information that suggests that his or her fitness has been restored.

Reducing Disability by Cognitive Rehabilitation

When neuropsychological assessment indicates that impairments and consequent disabilities exist, then the forensic neuropsychologist should be a resource for determining ways to rehabilitate the individual. If a plan of treatment can be developed to reduce a person's disability, or if the person's environment can be changed to reduce a handicap, then the person will have a better chance of returning to productive activity. As the AMA Guides note, an individual with an impairment who is able to accomplish a specific task (e.g., his/her job) is not disabled with respect to that task. Damages would be reduced accordingly.

Cognitive rehabilitation is a methodology that can reduce impairment, and thereby, reduce disability. Cognitive rehabilitation is the process by which an individual's acquired cognitive deficits, secondary to brain trauma or a neurological condition, are ameliorated. It is widely agreed that treatment must be tailored to each individual case (Raskin & Gordon, 1992). Some general principles regarding cognitive rehabilitation, with which the reader should be familiar, include the following.

Many methods have been developed to address acquired cognitive deficits including: (a) process-specific rehabilitation, such as attention process training (Sohlberg & Mateer, 1989a), (b) skills-based training, such as prospective memory training (Mayer, Keating & Rapp, 1986), (c) compensatory strategy training, such as use of a memory book system (Sohlberg & Mateer, 1989b), and (d) metacognitive training, such as providing rehabilitation interventions to improve a person's awareness of deficits and ability to self-monitor (Bewick et al., 1995). These methods and strategies are all incorporated into the comprehensive neurorehabilitation program Brainwave-R (Malia, Bewick, Raymond, & Bennett, 1997).

In general, for each patient, combining cognitive rehabilitation methods is the most effective treatment approach. Regardless of what approaches and materials are used in cognitive rehabilitation, the therapist must plan, from the beginning, ways to ensure that generalization of skills acquired during therapy will transfer to real-world activities. Sohlberg and Raskin (1996) describe five principles that they believe will promote generalization, including: (a) actively plan for and program generalization from the beginning of the treatment process, (b) identify naturally occurring reinforcers in the person's normal environment that will maintain the newly acquired (or reacquired) cognitive skill or process, (c) use training situations that are common to both the training environment and the real world, (d) use sufficient examples when conducting therapy, and (e) select methods for measuring generalization from the clinic to the real world to evaluate efficacy of the therapy procedures.

Using this framework in our own programs, we generally divide a cognitive rehabilitation session into thirds. The first part of the session is devoted to metacognitive training, the next portion of the session addresses skills-based training and compensatory strategies, and the last part of the session involves process-specific rehabilitation. When conducted appropriately, cognitive rehabilitation does facilitate recovery. As should be apparent to the reader, "conducted appropriately" is far removed from lining people up in front of computers in which the patient's task is to complete repetitive drills. Whereas the efficacy of cognitive rehabilitation will continue to be debated (as has been the value of rehabilitation in general), a number of published reports have demonstrated the benefits of this therapeutic intervention (e.g., Ben-Yishay & Diller, 1993; Cicerone, 1999; Ho & Bennett, 1997; Malia, Raymond, Bewick, & Bennett, 1998; Sohlberg & Mateer, 1987).

In our clinics, outpatient cognitive rehabilitation is provided by cognitive rehabilitation, speech/language, and/or occupational therapists. The advantage of neuropsychological assessment in planning a formal cognitive rehabilitation program is that test results can be used to specify the nature of the acquired cognitive impairments that are the basis for the patient's disabilities. This can be illustrated by two cases of patients with a presenting complaint of being unable to remember recent events.

For example, a client with mild–moderate overall cognitive impairment due to a TBI may complain of problems with everyday forgetfulness. Assessment findings could indicate normal consolidation and retrieval abilities, yet significantly impaired attention and concentration skills. In this situation, the memory problems are not primary, and improvements in everyday memory functions will be realized if the patient is provided therapy to improve awareness of deficits and situations in which memory problems occur (metacognitive training), strategies to remember what needs to be done each day (prospective memory skills-based training), remediation therapy to improve attention/concentration skills (attention process training), and a memory book system (compensatory strategy training).

A different patient who suffered a hypoxic brain injury might similarly complain of everyday forgetfulness, but in this case, the client could demonstrate normal performance on tests of attention and concentration, but severely impaired ability with respect to adding new information to memory. During testing, it could be observed on the CVLT that the person's trial-to-trial performance never improved, and recall after each trial was never greater than one's predicted working memory span. Recall of the list after interference was negligible. Such a person has a primary memory deficit. The focus of therapy in this latter case would be on metacognitive training, skills-based training, and especially compensatory strategies.

Skills-based training and compensatory strategy training vary greatly, depending on the typical demands that a client must face in returning to IADL, as well as work or school. For example, a receptionist would need to learn skills to filter out distractions in the work environment, stay on task until an activity is completed, double-check the accuracy of messages, and improve organization.

A student, in contrast, would need to learn strategies to improve taking notes during lectures and reading assignments, study skills, and test taking. For students, strategies can be provided to teachers regarding modifications to normal classroom activities so that the student's ability to meet the demands of the academic environment is enhanced. For the college student, we have asked the college's disabled students support services to provide note takers, record textbooks on audio tape, and provide a quiet, non-distracting environment with a reader for the student taking an exam. The neuropsychological test data can be used to verify the student's complaints and provide justification for such support. Making such recommendations is dependent on the neuropsychologist being able to predict the ecological significance of the neuropsychological testing results.

When therapy goals are primarily addressed by speech and language therapy, due to acquired communication deficits, the neuropsychologist can recommend metacognitive, process, and skills-based treatments to facilitate speed and efficiency of processing, attention, and self-monitoring. Combined with speech and language therapy, these interventions will promote recovery in areas such as word finding, tracking conversations, understanding what is read, verbal expression, and one's ability to write in an organized, sequential, and cohesive fashion.

When therapy goals are predominantly being met by occupational therapy, similar neuropsychological assessment-based cognitive interventions will facilitate return to normal IADL. For example, improvements in attention and concentration can facilitate the use and effectiveness of compensatory strategies acquired in occupational therapy for improving home organization, maintaining one's checkbook, staying with a task until it is completed, cooking, grocery shopping, driving, and employment-related activities. These are a few examples of how forensic neuropsychologists use neuropsychological assessment in developing and providing valuable suggestions to reduce the disability resulting from neurologically based impairments (Bennett, Dittmar, & Ho, 1997).

References

Allen, L. M., Conder, R. L., Green, P., & Cox, D. R. (1997). *CARB 97 manual for the computerized assessment of response bias.* Durham, NC: CogniSyst.

Anfang, S. A., Faulkner, L. R., Fromson, J. A., & Gendel, M. H. (2005). The American Psychiatric Association's resource document on guidelines for psychiatric fitness-for-duty evaluations of physicians. *Journal of the American Academy of Psychiatry and the Law, 33*, 85–88.

American Medical Association. (1993). *Guides to the evaluation of permanent impairment* (4th ed.). Chicago: Author.

Americans with Disabilities Act of 1990. Public Law 101-336, 42 U.S.C & 12101 et seq. (2008).

Ben-Yishay, Y., & Diller, L. (1993). Cognitive remediation in traumatic brain injury: Update and issues. *Archives of Physical Medicine and Rehabilitation, 74*, 204–213.

Bennett, T. L. (1988). Use of the Halstead-Reitan neuropsychological test battery in the assessment of head injury. *Cognitive Rehabilitation, 6*(3), 18–24.

Bennett, T. L., Dittmar, C., & Ho, M. (1997). The neuropsychology of traumatic brain injury. In A. M. Horton, Jr., D. Wedding, & J. Webster (Eds.), *The neuropsychology handbook: Behavioral and clinical perspectives* (2nd ed., Vol. 2, pp. 123–172). New York: Springer Publishing Company.

Bennett, T. L., & Moore, C. (1997). Living with amnesia: The case of Mike S. *Bulletin of the National Academy of Neuropsychology, 13*, 14–17.

Bennett, T. L., & Raymond, M. J. (2008). The neuropsychology of traumatic brain injury. In A. M. Horton, Jr., D. Wedding, & J. Webster (Eds.), *The neuropsychology handbook* (3rd ed., Vol. 3, pp. 533–570). New York: Springer Publishing Company.

Bennett, T. L., Raymond, M. J., Malia, K. B., Bewick, K. C., & Linton, B. S. (1998). Rehabilitation of attention and concentration deficits following brain injury. *Journal of Cognitive Rehabilitation, 16*(2), 8–13.

Bewick, K. C., Raymond, M. J., Malia, K. B., & Bennett, T. L. (1995). Metacognition as the ultimate executive: Techniques and tasks to facilitate executive functions. *NeuroRehabilitation, 5*, 367–375.

Binder, L. M. (1993). An abbreviated form of the Portland Digit Recognition Test. *Clinical Neuropsychologist, 7*, 104–107.

Bush, S. S., Ruff, R. M., Troster, A. I., Barth, J. T., Koffler, S., Plisken, N., et al. (2005). Symptom validity assessment: Practice issues and medical necessity. NAN policy and procedures committee. *Archives of Clinical Neuropsychology, 20*(4), 419–426.

Cicerone, K. D. (1999). Efficacy of cognitive rehabilitation in the treatment of mild brain injury. In M. J. Raymond, T. L. Bennett, L. C. Hartlage, & C. M. Cullum (Eds.), *Mild brain injury: A clinician's guide* (pp. 231–253). Austin, TX: Pro-Ed.

Dart, J., & West, J. (1995). Americans with disabilities act. *Encyclopedia of disability and rehabilitation* (pp. 47–53). New York: MacMillan.

Goldstein, K. (1942). *Aftereffects of brain injury in war.* New York: Grune and Stratton.

Green, P., Allen, L. M., & Astner, K. (1996). *The word memory test: A user's guide to the oral and computer-administered forms, US version 1.1.* Durham, NC: CogniSyst.

Heaton, R. K., & Pendleton, M. G. (1981). Use of neuropsychological tests to predict adult patients' everyday functioning. *Journal of Consulting and Clinical Neuropsychology, 49*, 807–821.

Ho., M., & Bennett, T. L. (1997). Efficacy of neuropsychological rehabilitation for mild-moderate traumatic brain injury. *Archives of Clinical Neuropsychology, 12*, 1–11.

Kay, T., & Silver, S. M. (1989). Closed head trauma: Assessment for rehabilitation. In M. D. Lezak (Ed.), *Assessment of the behavioral consequences of head trauma* (pp. 145–170). New York: Alan R. Liss.

Malia, K. B., Bewick, K. C., Raymond, M. J., & Bennett, T. L. (1997). *Brainwave-R: Cognitive strategies and techniques for brain injury rehabilitation.* Austin, TX: Pro-Ed.

Malia, K. B., Raymond, M. J., Bewick, K. C., & Bennett, T. L. (1996). A comprehensive approach to memory rehabilitation following brain injury. *Journal of Cognitive Rehabilitation, 14*(6), 18–23.

Malia, K. B., Raymond, M. J., Bewick, K. C., & Bennett, T. L. (1998). Information processing deficits and brain injury: Preliminary results. *NeuroRehabilitation, 11*, 239–247.

Mayer, N., Keating, D., & Rapp, D. (1986). Skills, routines, and activity patterns of daily living: A functional approach. In B. P. Uzzell & Y. Gross (Eds.), *Clinical neuropsychology of intervention* (pp. 205–222). Boston: Martinus Nijhoff.

Prigatano, G. P. (1986). *Neuropsychological rehabilitation after brain damage.* Baltimore: Johns Hopkins University Press.

Raskin, S., & Gordon, W. (1992). The impact of different approaches to remediation on generalization. *NeuroRehabilitation, 2*, 38–45.

Raymond, M. J., Bennett, T. L., Hartlage, L. C., & Cullum, C. M. (1999). *Mild traumatic brian injury: A clinician's guide.* Austin, TX: Pro-Ed.

Raymond, M. J., Bennett, T. L., Malia, K. B., & Bewick, K. C. (1996). Rehabilitation of visual processing deficits. *NeuroRehabilitation, 6*, 229–240.

Reitan, R. M., & Wolfson, D. (1993). *The Halstead-Reitan neuropsychological test battery: Theory and clinical interpretation* (2nd ed.). Tucson, AZ: Neuropsychology Press.

Rentz, D. M. (2006, June/July). Neuropsychological testing of physicians. *Vital signs.* Retrieved June 15, 2007, from http://www.MassachusettsMedical Society.org

Sbordone, R. J. (1996). Ecological validity: Some critical issues for the neuropsychologist. In R. J. Sbordonne & C. J. Long (Eds.), *Ecological validity of neuropsychological testing* (pp. 15–41). Delray Beach, FL: GR Press/St. Lucie Press.

Sbordone, R. J., & Long, C. J. (Eds.). (1996). *Ecological validity of neuropsychological testing.* Delray Beach, FL: GR Press/St. Lucie Press.

Slick, D. J., Hopp, G., Strauss, E., & Thompson, G. (1997). *The Victoria Symptom Validity Test.* Odessa, FL: PAR.

Sohlberg, M. M., & Mateer, C. (1987). Effectiveness of an attention training program. *Journal of Clinical and Experimental Neuropsychology, 9,* 117–130.

Sohlberg, M. M., & Mateer, C. (1989a) *Introduction to cognitive rehabilitation: Theory and practice.* New York: Guilford Press.

Sohlberg, M. M., & Mateer, C. (1989b). Training use of compensatory memory books: A three stage behavioral approach. *Journal of Clinical and Experimental Neuropsychology, 11,* 871–891.

Sohlberg, M. M., & Raskin, S. A. (1996). Principles of generalization applied to attention and memory interventions. *Journal of Head Trauma Rehabilitation, 11,* 65–78.

Tombaugh, T. N. (1996). *Test of memory malingering.* North Tonawanda, NY: Multi-Health Systems.

United Stated Department of Health, Education, and Welfare. (1977). Nondiscrimination on the basis of handicap. *Federal Register, 42,* 22679–22694.

Wettstein, R. M. (2005). Commentary: Quality improvement and psychiatric fitness-for-duty evaluations of physicians. *Journal of the American Academy of Psychiatry and the Law, 33,* 92–94.

Wilson, B. A. (1997). Cognitive rehabilitation: How it is and how it might be. *Journal of the International Neuropsychological Society, 3,* 487–496.

Wilson, B. A., Alderman, N., Burgess, P. W., Emslie, H., & Evans, J. J. (1996). *Behavioral assessment of the dysexecutive syndrome.* Bury St. Edmunds, U.K.: Thames Valley Test Company.

Wilson, B. A., Cockburn, J., Baddeley, A., & Hiorns, R. (1989). The development and validation of a test battery for detecting and monitoring everyday memory problems. *Journal of Clinical and Experimental Neuropsychology, 11,* 855–870.

World Health Organization. (1980). *International classification of impairments, disabilities, and handicaps: A manual of classification relating to the consequences of disease.* Geneva, Switzerland: Author.

Ylvisaker, M., & Szekeres, S. F. (1989). Metacognition and executive impairments in head injured children and adults. *Topics in Language Disorders, 9,* 34–49.

Forensic Neuropsychology and the Older Client

21

Kevin Duff

To paraphrase the advice of a number of prominent forensic neuropsychologists, good forensic practice starts with good clinical practice. Conducting comprehensive evaluations with reliable and valid instruments, keeping conclusions consistent with the observed data, and staying aware of current and relevant literature can make the defense of your findings and conclusions in the courtroom easier. However, good clinical practice (and therefore, good forensic practice) can be more challenging when working with older adults. This chapter will review some of the potential pitfalls of conducting forensic evaluations with older clients, as well as some of the special requests that might be made in these cases.

Normative Issues and the Older Client

While testifying at the competency hearing of your 82-year-old client, the following exchange occurs:

Attorney: In your report, you noted that the client's memory was "low average." What is that based on?

Neuropsychologist: In the course of my evaluation, I administered portions of the Wechsler Memory Scale (WMS)–Third Edition. One subtest from that test is the Word Lists subtest. In this subtest, a patient learns a list of 12 words across 4 learning trials. After 30 minutes, the patient is asked to recall as many words from that list as he can. My client's performance on that delayed recall trial was at the 16th percentile compared with age-matched peers, which is in the low average range.

Attorney: So after a 30-minute delay, how many words did your client recall from the list?

Neuropsychologist: None.

Attorney: None?

Neuropsychologist: None.

Attorney: Recalling no words after 30 minutes is low average?

Neuropsychologist: That's correct.

Attorney: Could your client get any worse than low average?

Neuropsychologist: No, I suppose not.

Advancing age has been widely accepted as a moderating factor in neuropsychological functioning. Several large-scale longitudinal studies, including the Seattle Longitudinal Study (Schaie, 1996), Victoria Longitudinal Study (Hertzog, Dixon, Hultsch, & MacDonald, 2003), and Berlin Aging Study (Baltes & Mayer, 1999), have tracked the cognitive abilities of adults from their 20s to their 100s. These studies have consistently demonstrated that certain cognitive abilities decline during the sixth, seventh, and eighth decades of life, whereas other cognitive abilities remain quite stable across time. For example, in a review of the findings from his Seattle Longitudinal Study, Schaie (2005) noted that the cognitive constructs of perceptual speed and numerical ability steadily decline from 25 to 88 years old (see Figure 21.1). Other cognitive abilities, like verbal ability, inductive reasoning, and verbal memory, start their decline at a much later point, around age 53. Modest declines are eventually observed on these abilities into the 70s and 80s.

Despite these clear results, normative data for some neuropsychological measures remain poor at the higher ends of the age spectrum, as reflected in the previous case vignette. For example, the Trail Making Test is one of the most widely used neuropsychological measures that investigates visual scanning, processing speed, and set shifting. However, for clients in their 70s, 80s, or beyond, normative data might be suboptimal for making clinical and forensic determinations. In one of the better studies, Tombaugh (2004) reports age- and education-corrected normative data on community-dwelling adults. Whereas individuals in their 70s and early 80s are well represented (e.g., 70–74-year-olds $n = 106$; 75–79-year-olds $n = 108$; 80–84-year-olds $n = 118$), older octogenarians are not (85–89-year-olds $n = 29$). In another study, perhaps the best-known study of older adults in neuropsychology, the Mayo's Older American Normative Studies (MOANS) also have relatively few older individuals contributing to their Trail Making Test norms (e.g., 70–74-year-olds $n = 57$; 75–79-year-olds $n = 53$; 80–84-year-olds $n = 27$;

21.1

Age-related changes in cognitive variables across adulthood.

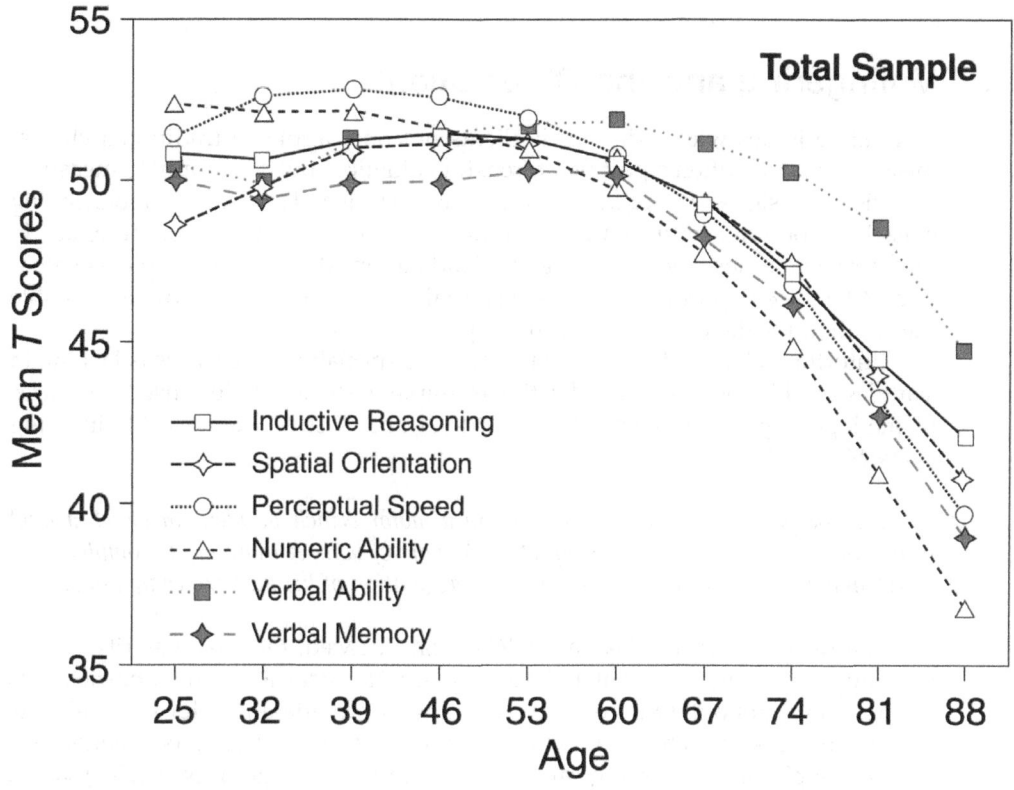

Note. Reprinted with permission from Schaie (2005).

85–89-year-olds $n = 17$; 90–94-year-olds $n = 5$) (Ivnik, Malec, Smith, Tangalos, & Petersen, 1996).

By highlighting the relatively small sample sizes of these studies, I am not trying to criticize their work. Both studies are among the best examples of normative data for older adults currently available. But neuropsychologists who use these (or smaller) normative sets with older clients should be aware of their limitations, both in clinical and forensic settings.

Another limitation in these normative data for older adults is their poorer psychometric properties. As reflected in the case example, "low average" is the worst performance possible on the WMS-III Word Lists II for 80–84 year olds. According to the WMS-III manual, individuals age 65 years or older can recall no words after a 30-minute delay and still achieve a corrected score between the 9th–16th percentiles. Unfortunately, this is not specific to the WMS-III. In our work on normative data on the Repeatable Battery for the Assessment of Neuro-psychological Status (RBANS), we found that 6.7% of 718 community-dwelling elders failed to recall even a single word on the delay portion of a list-learning task (Duff, Patton, Schoenberg, Mold, Scott, & Adams, 2003). Unfortunately, a number of cognitive tests suffer from floor effects in the elderly, and clinicians, especially those doing forensics work, need to be aware of these limitations in the instruments they use.

Malingering and the Older Client

Normative issues with older adult clients not only apply to traditional clinical measures that are often a part of a forensic evaluation, but also apply to measures specifically designed for forensic evaluations. Specialized measures for identifying biased responding, symptom exaggeration, or malingering are commonplace in forensic evaluations, and their absence could be considered an incomplete evaluation. When used appropriately, these specialized measures can provide valuable information for the clinician, attorneys, judge, and jury.

Unfortunately, validation of many of these specialized measures is lacking in samples of older adults. Consider this example with two widely used measures of malingering: Word Memory Test (WMT) and Test of Memory Malingering (TOMM).

Your 68-year-old client was involved in a motor vehicle accident in which a mild traumatic brain injury (TBI) is suspected. As part of your evaluation, he completes the WMT and TOMM to assess for symptom exaggeration of his memory complaints.

In a review of 11 articles on the WMT on PubMed, the vast majority do not seem appropriate for the client in the example, as the mean age of their participants is under 45 years old. Only one study seems to provide any relevant guidance. Merten, Bossink, & Schmand, 2007 presented data from two experiments: one with a sample of 48 neurological patients with a mean age of 56.4 (13.1) years, and another with a sample of 20 patients with Alzheimer's disease and 14 elderly controls (mean ages 73.4 [4.8] and 76.6 [6.7], respectively). In their younger cohort of neurological patients, those with clinically obvious cognitive impairments passed the WMT around 50% of the time, whereas those without clinically obvious cognitive impairments passed the WMT nearly 100% of the time. In Merten et al.'s older cohort, patients with Alzheimer's disease passed the WMT 5–10% of the time, whereas healthy elders passed it 100% of the time. Although one should be cautious in interpreting the results of a single study, it appears that the performances on the WMT in those without obvious cognitive impairments and in healthy elders should be near perfect. However, to the degree that the client in the example has some mild cognitive deficits or frank dementia, the results of Merten et al. cast doubts on the interpretability of a failed WMT.

In a similar review of articles on the TOMM on PubMed, several were identified that could offer guidance in the current case example. Ashendorf, Constantinou, and McCaffrey (2004) examined 197 community-dwelling older adults (mean age = 64.6 [5.5]) and found that neither depression nor anxiety significantly affected TOMM performances in these subjects, with all passing Trial 2. Teichner and Wagner (2004) studied a sample of 78 patients referred for a neuropsychological evaluation with a mean age of 70.5 (8.5) years. Patients classified as cognitively normal passed Trial 2 of the TOMM 100% of the time. Patients classified as cognitively impaired but not demented passed the TOMM 92% of the time. Patients classified as demented, however, passed the TOMM only 24% of the time. Merten et al. (2007) also compared demented and intact elders on the TOMM, and found that 70% of patients diagnosed with Alzheimer's disease passed Trial 2 of the TOMM, and that 100% of healthy elders passed that measure. Finally, O'Bryant et al. (2008) observed that 100% of 306 community-dwelling older adults (mean age = 63.9 [5.9]) passed Trial 2 of the TOMM. Although these four studies have their limitations, they appear to present a more convincing argument that the TOMM is relatively unaffected by older age (as well as depression and anxiety, and perhaps Alzheimer's disease).

The case example was not presented to identify either the WMT or the TOMM as the superior measure of effort. It was presented to suggest that, as with traditional clinical neuropsychological measures, the decision of which symptom validity measures to use with older adults should be informed by the literature. Forensic neuropsychologists should make those decisions wisely. It is also important to continue to expand research on normative data for older adults on these measures, as well as for older patients with actual TBIs.

Postconcussive Syndrome and the Older Client

The first two potential pitfalls in conducting forensic evaluations with older clients addressed individual tests, whether traditional clinical measures or specialized forensic tools. This third potential pitfall relates to the interpretation of a general neuropsychological pattern. Although any pattern could be applicable, the following example will concern postconcussive syndrome.

While testifying in the case of your 75-year-old client, whom you diagnosed with a mild TBI after a fall in the courtyard of his retirement facility, the following exchange occurs:

Defense Attorney:	*Following your examination of the plaintiff, you diagnosed him with "postconcussive syndrome." How did you make that determination?*
Neuropsychologist:	*During my clinical interview of the patient, he endorsed headaches, dizziness, anxiety, insomnia, poor concentration, and fatigue. These symptoms are typical for postconcussive syndrome, which can be a result of a mild traumatic brain injury.*
Defense Attorney:	*Are you aware that more than 25 studies have been published in the past 10 years on postconcussive syndrome and the average age of the subjects in those studies is less than 40?*
Neuropsychologist:	*No, I didn't know that.*
Defense Attorney:	*Did you know that only 1 study published in the past 10 years on postconcussive syndrome actually looked at the effects of age on these symptoms?*
Neuropsychologist:	*No.*

Defense Attorney:　　As you were unaware of that single study on aging effects of postconcussive symptoms, I suppose you do not know how postconcussive syndrome looks in a 75-year-old, like the plaintiff.
Neuropsychologist:　　No, I suppose I don't.

Because TBIs are most common in younger adults, it is not surprising that most of the research on this condition uses younger samples. Similarly, neuropsychology's knowledge of patterns associated with TBI (e.g., postconcussive syndrome, test profiles, recovery trajectories) is based on patterns of patients in their 20s, 30s, and 40s. However, your conclusions (and confidence) might weaken if presented with cross-examination questions in the previous example.

From 1998–2008, 23 empirical articles were listed on PubMed that focused on post-concussive symptoms. Of these, 8 had samples with mean ages in the late teens and 20s, 9 had samples with mean ages in the 30s, and 5 had mean ages in the 40s. Only one study (Butterworth, Anstey, Jorm, & Rodgers, 2004) presented data for a group of older participants. In this longitudinal study of health in Australia, three community-dwelling adult samples were studied: those in their 20s, 40s, and 60s. Head injury with loss of consciousness for 15 or more minutes and symptoms of post-concussive syndrome were assessed via a questionnaire. Although there were several interesting findings in this study, the most relevant to the case example was that head injury, even after controlling for cohort age, was related to post-concussive symptoms. If the neuropsychologist in the example above had been aware of this study, then he/she could have successfully rebutted the defense attorney's questions.

As noted earlier, this case example focuses on post-concussive syndrome in older adults, but it could have easily addressed cognitive profiles, expected recovery and rehabilitative gains, or functional disabilities associated with TBIs in patients over 65 years of age. Sadly, there is a general lack of research on older adults with head injuries, and this is a gap that needs to be filled. Validation (or refutation) of research findings in younger adults with head injuries is needed to better diagnosis, treat, and testify on behalf of these elderly individuals.

Neuroimaging and the Older Client

In reviewing the medical records on your 60-year-old client who sustained a mild TBI due to a motor vehicle accident, you come across the radiologist's report from neuroimaging two weeks post-accident. The report mentions mild temporal lobe atrophy, particularly of the hippocampal grey matter. Decreased white matter in this same region is also noted. How much should you make of these neuroimaging findings in this case?

Neuroimaging has advanced as a diagnostic procedure in the evaluation of brain disorders and dysfunctions over the past 10 years. As reviewed by Hoskins, Roth, and Giancola (in chapter 7 of this book), structural (e.g., computed tomography [CT], magnetic resonance imaging [MRI], diffusion tensor imaging [DTI]) and functional (e.g., functional MRI [fMRI], positron emission tomography [PET], single photon emission computed tomography [SPECT]) imaging studies can be used to objectively document that some damage to the brain has occurred, and often compliment the results of neuropsychological testing. As research with these radiological procedures progresses, characteristic profiles appear to reflect various disease states. This is particularly true in TBI.

In both children and adults, TBI has been linked to a number of abnormalities identified on neuroimaging. For example, hippocampal atrophy has been widely documented as a result of acquired brain injuries. Compared with healthy controls, individuals with TBIs show reduced hippocampal volumes on neuroimaging (Bigler et al., 1997; Tate & Bigler, 2000). The amount of hippocampal atrophy appears to be related to injury severity, so that individuals who sustain moderate-to-severe head injuries have more atrophy than those who sustain milder injuries (Jorge, Acion, Starkstein, & Magnotta, 2007; Tasker et al., 2005). Compared with other regions in the brain, Wilde et al. (2007) observed that the hippocampus is the most vulnerable brain structure in children suffering TBIs.

Another relatively robust neuroimaging finding in TBI is a disturbance of cerebral white matter. On traditional MRI, white matter loss has been observed in children and adults with TBIs (Bigler, Anderson, & Blatter, 2002; Mathias et al., 2004; Tasker et al., 2005). More recently, DTI has been used to identify abnormalities in the white matter tracts of the brain. DTI yields a measure of fractional anisotropy (FA), which assesses the presumed integrity/connectivity of white matter tracts. Poorer FA is typically associated with poorer integrity of the white matter. As with hippocampal volumes, reduced FA has been found in patients with TBIs (Benson et al., 2007; Wilde et al., 2006), related to poorer cognitive functioning in these patients (Wozniak et al., 2007), related to brain-injury severity (Kraus, Susmaras, Caughlin, Walker, Sweeney, & Little, 2007), and longitudinally worsens over the first year after a brain injury (Bendlin et al., 2008).

Taken together, these two brief synopses of the neuroimaging findings on TBI might lead one to conclude that the case above has objective "proof" of brain damage. However, this might not be the case, as normal and abnormal aging is also linked with a variety of neuroimaging findings, including reduction of hippocampal volumes and white matter disruptions. For example, in a sample of 511 non-demented older adults (mean age = 73), Hackert, den Heijer, Oudkerk, Koudstaal, Hofman, and Breteler (2002) observed that increasing age was associated with decreasing size of the head, body, and tail of the hippocampus bilaterally. In conditions linked to abnormal cognitive aging (e.g., mild cognitive impairment, Alzheimer's disease), reductions in hippocampal volumes, both cross-sectionally and longitudinally, have been widely reported (Kantarci & Jack, 2003). White matter abnormalities are also often commonly found in individuals with advancing age. Gunning-Dixon, Brickman, Cheng, and Alexopoulos (2008) reviewed neuroimaging studies in normal and abnormal aging, and found that cerebral white matter decreases across the normal lifespan, and it is even more disrupted in certain dementia illnesses.

As should not be surprising to most neuropsychologists, neuroimaging, like many other diagnostic tests, has reasonable sensitivity but lacks specificity. Both TBIs and normal and abnormal aging are associated with hippocampal atrophy and white matter dysfunction (as well as other neuroimaging markers of dysfunction). Given the lack of research explicitly examining TBIs in older adults, it remains unclear whether these two conditions have additive or synergistic effects, such that older adults with brain injuries might have more hippocampal reductions and white matter abnormalities than either condition alone. Until more definitive research is available, forensic neuropsychologists are advised to keep the value of neuroimaging findings in perspective when rendering an opinion on older patients.

Assessing Capacity and the Older Client

The legal system is often concerned with competency, which refers to the mental capacity of an individual to participate in legal proceedings. Neuropsychologists can render opinions on this matter. However, neuropsychology has a greater opportunity to assist the trier of fact with opinions about capacity, which relates to judgments about a client's ability to perform certain activities, including managing finances, making medical decisions, or driving.

As reviewed by Franzen (in chapter 9 of this book), capacity can be a reasonably complicated determination. Capacity is not a general term, and it should be viewed very specifically (Kapp, 2001; Sullivan, 2004). For example, one should not be viewed as having capacity or lacking capacity. Capacity likely varies in degrees (e.g., different individuals can have different levels of capacity). Capacity likely varies in situations (e.g., capacity to manage medications does not ensure capacity to manage finances). Capacity likely varies across time (e.g., lacking capacity currently does not mean that one will always lack capacity). Given that the concept of capacity is so varied, the assessment of capacity is similarly varied. This section will review several common questions of capacity as they relate to the older client.

Capacity to Manage Finances

You have received the following outpatient referral: An 86-year-old widowed male was referred to evaluate his capacity to manage his finances. His adult children, who live in another state, are concerned that he is forgetful and might be mismanaging his finances. They report that he has forgotten to pay bills, made some poor investment choices, and given modest sums of money to questionable charities in the past year. In talking with the client, he has plausible explanations for his behaviors (e.g., he recently moved but some bills were not forwarded in time, he took a chance on a risky investment, his children don't understand that this charity does good work). Premorbid intellect was estimated to be in the average range (~50th percentile), and current IQ was comparable. Attention was grossly intact compared with age-matched peers (e.g., WAIS-III Digit Span = 37th percentile, WAIS-III Digit Symbol = 25th percentile). Arithmetic skills generally met expectations (WRAT-4 Mathematics = 61st percentile, WAIS-III Arithmetic = 25th percentile). Reasoning tended to be borderline to low average (WAIS-III Comprehension = 16th percentile, WAIS-III Similarities = 9th percentile, WAIS-III Matrix Reasoning = 9th percentile). Learning and memory were also borderline (WMS-III Word Lists I = 9th percentile, Word Lists II = 9th percentile). From this limited evaluation, what do you conclude about this client's capacity to manage his own finances?

Marson et al. (2000) outlined a three-part model of financial capacity: (a) declarative knowledge about financial information, (b) procedural knowledge about how financial matters work, and (c) reasoning and judgment to make financial decisions. In the previous case example, there are test results that could be applied to this model. For example, declarative knowledge could be viewed as "intact" based on reasonable answers during the clinical interview and low average scores on the Comprehension subtest of the WAIS-III, particularly if the financial items were adequately answered. Procedural knowledge also seems "intact" based on low-average to average performances on measures of oral and written arithmetic. Regarding reasoning and judgment, there might be some doubt. Both Similarities and Matrix Reasoning subtests fell in the borderline range, which appears to be below expectations. His family questions his judgment. Depending on the adequacy of the explanations about his recent financial problems (i.e., missed bills, risky investment, gifts to charities), you might view his decisions as demonstrating adequate judgment. Recall that capacity varies in degree, so you do not have to decide that the client demonstrated the best judgment, only adequate judgment. Although not part of the formal model, the client's lower than expected performances on tasks of learning and memory might also factor into your decision about capacity, as these relative weaknesses could lead to problems with many instrumental activities of daily living, including managing finances.

Finally, although this example used standard neuropsychological measures to make the determination of financial capacity, there are other alternatives. For example, Marson and colleagues (2000) developed the Financial Capacity Instrument (FCI) based on their theoretical model of this ability. The FCI assesses 6 financial domains (e.g., basic money skills, cash transactions, bank statement management) with 14 behaviorally based tasks (e.g., counting coins, making a 3-item grocery purchase, explaining parts of a bank statement, rationale for making investment decisions). With the exception of very basic financial abilities, patients with mild Alzheimer's disease perform more poorly than age-matched peers on most complex financial tasks on the FCI. Tools like the FCI can augment a neuropsychological evaluation when a question of financial capacity is asked.

Capacity to Make Medical Decisions

You have received the following inpatient referral: A 64-year-old single homeless female was referred to evaluate her capacity to make medical decisions. She was admitted to the hospital a week ago with an infected blister on her foot, a likely complication of her diabetes. The infection has become gangrenous, and the doctors want to amputate her foot. She refuses this procedure. In talking with the client, she understands that her foot is "not well" and needs some medical attention. However, she notes that cutting off her foot would leave her unable to get around, earn money, and survive. She hopes that "some medicine" will work instead. When you try to explain that her doctors think an amputation is the best option, she refuses to talk to you any further. From this limited evaluation, what do you conclude about this client's capacity to make her own medical decisions?

Unfortunately, the case example did not generate any cognitive data to use in the evaluation of this specific capacity. However, medical decision making has been one of the most widely studied types of capacity/competency, and cognitive data is not necessary to render an opinion. Appelbaum (2007) notes four areas to assess when determining a client's ability to make medical decisions, including treatment choices. First, the client must communicate a choice (i.e., indicate what he or she wants to do in this situation). In the case example, the client has clearly indicated that she does not want to have her foot amputated, so she "passes" this criterion. An inability to make a choice (e.g., wavering between options, being unable to make a decision) is the only way to "fail" this criterion. A bad choice is still a choice. Second, the client must understand information relevant to the choice. He or she must understand the medical condition, the proposed treatment options and alternatives, and the risks and benefits of those options. Depending on the complexity of the medical conditions and its treatments, this might be a very complicated set of discussions. It is likely to be moderated by a host of individual differences between clients (e.g., education, occupation, life experiences). However, this is also an area that could be improved with remediation. A client should not "fail" this criterion because his/her care providers have not taken the time to adequately describe the medical condition and its treatment options. Books, brochures, or videos might be used to educate the client about his/her condition. In the case example, the client demonstrates some understanding of her condition (e.g., her foot is "not well" and needs medical attention). However, she also seems to be lacking an understanding of other key components of her situation and choice. The third criterion for medical decision making is an appreciation of the situation and its consequences. Clients need to be able to recognize their condition and the possible consequences of the treatment options. Impaired insight, which can occur in a number of neuropsychological conditions, can lead to a failure of this criterion. Furthermore, a poor understanding of inevitable outcomes of the choice can also exclude one's capacity to make medical decisions. In the case example, the client does understand some of the outcomes of having her foot amputated. As a homeless woman, she seems to clearly appreciate the downsides of being physically disabled as a result of this treatment. However, she does not appear to appreciate the consequences of not following this treatment recommendation. If she had noted that the infection could spread and death could occur, then she would have demonstrated her knowledge of the condition and its consequences. Finally, capacity to make medical decisions relies on sound reasoning about the treatment options. Can the client engage in a rational and logical discussion about the various choices? This criterion is not concerned with which choice was made, but how was the choice made. This criterion allows clients to make bad choices, as long as they make them in a reasonably sound manner. In the case example, the interview ended before this information could be gathered. In this case and others, clients must demonstrate that they "pass" all criteria—choice, understanding, appreciation, reasoning—to be deemed capable of making medical decisions. The "failure" of any one criterion is all that is needed to determine incapacity in these situations. Nonetheless, it is worth reiterating that capacity should be viewed as very specific. In the case example above, this woman's incapacity to make medical decisions about her foot amputation should necessarily be used to say that she cannot make any medical decisions for herself.

Although much of the information needed to determine medical decision-making capacity can be gathered during a clinical interview, a formal measure is available to guide clinicians through the process. The MacArthur Competence Assessment Tool–Treatment (MacCAT-T) (Grisso, Appelbaum, & Hill-Fotouhi, 1997) assesses these same four criteria of decision making, and has been shown in several studies to evaluate a client's ability to consent to medical and psychiatric treatments. Another measure that taps medical decision-making abilities is the Capacity to Consent to Treatment Instrument (CCTI) (Marson, Ingram, Cody, & Harrell, 1995). This measure requires clients to answer questions relating to two clinical vignettes. The questions address the same concepts measured in the Mac-CAT-T, but the CCTI has been more extensively studied in older adults with and without cognitive impairments. Of course, neuropsychological measures can also be used to inform care providers about a client's ability to make medical decisions (Dymek, Atchison, Harrell, & Marson, 2001; Gurrera, Moye, Karel, Azar, & Armesto, 2006).

Capacity to Drive

You have received the following outpatient referral: An 81-year-old widowed female was referred to evaluate her capacity to drive. She lives in a rural community with no public transportation options. She only drives into town a couple times a week for church, groceries, and the bank. She denied any recent accidents or traffic violations. Her adult children, however, are concerned that her reaction time has significantly slowed, she becomes easily distracted when driving, and are worried when she drives her grandchildren to the store. Premorbid intellect was estimated to be in the low average range (20th percentile), and current IQ was comparable. Attention was slightly below expectations compared with age-matched peers (e.g., WAIS-III Digit Span = 16th percentile, Trail Making Test Part A = 10th percentile, WAIS-III Digit Symbol = 9th percentile). Visuospatial skills were a relative strength (WAIS-III Picture Completion = 25th percentile, WAIS-III Block Design = 50th percentile, Rey Complex Figure Copy = 47th percentile). Executive functioning tended to be borderline to low average (Trail Making Test part B = 8th percentile, WAIS-III Similarities = 9th percentile, WAIS-III Comprehension = 16th percentile). Learning and memory were low average (WMS-III Word Lists I = 16th percentile, Word Lists II = 25th percentile). From this limited evaluation, what do you conclude about this client's capacity to drive?

Driving is a complex behavioral task that requires some level of cognitive functioning. Therefore, it is not surprising to have neuropsychologists weighing in on this particular type of capacity. Fortunately, driving has been widely studied in older adult populations, and there is a lot of literature on which to base opinions.

In a meta-analysis on the relationship between neuropsychological measures and driving abilities in dementia patients, Reger, Welsh, Watson, Cholerton, Baker, and Craft (2004) found that driving was related to performances on many cognitive tasks. This was particularly true for on-road driving tests, and when control subject performances were considered in the analyses. When control subjects were excluded from the analyses (presumably a more conservative test of the relationship), two cognitive domains continued to demonstrate relationships with on-road driving tests: visuospatial skills and attention/concentration. When other measures of driving abilities were considered (e.g., non-road tests, caregiver reports), visuospatial skills and general mental status scores were most related to driving. Overall, the authors concluded that visuospatial skills (e.g., Block Design, Picture Completion, Hooper Visual Organization Test) were most robustly related to driving, even though the magnitude of the relationships tended to be modest. Other recent reviews have similarly reported modest relationships between cognitive tests and driving abilities in the elderly (Brown & Ott, 2004; Withaar, Brouwer, & van Zomeren, 2000).

In the previous case example, is there sufficient evidence to say that capacity to drive is impaired? One complication in this case example is that premorbid and current intellect is low average, so the interpretation of other scores must consider this lower theoretical starting point. For example, as premorbid intellect is estimated to be at the 20th percentile, is a Digit Symbol score at the 9th percentile a decline? At this point in a normal distribution, only 1/2 standard deviation separates the 9th and 20th percentiles (−1.33 and −0.83, respectively). A second complication in the current case is that no scores fall into the "impaired" range (i.e., = 5th percentile). If nothing is technically impaired, can you make a determination of incapacity? Finally, the client's highest performing cognitive domain is visuospatial skills, which based on the results of Reger et al. (2004) is the domain most strongly linked with driving abilities. Can you suggest incapacity in the face of the current literature?

To reiterate, capacity is not an all-or-none situation. Capacity varies by degrees, situations, and across time. In this case (and any case), it is unwise to conclude that your client is "safe to drive," because most assessment methods are not specifically designed to provide that information. And even if there were methods designed to provide that level of specific information, it is unlikely that any of these methods would be accurate 100% of the time. When making determinations about driving (and other types of capacity), a more prudent recommendation might relate to the client's risk of engaging in this particular activity. For example, you might conclude that the client in the case example is at "no elevated risk" when operating a motor vehicle. More conservatively, you might place her risk as "mild" and recommend a road test to further evaluate the concerns raised by her children. Other cases with more serious cognitive impairments might lead to "heightened," "significant," or "severe" risk, and a direct recommendation to stop driving might be included.

Conclusions

As noted at the beginning of the chapter, good forensic practice starts with good clinical practice. However, good clinical (and forensic) practice can be more challenging when working with older adults, due to poorer normative data on this group on standard neuropsychological measures and those assessing effort, limited research on head injuries and their related symptoms (e.g., post-concussive syndrome) in the elderly, the overlap of neuroimaging findings in patients with TBIs and those with normal and abnormal aging, and the difficulties in determining capacity to perform certain daily functions (e.g., make medical decisions, manage finances, drive) in this later-life cohort. Although some of these pitfalls in working with the older client were briefly reviewed in this chapter, the goal was not to discourage this type of practice. Quite to the contrary, forensic practice with older adults is likely to be a growing segment of neuropsychological practice over the next 10–20 years as the United States (and world) population ages. Clinicians who undertake this type of practice should be aware of these potential pitfalls as they assist the trier of fact, and attempt to expand our knowledge base on forensic evaluations with older clients.

References

Appelbaum, P. S. (2007). Clinical practice. Assessment of patients' competence to consent to treatment. *New England Journal of Medicine, 357*, 1834–1840.

Ashendorf, L., Constantinou, M., & McCaffrey, R. J. (2004). The effect of depression and anxiety on the TOMM in community-dwelling older adults. *Archives of Clinical Neuropsychology, 19,* 125–130.

Baltes, P. B., & Mayer, K. U. (1999). *The Berlin aging study: Aging from 70 to 100.* Cambridge, UK: Cambridge University Press.

Bendlin, B. B., Ries, M. L., Lazar, M., Alexander, A. L., Dempsey, R. J., Rowley, H. A., et al. (2008). Longitudinal changes in patients with traumatic brain injury assessed with diffusion-tensor and volumetric imaging. *Neuroimage, 42,* 503–514.

Benson, R. R., Meda, S. A., Vasudevan, S., Kou, Z., Govindarajan, K. A., Hanks, R. A., et al. (2007). Global white matter analysis of diffusion tensor images is predictive of injury severity in traumatic brain injury. *Journal of Neurotrauma, 24,* 446–459.

Bigler, E. D., Anderson, C. V., & Blatter, D. D. (2002). Temporal lobe morphology in normal aging and traumatic brain injury. *American Journal of Neuroradiology, 23,* 255–266.

Bigler, E. D., Blatter, D. D., Anderson, C. V., Johnson, S. C., Gale, S. D., Hopkins, R. O., et al. (1997). Hippocampal volume in normal aging and traumatic brain injury. *American Journal of Neuroradiology, 18,* 11–23.

Brown, L. B., & Ott, B. R. (2004). Driving and dementia: A review of the literature. *Journal of Geriatric Psychiatry and Neurology, 17,* 232–240.

Butterworth, P., Anstey, K., Jorm, A. F., & Rodgers, B. (2004). A community survey demonstrated cohort differences in the lifetime prevalence of self-reported head injury. *Journal of Clinical Epidemiology, 57,* 742–748.

Duff, K., Patton, D., Schoenberg, M. R., Mold, J., Scott, J. G., & Adams, R. L. (2003). Age- and education-corrected independent normative data for the RBANS in a community dwelling elderly sample. *Clincal Neuropsychologist, 17,* 351–366.

Dymek, M. P., Atchison, P., Harrell, L., & Marson, D. C. (2001). Competency to consent to medical treatment in cognitively impaired patients with Parkinson's disease. *Neurology, 56,* 17–24.

Grisso, T., Appelbaum, P. S., & Hill-Fotouhi, C. (1997). The MacCAT-T: A clinical tool to assess patients' capacities to make treatment decisions. *Psychiatric Services, 48,* 1415–1419.

Gunning-Dixon, F. M., Brickman, A. M., Cheng, J. C., & Alexopoulos, G. S. (2008). Aging of cerebral white matter: A review of MRI findings. *International Journal of Geriatric Psychiatry, 46*(2), 34–41.

Gurrera, R. J., Moye, J., Karel, M. J., Azar, A. R., & Armesto, J. C. (2006). Cognitive performance predicts treatment decisional abilities in mild to moderate dementia. *Neurology, 66,* 1367–1372.

Hackert, V. H., den Heijer, T., Oudkerk, M., Koudstaal, P. J., Hofman, A., & Breteler, M. M. (2002). Hippocampal head size associated with verbal memory performance in nondemented elderly. *Neuroimage, 17,* 1365–1372.

Hertzog, C., Dixon, R. A., Hultsch, D. F., & MacDonald, S. W. (2003). Latent change models of adult cognition: Are changes in processing speed and working memory associated with changes in episodic memory? *Psychology and Aging, 18,* 755–769.

Ivnik, R. J., Malec, J. F., Smith, G. E., Tangalos, E. G., & Petersen, R. C. (1996). Neuropsychological tests' norms above age 55: COWAT, BNT, MAE Token, WRAT-R Reading, AMNART, STROOP, TMT, and JLO. *Clinical Neuropsychologist, 10,* 262–278.

Jorge, R. E., Acion, L., Starkstein, S. E., & Magnotta, V. (2007). Hippocampal volume and mood disorders after traumatic brain injury. *Biological Psychiatry, 62,* 332–338.

Kantarci, K., & Jack, C. R., Jr. (2003). Neuroimaging in Alzheimer disease: An evidence-based review. *Neuroimaging Clinics of North America, 13,* 197–209.

Kapp, M. B. (2001). Legal interventions for persons with dementia in the USA: Ethical, policy and practical aspects. *Aging & Mental Health, 5,* 312–315.

Kraus, M. F., Susmaras, T., Caughlin, B. P., Walker, C. J., Sweeney, J. A., & Little, D. M. (2007). White matter integrity and cognition in chronic traumatic brain injury: A diffusion tensor imaging study. *Brain, 130,* 2508–2519.

Marson, D. C., Ingram, K. K., Cody, H. A., & Harrell, L. E. (1995). Assessing the competency of patients with Alzheimer's disease under different legal standards. A prototype instrument. *Archives of Neurology, 52,* 949–954.

Marson, D. C., Sawrie, S. M., Snyder, S., McInturff, B., Stalvey, T., Boothe, A., et al. (2000). Assessing financial capacity in patients with Alzheimer disease: A conceptual model and prototype instrument. *Archives of Neurology, 57,* 877–884.

Mathias, J. L., Bigler, E. D., Jones, N. R., Bowden, S. C., Barrett-Woodbridge, M., Brown, G. C., et al. (2004). Neuropsychological and information processing performance and its relationship to white matter changes following moderate and severe traumatic brain injury: A preliminary study. *Applied Neuropsychology, 11,* 134–152.

Merten, T., Bossink, L., & Schmand, B. (2007). On the limits of effort testing: Symptom validity tests and severity of neurocognitive symptoms in nonlitigant patients. *Journal of Clinical and Experimental Neuropsychology, 29*, 308–318.

O'Bryant, S. E., Gavett, B. E., McCaffrey, R. J., O'Jile, J. R., Huerkamp, J. K., Smitherman, T. A., et al. (2008). Clinical utility of trial 1 of the test of memory malingering (TOMM). *Applied Neuropsychology, 15*, 113–116.

Reger, M. A., Welsh, R. K., Watson, G. S., Cholerton, B., Baker, L. D., & Craft, S. (2004). The relationship between neuropsychological functioning and driving ability in dementia: A meta-analysis. *Neuropsychology, 18*, 85–93.

Schaie, K. W. (1996). *Intellectual development in adulthood: The Seattle longitudinal study.* Cambridge, UK: Cambridge University Press.

Schaie, K. W. (2005). *Developmental influences on adult intelligence.* New York: Oxford University Press.

Sullivan, K. (2004). Neuropsychological assessment of mental capacity. *Neuropsychology Review, 14*, 131–142.

Tasker, R. C., Salmond, C. H., Westland, A. G., Pena, A., Gillard, J. H., Sahakian, B. J., et al. (2005). Head circumference and brain and hippocampal volume after severe traumatic brain injury in childhood. *Pediatric Research, 58*, 302–308.

Tate, D. F., & Bigler, E. D. (2000). Fornix and hippocampal atrophy in traumatic brain injury. *Learning and Memory, 7*, 442–446.

Teichner, G., & Wagner, M. T. (2004). The test of memory malingering (TOMM): Normative data from cognitively intact, cognitively impaired, and elderly patients with dementia. *Archives of Clinical Neuropsychology, 19*, 455–464.

Tombaugh, T. N. (2004). Trail making test A and B: Normative data stratified by age and education. *Archives of Clinical Neuropsychology, 19*, 203–214.

Wilde, E. A., Bigler, E. D., Hunter, J. V., Fearing, M. A., Scheibel, R. S., Newsome, M. R., et al. (2007). Hippocampus, amygdala, and basal ganglia morphometrics in children after moderate-to-severe traumatic brain injury. *Developmental Medicine and Child Neurology, 49*, 294–299.

Wilde, E. A., Chu, Z., Bigler, E. D., Hunter, J. V., Fearing, M. A., Hanten, G., et al. (2006). Diffusion tensor imaging in the corpus callosum in children after moderate to severe traumatic brain injury. *Journal of Neurotrauma, 23*, 1412–1426.

Withaar, F. K., Brouwer, W. H., & van Zomeren, A. H. (2000). Fitness to drive in older drivers with cognitive impairment. *Journal of the International Neuropsychological Society, 6*, 480–490.

Wozniak, J. R., Krach, L., Ward, E., Mueller, B. A., Muetzel, R., Schnoebelen, S., et al. (2007). Neurocognitive and neuroimaging correlates of pediatric traumatic brain injury: A diffusion tensor imaging (DTI) study. *Archives of Clinical Neuropsychology, 22*, 555–568.

Providing Forensic Neuropsychological Services to Children and Youth

22

Doris Shui Ying Mok
Rik Carl D'Amato
Deborah Witsken

Introduction

Forensic child neuropsychology is the application of the science of human understanding about brain-behavior relations applied to the practice of serving children and youth in the criminal justice system. Movies and television have popularized this study, and new training programs, books, articles, and journals have recently been developed in the area (Horton & Wedding, 2007; Lezak, Howieson, Loring, Hannay, & Fischer, 2004; Witsken, D'Amato, & Hartlage, 2008). To practice in this area requires highly specialized training in clinical child neuropsychology, forensic psychology, family psychology, neurodevelopment, and school psychology.

As the practice of forensic psychology expanded dramatically in the 1980s, Rosen (1983) advocated that a special model of forensic training for children is necessary, highlighting three major areas of education. He advocated that the forensic child psychologist: (a) needs to understand the legal system and its nomenclature. This includes understanding legal concepts (e.g., insanity versus psychosis) and legal theories, having the ability to identify the specific legal questions to be addressed, and being able to select the most appropriate assessment instruments available, It is also critical to be able to use relevant research evidence and communicate findings effectively in the form of a neuropsychological report that can be understood by the court; (b) must be familiar with the structure of the legal system; the most relevant being the referral process, the different court settings and how they interact, and how to construct relevant recommendations and dispositions; and (c) should have received specialized training in forensic assessment based on an understanding of neurodevelopment, family systems, and an ecological neuropsychological and educational assessment model.

As previously stated, forensic psychology has grown rapidly, with many subspecialties arising, one of which is *forensic child neuropsychology*. Hartlage and Long (2008) and Witsken et al. (2008) have addressed the history, training, and credentialing of neuropsychology as a professional psychological specialty, and highlighted the training and professional context of clinical child neuropsychology. These authors have said that child neuropsychology focuses primarily on brain–behavior relationships, with other factors viewed as secondary; neuropsychological assessment findings can benefit many disciplines in different systems, such as education and learning, medical intervention of neurological disorders, and others. But the legal system is one that increasingly has begun to use expertise from child clinical neuropsychologists (Witsken et al., 2008; Titus & Dean, 2003).

Skills Needed for Successful Practice

As clinicians enter into the forensic arena, more specialized skills are required. It is noted that the psychodiagnostic assessment model proposed by Rosen (1983) may not be sufficient in today's courtroom. The traditional clinical model focuses on a clinical case study of the child, in which the child neuropsychologist conducts assessments and interprets neuropsychological testing findings in light of multiple sources of data, making a diagnosis and providing a prognosis. He/she would usually interview the child, parents/caretakers, and relevant third parties, collect archival data such as development history, psychosocial history, school/education history, medical/psychiatric history, and family history, and examine environmental contextual such as the home, school, and community (e.g., see D'Amato, Crepeau-Hobson, Huang, & Geil, 2005; McCaffrey, Horwitz, & Lynch, 2008). But the clinical model often finds fault with the child before fully exploring many systemic-related variables. The legal context and forensic model requires the child neuropsychologist to also assess and address specific legal matter, such as competency to stand trial, amenability to evidence-based treatment, competency to testify as a witness, and so on. Although the processes of collecting data and conducting assessments are very similar, the legal context requires a more thorough understanding of the child and his or her world in light of the court system and legal concepts.

This chapter focuses on child forensic neuropsychology, with a significant portion devoted to neuropsychological assessment areas and related tools. Individual practitioners often offer decisions that are not data- or evidence-based, and our hope is to offer an approach to assessment (including measures) that enable child clinical neuropsychologists to improve in this regard. After a discussion of how to appropriately examine children, youth, families, schools, teachers, and other related personnel for forensic practice, four relevant areas of forensic psychology are discussed: delinquents in juvenile courts, child abuse and neglect victims (through the child protective systems in dependency and juvenile courts), custody issues in divorce and family court, and education and rehabilitation related to personal injury in civil court. In each section, specific legal concepts and theories, as well as relevant legal questions requiring assessment, will be addressed.

A developmental perspective is crucial in child neuropsychology. Children are not just small adults (Root, D'Amato, & Reynolds, 2005). Developmental neuropsychology examines a variety of subjects, such as changes in cognitive function, brain structure development across time, early cognitive behaviors in normal and brain-damaged children, plasticity and recovery of function after brain injury, the development of complex cognitive and motor skills, and specific and nonspecific disturbances (e.g., learning disabilities, mental retardation, schizophrenia, stuttering, and developmental aphasia, etc.). One main assumption is that a child's brain is different from an adult brain, characterized by growth and organization. The forensic child neuropsychologist should be prepared to address the anatomical development of the brain, as well as the behavioral correlates of brain growth (Riccio & Pizzitola-Jarratt, 2005; Willis, 2005).

Rationale for a Developmental Neuropsychological Approach to Forensic Practice

Support for applying a neurodevelopmental perspective to child forensic practice makes empirical sense (Titus & Dean, 2003; Traughber & D'Amato, 2005). Commonly reported (e.g., see Reynolds & Fletcher-Janzen, 2008; D'Amato & Hartlage, 2008) research-based factors that advocate for such a view (reprinted from Root et al., 2005, and Witsken, Stockel, and D'Amato, 2008) include:

- growing evidence that behavior and neurology are inseparable, including recognition that neurological factors have been found to underlie many learning and behavior problems once assumed to be strictly behavioral (Hynd & Willis, 1988);
- knowledge of brain development that is sequential and predictable (Willis, 2005);
- the long-term effects of brain injury on children's behavior and ability to learn (Teeter & Semrud-Clikeman, 2007);
- vulnerability of the developing brain to genetic and environmental conditions potentially resulting in severe childhood disorders (Riccio & Pizzitola-Jarratt, 2005);
- the impact of neuropsychological trauma in the highly plastic developing brain, potentially impacting both damaged and functional areas of the brain as the brain reorganizes and develops (Gaddes & Edgell, 1994);
- indications that some children who do not initially demonstrate behavioral indications of neuropsychological damage may develop problems as their brains mature (Root et al., 2005);
- increasing numbers of children are exposed to drugs and environmental neurotoxins with known and unknown neuropsychological consequences (D'Amato, Fletcher-Janzen, & Reynolds, 2005);

■ knowledge that a number of community problems (e.g., malnutrition) have neuropsychological consequences (D'Amato, Chittooran, & Whitten, 1992);

■ information demonstrating that neuropsychological prevention activities like perinatal education can have lifelong consequences for children (Dean & Davis, 2007);

■ evidence-based data indicating that neuropsychological interventions have changed the brain after individuals have learned to read (Shaywitz, 2003);

■ the advent of brain-based classroom strategies and teaching approaches that connect the needs of the students to classroom organization and teaching styles (Chittooran & Tait, 2005; Sousa, 2005; Work & Choi, 2005).

One area frequently requiring expertise from child neuropsychologists is early brain injury and behavior. Concepts such as critical periods of development, plasticity, and recovery of functions are central themes. Critical periods refer to early periods of development that are sensitive periods for development of specific behaviors or functions (D'Amato, Fletcher-Janzen, et al., 2005). This includes attachment and the development of basic social relationships, learning, development of motor and language skills, and so on. (Root et al., 2005; Witsken, Stoeckel, & D'Amato, 2008). Plasticity and recovery of functions are two key assumptions of the child's brain. Plasticity was first systematically examined by Kennard's studies (1942, cited by Stiles, 2000) on the resiliency of the brain after early injury, finding recovery of function to be inversely related to age of injury. The assumption is that different brain regions are genetically pre-specific for particular functions; however, alternative patterns of reorganization are possible when one region is damaged. As the brain matures, neural resources available for such reorganization become limited. Substantial research data in the literature document that focal brain injury in childhood is less detrimental than comparable injury in adulthood; an outcome often attributed to the brain's capacity for plastic reorganization (Lezak et al., 2004; Stiles, 2000). Nevertheless, this is a complex area that is not agreed upon by all researchers. For instance, researchers disagree on the extent of plasticity, with some viewing it as primarily a systemic response to injury, with others conceptualizing it as a central feature of normal brain development and neural functioning, noting some level of neural plasticity in adults, as well (D'Amato, Fletcher-Janzen, et al., 2005; Stiles, 2000).

Related to plasticity is the construct of preferential preservation of language and the notion of crowding. It has been observed that children with a left hemispheric injury may display perceptual deficits in the right hemisphere, whereas language functions remain intact. The crowding hypothesis proposes that the reorganization compensates for the loss of language functions and uses up neural resources normally reserved for perceptual functions, in order to preserve language (Satz, Strauss, Hunter, & Wada, 1994). Indeed, Satz et al. reviewed studies and re-examined the crowding hypothesis in a group of epileptic patients; they concluded that the crowding effect depends not only on inter-hemispheric speech transfer, but also on the age of injury (e.g., lesions occurring in the pre- or perinatal period). Right-hemisphere speech dominance alone does not sufficiently explain this phenomenon, and as such, an interaction of factors must be examined (Lezak et al., 2004).

Moreover, Kolb and Fantie (2008) summarized research studies in this area in an attempt to draw some helpful conclusions related to neurodevelopmental foundations. Although clearly not without some significant related controversy in a few of their items (e.g., see D'Amato, Fletcher-Janzen, et al., 2005; Horton & Wedding, 2007; Titus & Dean, 2003;), they have offered ten conclusions: (a) children show noteworthy recovery of language functions after early injury to known language areas, although they still have continuing linguistic impairments; (b) perinatal lesions of either the left or right hemisphere result in significant language deficits, a phenomena quite different from what is observed in adults; (c) children with focal right- or left-hemisphere injury show deficits in spatial processing, although these functions improve as the children develop; (d) focal damage in perinatal injury tends to have better outcomes than diffuse damage at similar ages; (e) recovery from early cortical injury is task-specific, such as in language, although compensation for non-language functions is not as extensive; (f) delayed effects of perinatal lesions are common; with deficits emerging many years later, sometimes not until puberty when higher order skills are required and thus assessed; (g) general intelligence is compromised by early cerebral injuries, especially for children with seizure disorders; (h) recovery from bilateral versus unilateral injuries is less; children with bilateral injuries have worse functional outcomes than children with a complete hemisphere removed; (i) descending motor pathways can be reorganized following early damage, and this reorganizing may be functionally significant; (j) the effects of early injury vary with age; with precise age at injury critical in predicting functional outcomes (refer to Kolb & Fantie, 2008, for details).

Training in Forensic Child Neuropsychology

The forensic neuropsychologist should be extremely familiar with the developmental aspects of the child's brain and related behavioral correlates. Findings from recent research should be reviewed and applied to address the specific disorders under examination (i.e., traumatic brain injury [TBI], epilepsy, abnormal neural structure, etc.), while concomitantly considering a host of relevant factors impacting the functional–behavioral outcomes (Reynolds & Fletcher-Janzen, 2008). Cutting-edge chapters are available from a great variety of handbooks, such as Horton and Weddings' (2007) *Handbook of Neuropsychology*; D'Amato, Fletcher-Janzen, and Reynolds' (2005) *Handbook of School Neuropsychology*; Reynolds and Fletcher-Janzen's (2008) *Handbook of Clinical Child Neuropsychology*. Professional associations offer journals with the latest research, seminars are offered yearly at annual professional conferences, and many universities offer classes in the area of neuropsychology, child development, and the law. However, psychologists and neuropsychologists alike are reminded that they should never practice in an area in which they have not been trained, and reading a comprehensive up-to-date handbook or completing an in-depth course does not equip one to offer forensic neuropsychological services. In general, clinical neuropsychological trainers advocate that specific neuropsychological course work, practica, research, a dissertation, and predoctoral internships and postdoctoral fellowships all must be part of a clinical neuropsychological training program. Most suggest following the "Houston" guidelines, and additional discussion of these requirements can be found in Witsken, D'Amato, et al. (2008).

Neuropsychological Assessment in Child Forensic Neuropsychology

In forensic practice, the neuropsychologist must deal with child outcomes. Figure 22.1 demonstrates how the clinical forensic child neuropsychologist must *reconcile* all of the factors of the child from his or her environment (e.g., home situation, nutrition, school, and classroom) with the biogenetic or neurological functions within the child himself or herself (e.g., motor skills, hearing, walking, talking, cerebral processing). It is only through the reconciliation of these two causal factors that the uniqueness of the child can be understood, and child outcome behaviors can be observed (e.g., academic achievement, social achievement; Hartlage & D'Amato, 2007). Child forensic neuropsychologists have unique training that enables them to collect and interpret data to investigate the interaction of neurocognitive, biogenetic, neurochemical, psychosocial, and environmental factors to understand a child's behavior (D'Amato, Crepeau-Hobson, Huang, & Geil, 2005; Teeter & Semrud-Clikeman, 2007). This facilitates the ability to study how abnormalities or complications in brain development interact with environmental factors in various childhood disorders, how disorders develop over time depending on the nature and severity of the neuropsychological impairment, the long-term consequences of brain injuries in children, the increased risks for psychiatric disorders in children depending on the impact of abnormalities in brain functioning, and early prediction and treatment of learning and reading disabilities (Hartlage & D'Amato, 2007; Hartlage & Long, 2008; Shaywitz, 2003; Teeter & Semrud-Clikeman, 2007).

Practitioners working with children and young adults are faced with increasing numbers of children with a wide range of severe and unusual neurological disorders (Root et al., 2005). Forensic neuropsychologists must be able to describe to judges, juries, and related personnel how a child's particular neuropsychological profile may affect behavior and learning. Most importantly, neuropsychologists must be able to translate this knowledge into practical, effective interventions that are realistic, functional within the context of the child's life, and within the court's jurisdiction (D'Amato, Crepeau-Hobson, et al., 2005; D'Amato, Fletcher-Janzen, et al., 2005).

Forensic Child Neuropsychology and Essential Areas to Evaluate

A forensic neuropsychological framework requires child practitioners to consider a wider range of functions that are known to influence behavior (Greiffenstein & Cohen, 2005; Rhodes, D'Amato, & Rothlisberg, 2008; Spooner & Pachana, 2006). An understanding of the complexity of the field is critical, because forensic neuropsychological examinations focus on the acquisition of data from some areas that overlap with school psychology and/or special education (e.g., cognitive abilities), and from other areas that are unique to the practice of neuropsychology (e.g., motor skills, sensory abilities). An ecologically based forensic neuropsychological approach should focus on what the child *can do* rather than what he or she cannot do (Reynolds, 1981, 1986; Telzrow, 1985). Such an approach must also focus on

22.1

Factors that serve as the foundation of child outcomes.

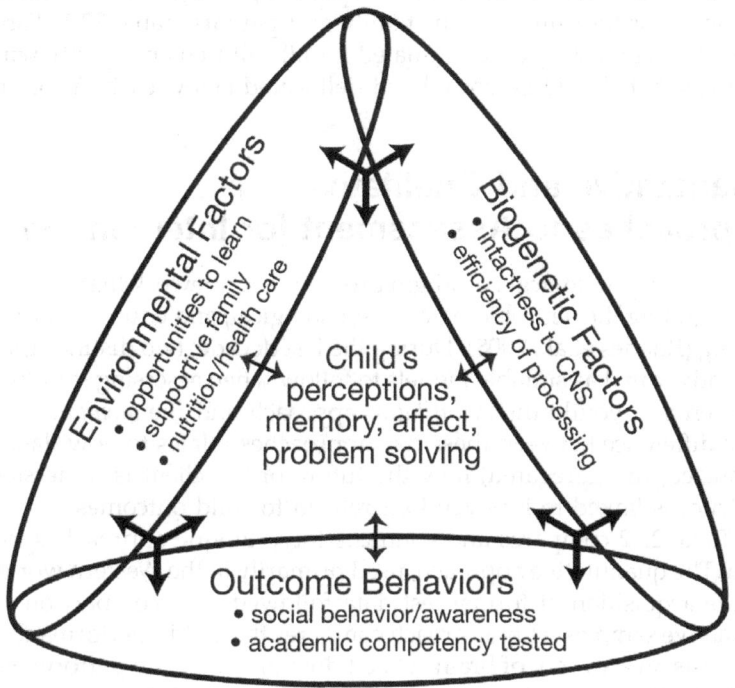

Adapted from D'Amato, Rothlisberg, and Leu Work (1999).

the best environment for the child in both living and learning. The evaluation must consider the match between the child and his or her instructional environment, while at the same time focusing on parents, relatives, and friends (Chittooran & Tait, 2005; D'Amato, Rothlisberg, & Work, 1999). The long-term needs of the child must be considered, and should emphasize the contribution of the child's total ecology to his or her ability to succeed and thrive in life (Conoley & Sheridan, 2005; Long & Collins, 1997; Spooner & Pachana, 2006).

There has never been clear agreement concerning the specific areas that a comprehensive neuropsychological examination should cover (Lezak et al., 2004; Titus & Dean, 2003). Whereas some have argued for a few critical areas, others (such as Luria) have advocated for as many as 30 areas to be evaluated (e.g., Glozman, 1999; Korkman, 1985). Neuropsychological domains or systems commonly assessed should include: (a) sensory and perceptual systems, (b) motor functions, (c) intelligence/cognitive abilities, (d) executive functioning/attention, (e) memory, (f) communication/language skills, (g) academic achievement, (h) personality/behavior/family, and (i) educational/classroom environment (D'Amato et al., 1999). Within a forensic setting, this information may be used to assess not only the functional integrity of the brain, but also to understand the educational and psychosocial impact of neurological and neuropsychological abilities or disabilities on daily living, schooling, future educational programming, and/or employment. Ultimately, the goal of forensic child neuropsychological services is to understand the world of the child, monitor changes if present, and most importantly, facilitate treatment planning that produces measurable desired outcomes for the child and/or family and parents. Table 22.1 displays the nine major areas that should be evaluated for all children and youth, with the specific subareas that should be considered delineated below each major area.

Quantitative and Qualitative Approaches to Assessment for Intervention

The neuropsychological paradigm provides a framework that assists practitioners in integrating the neurobiological, psychological, and educational aspects of functioning (Rhodes et al., 2008). During the last decade, two distinct approaches have been advocated as suitable models to follow when assessing for intervention with children and youth: the *quantitative* approach and the *qualitative* approach. The basic difference between these two approaches relates to how data are collected, organized, or aggregated, how the future of the client is understood, and how evidence is linked to interventions related to child outcomes.

Table 22.2 compares and contrasts these unique approaches to serving children. The quantitative approach, used primarily in the Western world, has focused on the acquisition of formal test data followed by a comparison of scores with normative samples. This approach compares the child's performance on standardized tests, in a variety of brain-related domains, with the performances of normal students. This comparison determines whether child functioning is below average, average, or above average in a number of areas. Standardized tests can offer the uninitiated practitioner a helpful set of tasks to evaluate and understand important neuropsychological abilities (Telzrow, 1985). If an appropriately selected neuropsychology battery is administered, most essential areas will likely be evaluated.

For many practitioners who use uniform assessments, such tests are selected because they evaluate core neuropsychological abilities that should be evaluated within a traditional assessment. From a quantitative view, child data are generated and used primarily for four comparisons: (a) How does a child's performance compare to that of others in the class, in the community, or in the state/nation? (b) What are the child's unique patterns of performance, including strengths and weaknesses? (c) When right hemispheric abilities (i.e., including sensory/motor processes) are compared with left hemispheric abilities, do unique patterns emerge that reveal significant processing styles? (d) Does an analysis of displayed signs and symptoms suggest problems related to a specific disorder (e.g., a nonverbal learning disorder) or the potential course of a disorder? Of course, all of these questions must be considered in light of the reason for forensic referral.

The qualitative approach focuses on the uniqueness of the individual under study and seeks to match the procedures used with the distinctive profile of the client. Although some practitioners in the United States have followed this method, A. R. Luria is the best-known leader in providing such individually focused services (Luria, 1966, 1970, 1980). Glozman (1999) has indicated that "Luria's

22.1 Areas That Should Be Formally and Informally Assessed in a Comprehensive Forensic Child Neuropsychological Evaluation

1. Perceptual/Sensory
- ✓ Visual
- ✓ Auditory
- ✓ Tactile/kinesthetic
- ✓ Integrated

2. Motor Functions
- ✓ Strength
- ✓ Speed coordination
- ✓ Lateral preference
- ✓ Strength

3. Intelligence/Cognitive Abilities
- ✓ Verbal functions
- ✓ Language skills
- ✓ Concepts/reasoning
- ✓ Numerical abilities
- ✓ Integrative functioning
- ✓ Nonverbal functions
- ✓ Receptive perception
- ✓ Expressive perception
- ✓ Abstract reasoning
- ✓ Spatial manipulation
- ✓ Construction
- ✓ Visual
- ✓ Integrative functions

4. Executive Functioning/Attention
- ✓ Problem solving
- ✓ Sustained attention
- ✓ Inhibition
- ✓ Shifting set

5. Memory
- ✓ Short-term memory
- ✓ Long-term memory
- ✓ Working memory
- ✓ Retrieval fluency

6. Communication/Language Skills
- ✓ Phonological processing
- ✓ Listening comprehension
- ✓ Expressive vocabulary
- ✓ Receptive vocabulary
- ✓ Speech/articulation
- ✓ Pragmatics

7. Academic Achievement
- ✓ Preacademic skills
- ✓ Academic skills
- ✓ Reading decoding
- ✓ Reading fluency
- ✓ Reading comprehension
- ✓ Arithmetic facts/calculation
- ✓ Social studies
- ✓ Language arts
- ✓ Science
- ✓ Written language

8. Personality/Behavior/Family
- ✓ Adaptive behavior
- ✓ Daily living
- ✓ Development
- ✓ Play/leisure
- ✓ Environmental/social
- ✓ Attachment
- ✓ Parenting skills
- ✓ Family interpersonal style
- ✓ Peers
- ✓ Community
- ✓ Student coping/tolerance

9. Educational/Classroom Environmental
- ✓ Learning environment fit
- ✓ Peer reactions
- ✓ Community reactions
- ✓ Teacher/staff knowledge
- ✓ Learner competencies
- ✓ Teacher/staff reactions
- ✓ Classroom dispositions
- ✓ School environment

Adapted from Witsken, Stockel, and D'Amato, 2008.

	Contrasts Between Lurian/Eastern Qualitative Approach and North American/Western Quantitative Approach to Neuropsychological Practice

22.2

Lurian/Eastern Qualitative Approach	North American/Western Quantitative Approach
Theory-driven	No overall a priori theory; data-driven
Attempts to support or confirm a theory	Attempts to disconfirm specific hypotheses
Synthetic	Analytical
Observation-oriented	Evaluation-oriented
Single-case-oriented	Group comparison-oriented
Describes behaviors	Evaluates behaviors
Subjective	Objective
Looks for patterns of functioning	Looks for differential diagnosis
Qualitative in nature	Quantitative in nature
Flexible	Fixed
Process-oriented	Product-oriented
Focuses on individualized activities	Focuses on multiple tests/procedures
Links behavioral data to functioning	Links psychometric data to diagnosis
Considers the functional system	Considers discrete brain-related areas
Clinical–theoretical	Actuarial–standardized

Adapted from Davis, Johnson, and D'Amato (2005), Witsken, Stoeckel, and D'Amato (2008), and Tupper (1999).

neuropsychological assessment is recognized today by the world's scientific community to be the most comprehensive and flexible method of neuropsychological evaluation available, which is also based on an understanding of the factors underlying complex psychological activities" (p. 23).

A few seasoned neuropsychological practitioners have offered models of assessment that evaluate curriculum-related processing skills to evaluate student educational difficulties (D'Amato et al., 1999; Glozman, 1999; Sousa, 2005). Sample tasks that could be used in a neuropsychologically based forensic child-assessment model have been offered by Gaddes and Edgell (1994) and Luria (1970). Gaddes and Edgell offer tasks to evaluate auditory processes and aphasic signs in oral speech (17 questions; p. 411), visual processes (13 questions; pp. 411–412), tactile processes (6 questions; p. 412), motor-expressive processes (6 questions; pp. 412–413), and auditory processes abilities (6 questions; p. 411). It is obvious that an analysis such as this can provide a wealth of educational information while concomitantly offering clear details related to the type of intervention that should be provided. It is important to use the child's strengths to support his or her needs. Luria (1970) has provided his list of evaluation activities to assess the neuropsychological processes that underlie arithmetic (Gaddes & Edgell, 1994). For example, his steps include asking the student: (a) to count aloud (to check memory of number in the correct sequence), (b) to recognize quantities, (c) to read and write single digits, and (d) to read and write multidigit numbers (Luria, 1970, p. 358, as cited in Gaddes & Edgell, 1994, p. 419).

Both the Qualitative and the Quantitative approach to neuropsychological assessment should be used in child forensic assessment. *In fact, it would appear critical to use instruments or procedures from both camps if we are to fully understand the psychological and educational issues that form the foundation of a child's life.* A single approach in isolation does not allow sufficient depth to understand a child and his or her family. Similarly, when conducting emotional assessments, it is vital to use both objective and projective personality measures in tandem if we are to understand the taproot of the child's personality.

Issues and Answers Related to Forensic Child Practice

Juvenile Delinquents

Several authors have highlighted the changes in the legal system for juveniles, noting a shift from the rehabilitation perspective toward a more adversarial and punitive system (Grisso, 2003; Melton, Petrila, Poythress, Slobogin, Lyons, & Otto, 2007). Early on, training in forensic child psychology emphasized clinical assessment (Rosen, 1983), which worked well with a court system that focused only on child study. In recent years, the court system has evolved from primarily providing psychological evaluations for treatment and rehabilitation of delinquents to an increasingly adversarial and punitive approach resembling adult criminal courts (Grisso, 2003; Melton et al.).

Given these changes, the forensic practitioner is often called to perform assessments to answer specific questions that are more forensic than clinical in nature. The key forensic assessment issues relevant to delinquents are as follows: (a) the ability of the youth to understand Miranda rights and waive constitutional rights including self-incrimination, (b) the assessment of potential danger to the community, from the youth, associated with pre-trial and post-trial detainment, (c) the amenability to treatment and appropriateness of transfer to criminal court, and (d) the competence to stand trial in ways that meet legal standards of fairness (Grisso, 2003). The child neuropsychologist must become familiar with these concepts and understand these specific legal issues from the mental health practitioner's perspective. In the last few years, these issues have been regularly discussed, and a number of outstanding resources are available (e.g., see Grisso, 2004; Grisso, Vincent, & Seagrave, 2005; Sparta & Koocher, 2006).

Assessment Instruments Developed for Use in the Forensic Area

Psychology has begun to focus on *evidence-based* services, and the forensic area has followed suit (Traughber & D'Amato, 2005). Thus, a number of related assessment instruments have been developed for child, youth, parents, and families (Rhodes et al., 2008). Instruments have been developed to assess these legal concepts, and research has begun to be conducted (e.g., Long & Collins, 1997; Traughber & D'Amato). These instruments fall into a number of areas, such as those used to evaluate child attachment, school progress, self-concept, parent–child relationships, Miranda rights, and violence. A potpourri of these instruments is discussed in the forthcoming sections.

Instruments for *Assessing Understanding and Appreciation of Miranda Rights* has been developed by Grisso (1998), and research data have provided support for its validity and clinical utility (Viljoen, Zapf, & Roesch, 2007). Researchers have also examined youths' ability to understand and waive Miranda rights. Roesch, McLachlan, and Viljoen (2008) examined relevant developmental considerations, including a child's tendency to yield to interrogation pressure and make a confession. In this regard, competency to stand trial must be evaluated if accurate information is to be collected, and most certainly this is related to developmental maturity. Studies on normal urban youth have indicated that the majority of youth do not understand basic court proceedings, as assessed by the *Georgia Court Competence Test* (Dreyer & Hart, 2008). Researchers' data from 1,357 forensic evaluations in Florida indicated that the majority of evaluations were inadequate and failed to identify the source of the noted incapacity or whether commitment criteria were met (Christy, Douglas, Otto, & Petrila, 2004). So, too, Evans (2003) emphasized that the assessment of cognitive capacity, such as intelligence, is *not* a sufficient indicator of competency to stand trial for youth. A variety of tests and competency indicators, such as the *MacArthur Competence Assessment Tool-Criminal Adjudication* (Hoge et al., 1997), should be considered. It is also important to evaluate sociocultural, ethnic, educational, and linguistic factors when assessing children, youth, parents, and families (Grisso et al., 2003; Hess & Rhodes, 2005).

Violence risk assessment is an area in which psychology has much to contribute. Studies on psychopathy first began with adults, and have gradually been extended to youth (Monahan, 2003). The forensic child neuropsychologist should be aware of the research literature on psychopathy and relevant assessment tools that are available. A few instruments have been developed to assess psychopathy among youth: *The Structured Assessment of Violence Risk in Youth* consists of three risk domains (historical, social/contextual, and individual/clinical factors), the *Assessing Risk for Violence Version II* (HCR-20), and the *Hare Psychopathy Checklist: Youth Version* (includes a semi-structured interview and collateral interview). Skeem and Petrila (2004) summarized some essential topics on the subject, indicating that it is important to review the psychometrics of juvenile psychopathy measures, it is necessary to understand the relationship between psychopathology and treatment progress, and it is critical to use valid instruments when assessing psychopathy in youth. Other researchers (e.g., Vincent, 2006) have reviewed the utility and limitations of psychopathy in this population, and have provided alternative tools for assessing violent risk in youth.

Obviously, the advent of recent school, university, and societal violence has shown a critical gap between what is known in the field of psychology and what is practiced in society (Root et al., 2005). One author has argued convincingly that we do not use the information that we already have available to us—such as case-history information and current school-functioning information. Dr. Kelly Zinna, a famous psychologist in the field of school violence, has indicated that "we do not need more metal detectors in our schools, we need more mental detectors" (Zinna, 2004).

It is imperative that neuropsychological variables be considered when planning or making juvenile justice policy decisions (e.g., see Wynkoop, 2008). For example, Kelly, Richardson, Hunter, and Knapp's (2002) study compared male adolescent sex offenders and matched controls, and this research revealed the importance of completing comprehensive neuropsychological examinations, including assessment of executive functioning and attention. In a similar study, Hulac, McConnell, Zafiris, Schrader, Manteris, and D'Amato (2008) evaluated the executive functioning of female adolescents placed in a residential treatment center, and they also found significant impairment in attentional abilities.

Schamber, Schrader, Zafiris, McConnell, Manteris, and D'Amato (2008) evaluated a similar group of emotionally disturbed children, but this time evaluated each child's ability to process executive functions. They also found that these children lacked skills that could be called frontal lobe functions. Martinez, Bjoraker, and D'Amato (2007) found communication problems using neuropsychological instruments with emotionally disturbed adolescents. Although certainly not causal, it seems like minor neuropsychological problems often lead to more significant issues that link to involvement in the juvenile justice system. It would seem as though prevention based on evidence-based interventions would be the key to stopping this circular process of neuropsychological impairment leading to juvenile justice system involvement (Root et al., 2005; Witsken, D'Amato, et al., 2008).

The forensic neuropsychologist has expertise particularly in the assessment of pre-existing conditions related to TBI, attention-deficit/hyperactivity disorder (ADHD), impulse control disorders, mood disorders, anxiety disorders, conduct disorders, aggressive behavior, and many additional disorders. He or she may be called as an expert witness addressing neuropsychological aspects of any of these conditions (Blau, 1998). For that reason, it becomes critical to understand the areas of expertise that one may possess. In addition to standard neuropsychological assessments, Wynkoop (2008) also emphasized that malingering measures used in adult assessment should be developed and used with the youth adult population. For a comprehensive review, see Tramontana, Hooper, Watts-English, Ellison, and Bethea (2008), who reviewed evidence that supports the prevalence of brain dysfunction in childhood psychopathology, and provided a summary of research findings related to specific disorders. In a related article, Mittenberg, Patton, Canyock, and Condit (2002) discussed malingering base rates and symptom exaggeration.

Case Example #1

Michael Marino was 15 years old when he was caught physically assaulting a peer who had bullied him at school for some time. Several witnesses observed the assault and Michael was immediately arrested and detained by the police. The case drew media attention because the victim was a popular football player in the local small town and he suffered significant trauma. The defense strategy focused on Michael's impulse-control difficulties related to his attention deficit/hyperactivity disorder (ADHD) and requested a psychological evaluation for Michael. Dr. Mary Cook, a forensic child neuropsychologist, was appointed by the court to conduct an independent medical evaluation, with both the prosecution and the defense team recognizing her expertise in the field. Dr. Cook reviewed Michael's records and found that Michael had recently switched from Ritalin to Adderall for his condition at the time of the incident. Michael also had a history of traumatic brain injury (TBI), and first received special education services under the Individuals with Disability Education Act (IDEA) category of "Other Health Impairment" (OHI) beginning in an early intervention pre-school program; however, details of the brain injury were not known. Michael's intelligence was found to be in the borderline range. Dr. Cook requested archival medical records to further examine Michael's history of brain injury, his medication history, and other relevant educational records.

Dr. Cook conducted neuropsychological testing that thoroughly addressed Michael's domains of functioning; in particular, assessment data related to attention and executive functioning, language and communication, memory, auditory and visual processing, planning and organization, foresight, concept formation, and problem solving. Dr. Cook focused on behavior, emotions, and personality to shed light on Michael's circumstances in this case. Dr. Cook's evaluation and findings from the neuropsychological report addressed other clinical and legal issues, informing the court about several areas. Clinically, the report addressed issues related to the physiological, psychological, and behavioral consequences of Michael's TBI; it re-examined the appropriateness of the ADHD diagnosis and medication prescribed in light of Michael's brain injury, and discussed the psychosocial consequences of the condition in the context of Michael's home and school environment. Moreover, the report also addressed specific legal issues, such as the impact of Adderall on Michael at the time of the offense, his competency to waive Miranda rights given his significant cognitive deficits in verbal comprehension and reasoning, and his obvious lack of knowledge regarding court proceedings indicated in the assessment. The report provided information concerning Michael's risk of potential violence, his need for educational treatment, and placement recommendations. Dr. Cook's comprehensive evaluation and her ability to use the data to address relevant clinical and legal questions educated the court on how to use expertise from a forensic child neuropsychologist to assist in decision making for the juvenile offender.

Child Abuse and Neglect

Child abuse and neglect is an area that has received significant attention from multiple disciplines. Psychologists may also serve different roles in the court (Melton et al., 2007); they may be involved in the investigation process, such as the forensic interviewing of a young child to examine the occurrence of mal-treatment. At times, a child's statement may be obtained through a mental health professional and used in the court. A neuropsychologist may be assessing the child's competency to testify as a witness, or examining and reporting issues related to memory and suggestibility as an expertise witness. Forensic child neuropsychologists may provide expert testimony on a variety of subjects, such as

the characteristics of maltreated children or child abusers, the long-term consequences of psychological injury resulting from abuse, mental health diagnoses
such as posttraumatic stress disorder (PTSD), and others (Larrabee, 2005). They
may also be involved in custody evaluations and termination of parental rights.
The forensic neuropsychologist needs to be aware of the complexity of these roles
that may involve the child protective system, the family court, the civil court, and
the criminal court. Neuropsychologists should be aware of the legal and ethical
issues and professional liability in handling forensic cases in the area of child
abuse and neglect (Reynolds & Fletcher-Janzen, 2008).

The forensic neuropsychologist should be aware of the legal definition of
child maltreatment related to physical abuse, physical neglect, sexual abuse, and
emotional abuse and neglect, which can be quite different from the broader definitions used in the social sciences. Obviously, familiarity with the wealth of research
on these subjects, as well as how they can be appropriately applied to the forensic
context, is required if one is to proceed successfully. An example would be the
Child Abuse Potential Inventory (CAP), which has been used extensively in the
research literature, but is not recommended as a clinical instrument due to the
high false-positive rates (Melton et al., 2007). Another controversial tool is the
use of anatomically detailed dolls, specifically in the evaluation of child sexual
abuse, and whether questions generated are leading to young children, who
are highly suggestible. Caution is also needed in applying research studies on
suggestibility and memory processes in relatively benign experimental settings
to the forensic setting (Sparta, 2003).

A major area requiring expertise from the forensic neuropsychologist is the
assessment of brain injury resulting from physical abuse and physical neglect
(Reynolds & Fletcher-Janzen, 2008). Another area is the assessment of childhood
trauma and the long-term consequences of physical, emotional, and sexual abuse.
In cases of child abuse and neglect, the assessment and reporting of findings
go beyond the practice of neuropsychological assessment (e.g., see American
Psychological Association [APA] ethical guidelines, currently available online,
2002). The child neuropsychologist needs to distinguish between non-interper-
sonal forms of trauma (e.g., accidents, witnessing fire, earthquakes) and interpersonal forms of trauma (e.g., sexual/physical abuse, witnessing domestic violence,
exposure to parental conflict in divorce) as well as single, sudden, and unexpected
incidents versus long-term repeated exposure to traumatic stressors (Sparta, 2003).

Differential diagnoses of mood disorders, ADHDs, and adjustment disorders
are necessary, as symptom presentations may be similar to PTSD, often complicated by comorbidity. The American Academy of Child and Adolescent Psychiatry
(1998) noted that diagnostic criteria for PTSD based on the *Diagnostic and Statistical
Manual of Mental Disorders* (*DSM-IV-TR*; American Psychiatric Association, 2000)
is not developmentally sensitive, and relies heavily on the child's ability to report
or describe certain symptoms. Differential diagnoses can be particularly challenging when the child is limited by language and cognitive abilities to describe his/
her experiences, and parents cannot provide a reliable source of information.
Cross-cultural issues complicate the process even further (e.g., see Hess & Rhodes,
2005). The neuropsychologist should also be familiar with the characteristics of
PTSD. In addition to using standard clinical assessment tools for children like the
Behavior Assessment System for Children-2 (BASC-2), specific trauma-assessment
instruments are available, and include the *Trauma Symptom Checklist for Children*,

the *Clinician-Administered PTSD Scale for Children*, the *Child Dissociation Checklist*, the *Child Posttraumatic Stress Reaction Index*, the *Children's Impact of Traumatic Events Scale*, *Child Rating Scales of Exposure to Interpersonal Abuse*, *When Bad Things Happen Scale*, *The Child's Reaction to Traumatic Events Scale*, and so on. Sparta (2003) provides a brief review and summary of the scales cited to guide clinicians in selecting appropriate instruments. When assessing for the effects of childhood trauma, the characteristics of stress, individual variables of the child (i.e., temperament, attachment, reactivity, protective factors), the child's subjective response to stress, and the response of others to the victim should also be considered (Sparta). It is important to understand trauma as part of the developmental pathological process, with potential future disruptions in functioning quite probable. Assessment of biological reactions, comorbidity, and pre-existing dysfunctions (including factors mediating traumatic response), should all be evaluated and seen as extremely relevant.

Case Example #2

Dr. Roberta Lee was retained by an attorney to review a court case concerning Crystal Flute, an alleged victim of child sexual abuse. Crystal had been diagnosed with epilepsy and had reported episodes of "memory blackouts." Crystal disclosed child sexual abuse by her father after her parents filed for divorce. Her father accused the mother of a malicious attempt to manipulate his daughter by implanting false memories and alienating Crystal from him.

In this referral, Dr. Lee did not complete an independent evaluation of Crystal Flute. She served the court as an expert witness providing scientific information on the neuropsychological aspects of epilepsy. Dr. Lee was also asked to address memory issues unique to epileptic patients and trauma victims. Dr. Lee summarized research findings on memory and answered specific questions related to suggestibility, accuracy of memories, the impact of stress on memory, delayed recall of traumatic events, and so on. She was also asked about standard interview protocol for alleged victims of sexual abuse, and controversies regarding the interpretation of findings on projective drawings in sexual abuse victims (i.e., genitalia on human figures). In this case, Dr. Lee's expert testimony was primarily based on research findings. She was cautious in acknowledging disagreements in both the scientific and professional community on issues regarding childhood memories, child statements, and others. Dr. Lee was also careful to clarify what the scientific data did and did not mean. Dr. Lee did not answer any questions related to Crystal, because she did not conduct an evaluation on her. In this case, the child forensic neuropsychologist's training offered expertise on neuropsychological correlates of epilepsy, as well as scientific research data on child sexual abuse.

Divorce and Custody

Mental health professionals also find themselves in a variety of roles in the family court system. Walker and Shapiro (2003) have summarized these roles into four major categories: (a) the psychological evaluator who assists the court in fact finding, (b) the expert witness who provides expert opinions about the meaning of facts based on clinical and empirical data, (c) the forensic evaluator who assists the court in understanding specific issues and answering specific questions such as mental state, amount of psychological damage, custodial arrangements, and so on., and (d) the consultant who assists attorneys in trial strategies or case conceptualization and management. In divorce and family court cases, the mental health professional should first clarify his/her role, which may vary from court to court. The neuropsychologist may find himself/herself in multiple roles, such as being the evaluator and investigator, as well as the mediator and interventionist (Melton et al., 2007). Potential conflicts of interest arising from multiple roles may violate the APA Ethical Principles of Psychologists and Code of Conduct (2002). Glassman's (1998) analysis of common ethical pitfalls in custody evaluations provides valuable insights. Clinicians specializing in this area should realize that malpractice lawsuits and complaints to the licensing board against the psychologist are not uncommon.

Neuropsychologists should receive specialized training in custody evaluations to acquire skills, training, and knowledge associated with this specialty. They should be familiar with relevant guidelines. Guidelines provide the forensic neuropsychologist pertinent information on custody evaluations. In addition, the APA Press has published two relevant and resourceful books, *Divorce Wars: Interventions with Families in Conflict* (Ellis, 2000) and *Family Evaluation in Custody Litigation* (Benjamin & Gollan, 2003).

Evaluators need to become familiar with research studies and empirical findings on a wide variety of relevant topics, ranging from parenting practices, child development, mental disorders, the impact of marital conflict/divorce on children's adjustment, economics after remarriage (i.e., economic decline for single parents), to more specialized issues such as the parental alienation syndrome (e.g., see Gardner, Sauber, & Lorandos, 2006). Moreover, Galatzer-Levy, Kraus, and Galatzer-Levy's (2007) *The Scientific Basis of Child Custody Decisions*, offers in-depth discussions on the use of scientific evidence in court, covering topics such as the impact of divorce on children, the contribution of psychological tests, valid observation methods for families, considerations of parental psychopathology, and other pertinent topics.

Understanding state family laws and stipulations and their applications in the local context are another essential subject. Local courts may adopt different standards for resolution of custody disputes—Melton et al. (2007) provide an excellent summary of the different standards. Traditionally the "tender years presumption" favors maternal custody, especially for young children in their development years. Recently, the "best interests of the child" standard has been adopted in most states, with each court providing some guidelines on factors determining "best interests." The "least detrimental alternative" and "primary-caretaker" standards both favor one parent taking primary care responsibilities; lastly, joint custody has become increasingly popular in the United States. Special population issues such as gay and lesbian parents, grandparents, and other third parties, such as step-parents and adoptive parents increase the complexity of these standards (Melton et al., 2007). Psychologists who perform custody evaluations need to become familiar with these standards and how they are applied in different courts.

Forensic custody evaluations generally involve the assessment of the following areas: (a) the relationship (and attachment) between the child and the parents, siblings, relatives, and significant persons, (b) the mental and physical health of the child and all parties, and (c) placement and visitation recommendations. Custody evaluations should include comprehensive observation and interviewing of parents and children, as well as relevant third parties, gathering of archival data (such as predivorce emotional and behavioral functioning), general psychological and educational testing, and administration of specialized tests. In addition to the assessment tools outlined earlier in this chapter, neuropsychologists are advised to follow the published guidelines on relevant areas of assessment in custody evaluation.

In assessing parent–child relationships, as previously discussed, both quantitative and qualitative data should be obtained. This may include parenting style, parent–child interactions, caretaking responsibilities, parenting practices such as discipline, attachment and bonding, and many others. It is recommended that semi-structured interviews and standardized formats of observation be used to systematically document parent–child relationships. Instruments such as the *Ackerman-Schoendorf Scales of Parent Evaluation of Custody* (ASPECT, Ackerman & Schoendorf, 2005) and the *Uniform Child Custody Evaluation System* (UCCES, Munsinger & Karlson, n.d.) made available from commercial test publishers provide standardized packages of assessment tools. Psychologists should, however, carefully review the validity of these instruments and empirical research data supporting these measures. Although these instruments may facilitate data collection, they may not have the reliability and validity to be used as formal indices in a court of law (Melton et al., 2007). As always, extreme care should be used when selecting instruments, and a review of reliability and validity should always be undertaken.

In assessing the mental and physical health of the child and all parties, the forensic neuropsychologist often provides expertise in specialized neuropsychological testing, assessing children with special medical and mental health needs. This may include children with epilepsy, neurological disorders, and other medical conditions requiring neuropsychological assessment, as well as other psychological disorders, such as ADHD, learning disorders, and so on (D'Amato, Fletcher-Janzen, et al., 2005). Other areas of assessment may include neuropsychological consequences of any history of child abuse and neglect, domestic violence, and other victimization issues resulting in psychological damage, which have been discussed in the previous sections. Brain damage does not always have to come from family members or other individuals. For instance, a child could become neuropsychologically impaired after consuming chemicals (D'Amato et al.). Parents with special medical or mental conditions may not be able to adequately care for their children. Assessment of parents or adult caretakers with medical or mental conditions may also include neuropsychological assessment test data in relation to the assessment of parenting capacities and limitations. In assessing for and providing recommendations on placement and custody arrangements, the forensic neuropsychologist needs to follow court guidelines on the standards adopted and integrate quantitative and qualitative assessment data of involved parties, as well as relevant research data on themes, in an effort to offer appropriate conclusions to the judge or court.

Case Example #3

Jacob Goldberg's parents were filing for divorce. His father was moving out of state to start a new life. His mother had been primarily a homemaker and Jacob's primary caretaker. Jacob had a brain tumor when he was 4 years old, resulting in the removal of part of his frontal lobe. He also had other medical complications. The health insurance carrier was based on his father's employment, and therefore, his father's moving out of state was a major concern relating to health care for Jacob.

Dr. B. Brian Bradford was a clinical neuropsychologist working at the Children's Hospital. He had followed up with Jacob for the previous 3 years. In this case, Dr. Bradford's primary role was not as custody evaluator. He was careful to draw boundaries on his expertise on rehabilitation as a child neuropsychologist. He did not assess the parents' relationship with Jacob and their parenting practices, and thus, he refrained from commenting on parenting capacities. He provided the court information on Jacob's medical condition, his past treatment, his prognosis, and future treatment needs. He focused on Jacob's strengths and needs and identified the supports needed to care for him, portraying the placement that was in Jacob's best interest. Based on Dr. Bradford's recommendations, the two parties agreed to proceed to mediation and negotiate the best custody arrangements for Jacob to ascertain how he could receive the medical care for optimal rehabilitation.

Personal Injury: Education and Rehabilitation Issues

The fourth area in forensic assessment pertains to education and rehabilitation issues for children with disabilities. In this section, our focus is on personal injuries of children in civil cases. The forensic neuropsychologist is usually involved in assessing for alleged damages; nevertheless, it is not uncommon that the neuropsychologist may be asked to address liability issues and responsibility of the plaintiff. It is, therefore, important to understand concepts such as proximate cause, which means whether one can reasonably foresee that one event causes another, and whether an unbroken sequence of events resulted in injury (Melton et al., 2007). (Interested readers should refer to Melton et al. [2007] for definition criteria on torts and an overview of related concepts in civil lawsuits.) Liability and responsibility issues are often complex. McCaffrey, Horwitz, and Lynch (2008) demonstrated all the facets to be considered in understanding the toxic effects of lead on children. Again, the child forensic neuropsychologist needs to be very familiar with the research literature and related scientific data (Reynolds & Fletcher-Janzen, 2008).

The most common scenario for the neuropsychologist involved in litigation is to provide information concerning the presence or absence, severity, causation, and sequelae of brain injury (Hartlage & D'Amato, 2007). Stanford and Dorflinger (2009) summarized research findings associated with the unique mechanisms and outcomes in pediatric brain injury. They discussed some of the difficulties in assessing parameters of injury, such as a poor witness account of loss of consciousness, the need to modify the coma scale for a nonverbal child, difficulty in assessing amnesia due to language limitations, different expression of injury in children, and others. The child's individual characteristics, the family context, the social circumstances, the preinjury skills the child had, the flexibility of the academic environment in providing support, and familial/environmental resources available for intervention all interact to impact the child's neuropsychological outcome.

The child neuropsychologist provides clinical expertise in the assessment of brain injury and its neurobehavioral sequelae. In addition to assessing for impairments in the various domains, the neuropsychologist also provides treatment recommendations and environmental supports that would ease the impact of the disability, and assist in adjustment at home and in school (Conoley & Sheridan, 2005). Moreover, Kade and Fletcher-Janzen (2008) summarized brain-injury rehabilitation of children and youth from a neurodevelopmental perspective. The forensic neuropsychologist is expected to understand two systems when addressing treatment issues for children and youth: the education system through the IDEA and the government system through the Americans with Disabilities Act (ADA). The IDEA details how states and public agencies must provide early intervention, special education, and related services to infants, toddlers, children, and youth with disabilities (U.S. Department of Education, n.d.). The ADA prohibits discrimination on the basis of disability in employment (Title I), state and local government (Title II), public accommodations (Title III), commercial facilities, transportation, and telecommunications. The forensic neuropsychologist may also be assessing for eligibility for disability services, as well as addressing legal consequences related to any violation of rights.

Case Example #4

Jose Lopez was hit by a car when riding his bicycle at home. He was immediately sent to the hospital by the driver, who was vague in reporting whether Jose lost consciousness. Jose was eager to deny injuries, for fear of being restrained from playing the final football game of the season on the upcoming weekend. Due to a lack of highly noticeable signs and symptoms, the physicians did not carefully monitor his symptoms or screen for more serious injuries. Jose was released to his parents without follow-up. He had a serious injury during the football game, lost consciousness, and was sent back to the hospital. This time he was hospitalized due to more severe symptoms and given a computed tomography (CT) scan. Jose continued to exhibit psychological symptoms in the coming months; he became easily tired and irritable, and he felt depressed. Jose had difficulty concentrating at school, and his academic performance suffered significantly. A preliminary school evaluation indicated significant cognitive deficits with a great deal of scatter between scores, and Jose was referred for a comprehensive neuropsychological assessment. The family sued for damages from the driver causing the initial accident, as well as suing the medical hospital for negligence. The case involved several parties (insurance companies) and teams of attorneys. An agreement was made, and a physician was retained as an expert to address medical issues related to the TBI and medical intervention. Dr. Chitto was retained to provide a neuropsychological assessment, as she had expertise in sports-related TBIs. She also worked closely with a neurologist with expertise in sports medicine. In addition to conducting a neuropsychological assessment on Jose and reporting any noted impairments and deficits, Dr. Chitto thoroughly addressed Jose's treatment and rehabilitation needs. She clearly articulated a developmental perspective, explaining adolescent brain development and long-term consequences of Jose's mild TBI. Dr. Chitto identified services potentially available through public education (e.g., individualized education program at school), as well as those to be supplemented through private funds from compensation. In this case, liability and responsibility issues were mostly addressed by the medical expert. Dr. Chitto worked effectively, using her expertise in clinical child forensic neuropsychology.

Summary

The expertise of the child forensic neuropsychologist is in increasing demand in today's litigious society and courts. This chapter has illustrated some of the complexities in conducting forensic evaluations for children and youth in various legal contexts. As Hartlage and Long (2008) have advocated, formal training in clinical child neuropsychology, including coursework, practicum, internships, and postdoctoral training fellowships, is necessary to develop proficiency in an area as specialized as forensic child neuropsychology. We have noted that forensic child neuropsychological assessments require additional advanced clinical training, which is not usually available, even in APA-accredited psychology programs and internships or postdoctoral training fellowships. Scholarly efforts exploring this area must be cultivated if we are to adequately prepare professionals to meet this demand. Professional associations should develop practice guidelines and articulate the many ethical issues involved in these clinical practice issues.

The forensic child neuropsychologist needs to be familiar with developmental neuropsychology and general neuropsychological assessment tools, as well as special instruments and measures designated to address specific legal concepts, such as competency to stand trial, psychopathy and violent risk, best interests in child custody, and many others. He or she needs to be knowledgeable in both research and clinical practice in the forensic area in order to best serve children and youth in legal settings.

Acknowledgment

Parts of this chapter are adapted from an earlier (2008) work entitled "Leading Educational Change Using a Neuropsychological Response-to-Intervention

Approach: Linking Our Past, Present, and Future" by Deborah Witsken, Amanda Stoeckel, and Rik Carl D'Amato, published in *Psychology in the Schools, 45*(9), 781–811.

References

Ackerman, M. J. & Schoendorf, M. (2005). The Ackerman-Schoendorf scales for parent evaluation of custody (ASPECT): A review of research and update. *Journal of Child Custody, 2*(1–2), 179–193.

American Psychiatric Association. (2000). *Diagnostic and statistical manual of mental disorders* (4th ed., text rev.). Washington, DC: American Psychiatric Press.

American Psychological Association. (2002). Ethical principles of psychologists and code of conduct. *American Psychologists, 57*(12), 1060–1073.

Benjamin, G. A. H., & Gollan, J. K. (2003). *Family evaluation in custody litigation: Reducing risks of ethical infractions and malpractice.* Washington, DC: American Psychological Association.

Blau, T. H. (1998). *The psychologist as an expert witness* (2nd ed.). New York: Wiley.

Chittooran, M. M., & Tait, R. C. (2005). Understanding and implementing neuropsychologically based written language interventions. In R. C. D'Amato, E. Fletcher-Janzen, & C. R. Reynolds (Eds.), *Handbook of school neuropsychology* (pp. 777–803). Hoboken, NJ: Wiley.

Christy, A., Douglas, K. S., Otto, R. K., & Petrila, J. (2004). Juveniles evaluated incompetent to proceed: Characteristics and quality of mental health professionals' evaluations. *Professional Psychology: Research and Practice, 35*(4), 380–388.

Conoley, J. C., & Sheridan, S. M. (2005). Understanding and implementing school–family interventions after neuropsychological-impairment. In R. C. D'Amato, E. Fletcher-Janzen, & C. R. Reynolds (Eds.), *Handbook of school neuropsychology* (pp. 721–737). Hoboken, NJ: Wiley.

D'Amato, R. C., Chittooran, M. M., & Whitten, J. C. (1992). The neuropsychological consequences of malnutrition. In L. C. Hartlage, D. I. Templer, & W. G. Cannon (Eds.), *Preventable brain damage: Brain vulnerability and brain health* (pp. 193–213). New York: Springer-Verlag.

D'Amato, R. C., Crepeau-Hobson, F. C., Huang, L. V., & Geil, M. (2005). Ecological neuropsychology: An alternative to the deficit model for conceptualizing and serving students with learning disabilities. *Neuropsychology Review, 15*(2), 97–103.

D'Amato, R. C., Fletcher-Janzen, E. & Reynolds, C. R. (Eds.). (2005). *Handbook of school neuropsychology.* Hoboken, NJ: Wiley.

D'Amato, R. C., Rothlisberg, B. A., & Work, P. H. L. (1999). Neuropsychological assessment for intervention. In C. R. Reynolds & T. B. Gutkin (Eds.), *The handbook of school psychology.* Hoboken, NJ: Wiley.

Davis, A. S., Johnson, J., & D'Amato, R. C. (2005). Evaluating and using long-standing school neuropsychological batteries: The Halstead-Reitan and the Luria-Nebraska neuropsychological batteries. In R. C. D'Amato, E. Fletcher-Janzen, & C. R. Reynolds (Eds.), *Handbook of school neuropsychology* (pp. 264–286). Hoboken, NJ: Wiley.

Dean, R. S., & Davis, A. S. (2007). Relative risk of perinatal complications in common childhood disorders. *School Psychology Quarterly, 22*, 13–25.

Dreyer, C. S., & Hart, K. J. (2008). Competence to stand trial-related skills in a sample of urban youth. *American Journal of Forensic Psychology, 26*(2), 5–23.

Ellis, E. M. (2000). *Divorce wars: Interventions with families in conflict.* Washington, DC: American Psychological Association.

Evans, T. M. (2003). Juvenile competency to stand trial: Problems and pitfalls. *American Journal of Forensic Psychology, 21*(2), 5–18.

Gaddes, W. H., & Edgell, D. (1994). *Learning disabilities and brain function: A neuropsychological approach* (2nd ed.). New York: Springer-Verlag.

Galatzer-Levy, R. M., Kraus, L., & Galatzer-Levy, J. (Eds.). (2007). *The scientific basis of child custody decisions* (2nd ed.). New York: Wiley.

Gardner, R. A., Sauber, S. R., & Lorandos, D. (Eds.). (2006). *The international handbook of parental alienation syndrome: Conceptual, clinical and legal considerations.* Springfield, IL: Charles C Thomas.

Glassman, J. B. (1998). Preventing and managing board complaints: The downside risk of custody evaluation. *Professional Psychology: Research and Practice, 29*(2), 121–124.

Glozman, J. M. (1999). Quantitative and qualitative integration of Lurian procedures. *Neuropsychology Review, 9*(1), 23–32.

Greiffenstein, M. F., & Cohen, L. (2005). Neuropsychology and the law: Principles of productive attorney–neuropsychologist relations. In G. Larrabee (Ed.), *Forensic neuropsychology: A scientific approach* (pp. 29–91). New York: Oxford University Press.

Grisso, T. (1998). *Instruments for assessing understanding & appreciation of Miranda rights.* Sarasota, FL: Professional Resource Press/Professional Resource Exchange.

Grisso, T. (2003). Forensic evaluation in delinquency cases. In A. M. Goldstein (Ed.), *Handbook of psychology: Vol. 11. Forensic psychology* (pp. 315–334). Hoboken, NJ: Wiley.

Grisso, T. (2004). *Double jeopardy: Adolescent offenders with mental disorders.* Chicago: University of Chicago Press.

Grisso, T., Steinberg, L., Woolard, J., Cauffman, E., Scott, E., Graham, S., et al. (2003). Juveniles' competence to stand trial: A comparison of adolescents' and adults' capacities as trial defendants. *Law and Human Behavior, 27*(4), 333–363.

Grisso, T., Vincent, G., & Seagrave, D. (2005). *Mental health screening and assessment in juvenile justice.* New York: Guilford Press.

Hartlage, L. C., & D'Amato, R. C. (2007). Understanding the etiology of psychiatric and neurologic disorders in neuropsychiatry. In A. MacNeill Horton, Jr., & D. Wedding (Eds.), *The neuropsychology handbook* (3rd ed., pp. 87–108). New York: Springer-Verlag.

Hartlage, L. C., & Long, C. J. (2008). Development of neuropsychology as a professional psychology specialty: History, training and credentialing. In C. R. Reynolds & E. Fletcher-Janzen (Eds.), *Handbook of clinical child neuropsychology* (pp. 3–18). New York: Springer Science.

Hess, R. S., & Rhodes, R. L. (2005). Providing neuropsychological services to culturally and linguistically diverse learners. In R. C. D'Amato, E. Fletcher-Janzen, & C. R. Reynolds (Eds.), *Handbook of school neuropsychology* (pp. 637–662). Hoboken, NJ: Wiley.

Hoge, S. K., Bonnie, R. J., Pothyress, N., Monahan, J., Eisenberg, M., & Feucht-Haviar, T. (1997). The MacArthur adjudicative competency study. Development and validation of a research instrument. *Law and Human Behavior, 21,* 141–170.

Horton, A. M., & Wedding, D. (2007). *The neuropsychology handbook* (3rd ed.). New York: Springer-Verlag.

Hulac, D. M., McConnell, E. D., Zafiris, C. M., Schrader, A. G., Manteris, E. M., & D'Amato, R. C. (2008). *Understanding executive functioning in female adolescents using the BRIEF.* Poster/paper presented at the 36th Annual Convention of the International Neuropsychological Society, Buenos Aires, Argentina.

Hynd, G. W., & Willis, W. G. (1988). *Pediatric neuropsychology.* Orlando, FL: Grune & Stratton.

Kade, D., & Fletcher-Janzen, E. (2008). Brain injury rehabilitation of children and youth: Neuropsychological perspectives. In C. R. Reynolds & E. Fletcher-Janzen (Eds.), *Handbook of clinical child neuropsychology* (pp. 427–458). New York: Springer Science.

Kelly, T., Richardson, G., Hunter, R., & Knapp, M. (2002). Attention and executive function deficits in adolescent sex offenders. *Child Neuropsychology, 8*(2), 138–143.

Kolb, B., & Fantie, B. D. (2008). Development of the child's brain and behavior. In C. R. Reynolds & E. Fletcher-Janzen (Eds.), *Handbook of clinical child neuropsychology* (pp. 19–46). New York: Springer Science.

Korkman, M. (1985). NEPSY: An adaptation of Luria's investigation for young children. *Clinical Neuropsychologist, 4,* 375–392.

Larrabee, G. (2005). (Ed.). *Forensic neuropsychology: A scientific approach.* New York: Oxford.

Lezak, M. D., Howieson, D. B., Loring, D. W., Hannay, J. H., & Fischer, J. S. (2004). *Neuropsychological assessment* (4th ed.). New York: Oxford.

Long, C. J., & Collins, L. F. (1997). Ecological validity and forensic pediatric neuropsychological assessment. In R. J. McCaffrey, A. D. Williams, J. M. Fisher, & L. C. Lang (Eds.), *The practice of forensic neuropsychology: Meeting challenges in the courtroom* (pp. 153–164). New York: Plenum.

Luria, A. R. (1966). *Higher cortical functions in man.* New York: Basic Books.

Luria, A. R. (1970). *The working brain.* New York: Basic Books.

Luria, A. R. (1980). *Higher cortical functions in man* (2nd ed.). New York: Basic Books.

Martinez, J., Bjoraker, K., & D'Amato, R. C. (2007). *Examining the neuropsychological abilities of students with and without emotional disorders using the NEPSY.* Poster/paper presented at the 27th Annual Convention of the National Academy of Neuropsychologists, Scottsdale, AZ.

McCaffrey, R. J., Horwitz, J. E., & Lynch, J. K. (2008). Child forensic neuropsychology: A scientific approach. In C. R. Reynolds & E. Fletcher-Janzen (Eds.), *Handbook of clinical child neuropsychology* (pp. 729–744). New York: Springer Science.

Melton, G. B., Petrila, J., Poythress, N. G., Slobogin, C., Lyons, P. M., & Otto, R. K. (2007). *Psychological evaluations for the courts: A handbook for mental health professionals and lawyers* (3rd ed.). New York: Guilford.

Mittenberg, W., Patton, C., Canyock, E. M., & Condit, D. C. (2002). Base rates of malingering and symptom exaggeration. *Journal of Clinical and Experimental Neuropsychology, 24*, 1094–1102.

Monahan, J. (2003). Violence risk assessment. In A. M. Goldstein (Ed.), *Handbook of psychology: Vol. 11. Forensic psychology* (pp. 527–540). Hoboken, NJ: Wiley.

Munsinger, H. L., & Karlson, K. W. (n.d.). *Uniform child custody evaluation system (UCCES)*. Retrieved January 21 2008, from http://www3.parinc.com/products/product.aspx?Productid=UCCES

Reynolds, C. R. (1981). Neuropsychological assessment and the habilitation of learning: Considerations in the search for the aptitude x treatment interaction. *School Psychology Review, 10*(3), 343–394.

Reynolds, C. R. (1986). Transactional models of intellectual development, yes. Deficit models of process remediation, no. *School Psychology Review, 15*, 256–260.

Reynolds, C. R., & Fletcher-Janzen, E. (2008). (Eds.). *Handbook of clinical child neuropsychology* (3rd ed.). New York: Plenum.

Rhodes, R. L., D'Amato, R. C., & Rothlisberg, B. A. (2008). Utilizing a neuropsychological paradigm for understanding educational and psychological tests. In C. R. Reynolds & E. Fletcher-Janzen (Eds.), *Handbook of clinical child neuropsychology* (3rd ed., pp. 106–133). New York: Plenum.

Riccio, C. A., & Pizzitola-Jarratt, K. (2005). Abnormalities of neurological development. In R. C. D'Amato, E. Fletcher-Janzen, & C. R. Reynolds (Eds.), *Handbook of school neuropsychology* (pp. 61–85). Hoboken, NJ: Wiley.

Roesch, R., McLachlan, K., & Viljoen, J. L. (2008). The capacity of juveniles to understand and waive arrest rights. In R. Jackson (Ed.), *Learning forensic assessment* (pp. 265–289). New York: Routledge/ Taylor & Francis Group.

Root, K. A., D'Amato, R. C., & Reynolds, C. R. (2005). Providing neurodevelopmental, collaborative, consultative, and crisis intervention school neuropsychology services. In R. C. D'Amato, E. Fletcher-Janzen, & C. R. Reynolds (Eds.), *Handbook of school neuropsychology* (pp. 15–40). Hoboken, NJ: Wiley.

Rosen, R. H. (1983). The need for training in forensic psychology. *Professional Psychology: Research and Practice, 14*, 481–489.

Satz, P., Strauss, E., Hunter, M., & Wada, J. (1994). Re-examination of the crowding hypothesis: Effects of age of onset. *Neuropsychology, 8*(2), 255–262.

Schamber, C. R., Schrader, A. G., Zafiris, C. M., McConnell, E. D., Manteris, E. M., & D'Amato, R. C. (2008). *Evaluating the executive functions of children who have experienced a trauma using selected subtest from the Delis Kaplan executive function system.* Poster/paper presented at the 36th Annual Convention International Neuropsychological Society, Buenos Aires, Argentina.

Shaywitz, S. (2003). *Overcoming dyslexia: A new and complete science-based program for reading problems at any level.* New York: Alfred A. Knopf.

Skeem, J. L., & Petrila, J. (2004). Juvenile psychopathy: Informing the debate. *Behavioral Sciences & the Law, 22*(1), 1–4.

Sousa, D. A. (2005). *How the brain learns* (3rd ed.). Thousand Oaks, CA: Corwin Press.

Sparta, S. N. (2003). Assessment of childhood trauma. In A. M. Goldstein (Ed.), *Handbook of psychology: Vol. 11. Forensic psychology* (pp. 209–231). Hoboken, NJ: Wiley.

Sparta, S. N., & Koocher, G. P. (Eds.). (2006). *Forensic mental health assessment of children and adolescents.* New York: Oxford.

Spooner, D. M., & Pachana, N. A. (2006). Ecological validity in neuropsychological assessment: A case for greater consideration in research with neurologically intact populations. *Archives of Clinical Neuropsychology, 21*, 327–337.

Stanford, L. D., & Dorflinger, J. M. (2009). Pediatric brain injury: Mechanisms and amelioration. In C. R. Reynolds & E. Fletcher-Janzen (Eds.), *Handbook of clinical child neuropsychology* (3rd ed., pp. 169–186). New York: Springer Science.

Stiles, J. (2000). Neural plasticity and cognitive development. *Developmental Neuropsychology, 18*(2), 237–272.

Teeter, P. A., & Semrud-Clikeman, M. (2007). *Child neuropsychology: Assessment and intervention for neurodevelopmental disorders* (2nd ed.). New York: Springer-Verlag.

Telzrow, C. F. (1985). The science and speculation of rehabilitation in developmental neuropsychological disorders. In L. C. Hartlage & C. F. Telzrow (Eds.), *The neuropsychology of individual differences: A developmental perspective* (pp. 271–307). New York: Plenum.

Titus, J. B., & Dean, R. S. (2003). Forensic neuropsychology with children. In A. M. Horton & L. C. Hartlage (Eds.), *Handbook of forensic neuropsychology* (pp.425–456). New York: Springer-Verlag.

Tramontana, M. G., Hooper, S. R., Watts-English, T., Ellison, T., & Bethea, T. C. (2008). Neuropsychology of child psychopathology. In C. R. Reynolds & E. Fletcher-Janzen (Eds.), *Handbook of clinical child neuropsychology* (3rd ed., pp. 117–146). New York: Springer Science.

Traughber, M. C., & D'Amato, R. C. (2005). Integrating evidence-based neuropsychological services into school settings: Issues and challenges for the future. In R. C. D'Amato, E. Fletcher-Janzen, & C. R. Reynolds (Eds.), *Handbook of school neuropsychology* (pp. 827–857). Hoboken, NJ: Wiley.

Tupper, D. E. (1999). Introduction: Alexander Luria's continuing influence on worldwide neuropsychology. *Neuropsychology Review, 9*(1), 1–7.

Viljoen, J. L., Zapf, P.A., & Roesch, R. (2007). Adjudicative competence and comprehension of Miranda rights in adolescent defendants: A comparison of legal standards. *Behavioral Sciences & the Law, 25*(1), 1–19.

Vincent, G. (2006). Psychopathy and violence risk assessment in youth. *Child and Adolescent Psychiatric Clinics of North America, 15*(2), 407–428.

Walker, L. E. A., & Shapiro, D. L. (2003). *Introduction to forensic psychology: Clinical and social psychological perspectives.* New York: Kluwer Academic/Plenum Publishers.

Willis, G. W. (2005). Foundations of developmental neuroanatomy. In R. C. D'Amato, E. Fletcher-Janzen, & C. R. Reynolds (Eds.), *Handbook of school neuropsychology* (pp. 41–60). Hoboken, NJ: Wiley.

Witsken, D., D'Amato, R. C., & Hartlage, L. C. (2008). Understanding the past, present, and future of clinical neuropsychology. In L. C. Hartlage & R. C. D'Amato (Eds.), *Essentials of neuropsychological assessment: Rehabilitation planning for intervention* (2nd ed., pp. 1–30). New York: Springer-Verlag.

Witsken, D., Stoeckel, A., & D'Amato, R. C. (2008). Leading educational change using a neuropsychological response-to-intervention approach: Linking our past, present, and future. *Psychology in the Schools, 45*(9), 781–811.

Work, P. H. L., & Choi, H.-S. (2005). Developing classroom and group interventions based on a neuropsychological paradigm. In R. C. D'Amato, E. Fletcher-Janzen, & C. R. Reynolds (Eds.), *Handbook of school neuropsychology* (pp. 663–683). Hoboken, NJ: Wiley.

Wynkoop, T. F. (2008). Neuropsychology in the juvenile justice system. In R. L. Denney & J. P. Sullivan (Eds.), *Clinical neuropsychology in the criminal forensic setting* (pp. 295–325). New York: Guilford.

Zinna, K. (March, 2004). *Violence assessment and solutions for schools and industry.* Workshop presented to the College of Education and Behavioral Sciences, University of Northern Colorado, Greeley, CO.

Special Difficulties of Autism Spectrum Disorders in the Forensic Arena

23

Henry V. Soper
Dori Pelz-Sherman

Working with the autism spectrum disorders (ASDs) in the forensic arena can be very difficult, but very rewarding. In addition to all the other difficulties associated with being a forensic clinician, you have to have the additional knowledge of this curious disorder that has defied clear understanding for decades. A very nice novel by Mark Haddon (2003) gives us some great insights into the disorder, but a solid knowledge is needed to work with those with an ASD when forensic issues come up. Unless you are already pretty well versed in autism, when a question of an ASD arises in the forensic setting, it is wise to consult with someone, a forensic clinician preferably, who is knowledgeable about such disorders. A good, solid understanding of why the person did what they did is essential to an accurate case formulation. This case formulation would consist of aspects such as fitness to stand trial, including understanding the various features of the legal proceedings and the court procedures. Although it is certainly true that some such defendants are not fit to stand trial, others are. However, because of the unique aspects of ASDs, such decisions are not always easy to make. For example, does he or she understand the nature of the charges brought against him or her? Although the person may have a simplistic understanding, he/she may have no clue to the ramifications of the charges or his/her plea. Later, we will discuss the difficulties they have in telling right from wrong, and how erroneous presumptions about their behaviors can be made.

An individual with an ASD in the forensic arena poses many rather unusual and peculiar problems. First, this person does not operate in the world in the same manner as the rest of us. Such individuals simply do not think like the rest of the population. Their interpersonal perception of the world is totally different, and their logical operation, when it comes to social situations, differs distinctly from most of the rest of the population. Second, most of the people in the forensic arena, including the triers of fact, have no idea of the world such an individual lives in. Forensic neuropsychologists have difficulty conceiving and understanding the perspective of those with ASD, and they are very resistant to accepting that there are others who process information, especially social information, in such a different manner. This leaves them to try to understand the behaviors from their own perspective, what they would have been thinking if they performed these acts. There is a big jump from surmising how people with autism feel to understanding, based on results, an inability to process certain kinds of information. Such triers of fact can understand, to a certain extent, the world of a person who is blind, but not that of someone who is very restricted in appreciating or participating in close, reciprocal interpersonal interactions. This is simply beyond the ken of most people.

In discussing ASD, the *Diagnostic and Statistical Manual of Mental Disorders* (*DSM-IV-TR*; American Psychiatric Association, 2000) generally breaks them into three diagnoses: autism disorder, Asperger's disorder, and pervasive developmental disorder not otherwise specified (PDD-NOS). The PDD-NOS diagnosis is a bit problematic, in that it can include individuals not within ASD, but those within this diagnostic category who do show the core deficits are also termed "high-functioning autism" by Wing (1992) and others. (Wing also provides an excellent description and categorization of these individuals.)

The presumption in this chapter is that the ASDs lie along a spectrum, from more severe to less severe. The core feature of the ASDs consists of deficits in reciprocal interpersonal interaction. These stem from their inability to perceive of a point of view other than their own. Some have these deficits so severely that communication, especially verbal communication, is very difficult. Because of the unique lack of social perception of those with an ASD, many behaviors are not controlled by external pressures from others, and hence, they display behaviors in public that are considered inappropriate (e.g., stereotopies, preoccupations, inflexible adherence to routines or rituals). If language is impaired and the behavioral abnormalities are present, the diagnosis of autism is most often offered. If language is relatively normal but behavioral abnormalities are present, Asperger's syndrome is usually diagnosed. If there are none of the language or behavioral abnormalities, then PDD-NOS is offered as a diagnosis.

Because this is a neurological disorder, at the one end, it is not surprising that there is a high rate of other neurological disorders (such as mental retardation and epilepsy). At the other end, those who show no major impairment in the various areas of functioning might well carry no diagnosis until they get into trouble. This is discussed more fully in Soper, Canavan, and Wolfson (2008).

There are a few advances in the past several years that have greatly increased our understanding of the social deficits in ASD. One is the study of mirror neurons and related phenomena, and the other is the development of the concept of the theory of mind (e.g., Baron-Cohen, 1999).

Fogassi, Ferrari, Gesierich, Rozzi, Chersi, and Rizzolatti (2005) have found neurons in monkeys, mirror neurons, which respond in the same manner to the intentions of the monkey itself and to the perceived intention of an observed monkey. It is as if, in some ways, one monkey can feel for the other monkey based on its own experiences. A similar thing happens in humans (Oberman, Hubbard, McCleery, Altschuler, Ramachandran, & Pineda, 2005). A significant mu (8–13 Hz) suppression is observed either when people move their own hands or when they observe others moving their hands. However, this phenomenon does not exist among those with an ASD. Although they show significant mu suppression to self-performed hand movements, there is no such response to the same movements when performed by others. Although admittedly somewhat of a jump, it is easy to see why the authors would conclude that these results help to explain the deficits observed among those with ASDs in imitation, pragmatic language, theory of mind, and empathy. These results also support the contention that those with ASD have a severe neurobiologically based impairment in reading, or appreciating, the minds of others.

Baron-Cohen (1999) uses the term "mindblindness" to understand this aspect of the autism presentation. This term is particularly good because, like congenital blindness, the individual with ASD does not misunderstand or fail to interpret accurately what is going on in the mind of another. The person simply does not conceive that the other has a separate mind, and hence, thoughts. When they see someone walk into a room, they simply observe it, and do not think of what might be going on in the mind of that person. In part because of this, they also have difficulty making simple cause-and-effect interpretations. In this example, the person walks into the room behind the person with ASD and turns on the lights. The person with ASD may become upset at the sudden change in illumination, for they did not understand why it occurred. They did not make the connection between the person walking in and the lights going on or off. We all would feel a bit disturbed if lights suddenly went on or off and we had no explanation. In the circumstance just described, the person with ASD had no explanation because of his or her "mindblindness."

People with ASDs really cannot put their feet in the shoes of others, or view the world from the perspective of another. When asked to tell the story of Snow White and the Seven Dwarfs from Grumpy's perspective, they find it impossible. You get the story as they perceived it, even to the point of talking about the seven little miners. Fein (2006) points out that they find it effectively impossible to point something out that is of interest to another, but not to themselves. This situation also leaves them devoid of empathy. Lack of empathy in the forensic arena initially calls to mind sociopathy. Although those with an antisocial personality disorder also can be without empathy, the two situations are quite different. In the case of the antisocial person, he or she may well know that the other is suffering, but he/she does not use that to regulate his/her behavior. In addition, as Attwood (2007) says, with the antisocial, there is a superficial charm and a history of exploitation and manipulation. With ASDs, empathy is just lacking, due to the inability to appreciate the emotional position of another. In the case of some with an ASD, they simply cannot read the emotion of another. Given gross cues, such as laughing and crying, they can conclude that the person may be happy or sad, but the subtle expressions of facial and body language are not read, prosody seems to be poorly perceived at best, and the person does not have the foggiest idea what the other is feeling or that it could be different from what he or she is feeling. This also precludes true interpersonal feelings, such as love and hate. Family members are often very upset that there is no bereavement when someone presumed to be close to the individual dies. In addition, it makes true remorse impossible. The person is sorry for his/her actions because of the trouble he/she got into, but not because of the suffering he/she caused others. Although this is terra incognita to them, others may, and have, placed another interpretation on such lack of remorse.

From observations such as these, has come the concept of the Theory of Mind (e.g., Leslie, 1987). Most of us who watch someone working their way around an environment automatically think of what might be going on in that person's mind. In fact, we often attribute such minds, including thoughts and feelings, to most animals. We may feel that a dog can understand us and not only have feelings, but understand the feelings we have. In other words, there is a reciprocal relationship. However, were we to say that a stop light is out to get us by turning red every time we approach, it is clearly understood that this cannot literally be, and another interpretation is called for. One could also say that the stop light is mind blind, it cannot appreciate what is going on in the mind of "others," or even that others have a mind. Such "mindblindness" is discussed by Baron-Cohen (1999), as mentioned above, to explain why those with ASD not only are unable to have an appreciation for what is going on in the minds of others, but also they cannot imagine a mind different from their own. There is a presumption that others know what they know, somewhat like a collective fund of knowledge. For example, if they have found out that a box labeled cookies actually contains candies, they expect that others will also now know that there are candies there. When pressed later, they can appreciate that the other person would have no way of knowing that, but this appreciation is more through a mechanical determination than insight.

Given this quite different orientation to the world, one can see the difficulties of people with ASD when they get into legal difficulties. On the surface, they can resemble people without ASDs, but the inner differences, most often related to what got them into trouble in the first place, will also make it difficult for fair adjudication. For example, moral development is very primitive, due to their mindblindness and poor social responsivity. Although Kohlberg's (1976) moral stages do not fit exactly, such individuals would find it impossible to act beyond what he calls the preconventional stage. Taking into account the thoughts and feelings of others and acting for the greater good is beyond those who do not possess a theory of mind. It is a somewhat instrumental morality, in that they learn what is good and bad in a more rote manner, from punishment or direction. For example, you should not throw rocks at trucks because you will get punished, with no appreciation for the potentially devastating outcomes such behaviors could have on others.

In line with this, such individuals have little or no appreciation of the relative severity of such actions. This is directly related to their inability to appreciate the full effect of their actions on others. Higher functioning individuals do appreciate that their teasing has an effect, and that the other person is upset. However, they do not have an appreciation of how inappropriate their behavior is. One young lad was denied a significant trip with his classmates for his behavior, and as a result, verbally threatened to kill the school principal. In line with a zero-tolerance policy, he wound up in juvenile detention. There was never any danger, but he had no idea how his words could be taken by others (and he had never been diagnosed with an ASD). When seen later, he knew he should never have said such a thing, but he never really understood why. In a way, he knew he was not serious, so the others should have known it too (the collective knowledge).

Another adolescent with ASD became very excited when his father, a tele-vangelist, was "arrested" for speeding on the highway. He had images of his father being handcuffed and carted off to prison to serve a lengthy sentence. He, like so many with ASD, had no appreciation for the moral severity differences between going 8 miles over the speed limit, embezzlement of large sums of money, walking on the grass in a park against the posted regulations, and dropping an infant from a fifth-story window to get it to stop crying.

As an aside, North, Russell, and Gudjonsson (2008) present findings that suggest that those with ASDs are particularly vulnerable when questioned by the authorities because of a desire to please and avoid conflict. This would result in compliancy to suggestions even when they disagree. However, the participants in this study were not from forensic populations, and the generalizability to such situations may be questioned. In fact, one suspects that it is more likely that there will be insistence on the accuracy of even the most minor of details (as has been our experience) and little suggestibility.

Aggression

What is the nature of aggression seen in those with ASDs? We see a lot of aggression among those with both mental retardation and autism, and most of this is based on frustration. It is more of an indiscriminate lashing out. This form is closest to what has been called irritable aggression (Moyer, 1968). Often this frustration is based on confusion arising from not knowing what is going on, including not understanding changes in schedules. An inability to have empathy and a mindblindness contribute to this form of aggression. Lacking social skills and the ability to read facial expressions, they can find themselves in irresolvable, and hence, frustrating situations (Murrie, Warren, Kristiansson, & Dietz, 2002). Although fear-induced aggression can occur among lower functioning individuals, most often such a person will shrink away and become physically defensive. Among higher functioning people, the consequences of the aggression and the reaction of the victim are not taken into account, or at least not fully taken into account. An eight-year-old girl's arm was in a cast, and she would use this cast to beat her younger brother. At times, she did this when he irritated her, but at other times, there was no clear precipitant to the violence. In addition, often one or both parents were there when she did it. She was fully aware that if this persisted she would have to be removed from the family, something she certainly did not want to happen. However, she was unable to use this knowledge to control her behavior. Aspects of the psychological testing made it clear that she did not really make the connection between this behavior and her possible removal from the house. In this case, the authorities were not called in, but one could see that should she act in this manner toward someone outside her family, there could be a real problem. Performing such acts outside her family is not as outrageous as it might seem. When at the beach, she would often wander to the area of another family, sit down, reach into the cooler and pull out a sandwich, and start talking to them while eating it. One evening, she went into the house of a neighbor and made herself comfortable in the living room watching television. When the neighbors came home, she invited them to watch the program with her, telling them how great it was. Even though she was perfectly normal in looks and language, and of at least average intelligence, she was profoundly mindblind.

Empathy, Remorse, and Love

Saying that people with an ASD have no empathy makes it sound as though they are bad people, but this is not true. People with antisocial personality disorders usually lack empathy, and that is a bad thing because they use this lack as a method for violating the rights of others. They are, most often, fully aware of what they are doing and they have a good appreciation why it is wrong. Unlike the rest of us, they do not, or can not, use this information to control their behavior. Those with an ASD lack empathy for a different reason. They cannot appreciate that the others have feelings, wants, and desires, and that these can differ from their own wants, feelings, and desires. This blindness to the minds of others makes it impossible to have empathy. The people with antisocial personality disorders, though they cannot feel empathy for others, do have an idea how the others are feeling, and they just do not feel sorry or happy for them because of what they are going through. In the case of those with ASDs, they simply do not have any idea what the other is going through emotionally. It is as if the mirror neuron information is not getting through. Therefore, they have a lack of empathy.

Similarly, although those with ASDs can feel badly for what they have done, it is for instrumental reasons (such as getting punished). They cannot feel true emotional remorse for their actions. They cannot feel sorry for what they have put another through.

It should be clear by now that emotional attachment is impossible. Relatives of those with ASD often complain that the person did not grieve the loss of a parent or someone close to them. This can be very hard to deal with. Even when you explain that this is to be expected in someone with this kind of a disorder, the person responds that because there was so much love that went in one direction, there must have been some that went in the other. Sadly, there was none. We also see this in a person with an ASD whom we discuss later who moved away to go to college. This person never thought to call home or to call his "friends." He had a roommate for 3 years, but when asked later he had no idea what the person did for a living, or even whether he was also a student. He never thought to ask.

Although not strictly relevant to this chapter, those with an ASD do not have the capacity for love. In fact, when discussing this with those who are high functioning but with autism, they clearly do not understand the concept of love.

Inappropriate Behaviors

Often, when the person with an ASD feels detached and does not relate to the crime, he or she will smile during the telling of the story. This is in response to being the center of attention, rather than to the content of the story. However, to casual observer, it looks as if the person is smirking because of the crime, a behavior similar to what is often seen among serial killers. This is a potential liability should the person be called to the witness stand. The triers of fact would have no idea why the person is smiling, and, understandably, presume this is a sign of sociopathic behavior.

Similarly, at the time of arrest, the person, not understanding the big picture or the point of view of the arresting officers, can act vary inappropriately and even with violence. Along with their mindblindness comes a lack of normal pragmatics. They do not understand the context of the situation and, therefore, cannot act in accordance with the context. Inappropriate behaviors, such as yelling or throwing a fist, would naturally be misinterpreted by those in the area, including the arresting officers.

The Innocents

A common plight of those with an ASD in legal trouble is being talked into the situation by a "friend," often someone who threatens to withdraw the friendship if the person does not perform as requested. This situation is also discussed elsewhere in this chapter. The term "innocent," coined from Wing (1992), aptly describes those who are duped into getting involved, even though they may not know what they are doing is wrong, or they have no idea of the severity of the crime they are getting involved in. North et al. (2008) found that those with an ASD were far more compliant than matched controls. They suggest that this may lead such individuals to be relatively "easily led, manipulated or coerced into criminal activity by peers" (p. 331).

It has been our experience that quite frequently, our spectrum-disordered clients have become involved in overt crimes to help out a friend, either with no knowledge of the illegal aspect of the activity, to maintain the friendship against the threats of losing it if they do not perform in the desired way, or for the excitement of doing something with someone and the perception that they must be important to be included. The sad thing is that they can be induced into doing some pretty horrible things, like kidnap, rape, and murder, with the perception that if they are doing anything wrong, it is on a par with going slightly over the speed limit on the highway.

Related to this innocence is the social naiveté that Murrie et al. (2002) speak of. The severe impairments in social skills resulting from their inability to see the world from the eyes of another will result in an impoverished understanding of friendships and other relationships. Not only does this leave them vulnerable to maltreatment from others, but Murrie et al. cite examples such as the man who bought a large apartment expecting that it would immediately bring about a marriage. Another thought that he could attract a sexual partner by performing sex with an inflatable doll. They also mention the full and honest confessions, with no regard to self-preservation, of those with an ASD who are arrested. In fact, as mentioned elsewhere, they can become insistent that even the minutest detail be accurately represented.

Case Examples

In this next section, we will present a number of cases from the literature and our own experience. With each presentation, we will provide an explanation for the apparent criminal behavior in terms of autistic processes. Through these examples, we can see how the activity looked from the ASD person's point of view, and how the situation can be misunderstood by them, by the clinicians, and the triers of fact.

Mukaddes and Topcu (2006) report on a 10-year-old girl with autism who threw her 6-month-old sister out of a window, killing her. This child was quite compromised, with intellectual and communication impairments. She had a seizure disorder at age 3, though only one seizure after that. She was admittedly unwanted and unloved. She had been subjected to abuse by several people. She had minimal treatment for her condition. In addition, she had acted aggressively toward her infant sister for a month prior to the incident. In their formulation, the authors considered all these factors, though they ruled out the seizure disorder as contributing. They termed the action a homicide, though without prior planning. They stated, "Taken all together, it seems that a severe intellectual disability coupled with a lack of appropriate environment, supervision and treatment program as well as the existence of neglect and physical abuse in this case led to the homicidal act" (p. 474). Although the poor treatment may well have contributed to her general aggression, in her case, a simpler explanation may be appropriate. She had thrown things out the window before. Given that she is very autistic, has no empathy, has no idea of theory of mind, her action may well have been a reasonable method of getting rid of something that had been irritating her for a month, and in this case, the intent was to ease an irritation, much as someone might throw a bug out the window, or a piece of food that has gone bad. I rather suspect that the intent was not to kill anyone, but simply to cease the irritation.

At the state hospital, we had a young man of mild mental retardation and autism who was there because he had tossed an infant from a second-story balcony. When asked why he did it, he replied that he only wanted to see how high he would bounce. Although in this case, the infant did survive, it was clear that our patient had no appreciation for the potential severity of the outcomes of what he had done. In fact, because it was an infant, he did not even appreciate that it was a human being. To him it might as well have been a ball or pillow. There was no malicious intent in what he did. It was more akin to dropping a basketball from that height to see how far up it would bounce.

Mawson, Grounds, and Tantum (1985) present a case of an individual whom they diagnose with Asperger's syndrome who had a predilection for attacking sources of high-pitched noise. These included women (especially sopranos), infants, dogs, televisions, and radios. Knowing what we do now about these disorders, it is easy to see how the people, and even the dogs, would be put into the same category as the lifeless items, the television and the radio, and treated in that manner. One can understand someone smashing an irritating radio or television, especially if it did not belong to you. We hear of people who destroy dogs that irritate them. However, we would not think to end irritation from humans by putting an end to them. Yet, with his lack of theory of mind and his inability to take the perspective of another, to him the focus of the attack was to end the irritant, much as one might kill a wasp that is flying around you. (This individual also became infatuated with poisons, but did not understand why this would bother others. In fact, a part of the appeal may well have been the reaction of others.)

Everall and LeCouteur (1990) describe an adolescent diagnosed with Asperger's syndrome who repeatedly set fires, initially small ones, but later rather large and potentially dangerous ones. When finally confronted, he could not provide an explanation beyond that he liked fires. He also presented, not surprisingly, no evidence that he comprehended the seriousness or dangerousness of what he was doing. In addition, he seemed unconcerned about the aftermath of what he had done. However, he did admit to planning most of them. The authors state that he seemed to comprehend the meaning of right or wrong, but one suspects that this is based on a very primitive morality, that something is right or wrong because you are told it is, with little understanding of the moral basis. It seems that he was setting the fires because he enjoys them. The stimulation could be reinforcing in the same manner finger flicking is to others with an ASD. However, now he understands that if he is caught, he will be prevented from doing it. He does not, however, understand that he is placing others in danger or the distress that others can feel because of his actions. Although technically he may be violating the rights of others, he does not understand his situation in those terms. Although he understands that he should not do it, it is rather like going slightly over the speed limit on an empty highway.

One of our clients got into a lot of trouble because of his inability to understand how others might view his behavior. He presumed that everyone would view the situation as he did. He states that he had gotten quite drunk, and two males had stolen his bicycle and they would not return it unless he knocked on an identified dwelling's door and asked "for the guy who owns it." He knocked, was told someone is coming out, and to wait at the table. Then, in his own words:

I was waiting at the table for some time, at least 10 minutes. Then an older, slightly overweight man came out. He shook my hand and I asked him if he [had] a son and that's who I wanted to talk to. He said that he did have a son and knows that he had been involved in illegal activity. At this point, I pulled my closed knife from back pocket and placed it on the table and said that I wasn't there for anything violent. My reason for this was that I had not told the man anything other than I wanted to talk to son. When he said criminal activity, it caught me [off] guard and wondered what the heck was going on. It was at this time an officer arrived and picked up the closed knife and took me into custody.

His arrest report says something substantially different. It stated that he broke into a house and while there, he brandished a knife and would not leave. The resident of the dwelling reported that he entered the kitchen before showing the knife. Then a second person came up, and he brandished the knife at that person, too. Somehow one of the witnesses got hold of the knife before the police arrived, but there is no report of disarming or a fight for the knife. He was outside when the officers arrived. This arrest report version differs substantially from his. One can see how it is very self-serving to the residents of the house.

He says that he understands now what an error it was to show the knife, but at the time, he was simply trying to show that he was harmless, somewhat in the manner of a policeman who sets his pistol on the table to show that he is unarmed.

At the time, he expected that the man at the house would take the presentation as a sign that he was not looking for any trouble. He had no idea that it could be considered a threatening gesture, and that he would be accused of "brandishing" a knife. He does understand now that he should not have displayed the knife in that manner, but at the time, it seemed a reasonable thing to do.

Another man, 42 years old, was charged with grand theft and conspiracy to commit a crime. Apparently, two other people stole some copper wire/cable from a railroad trestle. One of them contacted our person to see about using his van to help them take the material to the recycle location. He agreed, but then he became bothered when it appeared that what they were doing might be illegal. At this point, he locked everyone out of his van. The other two tried to break in, causing the van's alarm system to go off. The police arrived, and arrested all three.

This man was certainly duped into becoming involved in something illegal, but this appears to be a common occurrence. In the words of Lorna Wing (1992), others recognize these people as "innocents" and use them to assist in criminal activities. The problems might be avoided if the autism spectrum handicap were known, and the gullibility anticipated. Such individuals really want to be a friend and have friends, and often either do not know the illegality of the acts they are asked to perform or appreciate the seriousness of the acts and the consequences.

In the case Wing (1992) presents, the individual had a job in which he counted and stored large sums of money. A "friend" asked him to keep back a certain sum, which later they shared. When caught, fortunately, the court realized that he had "no idea of the implications of his actions and had simply obeyed directions without question" (p. 136).

Years ago a man in his mid-20s with an ASD broke into a Catholic church and stole some candlesticks from the altar. His roommate told the staff about the theft, and, when confronted, he admitted to everything that he did. He did not understand what all the excitement was about. He was a member of another denomination, and thought he would be praised by them for what he had done, much like the pranks pulled around the Yale–Harvard and Army–Navy games. To him, what he had done was along the line of Army cadets stealing the Navy goat just before the game. A full explanation was offered, but he did not understand the gravity of what he had done. He did understand, now, however, that it was wrong. A very understanding priest resulted in no severe consequences, but it was still a very awkward situation for the board-and-care facility.

A much more tragic case occurred when a person with an ASD came under the influence of a clearly antisocial individual. This person was induced to help the other to go with him on a spree, a somewhat planned one, in which they kidnapped a young woman, raped her, and murdered her. Her only "crime" was to stop one evening at a stoplight on the way to visiting a friend. When asked to relate what happened, the person with ASD denied nothing, but told the full story. In relating the story, he told it much as one might tell of an evening of barhopping and incidental fights along the way. Although initially sitting in the car during the kidnapping, he was ordered out to help when the other was having difficulty. The young man said that even though he did not want to have sex with the girl, his "friend" basically coerced him into it by threatening to remove his friendship if he did not do it, and accusing him of not being a man. The same threat was effective in getting him to murder with the knife. Several times he was asked how the young girl felt during the ordeal, and it was clear that this had never occurred to him. When asked how he felt the victim felt, he stopped to think about it, and then said that because of the way she was grunting she must not have liked it. Even though this was well after the incident, he still did not know the victim's name.

At the conclusion of relating his story, he was asked what he expected to happen to him when he was arrested, and he replied that he thought he was going to have to pay a fine, because that is what had happened the last time. When asked about "last time," it turns out that the two of them had been arrested several years before for throwing rocks at trucks. This person knew that throwing rocks and kidnap and rape and murder were all wrong, but had no idea of the differences in the gravity of the offenses.

This young man clearly did not live in the same world as the rest of us. This is the person referred to earlier, who several years before had moved out of state to go to college, but when asked he had no idea what his roommate of that time did for a living, or even whether he was a student. Similarly, he never once called his antisocial "friend" the whole time he was gone. Literally, when out of his sight, you were out of his mind. In addition, I have always had the feeling that if he had connected with a minister or priest instead of an antisocial person, he might well be receiving community awards for cleaning up community parks, instead of spending the rest of his life in prison.

Resolutions

Those with ASDs have a number of hurdles to overcome in the courtroom. First, the diagnosis is usually not obvious, and those trying to convict can be very resistant to first, accepting the diagnosis at all, and second, to accepting it as a mitigating factor. It is not that these are bad people. It is that they are not clinicians, often do not appreciate the significance of the diagnosis, and the diagnosis does not fit their argument. In fact, the lack of empathy and remorse, if brought up, erroneously reinforces their idea of an antisocial factor. Unusual behavior in the courtroom, including on the stand, can be misinterpreted as supporting great culpability.

As mentioned by Attwood (2007), another possibility is that the legal team may elicit sympathy and compassion, resulting in relative leniency. On the other hand, regardless of the comprehension of the disorder, there could be concern for re-offending. The young man may have genuinely only been interested in how high the baby would bounce, with no appreciation of the effects that dropping it might have on its welfare. However, the triers of fact may be concerned that such obliviousness to the welfare of others can and probably will result in similar activities in the future, and therefore, long-term incarceration in a state hospital may be recommended.

Attwood (2007) states that the diagnosis often is more relevant to the sentencing, and less so to the more preliminary factors, such as fitness to plead. An appreciation of the level of moral reasoning can be helpful at this time, but of more value is a full explanation as to why he or she did what he or she did. Although the term "homicide" technically means one human taking the life of another human, usually there is an implied intent to kill. Terming dropping a baby out of a window to quiet her as a homicide (Mukaddes & Topcu, 2006) seems a bit inappropriate when one considers the idea of dropping an alarm clock that will not be quiet out of the window stop its noise. On the other hand, whether the individual with ASD understands it or not, she is still taking a human life, and this must be adjudicated.

Sentencing can be difficult. As Attwood says (2007), consideration should be made for the reasons for the offenses, the likelihood of victimization should the person be put in with other prisoners, and the availability of programs to reduce the chance of re-offending. Such programs would include anger management and social skills training, as well as help with depression, anxiety, or any other disorder the person with the ASD might be suffering from. He also suggests encouraging friendships with appropriate peers, and this should be emphasized. Because such individuals so often become "innocents" and not see the trouble someone else is getting them into, parents, relatives, guardians, and others should be made aware of this complication, and exert some control over the people with whom the person with an ASD interacts. In fact, if people were more aware of this potential problem, there might be far fewer people with ASDs who come into the penal system. The problem is that so many with an ASD look so normal at first, and yet, without a theory of mind, they live in a world quite different from that of others, and hence, the rules of logic and morality are substantially different.

Acknowledgment

The authors would like to thank Hugo M. Doig, Teri McHale, Lisa V. Kandra, Jodi J. Deluca, and Katherine Tong for their assistance with this manuscript.

References

American Psychiatric Association. (2000). *Diagnostic and statistical manual of mental disorders* (4th ed., text revision). Washington, DC: American Psychiatric Press.

Attwood, T. (2007). *The complete guide to Asperger's syndrome*. London: Jessica Kingsley.

Baron-Cohen, S. (1999). *Mindblindness: An essay of autism and theory of mind*. Cambridge, UK: IT Press.

Everall, I. P., & LeCouteur, A. (1990). Firesetting in an adolescent boy with Asperger's syndrome. *British Journal of Psychiatry, 157,* 284–287.

Fein, D. (2006, March). *Recovery in autism: A neuropsychological analysis*. Paper presented at the 16th Annual Nelson Butters' West Coast Neuropsychology Conference: Advances in Pediatric Neuropsychology: From Toddlers through School-Aged Children, San Diego, CA.

Fogassi, L., Ferrari, P. F., Gesierich, B., Rozzi, S., Chersi, F., & Rizzolatti, G. (2005). Parietal lobe: Action organization to intention understanding. *Science, 308,* 662–667.

Haddon, M. (2003). *The curious incident of the dog in the night-time*. New York: Vintage.

Kohlberg, L. (1976). Moral stages and moralization: The cognitive-developmental approach. In J. Lickona (Ed.), *Moral development behavior: Theory, research and social issues*. New York: Holt, Reinhart and Winston.

Leslie, A. (1987). Pretense and representation: The origins of "theory of mind." *Psychological Review, 94,* 412–426.

Moyer, K. E. (1968). Kinds of aggression and their physiological basis. *Communications in Behavioral Biology, 2A,* 65–87.

Mukaddes, N. M., & Topcu, Z. (2006). Case report: Homicide by a 10-year-old girl with autistic disorder. *Journal of Autism and Developmental Disorders, 36*(4), 471–474.

Murrie, D. C., Warren, J. I., Kristiansson, M., & Dietz, P. E. (2002). Asperger's syndrome in forensic settings. *International Journal of Forensic Mental Health, 1*(1), 59–70.

North, A. S., Russell, A. J., & Gudjonsson, G. H. (2008). High functioning autism spectrum disorders: An investigation of psychological vulnerabilities during interrogative interview. *Journal of Forensic Psychiatry and Psychology, 19*(3), 323–334.

Oberman, L. M., Hubbard, E. M., McCleery, J. P., Altschuler, E. L., Ramachandran, V. S., & Pineda, J. A. (2005). EEG evidence for mirror neuron dysfunction in autism spectrum disorders. *Cognitive Brain Research, 24*(2), 190–198.

Soper, H. V., Canavan, F., & Wolfson, S. S. (2008). Neuropsychology of autism spectrum disorders. In A. M. Horton & D. Wedding (Eds.), *Neuropsychology handbook* (3rd ed., pp. 681–703). New York: Springer Publishing Company.

Wing, L. (1992). Manifestations of social problems in high-functioning autistic people. In E. Schopler & G. B. Mesibov (Eds.), *High-functioning individuals with autism*. New York: Plenum.

Neuropsychology of Substance-Use Disorders in Forensic Settings

24

Daniel N. Allen
Griffin P. Sutton
Bradley C. Donohue
Michael Haderlie

Overview

Substance-use disorders occur at a high rate in the United States (14.6% lifetime prevalence; Kessler, Berglund, Demler, Jin, Merikangas, & Walters, 2005), and males are affected two to three times more often than females. The total cost of drug and alcohol abuse to society is enormous. From a monetary perspective, estimated costs of illicit drug abuse were $97.7 billion for 1992 (National Institute on Drug Abuse, 1998). Furthermore, these costs have increased over the years. Substance abusers have been found to be nearly four times more likely to be involved in work-related accidents, and are five times more likely to file workers' compensation claims, than those who do not use illegal drugs (Substance Abuse and Mental Health Services Administration, 2002). The magnitude of the problem becomes clearer when one considers that in 2001, approximately 76% of those who used drugs and about 80% of adults judged to be "heavy" or "binge" alcohol users were employed either full time or part time (Substance Abuse and Mental Health Services Administration, 2002), and these individuals evidence higher rates of workplace accidents (Elliott & Shelley, 2006). The monetary costs of drug abuse from the years 1992 to 2002, according to the categories of health care expenditures and productivity losses and other impacts, increased by $73 billion (Office of National Drug Control Policy, 2005), and the cost of drug abuse treatment accounted for approximately 4% of state-administered mental health spending in 1991, and increased to approximately 15% in 2001 (Buck & Mark, 2006). These estimates, however, do not reflect the interpersonal, intrapersonal, and psychosocial costs associated with drug and alcohol abuse that are difficult to quantify, but are also devastating.

A substantial portion of these costs results from the association between substance abuse and criminality. It is estimated that the total number of individuals incarcerated in federal prisons, state prisons, and jails for drug-related offenses, such as possession and trafficking, has increased from 38,680 in 1972 to 480,519 in 2002 (Caulkins & Chandler, 2006). Additionally, approximately 64% of male arrestees had used cocaine, marijuana, methamphetamine, opiates, or phencyclidine (PCP) at the time of their arrest, with estimates as high as 80% in some states (Arrestee Drug Abuse Monitoring Program, 2003). Male arrestees tested positive most often for marijuana (approximately 40%), cocaine (31%), methamphetamine (< 1–36% depending on the area of the country, with the highest percentages in the western part of the United States), and opiates (< 7–21%). Women, on the other hand, were more likely to test positive for cocaine at time of arrest, though the overall prevalence of recent drug use was less than that of men, by about 11%. The prevalence of substance abuse and dependence ranges between 10–48% in male prisoners, and from 30% to 60% in female prisoners (Fazel, Bains, & Doll, 2006). Interestingly, early age of onset (< 16 years) of a substance-use disorder is associated with as much as a four times higher risk of later incarceration (Slade, Stuart, Salkever, Karakus, Green, & Ialongo, 2008).

Not only is substance use higher among those who are arrested or incarcerated, but substance use also appears to be a major contributor to the commission of criminal offenses (Sullivan & Hamilton, 2007). For individuals in residential treatment sites, 41% had been involved in at least one violent incident within the prior 30 days, of which 40% occurred following alcohol or drug use (Mericle & Havassy, 2008). Similarly, alcohol use is involved in approximately half of all homicides and half of all driving fatalities in the United States (California Department of Alcohol & Drug Problems, 2004; Office of National Drug Control Policy, 2005).

Alcohol and drug use also play a significant role in domestic violence, including physical, sexual, psychological, and emotional abuse (Coker, Smith, McKeown, & King, 2000; Holtzworth-Munroe, Meehan, Herron, Rehman, & Stuart, 2000) in both perpetrators and victims (Moore & Stuart, 2004). Incarcerated men who are violent toward their partners are particularly likely to abuse drugs, compared with those inmates who have not maltreated their partners (Logan, Walker, & Leukefeld, 2001). Illicit drug use also predicts victimization in women (Testa, Livingston, & Leonard, 2003), such that victims of intimate partner violence are more likely to use substances, with the prevalence of alcohol and drug abuse approximately 19% and 9%, respectively (Golding, 1999). Self-reported drug use (especially stimulant and marijuana use) is a stronger predictor of intimate partner violence than self-reported alcohol use (Stuart et al., 2008), with cocaine use also being a significant risk factor for intimate partner violence (Chase, O'Farrell, Murphy, Fals-Stewart, & Murphy, 2003). Similarly, severe alcohol and drug abuse distinguishes between men who commit intimate partner violence and men who do not (Chase et al.).

Child maltreatment (i.e., neglect and abuse) is also strongly associated with substance use and has neuropsychological implications. In a large group of children who had been exposed in utero to substances, 30% were later reported as being either abused or neglected (19.9% of which were substantiated claims), and the biological parents were found to be responsible for the maltreatment 88% of the time (Jaudes, Ekwo, & Van Voorhis, 1995). Furthermore, it is estimated that the percentage of parents involved in child welfare services who also have substance-use disorders is as high as 79% (Young, Boles, & Otero, 2007), and that childhood maltreatment and parental drug-use problems co-occur in 30–43% of child welfare cases (Murphy et al., 1991; Locke & Newcomb, 2003). From a neurocognitive perspective, children who are exposed to substances in utero are at increased risk for developmental delay and neurological abnormalities, which is particularly the case for those who develop fetal alcohol syndrome (FAS), which often results in severe neurocognitive deficits (Sari & Gozes, 2006).

Regarding other crimes committed, Campbell, Deck, and Krupski (2007) found that 42% of opiate users who had undergone substance-abuse treatment had been arrested within 3 years posttreatment for property crimes (the most common being theft), 26% for miscellaneous crimes (the most common being driving under the influence [DUI]), 26% for drug-related crimes (the most common being a felony violation of the Uniform Controlled Substance Act, committed by 32%), 11.7% for assault, 3.0% for robbery, 0.5% for sex-related crimes (the most common being rape, committed by 40%), and 0.3% for homicide (the most common being murder, committed by 57%). Sexual offenders score significantly higher on the Michigan Alcohol Screening Test (MAST) than nonsexual offenders, with the average score of the sex-offending group falling in the "problem drinking range" implicating the role of alcohol in at least some of these crimes (Abracen, Looman, Di Fazio, Kelly, & Stirpe, 2006). There is also an increased risk of arrest in individuals with bipolar disorder or schizophrenia and no substance abuse (Ekiran et al., 2006; McDermott, Quanbeck, & Frye, 2007).

Therefore, the linkage of substance use and abuse in criminal activities is clear. Indeed, neuropsychologists are expected to assess individuals with substance disorders and, in some cases, testify with regard to their cognitive functioning. The remainder of this chapter will review the neurocognitive and neurological deficits associated with alcohol and drug abuse, particularly in substances that are frequently encountered in forensic settings.

Diagnosis and Clinical Assessment of Substance-Use Disorders

The *Diagnostic and Statistical Manual of Mental Disorders, Fourth Edition, Text Revision* (*DSM-IV-TR*; American Psychiatric Association, 2000) delineates two categories of substance-related disorders: (a) substance-use disorders and (b) substance-induced disorders (American Psychiatric Association, 2000, pp. 191–295). Substance-use disorders include the subcategories of substance abuse and substance dependence, which are the most commonly diagnosed of the substance-related disorders. Substance abuse is diagnosed when, during a 12-month period, substance use leads to significant problems in at least one of the following four domains: (a) legal, (b) interpersonal, (c) work or school, or (d) hazardous behaviors. Legal problems are particularly relevant in the context of this chapter, and as previously discussed, can range from serious offenses, such as assault, robbery, rape, or DUI, to relatively minor offenses, such as urinating in an inappropriate public place or being arrested for disorderly conduct. The diagnosis of substance dependence is made when substance use causes three or more cognitive, behavioral, or physiological symptoms that occur within the same 12-month period. Symptoms may include unsuccessful attempts to "cut down," tolerance, withdrawal, and curtailment of social, occupational, and/or recreational activities in order to obtain, use, or recover from the effects of the substance. Physiological dependence as indicated by tolerance or withdrawal symptoms is not required to diagnose substance dependence, although it is often present. Although substance dependence is a more severe disorder than substance abuse, substance abuse is not a less severe form of dependence, but rather, they are distinct diagnostic entities with distinct symptoms; substance abuse does not typically progress into substance dependence, and as many as 34% of individuals with dependence diagnoses do not meet criteria for abuse (B. F. Grant et al., 2007).

Substance-induced disorders include intoxication and withdrawal, as well as a number of other disorders that resemble primary mental health disorders described elsewhere in the *DSM-IV-TR* (e.g., major depressive disorder), but unlike these primary disorders, their symptoms are due to the effects of alcohol or drugs. Of particular relevance to this chapter are the disorders alcohol-induced persisting dementia and alcohol-induced persisting amnestic disorder.

Accurate diagnosis of substance-related disorders requires a sound clinical history, which is often difficult to obtain because intoxication interferes with the ability to provide accurate historical accounts. Moreover, individuals who evidence cognitive impairments are more likely to deny substance use in contrast to their non-cognitively impaired counterparts (Burgard, Donohue, Azrin, & Teichner, 2000). Neurocognitive deficits may also impair accuracy in remembering previous patterns of substance use. Furthermore, those with substance-abuse disorders are often under social and legal pressures to deny or underreport the extent and negative consequences of their substance use. Given these challenges, specialized assessment methods are necessary to increase the likelihood of obtaining an accurate history of substance use and related problem behaviors, which is particularly important when recommendations to legal proceedings are required.

Structured interviews, such as the Time-Line Follow Back (TLFB) assessment procedure (Sobell, 1980), have demonstrated significant agreement between urinalysis testing (see the following), collateral, and self-reports of illicit drugs and alcohol for up to 6 months prior to evaluation (Donohue, Azrin, Strada, Silver, Teichner, & Murphy, 2004; Donohue, Hill, Azrin, Cross, & Strada, 2007). In the TLFB, the individual is prompted to indicate significant "memory anchor points" (e.g., birthdays, holidays, special events) on a calendar. The interviewee is then asked to indicate which days alcohol and illicit drug use were used on the calendar. The memory anchor points are particularly helpful for individuals with substance-induced cognitive impairments (Burgard et al., 2000). This scale has demonstrated psychometric support (Donohue et al., 2004, 2007), and has also been used to measure progress in therapy in substance-abusing and conduct-disordered adolescents recently referred to treatment by the courts, due to perpetration of criminal acts (Azrin, Donohue, Teichner, Crum, Howell, & DeCato, 2001). Thus, the TLFB is effective in delinquent youth within the juvenile justice system.

Some measures are also useful for identifying individuals at risk for substance-use disorders, including the Substance Abuse Subtle Screening Inventory-3 (SASSI; Miller, Roberts, Brooks, & Lazowski, 1997), which is widely used in judicial settings. Self-report measures like the SASSI are brief, evaluate a range of alcohol- and drug-use behaviors, often include validity scales to detect defensiveness, underreporting and deviant response styles, and use established cut-off scores to determine the level of risk for substance-use disorders. Although the SASSI and other similar measures cannot provide a comprehensive understanding of those factors that cause and maintain substance-use disorders, they are helpful in identifying individuals at risk for substance-use disorders. Also, instruments such as the SASSI do not establish the diagnosis of substance abuse or dependence, which requires further evaluation.

If it is important to establish a substance abuse or dependence diagnosis, the Structured Clinical Interview for *DSM-IV* (SCID; First, Spitzer, Gibbon, & Williams, 2002) may be used for this purpose. The SCID typically requires from 90 to 120 minutes to complete, and assesses various *DSM-IV* Axis I diagnoses. However, the substance-use disorders section can be used by itself, and completed in only 10 to 25 minutes if assessment time is limited. Once identified, measures such as the Addiction Severity Index (ASI; McLellan et al., 1992) may be used to assess the impact that substance-use disorders have on a variety of domains, such as medical status, employment status, family and social relationships, legal status, and psychiatric/psychological status.

Biological screening procedures provide an objective assessment of both alcohol and illicit drug use, and should be used whenever possible to support self- and collateral reports of substance use. For instance, hair follicle tests may be sent to laboratories for examination, and these tests typically are able to detect illicit drug use up to 3 or 4 months after use. These tests are increasingly being used in child welfare and judicial contexts, but are often cost-prohibitive. Therefore, urinalysis testing provides a cost-effective alternative, although with the exception of a small minority of drugs (e.g., marijuana, PCP), urinalysis testing procedures are able to detect substances that were used within 2 to 3 days of the test (Olmeztoprak, Donohue, & Allen, 2009). Furthermore, some drugs are detectable for only a few hours after substance use (e.g., alcohol, LSD). Despite this limitation, onsite urinalysis testing can be inexpensively accomplished using panel "dip tests" that allow immediate analysis for a variety of selected substances.

Individuals who are found to use drugs according to biological screening measures will often act surprised and deny substance use, claiming the tests are inaccurate. They may state positive tests for opiate drugs are due to ingesting poppy seeds from bagels, that positive marijuana results must have occurred from an earlier time period that was previously detected, or that marijuana was positive due to spending time in the car with others who were smoking the substance. Toxicologists are able to provide accurate detection windows, and answer questions about false negatives (i.e., testing indicates no use, although use has occurred in the recent past) and false positives (i.e., testing indicates use has occurred, although no use has occurred). They may be able to indicate that detection of opiates from poppy seeds is extremely unlikely; or that it is possible a second positive drug test may reflect drug use that occurred prior to a previous urinalysis testing if THC levels are lower in the second testing, and the second testing is within 1 or 2 weeks; or that a youth may have tested positive for marijuana without smoking marijuana, if in a car for an extended period of time with abundant amounts of marijuana being smoked. It should also be emphasized that biological screens are highly accurate (i.e., usually > 97%) if they are administered properly, substance use occurred during the appropriate detection window, and no adulterants were introduced into the specimen (e.g., water from the toilet or sink). Although some adulterants can mask detection, most are detectable. For instance, putting bleach on a finger and dipping it into the urine specimen or drinking excessive amounts of water will be indicated in testing. Some of the factors that decrease false negatives include being chronically obese, low activity levels, and heavy and chronic use of the respective substance (Olmeztoprak et al., 2009).

Biological tests for alcoholism include standard laboratory tests such as gamma-glutamyltransferase (GGT) and carbohydrate deficient transferrin (CDT), which are sensitive state indicators of heavy drinking. Liver function tests such as albumin (Alb), total bilirubin (TBIL), alanine aminotransferase (ALT), aspartate aminotransferase (AST), and alkaline phosphatase (ALP) are useful for documenting liver damage resulting from chronic and heavy alcohol use. Alcohol intoxication can also be identified through blood alcohol levels in a blood sample or by using a breathalyzer test, which can conveniently yield instant results (Allen & Holman, 2009).

Finally, review of medical records can assist in determining whether physical problems are consistent with substance use, or whether the individual has access to medications that have a high potential for abuse. Medical records may also be useful for determining the presence of comorbid psychiatric or medical disorders that may indirectly contribute to the pattern and severity of neurocognitive deficits in these patients.

Medical and Psychiatric Comorbidity

It is important to assess medical and psychiatric comorbidity in those with substance-use disorders, because these comorbid disorders often cause or contribute to the severity of neurocognitive deficits. Such evaluations may help clarify whether neurocognitive deficits are the result of the direct effects of substances on the brain, or arise from indirect effects associated with medical and psychiatric comorbidities (Allen & Knatz, 2009). The direct effects of substances on brain function result from the unique pharmacological properties of the substance. Drugs that are highly neurotoxic produce long-term deficits that are often associated with the amount of the substance used, and may not fully resolve even after long-term abstinence. During intoxication, alterations in neurocognitive function result from the direct effects (e.g., agonist or antagonist) of substances on neurotransmitter function. During withdrawal, deficits may also become evident because the chronic effects of substance use have caused up-regulation or down-regulation of various neurotransmitter systems. Neurocognitive deficits that arise as a result of these intoxication and withdrawal effects are typically transient in nature, and tend to resolve as intoxication and withdrawal symptoms resolve.

The brain can also be negatively affected through the indirect influences of substances by at least two mechanisms, and in these instances, the neurotoxic effects of the substances are not responsible for brain damage per se. First, some substances can damage organ systems other than the brain, which, in turn, compromise brain function. Hepatic encephalopathy resulting from cirrhosis of the liver, which is common in alcoholism (Tarter & Butters, 2001), is an example of this type of indirect effect. A second means by which substances can indirectly affect brain function is by causing or exacerbating neurological disorders. Possible disorders include, among others, infectious disease (e.g., human immunodeficiency virus, hepatitis), cerebrovascular accidents, traumatic brain injury (TBI) (Allen, Goldstein, Caponigro, & Donohue, 2009; Lange, Iverson, & Franzen, 2007), epileptic seizures, and disorders resulting from malnutrition (e.g., Wernicke-Korsakoff [W-K] syndrome; Victor, Adams, & Collins, 1989). These conditions may have either direct additive effects, or interactive effects on neurocognitive deficits. Recently, evidence of additive effects was reported for individuals who were both HIV seropositive and who had also been diagnosed with methamphetamine dependence, in that individuals affected by both conditions exhibited higher levels of neuropsychological impairment (Carey et al., 2006) and grey matter abnormalities as measured by magnetic resonance imaging (MRI) (Jernigan et al., 2005) than do comparable groups affected by either condition alone.

Similarly, among those diagnosed with substance-use disorders that may present in Court, the presence of comorbid mental and physical disorders are common, and often cause more severe neurocognitive impairments than the substance itself. For example, it has long been reported that substance-use disorders are highly comorbid in several psychiatric conditions such as anxiety, affective, and psychotic disorders (Alterman, 1985; B. F. Grant et al., 2004; Hubbard & Martin, 2001). Indeed, as many as 65% of individuals with schizophrenia have been diagnosed with a substance-use disorder (Cuffel, 1992; Mueser et al., 1990; Regier et al., 1990), and this comorbidity appears to have compounding and interactive effects on brain dysfunction. That is, the deficits observed in those with comorbid disorders is greater than what might be expected from the simple additive neurocognitive effects of one disorder to the other (Allen, 2004; Allen & Remy, 2000; Thoma et al., 2006), as well as causing an acceleration in age-associated cognitive decline (Allen, Goldstein, & Aldarondo, 1999; Mohamed, Bondi, Kasckow, Golshan, & Jeste, 2006). Other psychiatric disorders, such as major depressive disorder, attention-deficit/hyperactivity disorder, and various personality disorders have also been found to frequently co-occur in individuals who use substances and are incarcerated. As might be expected, the symptoms that characterize these psychiatric disorders often overlap with symptoms of substance intoxication and withdrawal, depending on the substances ingested. Thus, the causes of neurocognitive deficits that commonly occur in substance-use disorders can be quite complex, and psychiatric and medical evaluation may assist in determining those that result from the direct effects of substances on the brain, and those that are caused by other indirect mechanisms.

Neuropsychological Assessment

Neuropsychological screening instruments can be employed when it is not possible to conduct a comprehensive neuropsychological evaluation, including instruments such as the Cognistat (Kiernan, Mueller, Langston, & Van Dyke, 1987), Repeatable Battery for the Assessment of Neuropsychological Status (RBANS; Randolph, Tierney, Mohr, & Chase, 1998), and Neuropsychological Screening Battery (NSB; Heaton, Thompson, Nelson, Filley, & Franklin, 1990). These screening methods have both advantages and disadvantages. The advantages of Cognistat and RBANS include minimal training requirements, as well as brief administration time (i.e., < 30 minutes), which may be important when assessments are conducted in prisons or other forensic settings that provide only limited access to the test subject. However, neither has been extensively validated with individuals who have substance-use disorders. On the other hand, the NSB requires greater administration time, but reliably discriminates individuals with substance-use disorders from controls.

Cognistat assesses orientation, attention, language comprehension, language repetition, confrontational naming, construction, memory, calculation, verbal abstraction, and judgment. However, recent research suggests some items in this instrument may be culturally/ethnically biased, necessitating recommendations that the full Cognistat be administered when assessing substance-use disorders (Schrimsher, O'Bryant, Parker, & Burke, 2004). Performance is also influenced by age and education (Ruchinskas, Repetz, & Singer, 2001) with Construction and Memory appearing to be the most consistently impacted by age (Drane & Osato, 1997). Normative data is limited (Drane et al., 2003), which limits interpretation of Cognistat performance in the elderly and those with low levels of education.

The RBANS includes 12 subtests that allow for the assessment of immediate and delayed memory, visuospatial/constructional abilities, attention, and language. It was standardized on a nationally stratified sample of 540 adults and comes in two equivalent alternate forms, which is useful for repeated evaluations. Significant improvement in Immediate Memory and Attention were recently reported among a VA sample completing a 24-day substance-abuse treatment program (Schrimsher & Parker, 2008), although other information on its usefulness in the assessment of substance abuse is not available.

The NSB provides an assessment of attention, visual, and verbal learning and memory, psychomotor speed, language and reading comprehension, verbal fluency, and visuoconstructional ability, and is composed of a number of well-validated measures of ability including the Trail Making Test, Symbol Digit Modalities Test, Rey-Osterrieth Complex Figure, and others. It yields a total score that has been demonstrated to be sensitive to cognitive impairment in those with substance-use disorders (Fals-Stewart, 1996; Grohman & Fals-Stewart, 2004; O'Malley, Adamse, Heaton, & Gawin, 1992).

The subsequent sections focus on describing those neurocognitive deficits that are most consistently identified in substance abusers who have a history of being arrested. Alcohol is the most widely used of all substances, and its effects on brain function have received the most thorough evaluation and documentation. In addition to alcohol, this chapter focuses on cannabis, cocaine, amphetamines, opiates, benzodiazepines, and polysubstance use.

Assessment of Specific Substance-Use Disorders

As previously suggested, neurocognitive deficits that accompany substance-use disorders can be quite complex, with some being transient and others enduring in nature, and some resulting from direct effects and others from indirect effects. Furthermore, deficits resulting from the direct effects are often difficult to separate from those caused by coexisting psychiatric or medical disorders. As a result, careful consideration should be given to the selection of a battery of neuropsychological tests that are sensitive to the unique deficits associated with each substance. The following section delineates neurocognitive deficits that are specific to particular substances.

Ethanol

Ethanol, commonly referred to as "alcohol," is the most frequently used CNS depressant in the world, with as much as 90% of the United States adult population consuming alcohol at some point (American Psychiatric Association, 2000). A 2006 survey conducted by SAMSHA found that in the past month, 51% of individuals in the United States used alcohol, 23% had engaged in binge drinking (5 or more drinks on one occasion), and 7% were considered heavy drinkers (5 or more episodes of binge drinking in 1 month). Males have higher rates of problems resulting from alcohol use (60 versus 30%), and are more often diagnosed with alcohol-related disorders. Recent estimates indicate that lifetime risk for alcohol dependence is 5.4%, and alcohol abuse is 13.2% (Kessler et al., 2005). Individuals 21–25 years of age are the heaviest users, with 69% reporting use in the past month, 50% reporting at least one episode of binge drinking, and 17% classified as heavy alcohol users. Per capita consumption of alcohol in the United States is estimated to be at 2.24 gallons in 2005 (Kessler et al., 2005) (http://www.niaaa.nih. gov/Resources/GraphicsGallery/consfigs4text .htm). As indicated above, mental and physical disorders resulting from the excessive use of alcohol are also highly prevalent. Approximately 40% of the United States population will experience at least one alcohol-related accident, as much as 55% of all driving-related fatalities are associated with alcohol use, and more than 50% of all homicides are alcohol related, with either the perpetrator or the victim being intoxicated at the time of the murder.

Alcohol effects are primarily attributed to the potentiation of the action of gamma-aminobutyric acid (GABA), the major inhibitory neurotransmitter, at its receptor. Alcohol use also causes the release of dopamine indirectly through the ventral tegmental area and nucleus accumbens, and increases endorphine levels. Multiple neurocognitive deficits have been associated with alcohol abuse and dependence during intoxication, withdrawal, the acute phase of recovery (within 1 week following cessation of use), and all phases of the recovery process following cessation of use, including short-term recovery (within 5 weeks following cessation of use), and long-term recovery (13 months or more following cessation of use). Chronic excessive use can be associated with dementia and/or amnestic disorder.

Alcohol Intoxication and Withdrawal

The most common neurocognitive deficits occurring as a result of intoxication include memory (immediate and delayed), attention, executive abilities such as planning and behavioral control, and psychomotor function (Oscar-Berman & Marinkovi, 2007). Physiological symptoms include slurred speech, ataxia, incoordination, and nystagmus (involuntary eye movements), and psychological symptoms most often include mood instability.

Dramatic variation occurs in severity of alcohol-withdrawal symptoms from one individual to the next. During withdrawal, neurocognitive deficits can be severe, including deficits in intellectual functioning, memory, and visuospatial skills. Extreme cases of withdrawal can be characterized by frank delirium, often referred to as delirium tremens, during which alternations in consciousness occur. Delirium tremens is a substance-induced withdrawal delirium that can prove fatal, and requires immediate medical intervention. Common symptoms of this delirium include confusion, disorientation, anxiety and restlessness, agitation, irritability, emotional lability, depression, fatigue, heart palpitations, tachycardia, hypertension, diaphoresis, nausea and vomiting, paranoia, visual hallucinations (e.g., insects, snakes, rats, stereotypical "pink elephants"), auditory hallucinations, tactile hallucinations (sensation of something crawling on the skin), sensitivity to light, sound, and touch, fever, and seizures. This latter symptom can produce its own negative effects on neurocognitive functioning, and treatment with benzodiazepines or anti-seizure medications are typically used to decrease the likelihood of seizures during alcohol withdrawal. Therefore, it is important to carefully assess symptoms of alcohol withdrawal, particularly inmates who have been recently incarcerated. Improvements in cognitive function may be achieved by some individuals following the period of withdrawal simply due to abstinence itself, and for some, improved nutrition may contribute to recovery of cognitive function (G. Goldstein, 1987). Cognitive improvement occurs at a slower rate in older individuals, for whom improvements tend to occur within 3 to 4 weeks following cessation of use.

Neurocognitive Effects

With the cessation of alcohol use, there is marked spontaneous recovery of some neurocognitive abilities. Neuropsychological evaluation in the days immediately following cessation of use typically reveals impairment across most abilities (Pitel et al., 2007), including intelligence. As reviewed by Allen, Goldstein, and Seaton (1997), substantial spontaneous improvement occurs during the first week, with intellectual abilities often returning to normal levels. Whereas cognitive deficits do persist after the first week (Rourke & Grant, 1999; Sullivan, Rosenbloom, & Pfefferbaum, 2000), spontaneous improvement continues in the next 4 to 5 weeks, most notably in the areas of problem solving, abstraction, perceptual–motor skills, verbal memory (both short and long term), nonverbal memory (both short and long term), gait, balance, and visuospatial abilities (Schottenbauer, Momenan, Kerick, & Hommer, 2007). This improvement is particularly noticeable for individuals less than 40 years of age who have used alcohol less than 10 years (Eckardt, Stapleton, Rawlings, Davis, & Grodin, 1995). During the year following cessation of alcohol use, spontaneous recovery of function will continue to occur in those who remain abstinent, although this recovery occurs at a slower rate. Recovery also varies based on neurocognitive ability. Thus, improvements often continue to be made during this period, especially within the area of nonverbal learning and memory; these improvements, however, again depend on age, history of abuse, and any relapses of drinking (Rourke & Grant, 1999). Some neurocognitive domains that continue to remain problematic in the long term may include deficits in problem-solving skills, perceptual–motor abilities, contextual memory deficits, and visual learning and memory, particularly in older individuals (Sullivan, Shear, Zipursky, Sager, & Pfefferbaum, 1997).

Neuroimaging Findings

Neuroimaging findings using computed tomography (CT) and MRI in recently detoxified individuals have found evidence of cerebral atrophy with a reduction in tissue of both the cortex and the subcortex. Areas most susceptible to the detrimental effects of alcoholism include the cerebellum, limbic system, and frontal lobes (Oscar-Berman & Marinkovi, 2007). Similar to variances in deficits and improvements, this tissue reduction is often most severe in older individuals and in individuals with more extreme histories of abuse and/or dependence, with the more anterior regions of the brain appearing to be especially sensitive to the combined effects of aging and alcohol. Abstinence lasting at least 3 to 6 months may lead to some degree of improvement, especially in the subcortex. Finally, positron emission tomography (PET) studies have yielded evidence to suggest that neuropsychological impairment is associated with an overall decrease in the metabolism of glucose in the frontal cortex and subcortical structures.

Amnestic Disorder (Wernicke-Korsakoff Syndrome)

Another neurocognitive result of excessive alcohol use comes in the form of amnestic disorder, also known as W-K syndrome. The neurocognitive deficits associated with W-K are due to a thiamine (vitamin B1) deficiency that occurs due to poor nutrition, which is so often observed in individuals suffering from alcoholism. This deficiency leads to the occurrence of hemorrhages in the brain. Symptoms of W-K often include unsteady gait, nystagmus, ophthalmoplegia (i.e., partial or full paralysis of the eyes), and mental confusion. (Please note that these symptoms are due to the vitamin B1 deficiency, not to the presence of alcoholism per se; thus, similar symptoms may be observed in other individuals who are not abusers of alcohol or who are not alcoholics, but who may have a vitamin B1 deficiency for some other reason.) Together, this particular set of acute symptoms is known as Wernicke's encephalopathy. Interestingly, many of these symptoms can be improved upon the administration of large doses of thiamine, often within a span of 4 weeks. However, a lack of such vitamin administration may lead to coma and/or death. Many individuals who suffer from Wernicke's encephalopathy go on to develop Korsakoff's syndrome, whose most notable symptom is that of a severe memory deficit, primarily in the ability to learn new information. Other symptoms often associated with Korsakoff's syndrome include neurocognitive deficits in the domains of problem-solving skills and executive functioning, whereas retrograde memory and general levels of intelligence tend to be preserved.

Alcohol-Induced Persisting Dementia

Alcohol-induced persisting dementia is characterized by a constellation of symptoms that are the result of extensive alcohol abuse, last long after cessation of use, tend to be permanent, and often significantly interfere with day-to-day functioning. Specifically, symptoms may include neurocognitive deficits in the areas of memory, object recognition, and problem solving; preserved abilities may include language and orientation to time and place (that are not typically preserved in individuals suffering from dementia due to Alzheimer's disease).

Hepatic Encephalopathy

Approximately one third of those suffering from alcohol-use disorders also eventually suffer from cirrhosis of the liver, which may lead to hepatic encephalopathy and subsequent neurocognitive deficits. Symptoms commonly associated with hepatic encephalopathy due to alcohol use may include impaired short-term memory, hand–eye coordination, and eye tracking, as compared with individuals suffering from cirrhosis of the liver but not from alcohol-use disorders. Although some symptoms may improve following a liver transplant, memory impairment is usually permanent.

Traumatic Brain Injury

Another factor that must be considered is the increased incidence of TBI that occurs during intoxication, resulting from falls, fights, and other accidents. In fact, 35–50% of cases of TBI are alcohol related (Cowie, Brubaker, Lee, Lee, & Simons, 2005). Furthermore, 33–72% of those treated in emergency rooms have positive blood alcohol levels (Corrigan, 1995; Rimel & Jane, 1983). Some evidence suggests that those who are intoxicated at the time they sustain a TBI experience a greater degree of brain damage, as evidenced by poorer performance on neuropsychological tests after the traumatic experience. This increased impairment may simply represent pre-injury impairment associated with alcoholism, as up to one third of individuals intoxicated at the time of TBI have a diagnosis of alcohol dependence (Brismar, Engstrom, & Rydberg, 1983; O'Shanick, Scott, & Peterson, 1984). However, it may also be that the physiological mechanisms associated with alcohol intoxication, such as decreased respiration and decreased blood clotting, worsen the severity of brain damage. It is not yet clear how these mechanisms influence observed increases in neurocognitive dysfunction, or what severity of head injury is necessary in order for increased neurocognitive impairment to occur. However, there is some evidence to suggest additive impairment does not occur in cases of mild TBI (Lange et al., 2007; also see Allen et al., in press).

Cannabis

The cannabinoids are the most frequently abused illicit drugs, with smoking marijuana being the most common form of use. The lifetime prevalence rate for marijuana use in the United States is approximately 30%. Because of this, marijuana accounted for approximately 13% of all drug offenses at the state level in 1997 (Office of National Drug Control Policy, May 2005). The psychoactive agent in cannabinoids is delta-9-tetrahydrocannabinol, or THC, which is responsible for the characteristic symptoms of intoxication.

Intoxication and Withdrawal

Physiological symptoms of intoxication may include blood-shot eyes, an increased appetite, and a dry mouth. Psychological symptoms of intoxication may include impaired cognitive abilities (e.g., sensory perception, memory, and judgment), fluctuations in mood state (e.g., anxiety and/or euphoria), and psychotic symptoms (e.g., paranoia, grandiosity, and hallucinations). The *DSM-IV* does not include a diagnostic category for cannabis withdrawal, as it is uncertain whether there are withdrawal symptoms that occur with cessation of cannabis use. However, there is limited evidence that withdrawal symptoms may occur with very heavy and prolonged use. Withdrawal symptoms may be either physiological (i.e., nausea, tremor, and insomnia) or psychological (i.e., anxiety and irritability). Cannabis use is also associated with a number of negative outcomes, including poor social relationships, higher incidence of legal problems, lower employment status, poor work record, decreased motivation, apathy, affective blunting, and decreased libido.

Neurocognitive Effects

Neuropsychological deficits associated with cannabis use have been examined in relation to intoxication, short-term effects, and long-term effects. Intoxication causes cognitive deficits in the areas of problem solving, abstraction, attention, expressive and receptive language, and memory. Furthermore, neurocognitive impairments, especially in the areas of abstract reasoning and processing accuracy, may be associated with increased rates of attrition in treatment programs for marijuana-dependent individuals (Aharonovich, Brooks, Nunes, & Hasin, 2008). Following cessation of use, short-term deficits occur during the first 24 hours that include impairment in attention, executive functioning, mental calculations, immediate verbal recall, and complex reaction times (Iverson, 2003; Pope & Yurgelun-Todd, 1996). Though it appears that cannabis-use disorders do not lead to marked long-term neurocognitive deficits, subtle deficits may persist long after cessation of use in the areas of learning and memory (I. Grant, Gonzalez, Carey, Natarajan, & Wolfson, 2003). It is not clear, however, whether these deficits reflect neurological damage caused by cannabis, or whether they existed before cannabis use began.

Neuroimaging Findings

Neuroimaging studies suggest that cannabis use causes distinct functional abnormalities. Acute administration of cannabis is associated with increased regional cerebral blood flow (rCBF) in the cerebellum, which is consistent with a high concentration of cannabinoid C1 receptors in that region. Increased rCBF has also been reported in the orbitofrontal cortex, insula, and cingulate gyrus following acute intoxication (Matthew, Wilson, Coleman, Turkington, & DeGrado, 1997). Chronic users examined after short-term and long-term abstinence exhibit abnormal activation of the dorsolateral prefrontal cortex and left superior parietal cortex in response tasks requiring working memory (Jager, Kahn, Van Den Brink, Van Ree, & Ramsey, 2006; Loeber & Yurgelun-Todd, 1999). It also appears that, even after 25 days of abstinence, heavy use is associated with poorer performance on decision-making tasks accompanied by decreased activation in the left medial and orbital frontal cortex, as well as increased activation in the cerebellum (Bolla, Eldreth, Matochik, & Cadet, 2005). There is little evidence to suggest that cannabis abuse causes structural brain abnormalities.

Cocaine

Cocaine is a stimulant that is processed from the leaves of the coca plant. It is an alkaloid (benzoylmethyl ecgonine) that inhibits the reuptake of dopamine, norepinephrine, and serotonin, and thus has a powerful effect on the mesolimbic dopamine pathways, including the major reward pathways projecting from the ventral tegmental area to the nucleus accumbens. Recent estimates suggest that cocaine-related offenses account for approximately two thirds of drug-related incarcerations (Sevigny & Caulkins, 2004). Cocaine use is associated with increased risk for cerebrovascular accidents, due to its hypertensive and vasoconstrictive effects.

Intoxication and Withdrawal

Physiological effects of cocaine intoxication include tachycardia, hypertension, pupil dilation, and perspiration. Behavioral symptoms include hyperactivity, restlessness, and stereotyped behavior. Psychological symptoms commonly include euphoria, grandiosity, increased alertness, anxiety, and depression. Heavy chronic cocaine use results in physiological dependence. For those who are physiologically dependent, withdrawal can occur within hours after the cessation of use, and almost always occurs within 2 or 3 days following cessation of use. Withdrawal is often characterized by disrupted sleep, appetite, and psychomotor functioning, as well as feelings of depression, sadness, and anxiety. Although many of the symptoms abate after physiological withdrawal is complete (usually 1 to 5 days), some may last much longer, with some reporting anhedonic symptoms up to 10 weeks following cessation of heavy use.

Neuropsychological Effects

Cocaine use is associated with a number of neuropsychological and neurological abnormalities, although general intellectual functioning remains intact. These abnormalities vary in severity from one individual to the next, depending on a number of factors, including the duration and frequency of use, time since last use, and severity of withdrawal symptoms. Current use results in impaired attention, recall of verbal and visual information, and working memory (Simon, Domier, Sim, Richardson, Rawson, & Ling, 2002). Cocaine dependence is also associated with impairment in cognitive control, with more severe impairment predictive of more frequent dropout from treatment (Streeter et al., 2008). A recent quantitative review of the neuropsychological effects of cocaine use, indicated that attention, executive function, working memory, and declarative memory were the most frequently impaired following cessation of cocaine use (Jovanovski, Erb, & Zakzanis, 2005). These deficits were present after both short-term and long-term abstinence. Most of the participants in the studies examined by Jovanovski et al. were heavy users who were in various stages of remission, although many were no longer in withdrawal. Despite the presence of long-term deficits, some improvement in neurocognitive abilities occurs following cessation of use. Memory improves over the first 6 weeks of abstinence, with more gradual improvement later in recovery (6 weeks to 6 months) (Berry et al., 1993; Block, Erwin, & Ghoneim, 2002; Bolla, Funderberk, & Cadet, 2000; Di Sclafani, Tolou-Shams, Price, & Fein,

2002; Selby & Azrin, 1998; Van Gorp et al., 1999). However, it appears that little recovery occurs even after 6 months of sobriety for delayed memory, attention, executive function, or spatial processing.

Neuroimaging Findings

Much like the neuropsychological literature, neuroimaging studies suggest that the deleterious effects of cocaine use on brain function differ in relation to pattern and length of use. During cocaine intoxication, functional MRI (fMRI) indicates decreased function in the medial prefrontal cortex, amygdala, and temporal pole, as well as activation of the anterior cingulate gyrus, nucleus accumbens, hippocampal gyri, and lateral prefrontal cortex (Fein, Di Sclafani, & Meyerhoff, 2002; R. Z. Goldstein et al., 2004; Gottschalk, Beauvais, Hart, & Kosten, 2001; Holman et al., 1991). PET studies also indicate that intoxication is associated with decreased glucose metabolism throughout the brain (R. Z. Goldstein & Volkow, 2002). MRI findings report relatively consistent findings involving abnormalities in frontal and prefrontal cortices, including frontal and prefrontal gray-matter volume and cortical density reductions that include the anterior cingulate (Fein et al., 2002; Matochik, London, Eldreth, Cadet, & Bolla, 2003; O'Neill, Cardenas, & Meyerhoff, 2001), with SPECT and PET indicating reduced cerebral blood flow and glucose metabolism in these regions (e.g., Holman et al., 1991; Strickland et al., 1993; Weber et al., 1993). Abnormalities in the temporal and parietal cortices have also been identified, and altered myelin in the corpus callosum has also been identified in cocaine-dependent individuals (Moeller et al., 2007). Additionally, whereas some improvement occurs, decreased regional cerebral blood flow in the frontal lobes may persist for up to 4 months following cessation of cocaine use (Volkow et al., 1992), which is consistent with neuropsychological findings. These abnormalities appear to be related to both the dose and length of cocaine use.

Amphetamines

Amphetamines, including MDMA, are stimulant drugs with properties similar to cocaine. However, MDMA is described here independently, due to its hallucinogenic properties and differential neuropsychological effects. Sympathomimetic effects of amphetamines are generally more potent than are those resulting from cocaine use.

Intoxication and Withdrawal

Physiological effects associated with amphetamine intoxication reflect sympathetic nervous system arousal, and include increased blood pressure, heart rate, and body temperature, as well as tachycardia, cardiac arrhythmias, and pupillary dilation. As with cocaine, amphetamine use is associated with increased risk for cerebrovascular accidents, due to hypertensive and vasoconstrictive effects. Psychological symptoms of intoxication commonly include euphoria or anxiety, as well as decreased concentration, impaired judgment, and perceptual alterations. The neuropsychological effects of amphetamines have not received extensive examination; however, the limited research available indicates effects similar to those found in cocaine abuse. Primary deficits are noted in attention, executive function, and memory. Amphetamine intoxication is associated with general cognitive arousal and increased vigilance, without a corresponding improvement in cognition or memory, as well as impairment of delayed memory recall and attention (Dumont et al., 2008). Withdrawal symptoms, which generally occur within a few hours or days of amphetamine cessation, include fatigue, sleep disruption, increased appetite, and psychomotor agitation or retardation. Dysphoria and anhedonia are also common during withdrawal.

Neurocognitive Effects

During acute withdrawal, short-term deficits are noted in attention, psychomotor speed, verbal fluency, and verbal learning and memory (Kalechstien, Newton, & Green, 2003). Among individuals who are diagnosed as amphetamine-dependent, impaired verbal learning and memory, as well as impaired information-processing speed, are still present following 1 month of abstinence (Johanson et al., 2006). The noted verbal memory impairment appears to result from poor organizational strategies and limitations in general semantic relationships, and is, therefore, apparent on tasks requiring free recall, but may not be observed on recognition tasks (Woods et al., 2005). Prolonged amphetamine use is also associated with long-term neurotoxic effects. In heavy users, deficits in attention and motor abilities may persist even after 1 year of abstinence (Toomey et al., 2003).

Neuroimaging Findings

Recent evidence from PET has indicated potential nerve terminal degeneration in the striatum of methamphetamine users who had been abstinent for at least 30 days (Johanson et al., 2006). Neuroimaging studies of individuals who are methamphetamine-dependent have also indicated overall reductions in temporal lobe volume, hippocampal volumes, anterior cingulate grey matter, and prefrontal grey matter, as compared with normal controls (Bartzokis et al., 2000; Kim et al., 2006; Thompson et al., 2004). Conversely, increased volume has been noted in a number of structures, including the parietal cortex, the basal ganglia, and the nucleus accumbens, associated in each case with increased neurocognitive impairment (Jernigan et al., 2005; see also Thompson et al., 2004). The mechanisms accounting for such increases in volume are unclear, but may include astrocytosis, microgliosis, or premorbid neurodevelopmental conditions such as attention-deficit/hyperactivity disorder.

MDMA (3,4-Methylendioxymethamphetamine)

Intoxication and Withdrawal

The psychostimulant effects of MDMA (also known as "Ecstasy") are typically longer lasting than those of other amphetamines. As with other amphetamines, physiological effects of MDMA intoxication reflect sympathetic nervous system arousal. Additionally, some users (as many as 25%) experience intense negative reactions during intoxication, including severe anxiety.

Neurocognitive Effects

Various neurocognitive deficits are present directly following the cessation of MDMA use. Both occasional and chronic users exhibit impairments in verbal fluency and immediate and delayed prose recall, with acute effects lasting approximately 2 to 3 weeks (Bhattachary & Powell, 2001). MDMA use is also associated with various long-term neurocognitive deficits that are generally proportional to the amount and duration of use. In both occasional and heavy MDMA users, deficits have been found to persist up to 1 year post-abstinence (Parrot, 2001; Reneman, Booij, Majoie, van den Brink, & den Heeten, 2001). The largest neurocognitive effects appear to occur in the domains of learning and memory, particularly verbal memory (Kalechstein, de la Garza, Mahoney, Fantegrossi, & Newton, 2007). Additional deficits have been noted in the domains of executive function and planning, attention and vigilance, verbal fluency, psychomotor speed, and visual scanning. Task-switching abilities have been shown to be impaired proportionally with the level of lifetime usage, such that those having higher levels of lifetime usage demonstrate greater impairment on task-switching abilities (Dafters, 2006).

Neuroimaging Findings

Evidence for significant functional impairment following MDMA use has also been provided through neuroimaging findings (for a review, see Reneman et al., 2001). PET studies demonstrate that a single dose of MDMA increases regional cerebral blood flow in both the ventromedial and occipital cortices, the inferior temporal lobe, and the cerebellum; corresponding decreases are observed in the motor and somatosensory cortices, the temporal lobe, the cingulate cortex, the insula, and the thalamus. Chronic users evidence long-term changes in relation to neuronal pruning, as well as significant serotonergic abnormalities, with resultant changes in psychological functions such as behavior, mood, and sleep. For heavy users, global decreases in serotonin (5-HT) transporter densities are present primarily in the parieto-occipital, occipital, and sensory cortex, indicating serotonin neuronal injury. SPECT studies also demonstrate decreases in 5-HT transporter densities, as well as changes in postsynaptic 5-HT receptors indicative of down-regulation in most cortical regions, with the exception of demonstrated up-regulation in the occipital cortex. Similarly, electrophysiological evidence indicates 5-HT impairment associated with MDMA use, with greater impairment occurring with more frequent use (Croft, Klugman, Baldeweg, & Gruzelier, 2001).

Opioids

The opioid category of the *DSM-IV* includes natural (e.g., morphine), semi-synthetic (e.g., heroin), and purely synthetic (e.g., codeine and methodone) opioid agonists. Opioid-use disorders are less prevalent than are cannabis-, cocaine-, or alcohol-use disorders; however, some evidence suggests that the prevalence of heroin use is increasing. Heroin is the most frequently abused opioid, although other opioids are also commonly misused. Heroin use is associated with a number of medical, social, and psychiatric comorbidities including head trauma, poor school and/or occupational performance, and hyperactivity or attention problems.

Intoxication and Withdrawal

Opioid intoxication is characterized by significant behavioral and psychological changes. Common features include initial feelings of euphoria often followed by dysphoria, impaired judgment and attention, slurred speech, lethargy, and pupillary constriction. Some individuals experience hallucinations and delirium during opioid intoxication. Withdrawal symptoms typically occur within 24 hours following the last dose, and are characterized by feelings of anxiety, restlessness, and depression. Physical symptoms of withdrawal commonly include nausea, malaise, sweating, pupillary dilation, insomnia, and muscle aches. Most of these withdrawal symptoms peak within a few days and resolve within a week; however, some symptoms, such as dysphoria, can continue for several months following cessation of use.

Neurocognitive Effects

The neurocognitive deficits arising from opioid use have received relatively little research attention. The acute period following heroin administration is marked by impairment in attention and concentration, as well as long-term visual and verbal memory. Persisting verbal-memory deficits may be due to the activation of apoptotic pathways, and thus neuronal death, by opioids (Tramullas, Martínez-Cué, & Hurlé, 2008). Current opiod users demonstrate deficits in fine motor speed, visuospatial and visuomotor abilities, attention, verbal fluency, and memory, as well as more generalized cognitive impairment (I. Grant et al., 1978; Hill & Mikhael, 1979).

Opiod-dependent individuals who have been abstinent for relatively short periods (5–15 days) have demonstrated deficits in complex working memory, executive function, and fluid attention, as compared with controls. These effects vary with the number of days from withdrawal, and may have been due to temporary neural disruption (Rapeli et al., 2006). Extant studies have produced conflicting results with regard to the long-term effects of opiod use. The most consistently noted deficits involve executive functioning, impulse control, and nonverbal reasoning; these deficits have been found to persist for weeks to months in chronic users following opioid cessation (Lee & Pau, 2002; Pau, Lee, & Chan, 2002; Lyvers & Yakimoff, 2003). However, these results are somewhat inconsistent across studies, and such studies have not controlled for the influence of polydrug and/or alcohol use, or for comorbid psychiatric and medical disorders. Additionally, some preliminary results suggest that these deficits may resolve following 4 or more months of sustained abstinence (Gerra et al., 1998). As with other substance-use disorders, the neurocognitive deficits associated with opioid use appear to vary in relation to the duration and quantity of use.

Neuroimaging Findings

Research on the effects of opioid use on brain structure and function has produced discrepant results, which may be due to variability in imaging methods and sample selection. Although one CT study indicated no significant differences between heroin users and controls, structural MRI findings have indicated bilateral reductions in prefrontal cortex volume, with specific reductions in gray, but not white, matter (Liu, Matochik, Cadet, & London, 1998). Also, EEG findings suggest that opioid-dependent individuals experience disrupted functional connectivity, as compared with non-opioid-dependent individuals (Fingelkurts et al., 2006).

Infectious Diseases Including HIV and Hepatitis

Substances such as heroin and cocaine, which tend to be administered via intravenous injection, are associated with an increased risk of contracting infectious diseases, such as HIV and hepatitis, which can themselves cause neuropsychological impairment. Hepatitis can cause liver damage and, as in alcohol, if this damage is severe enough, it can lead to hepatic encephalopathy. For HIV, neurocognitive impairment is not restricted to dementia, but can include more subtle presentations of neurocognitive slowing, as well as neurocognitive-related motor dysfunction prior to the onset of AIDS. Individuals who are infected with HIV but are asymptomatic may also show a variable pattern of neuropsychological impairment, which can be attributed to one of two different patterns of progression that are known to occur. One involves a gradual increase in neurological dysfunction followed by an eventual presentation of AIDS dementia, whereas the other has a more sporadic course, in which there are several acute episodes of neurological disturbances that seem to remit between episodes. Although the type of asymptomatic presentation may vary, research suggests that those individuals who demonstrate impairment in any two domains of neurological functioning are more likely to experience functional difficulties in their everyday lives. Those otherwise asymptomatic individuals who demonstrate neuropsychological impairment tend to have greater difficulty in keeping and maintaining employment, and also show a decrease in driving abilities. Most importantly, they have a higher mortality rate, with those who also demonstrate a minor cognitive motor disorder having the highest mortality rate (I. Grant, Marcotte, Heaton, & the HNRC Group, 1999).

AIDS dementia is a rapidly progressive deterioration of cerebral functioning that, if left untreated, will become debilitating within 3 days to 2 months of the onset of the presenting symptoms. AIDS dementia can have a broad presentation that may include any or all of the following symptoms: general mental slowing; more obvious motor impairments, such as an altered gait, weakness, or motor-discoordination; emotional disturbances; and psychosis (Lezak, Howieson, & Loring, 2004). In the United States, however, current pharmacological treatment for AIDS has dramatically reduced the number of affected individuals who go on to develop dementia.

Benzodiazepines

Benzodiazepines are classified as sedative/hypnotics in the *DSM-IV*. These drugs are among the most widely prescribed medications in the world, and have a high potential for abuse due to their calming and sometimes euphoric effects. Due to higher prevalence rates in elderly populations of certain disorders (e.g., insomnia) that may warrant the prescription of benzodiazepines, elderly individuals receive almost 40% of all benzodiazepine prescriptions in the United States. Thus, although benzodiazepines are abused by individuals of all ages, higher rates of abuse of the drug have been found in elderly populations, as compared with other age groups. Furthermore, elderly individuals who abuse benzodiazepines have an increased risk for adverse reactions, such as delirium and confusion. It is, therefore, recommended that clinicians pay special attention to the assessment of benzodiazepine-use disorders in the elderly (for reviews, see Allen & Landis, 1997; Mort & Aparasu, 2002).

Intoxication and Withdrawal

Benzodiazepine intoxication effects include incoordination, ataxia, dysarthria, diplopia, and dizziness. Although benzodiazepines typically induce relaxation, calmness, and euphoria, feelings of depression and hostility may occur in some cases. Although chronic benzodiazepine use often leads to the development of tolerance, physiological dependence may occur after only a few days of use. Withdrawal symptoms may include irritability, anxiety, insomnia, sweating, muscle twitching or aching, concentration difficulties, depression, and derealization. Severe withdrawal symptoms such as delirium, confusion, and seizures have also been reported. It appears that the abrupt discontinuation of benzodiazepines with long half-lives (e.g., diazepam) increases the risk for seizures within 3 days of discontinuation. The discontinuance of shorter acting benzodiazepines, however, may cause more intense withdrawal symptoms.

Neuropsychological Effects

Neuropsychological deficits observed with benzodiazepine use depend upon the age of the user. Studies suggest that benzodiazepines have several acute cognitive effects on elderly individuals. Although these effects may be negligible (at least at low doses) in younger individuals, some research has demonstrated impaired episodic memory and visual perceptual abilities in young, healthy participants (Pompéia, Pradella-Hallinan, Manzano, & Bueno, 2008). Additionally, elderly individuals display cognitive impairment even at low doses, with impairments increasing as dose increases. However, these deficits appear to become less severe with chronic administration.

The half-life of the specific benzodiazepine also influences the type of neuropsychological deficits observed. Long-acting benzodiazepines are associated with multiple neurocognitive abnormalities, including impairments in immediate and delayed verbal recall, delayed visual recall, processing speed, and psychomotor functioning, as well as higher rates of intrusion errors on list-learning tasks. Short-acting benzodiazepines impair attention, as well as explicit, working, and semantic memory. Neuropsychological impairments typically subside rapidly once benzodiazepine use is discontinued. However, chronic long-term benzodiazepine users have been found to display impairment up to 6 months after discontinuation of use.

Neuroimaging Findings

Structural and functional neuroimaging studies have also been conducted with benzodiazepine users. Structural imaging (CT) studies have provided no evidence of anatomical differences between benzodiazepine users and controls. However,

PET studies suggest that regional cerebral glucose metabolism is reduced with benzodiazepine administration, and fMRI studies indicate similar decreases (Streeter et al., 1998).

Polysubstance Use

The majority of studies examining the neuropsychological effects of polysubstance use have examined individuals who meet criteria for the abuse of or dependence on more than one substance. It should be noted that this broad definition of polysubstance abuse is inconsistent with the polysubstance-dependence category of the *DSM-IV*, which, by definition, requires that no single substance meets criteria for substance dependence during a 1-year period of polysubstance use in which dependence criteria were met for substances overall. Individuals meeting dependence criteria for multiple substances would, therefore, receive multiple diagnoses of abuse and dependence, rather than a single diagnosis of polysubstance dependence, according to *DSM-IV* nomenclature.

Intoxication and Withdrawal

The intoxication and withdrawal effects of polysubstance use generally reflect the symptoms associated with the specific substances used. However, effects can be difficult to predict because they are not necessarily simply additive; interaction or potentiation effects may occur when multiple substances are used together. For example, concurrent use of benzodiazepines and alcohol produces symptoms of sedation and euphoria more intense than when either substance is used alone. Consideration of interaction effects is, therefore, essential when assessing individuals who use multiple substances.

Neurocognitive Effects

The prevalence of neurocognitive deficits is relatively high among polysubstance users; up to 50% of current users demonstrate deficits (I. Grant et al., 1978; I. Grant & Judd, 1976). The pattern of deficits, however, varies widely, depending on the specific substances used. The types of neurocognitive deficits observed in polysubstance users also vary with comorbid medical and psychiatric factors, which are often uniquely associated with particular substances (Carey et al., 2006). The most consistent general pattern of deficits associated with polysubstance use includes impairments in verbal and visual memory, motor ability, perceptual motor skills, visuospatial abilities, and problem-solving skills.

Neuroimaging Findings

As with intoxication and withdrawal effects and associated neuropsychological deficits, the structural and functional abnormalities associated with polysubstance use vary as a function of the individual substances used. Studies examining neurological effects of polysubstance use have, therefore, resulted in variable findings in regards to the range of brain structures implicated and the level of impairment, which has ranged from severe to benign. It should be noted that the combination of various substances may result in interactive effects to impairment. A frequently studied example is the common combination of cocaine and alcohol. Laboratory studies with animals and humans have identified a metabolite of cocaine derived from ethanol (cocaethylene), leading some to hypothesize that the combined effects of the two drugs would cause greater impairment than the use of either substance alone (e.g., McCance-Katz, Kosten, & Jatlow, 1994). This hypothesis has received equivocal support; some studies have shown greater neurocognitive impairment associated with cocaine–alcohol comorbidity (Bolla et al., 2000), but most have found no effect (e.g., Lawton-Craddock, Nixon, & Tivis, 2003), and still others have suggested better neurocognitive abilities in comorbid groups, compared with those with cocaine dependence alone (e.g., Robinson, Heaton, & O'Malley, 1999). The latter finding has been postulated to be due to alcohol's reduction of platelet aggregation, which may actually reduce the likelihood of cocaine-related cerebral vascular accidents (e.g., Robinson et al.), a common cause of neurocognitive dysfunction. Given this and other similar considerations, readers are encouraged to consult other sections of this chapter and additional resources to estimate the types of abnormalities that may occur in polysubstance use, based on the combination of specific substances.

Neurocognitive Deficits, Rehabilitation, and Recidivism

Researchers have become increasingly interested in the effects of neurocognitive deficits on the treatment of alcohol- and drug-use disorders (Aharonovich et al., 2006; Allen et al., 1997), given that the presence of neurocognitive deficits may interfere with treatment response. For instance, individuals who are cocaine-dependent and exhibit neurocognitive deficits have lower retention rates in substance-abuse treatment (Aharonovich et al.). Burgard et al. (2000) noted that standardized treatments were relatively ineffective with cognitively impaired individuals in a controlled treatment outcome study; in contrast to substance abusers who did not evidence cognitive impairments, the approximately one-dozen participants who were identified to be cognitively impaired or functioning in the Borderline range of intellectual functioning rarely completed treatment, and none achieved abstinence. Treatment response may also be mediated by the type of neurocognitive deficits present (and thereby differ, based upon the types of substances abused). For example, deficits in executive function may hinder the application of problem-solving strategies that have been indicated to: (a) assist substance abusers from acting upon their urges to use drugs, (b) curb derogatory comments when angry, and (c) resist temptations to be truant or absent from work or school (e.g., Azrin et al., 2001). Memory deficits have been associated with difficulties in learning and retaining psychoeducational information, rationales for treatment, logic and rule-governed behavior involved in cognitive therapies, and appreciation of consequences involved in contingency management strategies (see Burgard et al.). Despite such findings, the relationship between neurocognitive deficits and treatment outcome is complex. Neurocognitive impairment likely exerts both mediating and moderating effects, depending on the outcome domains, risk factors, and neurocognitive abilities under consideration (Bates, Bowden, &

Barry, 2002). Due to the varied effects of neurocognitive deficits upon the treatment of substance and alcohol abuse, neuropsychologists should consider the type and severity of such deficits when planning treatment for a given individual. When deficits are present, cognitive rehabilitation procedures may increase treatment efficacy by remediating associated impairment. Specific suggestions for the remediation of substance-induced deficits were provided by Bates and colleagues.

In addition to these effects on treatment outcome, substance-related cognitive impairment is also related to rates of recidivism. There have been two large-scale studies overseen by the Bureau of Justice Statistics (Beck & Shipley, 1989; Lanagan & Levin, 2002). The two studies documented recidivism rates for half (Beck & Shipley) to two thirds (Lanagan & Levin) of the individuals released from prison during that year. Beck and Shipley reported that, of the prisoners who were followed, 63% were rearrested within 3 years, 47% were reconvicted, and 41% were resentenced. In regards to substance use, 14% of the rearrests were for drug-related offenses. Moreover, of those who had been released following incarceration for a drug-related offense, 50% were rearrested, and 25% were rearrested for another drug-related offense. Similarly, Lanagan and Levin reported that, of those prisoners followed, 68% were rearrested within 3 years, 47% were convicted for a new crime, and 25% were sentenced to prison for a new crime. Regarding drug-related offenses, 30% of the rearrests were for drug-related offenses. Furthermore, of those who had been released following incarceration for a drug-related offense, 67% were rearrested, and 41% were rearrested for another drug-related offense. Substance use appears to increase rates of recidivism.

As might be expected, research has demonstrated an increased risk of recidivism in substance users who have demonstrated significant levels of cognitive impairment. Specifically, Ouimet and colleagues (Ouimet et al., 2007) found that at least two thirds of a group of individuals who had been convicted of at least two DUI charges demonstrated significant cognitive impairment in at least one area, with the majority of the participants demonstrating impairment in the areas of visuospatial construction abilities and visual memory. Furthermore, the investigators posed that such cognitive impairments and recidivism may be more strongly related to excessive alcohol use than to exposure to alcohol and head trauma, and that the demonstrated cognitive impairments may be common in DUI recidivists (Ouimet et al.). Additional research is needed that examines the interaction between type of offense, the substance associated with the offense, and patterns of neurocognitive deficits and sparing, before more definitive conclusions can be reached regarding the role of cognitive impairment in recidivism.

Case Examples

Given the ever-increasing number of individuals who are arrested and incarcerated for alcohol- and drug-related offenses, it is becoming more common for neuropsychologists who practice in forensic settings to evaluate cognitive deficits that are thought to be associated with substance use. Forensic neuropsychological evaluations may play a critical role in determining the disposition of substance abusers who present in judicial settings. The following brief vignettes may be of assistance in gaining an appreciation of some of the complexities of these cases.

Case Example: John

John is a 14-year-old Caucasian arrested for possession of marijuana while on school property. He had a 2-year history of "huffing" glue and inhaling various publicly available aerosol sprays. A few weeks before he was arrested, he broke his arm after falling off the roof of his girlfriend's house subsequent to inhaling Freon from the roof-mounted air conditioner. Hospital records indicated that this accident also resulted in a minor concussion. He presented to the judge with flat affect, and it often took him several seconds to respond to the judge's queries. His mother pleaded for the judge to consider inpatient treatment in lieu of incarceration, due to his having never been arrested. She indicated that she was unable to get him to complete two outpatient treatment programs, and thought a locked psychiatric hospital would provide him the structured environment he needed. Given his apparent difficulty in comprehending verbally presented information and slowed information processing, a neuropsychological evaluation was requested. Results indicated that John did indeed have significant verbal comprehension deficits, slowed information-processing speed, and deficits in executive function and attention. Because the evaluation was conducted several weeks after the initial charges were brought, it was suggested that some improvement in these abilities might occur. It was also suggested that these deficits should be considered in the treatment-planning process, as they would no doubt interfere with John's ability to benefit from treatment.

Case Example: Shaniqua

Shaniqua is a 40-year-old African American residing in a state penitentiary for the past 2 years due to possession of MDMA, who is eligible for parole. She had a 6-year history of abusing "crack" cocaine. During the time of this addiction, she reportedly used alcohol soon after the effects of her cocaine use "wore off" in order to avoid headaches and depressed feelings. She also had a history of being assaulted by several boyfriends, and four of these incidents resulted in her being hospitalized for physical injuries, including head injuries. On one occasion, after being assaulted by her boyfriend, she was found by her neighbor unconscious with a laceration in the left temporal region. She was transported to the hospital, where she regained consciousness after 2 days. She is the oldest of six children, and had completed 9 years of education prior to dropping out of school in order to work to support her family, and assist her mother in caretaking of her younger siblings. At her parole hearing, she provided a convincing argument to the parole board that she had not used any substances during her time in prison. She reported that she had received secretarial training in prison after passing her high school equivalency examination, and was ready to pursue gainful employment. She had no history of substance-abuse treatment. The Parole Board recommended an educational/neuropsychological examination given her history of TBI and substance use, to determine whether she was, in fact, capable of functioning independently and holding gainful employment. Neuropsychological evaluation revealed scores that were generally lower than the normative sample mean for a number of the tests, but these were deemed to be consistent with her level of education. Additionally, some evidence for mild impairment in verbal memory was present, which was attributed to TBI. Finally, given discrepancies between achievement and IQ test performance, a diagnosis of pre-existing verbal learning disability was made. Although these deficits were not considered severe enough to interfere with her ability to live independently, recommendation was made for additional assistance in securing and maintaining employment.

Concluding Remarks

The social and monetary costs associated with substance disorders are extremely high, relative to other disorders. Substance abuse and dependence are grossly overrepresented in forensic populations, relative to other *DSM-IV-TR* Axis I disorders. These disorders are notorious for diminishing treatment outcomes, increasing arrest and recidivism rates, and often resulting in both acute and long-term neuropsychological deficits that ultimately may influence forensic recommendations. Science has greatly enhanced our understanding of the patterns of neuropsychological deficits associated with substance use, abuse, and dependence. The corpus of research literature available for neurocognitive and neuroimaging research in substance abuse is centered on isolating specific brain structures associated with corresponding functional abnormalities and neurocognitive deficits. Although study results suggest associated deficits in cognition and behavior exist in substance abusers, the extent and manner by which substance use contributes to these problems is often unclear in clinical settings. However, it is quite clear that neurocognitive deficits in substance abusers can be attributed to multiple complicated factors that necessitate a multi-method approach to neuropsychological assessment, that includes evaluation of physical, psychiatric, and psychosocial functioning. Relevant to rehabilitation, there is some support to suggest substance-abusing individuals with neurocognitive deficits evidence poor attendance and outcomes in substance-abuse treatment programs, relative to those without such deficits. Indeed, treatment programs may need to be modified to manage cognitive deficits, such as avoiding complicated treatment rationales and cognitive therapies, and using stimulus-control strategies in which the environment is adjusted to facilitate opportunities to engage in non-drug associated activities, and inhibit time spent in drug-associated activities. Moreover, treatment outcome studies should begin to administer neuropsychological batteries to assist in determining which, if any, neuropsychological deficits compromise treatment outcomes and contribute to increased rates of arrest, incarceration, and recidivism.

Acknowledgment

This work was partially supported by funding from NIDA (grant number DA020548-01A1).

References

Abracen, J., Looman, J., Di Fazio, R., Kelly, T., & Stirpe, T. (2006). Patterns of attachment and alcohol abuse in sexual and violent non-sexual offenders. *Journal of Sexual Aggression, 12*, 19–30.

Aharonovich, E., Brooks, A. C., Nunes, E. V., & Hasin, D. S. (2008). Cognitive deficits in marijuana users: Effects on motivational enhancement therapy plus cognitive behavioral therapy treatment outcome. *Drug and Alcohol Dependence, 95*, 279–283.

Aharonovich, E., Hasin, D. S., Brooks, A. C., Liu, X., Bisaga, A., & Nunes, E. V. (2006). Cognitive deficits predict low treatment retention in cocaine dependent patients. *Drug and Alcohol Dependence, 81*, 313–322.

Allen, D. N. (2004). Substance abuse and schizophrenia [Abstract]. *Clinical Neuropsychologist, 18*, 162.

Allen, D. N., Goldstein, G., & Aldarondo, F. (1999). Neurocognitive dysfunction in patients diagnosed with schizophrenia and alcoholism. *Neuropsychology, 13*, 62–68.

Allen, D. N., Goldstein, G., Caponigro, J. M., & Donohue, B. (2009). The effects of alcoholism comorbidity on neurocognitive function following traumatic brain injury (TBI). *Applied Neuropsychology, 16*(3), 186–192.

Allen, D. N., Goldstein, G., & Seaton, B. E. (1997). Cognitive rehabilitation of chronic alcohol abusers. *Neuropsychology Review, 7*, 21–39.

Allen, D. N., & Holman, C. (2009). Alcohol testing. In G. L. Fisher & N. A. Roget (Eds.), *Encyclopedia of substance abuse prevention, treatment, and recovery* (pp. 56–62). Thousand Oaks, CA: Sage.

Allen, D. N., & Knatz, D. (2009). Neurocognitive effects of alcohol and other drugs. In G. L. Fisher & N. A. Roget (Eds.), *Encyclopedia of substance abuse prevention, treatment, and recovery* (pp. 639–646). Thousand Oaks, CA: Sage.

Allen, D. N., & Landis, R. K. B. (1997). Substance abuse in elderly individuals. In P. D. Nussbaum (Ed.), *Handbook of neuropsychology and aging* (pp. 111–137). New York: Plenum.

Allen, D. N., & Remy, C. J. (2000). Neuropsychological deficits in patients with schizophrenia and alcohol dependence [Abstract]. *Archives of Clinical Neuropsychology, 15*, 762–763.

Alterman, A. (Ed.). (1985). *Substance abuse and psychopathology.* New York: Plenum.

American Psychiatric Association. (2000). *Diagnostic and statistical manual of mental disorders* (4th ed., text rev.). Washington, DC: American Psychiatric Press.

Arrestee Drug Abuse Monitoring Program. (2003). *2000 arrestee drug abuse monitoring: Annual report* (research report, NCJ 193013). Washington, DC: U.S. Department of Justice, National Institute of Justice.

Azrin, N. H., Donohue, B., Teichner, G., Crum, T., Howell, J., & DeCato, L. (2001). A controlled evaluation and description of individual-cognitive problem solving and family-behavioral therapies in conduct-disordered and substance dependent youth. *Journal of Child and Adolescent Substance Abuse, 11*, 1–43.

Bartzokis, G., Beckson, M., Lu, P. H., Edwards, N., Rapoport, R., Wiseman, E., & Bridge, P. (2000). Age-related brain volume reductions in amphetamine and cocaine addicts and normal controls: Implications for addiction research. *Psychiatry Research: Neuroimaging, 98*, 93–102.

Bates, M. E., Bowden, S. C., & Barry, D. (2002). Neurocognitive impairment associated with alcohol use disorders: Implications for treatment. *Experimental and Clinical Psychopharmacology, 10*, 193–212.

Beck, A. J., & Shipley, B. E. (1989). *Bureau of Justice Statistics special report: Recidivism of prisoners released in 1983.* Washington, DC: Bureau of Justice Statistics (Publication No. NCJ-116261).

Berry, J., van Gorp, W. G., Herzberg, D. S., Hinkin, C., Boone, K., Steinman, L., & Wilkins, J. N. (1993). Neuropsychological deficits in abstinent cocaine abusers: Preliminary findings after two weeks of abstinence. *Drug & Alcohol Dependence, 32*, 231–237.

Bhattachary, S., & Powell, J. H. (2001). Recreational use of 3,4 methylenedioxymethamphetamine (MDMA) or 'ecstasy': Evidence for cognitive impairment. *Psychological Medicine, 31*, 647–658.

Block, R. I., Erwin, W. J., & Ghoneim, M. M. (2002). Chronic drug use and cognitive impairments. *Pharmacology, Biochemistry, and Behavior, 73*, 491–504.

Bolla, K. I., Eldreth, D. A., Matochik, J. A., & Cadet, J. L. (2005). Neural substrates of faulty decision-making in abstinent marijuana users. *Neuroimage, 26*, 480–492.

Bolla, K. I., Funderberk, F. R., & Cadet, J. L. (2000). Differential effects of cocaine and cocaine and alcohol on neurocognitive performance. *Neurology, 54*, 2285–2299.

Brismar, B., Engstrom, A., & Rydberg, U. (1983). Head injury and intoxication: A diagnostic and therapeutic dilemma. *Acta Chirugica Scandinavica, 149*(1), 11–14.

Buck, J. A., & Mark, T. L. (2006). State-administered spending on mental health services by type of service. *Psychiatric Services, 56*, 29.

Burgard, J., Donohue, B., Azrin, N. H., & Teichner, G. (2000). Prevalence and treatment of substance abuse in the mentally retarded population: An empirical review. *Journal of Psychoactive Drugs, 32,* 293–298.

California Department of Alcohol & Drug Programs. (2004). *Fact sheet: Driving under-the-influence (DUI) statistics.* Retrieved January 21, 2008, from www.adp.ca.gov

Campbell, K. M., Deck, D., & Krupski, A. (2007). Impact of substance abuse treatment on arrests among opiate users in Washington state. *American Journal on Addictions, 16,* 510–520.

Carey, C. L., Woods, S. P., Rippeth, J. D., Gonzalez, R., Heaton, R. K., Grant, I., & HIV Neurobehavioral Research Center (HNRC) Group (2006). Additive deleterious effects of methamphetamine dependence and immunosuppression on neuropsychological functioning in HIV infection. *AIDS and Behavior, 10,* 185–190.

Caulkins, J. P., & Chandler, S. (2006). Long-run trends in incarceration of drug offenders in the United States. *Crime & Delinquency, 52*(4), 619–641.

Chase, K. A., O'Farrell, T. J., Murphy, C. M., Fals-Stewart, W., & Murphy, M. (2003). Factors associated with partner violence among female alcoholic patients and their male partners. *Journal of Studies on Alcohol, 64,* 137–149.

Coker, A. L., Smith, P. H., McKeown, R. E., & King, M. J. (2000). Frequency and correlates of intimate partner violence by type: Physical, sexual, and psychological battering. *American Journal of Public Health, 90,* 553–559.

Corrigan, J. (1995). Substance abuse as a mediating factor in outcome from traumatic brain injury. *Archives of Physical Medicine and Rehabilitation, 76*(4), 302–309.

Cowie, S. E., Brubaker, J. R., Lee, D., Lee, R., & Simons, R. (2005) Documentation of substance abuse problems on Canadian trauma patients (abstract). *Journal of Trauma, 59*(2), 546

Croft, R. J., Klugman, A., Baldeweg, T., & Gruzelier, J. H. (2001). Electrophysiological evidence of serotonergic impairment in long-term MDMA ("ecstasy") users. *American Journal of Psychiatry, 158,* 1687–1689.

Cuffel, B. J. (1992). Prevalence estimates of substance abuse in schizophrenia and their correlates. *Journal of Nervous and Mental Disease, 180,* 589–592.

Dafters, R. I. (2006). Chronic ecstasy (MDMA) use is associated with deficits in task-switching but not inhibition of memory updating executive functions. *Drug and Alcohol Dependence, 83,* 181–184.

Di Sclafani, V., Tolou-Shams, M., Price, L. J., & Fein, G. (2002). Neuropsychological performance of individuals dependent on crack-cocaine or crack-cocaine and alcohol at six weeks and six months abstinence. *Drug and Alcohol Dependence, 66,* 161–171.

Donohue, B., Azrin, N. H., Strada, M. J., Silver, N. C., Teichner, G., & Murphy, H. (2004). Psychometric evaluation of self- and collateral timeline follow-back reports of drug and alcohol use in a sample of drug-abusing and conduct-disordered adolescents and their parents. *Psychology of Addictive Behaviors, 18,* 184–189.

Donohue, B., Hill, H. H., Azrin, N. H., Cross, C., & Strada, M. J. (2007). Psychometric support for contemporaneous and retrospective youth and parent reports of adolescent marijuana use frequency in an adolescent outpatient treatment population. *Addictive Behaviors, 32,* 1787–1797.

Dumont, G. J. H., Wezenberg, E., Valkenberg, M. M. G. J., de Jong, C. A. J., Buitelaar, J. K., van Gerven, J. M. A., et al. (2008). Acute neuropsychological effects of MDMA and ethanol (co-) administration in healthy volunteers. *Psychopharmacology, 197,* 465–474.

Drane, D. L., & Osato, S. S. (1997). Using the neurobehavioral cognitive status examination as a screening measure for older adults. *Archives of Clinical Neuropsychology, 12*(2), 139–143.

Drane, D. L., Yuspeh, R. L., Huthwaite, J. S., Klingler, L. K., Foster, L. M., Mrazik, M., & Axelrod, B. N. (2003). Healthy older adult performance on modified version of the Cognistat (NCSE): Demographic issues and preliminary normative data. *Journal of Clinical and Experimental Neuropsychology, 25*(1), 133–144.

Eckardt, M. J., Stapleton, J. M., Rawlings, R. R., Davis, E. Z., & Grodin, D. M. (1995). Neuropsychological functioning in detoxified alcoholics between 18 and 35 years of age. *American Journal of Psychiatry, 152,* 53–59.

Elliott, K., & Shelley, K. (2006). Effects of drugs and alcohol on behavior, job performance, and workplace safety. *Journal of Employment Counseling, 43,* 130–134.

Erkiran, M., Özünalan, H., Evren, C., Aytaçlar, S., Kirisci, L., & Tarter, R. (2006). Substance abuse amplifies the risk for violence in schizophrenia spectrum disorder. *Addictive Behaviors, 31,* 1797–1805.

Fals-Stewart, W. (1996). Intermediate length neuropsychological screening of impairment among psychoactive substance-abusing patients: A comparison of two batteries. *Journal of Substance Abuse, 8*(1), 1–17.

Fazel, S., Bains, P., & Doll, H. (2006). Substance abuse and dependence in prisoners: A systematic review. *Addiction, 10,* 181–191.

Fein, G., Di Sclafani, V., & Meyerhoff, D. J. (2002). Prefrontal cortical volume reduction associated with frontal cortex function deficit in 6-week abstinent crack-cocaine dependent men. *Drug and Alcohol Dependence, 68,* 87–93.

Fingelkurts, A. A., Kivisaari, R., Autti, T., Borisov, S., Puuskari, V., Jokela, O., & Khkönen, S. (2006). Increased local and decreased remote functional connectivity at EEG alpha and beta frequency bands in opioid-dependent patients. *Psychopharmacology, 188,* 42–52.

First, M. B., Spitzer, R. L., Gibbon, M., & Williams, J. B. W. (2002). *Structured clinical interview for DSM-IV-TR Axis I disorders, research version, patient edition (SCID-I/P).* New York: Biometrics Research, New York State Psychiatric Institute.

Gerra, G., Calbiani, B., Zaimovic, A., Sartori, R., Ugolotti, G., Ippolito, L., et al. (1998). Regional cerebral blood flow and comorbid diagnosis in abstinent opioid addicts. *Psychiatry Research: Neuroimaging, 83,* 117–126.

Golding, J. M. (1999). Intimate partner violence as a risk factor for mental disorders: A meta-analysis. *Journal of Family Violence, 14,* 99–132.

Goldstein, G. (1987). Recovery, treatment, and rehabilitation in chronic alcoholics. In O. A. Parsons, N. Butters, & P. E. Nathan (Eds.), *Neuropsychology of alcoholism: Implications for diagnosis and treatment* (pp. 361–377). New York: Guilford Press.

Goldstein, R. Z., Leskovjan, A. C., Hoff, A. L., Hitzemann, R., Bashan, F., Khalsa, S. S., et al. (2004). Severity of neuropsychological impairment in cocaine and alcohol addiction: Association with metabolism in the prefrontal cortex. *Neuropsychologia, 42,* 1447–1458.

Goldstein, R. Z., & Volkow, N. D. (2002). Drug addiction and its underlying neurological basis: Neuroimaging evidence for the involvement of the frontal cortex. *American Journal of Psychiatry, 159,* 1642–1652.

Gottschalk, C., Beauvais, J., Hart, R., & Kosten, T. (2001). Cognitive function and cerebral perfusion during cocaine abstinence. *American Journal of Psychiatry, 158,* 540–545.

Grant, B. F., Compton, W. M., Crowley, T. J., Hasin, D. S., Helzer, J. E., Li, T., et al. (2007). Errors in assessing DSM-IV substance use disorders. *Archives of General Psychiatry, 64*(3), 379–380.

Grant, B. F., Stinson, F. S., Dawson, D. A., Chou, S. P., Dufour, M. C., Compton, W., Pickering, R. P., et al. (2004). Prevalence and co-occurrence of substance use disorders and independent mood and anxiety disorders: Results from the national epidemiologic survey on alcohol and related conditions. *Archives of General Psychiatry, 61,* 807–816.

Grant, I., Adams, K. M., Carlin, A. S., Rennick, P. M., Judd, L. L., & Schoof, K. (1978). The collaborative neuropsychological study of polydrug users. *Archives of General Psychiatry, 35,* 1063–1074.

Grant, I., Gonzalez, R., Carey, C. L., Natarajan, L., & Wolfson, T. (2003). Non-acute (residual) neurocognitive effects of cannabis use: A meta-analytic study. *Journal of the International Neuropsychological Society, 9,* 679–689.

Grant, I., & Judd, L. (1976). Neuropsychological and EEG disturbances in polydrug users. *American Journal of Psychiatry, 133,* 1039–1042.

Grant, I., Marcotte, T. D., Heaton, R. K., & HIV Neurobehavioral Research Center Group. (1999). Neurocognitive complications of HIV disease. *Psychological Science, 10,* 191–195.

Grohman, K., & Fals-Stewart, W. (2004). The detection of cognitive impairment among substance-abusing patients: The accuracy of the neuropsychological assessment battery-screening module. *Experimental and Clinical Psychopharmacology, 12*(3), 200–207.

Heaton, R. K., Thompson, L. L., Nelson, L. M., Filley, C. M., & Franklin, G. M. (1990). Brief and intermediate length screening of neuropsychological impairment in multiple sclerosis. In S. M. Rao (Ed.), *Multiple sclerosis: A neuropsychological perspective* (pp. 149–160). New York: Oxford University Press.

Hill, S. Y., & Mikhael, M. A. (1979). Computerized transaxial tomographic and neuropsychological evaluations in chronic alcoholics and heroin abusers. *American Journal of Psychiatry, 36,* 598–602.

Holman, B. L., Carvalho, P. A., Mendelson, J., Teoh, S. K., Nardin, R., Hallgring, E., et al. (1991). Brain perfusion is abnormal in cocaine-dependent polydrug users: A study using technetium-99m-HMPAO and ASPECT. *Journal of Nuclear Medicine, 32,* 1206–1210.

Holtzworth-Munroe, A., Meehan, J. C., Herron, K., Rehman, U., & Stuart, G. L. (2000). Testing the Holtzworth-Munroe and Stuart (1994) batterer typology. *Journal of Consulting and Clinical Psychology, 68,* 1000–1019.

Hubbard, J. R., & Martin, P. R. (Eds.). (2001). *Substance abuse in the mentally and physically disabled.* New York: Marcel Dekker.

Iverson, L. (2003). Cannabis and the brain. *Brain, 126,* 1252–1270.

Jager, G., Kahn, R. S., Van Den Brink, W., Van Ree, J. M., & Ramsey, N. F. (2006). Long-term effects of frequent cannabis use on working memory and attention: An fMRI study. *Psychopharmacology (Berl), 185,* 358–368.

Jaudes, P. K., Ekwo, E., & Van Voorhis, J. (1995). Association of drug abuse and child abuse. *Child Abuse & Neglect, 19,* 1065–1075.

Jernigan, T. L., Gamst, A. C., Archibald, S. L., Fennema-Notestine, C., Mindt, M. R., Marcotte, T. D., et al. (2005). Effects of methamphetamine dependence and HIV infection on cerebral morphology. *American Journal of Psychiatry, 162,* 1461–1472.

Johanson, C., Frey, K. A., Lundahl, L. H., Keenan, P., Lockhart, N., Roll, J., et al. (2006). Cognitive function and nigrostriatal markers in abstinent methamphetamine abusers. *Psychopharmacology, 185,* 327–338.

Jovanovski, D., Erb, S., & Zakzanis, K. K. (2005). Neurocognitive deficits in cocaine users: A quantitative review of the evidence. *Journal of Clinical and Experimental Neuropsychology, 27,* 189–204.

Kalechstein, A. D., de la Garza, R., II, Mahoney, J. J., III, Fantegrossi, W. E., & Newton, T. F. (2007). MDMA use and neurocognition: A meta-analytic review. *Psychopharmacology, 189,* 531–537.

Kalechstein, A. D., Newton, T. F., & Green, M. (2003). Methamphetamine dependence is associated with neurocognitive impairment in the initial phases of abstinence. *Journal of Neuropsychiatry and Clinical Neuroscience, 15,* 215–220.

Kessler, R. C., Berglund, P., Demler, O., Jin, R., Merikangas, K. R., & Walters, E. E. (2005). Lifetime prevalence and age-of-onset distributions of DSM-IV disorders in the national comorbidity survey replication. *Archives of General Psychiatry, 62,* 593–602.

Kiernan, R. J., Mueller, J., Langston, J. W., & Van Dyke, C. (1987). The neurobehavioral cognitive status examination. *Annals of Internal Medicine, 107,* 481–485.

Kim, S. J., Lyoo, I. K., Hwang, J., Chung, A., Sung, Y. H., Kim, J., et al. (2006). Prefrontal grey-matter changes in short-term and long-term abstinent methamphetamine abusers. *International Journal of Neuropsychopharmacology, 9,* 221–228.

Lanagan, P. A., & Levin, D. J. (2002). *Bureau of Justice Statistics special report: Recidivism of prisoners released in 1994.* Washington, DC: Bureau of Justice Statistics (Publication No. NCJ-193427).

Landry, M. J. (2002). MDMA: A review of epidemiologic data. *Journal of Psychoactive Drugs, 34,* 163–169.

Lange, R. T., Iverson, G. L., & Franzen, M. D. (2007). Short term neuropsychological outcome following uncomplicated mild TBI: Effects of day-of-injury intoxication and pre-injury alcohol abuse. *Neuropsychology, 21,* 590–598.

Lawton-Craddock, A., Nixon, S. J., & Tivis, R. (2003). Cognitive efficiency in stimulant abusers with and without alcohol dependence. *Alcoholism: Clinical and Experimental Research, 27,* 457–464.

Lee, T. M. C., & Pau, C. W. H. (2002). Impulse control differences between abstinent heroin users and matched controls. *Brain Injury, 16,* 885–889.

Lezak, M. D., Howieson, D. B., & Loring, D. W. (with Hanay, H. J., & Fischer, J. S.). (2004). *Neuropsychological assessment* (4th ed.). New York: Oxford Press.

Liu, X., Matochik, J. A., Cadet, J. L., & London, E. D. (1998). Smaller volumes of prefrontal lobe in polysubstance abusers: A magnetic resonance imaging study. *Neuropsychopharmacology, 18,* 243–252.

Locke, T. F., & Newcomb, M. D. (2003). Childhood maltreatment, parental alcohol/drug-related problems, and global parental dysfunction. *Professional Psychology: Research and Practice, 34,* 73–79.

Loeber, R., & Yurgelun-Todd, D. A. (1999) Human neuroimaging of acute and chronic marijuana use: Implications for frontocerebellar dysfunction. *Human Psychopharmacology; Clinical and Experimental, 14*(5), 291–304.

Logan, T. K., Walker, R., & Leukefeld, C. G. (2001). Intimate partner and nonintimate violence history among drug-using, incarcerated men. *International Journal of Offender Therapy and Comparative Criminology, 45,* 228–243.

Lyvers, M., & Yakimoff, M. (2003). Neuropsychological correlates of opioid dependence and withdrawal. *Addictive Behaviors, 28,* 605–611.

Mathew, R. J., Wilson, W. H., Coleman, R. E., Turkington, T. G., & DeGrado, T. R. (1997). Marijuana intoxification and brain activation in marijuana smokers. *Life Science, 60,* 2075–2089.

Matochik, J. A., London, E. D., Eldreth, D. A., Cadet, J. L., & Bolla, K. I. (2003). Frontal cortical tissue composition in abstinent cocaine abusers: A magnetic resonance imaging study. *Neuroimage, 19,* 1095–1102.

McCance-Katz, E. F., Kosten, T. R., & Jatlow, P. (1994). Concurrent use of cocaine and alcohol is more potent and potentially more toxic than use of either alone—A multiple-dose study. *Biological Psychiatry, 44,* 250–259.

McDermott, B. E., Quanbeck, C. D., & Frye, M. A. (2007). Comorbid substance use disorder in women with bipolar disorder associated with criminal arrest. *Bipolar Disorders, 9*, 536–540.

McKetin, R., & Mattick, R. P. (1997). Attention and memory in illicit amphetamine users. *Drug and Alcohol Dependence, 50*, 181–184.

McLellan, A. T., Kushner, H., Metzger, D., Peters, R., Smith, I., Grissom, G., et al. (1992). The fifth edition of the addiction severity index. *Journal of Substance Abuse Treatment, 9*, 199–213.

McLellan, A. T., Luborski, L., Cacciula, J., Griffith, J., McGahan, P. & O'Brien, C. P. (1985). *Guide to the Addiction Severity Index: Background, administration and field testing results* (National Institute on Drug Abuse Treatment Research Report, DHHS Pub. No. (ADM) 85-1419). Washington, DC: Sup. of Docs. U.S. Government. Printing Office.

Mericle, A. A., & Havassy, B. E. (2008). Characteristics of recent violence among entrants to acute mental health and substance abuse services. *Social Psychiatry and Psychiatric Epidemiology, 42*, 392–402.

Miller, F. G., Roberts, J., Brooks, M. K., & Lazowski, L. E. (1997). *SASSI-3: A quick reference guide for administration and scoring.* Bloomington, IN: Baugh Enterprises.

Miller, N. S., Belkin, B. M., & Gold, M. S. (1991). Alcohol and drug dependence among the elderly: Epidemiology, diagnosis, and treatment. *Comprehensive Psychiatry, 32*, 153–165.

Moeller, F. G., Hasan, K. M., Steinberg, J. L., Kramer, L. A., Valdes, I., Lai, L. Y., et al. (2007). Diffusion tensor imaging eigenvalues: Preliminary evidence for altered myelin in cocaine dependence. *Psychiatry Research: Neuroimaging, 154*, 253–258.

Mohamed, S., Bondi, M. W., Kasckow, J. W., Golshan, S., & Jeste, D. V. (2006). Neurocognitive functioning in dually diagnosed middle aged and elderly patients with alcoholism and schizophrenia. *International Journal of Geriatric Psychiatry, 21*, 711–718.

Moore, T. M., & Stuart, G. L. (2004). Illicit substance use and intimate partner violence among men in batterers' intervention. *Psychology of Addictive Behaviors, 18*, 385–389.

Morgan, K., Dallosso, H., Ebrahim, S., Arie, T., & Fentem, P. H. (1988). Prevalence, frequency, and duration of hypnotic drug use among the elderly living at home. *British Medical Journal Clinical Research Education, 296*, 601–602.

Mort, J. R., & Aparasu, R. R. (2002). Prescribing of psychotropics in the elderly: Why is it so often inappropriate? *CNS Drugs, 16*, 99–109.

Mueser, K. T., Yarnold, P. R., Levinson, D. F., Singh, H., Bellack, A. S., & Kee, K. (1990). Prevalence of substance abuse in schizophrenia: Demographic and clinical correlates. *Schizophrenia Bulletin, 16*, 31–56.

Murphy, J. M., Jellinek, M., Quinn, D., Smith, G., Poitrast, F. G., & Goshko, M. (1991). Substance abuse and serious child mistreatment: Prevalence, risk, and outcome in a court sample. *Child Abuse & Neglect, 15*, 197–211.

National Institute on Drug Abuse. (2007). Retrieved January 21, 2008, from http://www.nida.nih.gov/Infofacts/costs.html

Office of National Drug Control Policy. (2001). *The economic costs of drug abuse in the United States: 1992-2002.* Washington, DC: Executive Office of the President (Publication No. 207303).

Office of National Drug Control Policy. (2005). *Who's really in prison for marijuana?* Washington, DC: Executive Office of the President.

Olmeztoprak, E., Donohue, B., & Allen, D. N. (2009). Urine toxicology testing. In G.L. Fisher & N. A. Roget (Eds.), *Encyclopedia of substance abuse prevention, treatment, and recovery* (pp. 982–985). Thousand Oaks, CA: Sage.

O'Malley, S., Adamse, M., Heaton, R. K., & Gawin, F. H. (1992). Neuropsychological impairment in chronic cocaine abusers. *American Journal of Drug and Alcohol Abuse, 18*, 131–144.

O'Neill, J., Cardenas, V., & Meyerhoff, D. (2001). Separate and interactive effects of cocaine and alcohol dependence on brain structures and metabolites: Quantitative MRI and proton MR spectroscopic imaging. *Addiction Biology, 6*, 347–361.

Oscar-Berman, M., & Marinkovi, K. (2007). Alcohol: Effects on neurobehavioral functions and the brain. *Neuropsychology Review, 17*(3), 239–357.

O'Shanick, G. J., Scott, R., & Peterson, L. G. (1984) Psychiatric referral after head trauma. *Psychiatric Medicine, 2*(2), 131–137.

Ouimet, M. C., Brown, T. G., Nadeau, L., Lepage, M., Pelletier, M., Couture, S., et al. (2007). Neurocognitive characteristics of DUI recidivists. *Accident and Analysis Prevention, 39*, 743–750.

Parrott, A. C. (2001). Human psychopharmacology of ecstasy (MDMA): A review of 15 years of empirical research. *Human Psychopharmacology, 16*, 557–577.

Pau, C. W. H., Lee, T. M. C., & Chan, S. F. (2002). The impact of heroin on frontal executive functions. *Archives of Clinical Neuropsychology, 17*, 663–670.

Paulus, M. P., Hozack, N. E., Zauscher, B. E., Frank, L., Brown, G. G., Braff, D. L., & Schuckit, M. A. (2002). Behavioral and functional neuroimaging evidence for prefrontal dysfunction in methamphetamine-dependent subjects. *Neuropsychopharmacology, 26,* 53–63.

Pitel, A. L., Beaunieux, H., Witkowski, T., Vabret, F., Guillery-Girard, B., Quinette, P., et al. (2007). Genuine episodic memory deficits and executive dysfunctions in alcoholic subjects early in abstinence. *Alcoholism: Clinical and Experimental Research, 31,* 1169–1178.

Pompéia, S., Pradella-Hallinan, M., Manzano, G. M., & Bueno, O. F. A. (2008). Effects of lorazepam on visual perceptual abilities. *Human Psychopharmacology: Clinical and Experimental, 23,* 183–192.

Pope, H. G., & Yurgelun-Todd, D. (1996). The residual cognitive effects of heavy marijuana use in college students. *Journal of the American Medical Association, 275,* 521–527.

Randolph, C., Tierney, M. C., Mohr, E., & Chase, T. N. (1998). The repeatable battery for the assessment of neuropsychological status (RBANS): Preliminary clinical validity. *Journal of Clinical and Experimental Neuropsychology, 20,* 310–319.

Rapeli, K., Kivisarri, R., Autti, T., Ǩähkönen, S., Puuskari, V., Jokela, O., et al. (2006). Cognitive function during early abstinence from opioid dependence: A comparison to age, gender, and verbal intelligence matched controls. *BMC Psychiatry, 6,* 9.

Regier, D. A., Farmer, M. E., Rae, D. S., Locke, B. Z., Keith, S. J., Judd, L. L., et al. (1990). Comorbidity of mental disorders with alcohol and other drug abuse. Results from the epidemiologic catchment area (ECA) study. *Journal of the American Medical Association, 264,* 2511–2518.

Reneman, L., Booij, J., Majoie, C. B. L. M., van den Brink, W., & den Heeten, G. J. (2001). Investigating the potential neurotoxicity of ecstasy (MDMA): An imaging approach. *Human Psychopharmacology, 16,* 579–588.

Rimel, R., & Jane, J. (1983). Characteristics of the head injured patient. In M. Rosenthal, E. R. Griffith, M. R. Bond, & J. D. Miller (Eds.), *Rehabilitation of the head injured adult* (pp. 9–21). Philadelphia: Davis.

Robinson, J. E., Heaton, R. K., & O'Malley, S. S. (1999). Neuropsychological functioning in cocaine abusers with and without alcohol dependence. *Journal of the International Neuropsychological Society, 5,* 10–19.

Rourke, S. B., & Grant, I. (1999). The interactive effects of age and length of abstinence on the recovery of neuropsychological functioning in chronic male alcoholics: A 2-year follow-up study. *Journal of the International Neuropsychological Society, 5,* 234–246.

Ruchinskas, R. A., Repetz, N. K., & Singer, H. K. (2001). The use of the neurobehavioral cognitive status examination with geriatric rehabilitation. *Rehabilitation Psychology, 46*(3), 219–228.

Sari, Y., & Gozes, I. (2006). Brain deficits associated with fetal alcohol exposure may be protected, in part, by peptides derived from activity-dependent neurotrophic factor and activity-dependent neuroprotective protein. *Brain Research Reviews, 52,* 107–118.

Schottenbauer, M. A., Momenan, R., Kerick, M., & Hommer, D. W. (2007). Relationships among aging, IQ, and intracranial volume in alcoholics and control subjects. *Neuropsychology, 21,* 337–345.

Schrimsher, G. W., O'Bryant, S. E., Parker, T. D., & Burke, R. S. (2004). The relation between ethnicity and Cognistat performance in males seeking substance use disorder treatment. *Journal of Clinical and Experimental Neuropsychology, 27,* 873–885.

Schrimsher, G. W., & Parker, J. D. (2008). Changes in cognitive function during substance use disorder treatment. *Journal of Psychopathology and Behavioral Assessment, 30*(2), 146–153.

Selby, M. J., & Azrin, R. L. (1998). Neuropsychological functioning in drug abusers. *Drug and Alcohol Dependence, 50,* 39–45.

Sevigny, E., & Caulkins, J. P. (2004). Kingpins or mules? An analysis of drug offenders incarcerated in federal and state prisons. *Criminology and Public Policy, 3,* 401–434.

Simon, S. L., Domier, C. P., Sim, T., Richardson, K., Rawson, R. A., & Ling, W. (2002). Cognitive performance of current methamphetamine and cocaine abusers. *Journal of Addictive Diseases, 21,* 61–71.

Slade, E. P., Stuart, E. A., Salkever, D. S., Karakus, M., Green, K. M., & Ialongo, N. (2008). Impacts of age of onset of substance use disorders on risk of adult incarceration among disadvantaged urban youth: A propensity score matching approach. *Drug and Alcohol Dependence, 95,* 1–13.

Sobell, M. B. (1980). Developing a prototype for evaluating alcohol treatment effectiveness. In L. C. Sobell, et al. (Eds.), *Evaluating drug and alcohol abuse effectiveness: Recent advances.* New York: Pergamon Press.

Spreen, O., & Strauss, E. (1998). *A compendium of neuropsychological tests: Administration, norms, and commentary* (2nd ed.). Oxford, UK: Oxford University Press.

Streeter, C. C., Ciraulo, D. A., Harris, G. J., Kaufman, M. J., Lewis, R. F., Knapp, C. M., et al. (1998). Functional magnetic resonance imaging of alprazolam-induced changes in humans with familial alcoholism. *Psychiatry Research, 82,* 69–82.

Streeter, C. C., Terhune, D. B., Whitfield, T. H., Gruber, S., Sarid-Segal, O., Silveri, M. M., et al. (2008). Performance on the Stroop predicts treatment compliance in cocaine-dependent individuals. *Neuropsychopharmacology, 33*, 827–836.

Strickland, T. L., Mena, I., Villanueva-Meyer, J., Miller, B. L., Cummings, J., Mehringer, C. M., et al. (1993). Cerebral perfusion and neuropsychological consequences of chronic cocaine use. *Journal of Neuropsychiatry and Clinical Neurosciences, 5*, 419–427.

Stuart, G. L., Temple, J. R., Follansbee, K. W., Bucossi, M. M., Hellmuth, J. C., & Moore, T. M. (2008). The role of drug use in a conceptual model of intimate partner violence in men and women arrested for domestic violence. *Psychology of Addictive Behaviors, 22*, 12–24.

Substance Abuse and Mental Health Services Administration. (2002). *Results from the 2001 national household survey on drug abuse.* Rockville, MD: Office of Applied Studies (Publication No. SMA 02-3758).

Sullivan, C. J., & Hamilton, Z. K. (2007). Exploring careers in deviance: A joint trajectory analysis of criminal behavior and substance use in an offender population. *Deviant Behavior, 28*, 497–523.

Sullivan, E. V., Rosenbloom, M. J., Lim, K. O., & Pfefferbaum, A. (2000). Longitudinal changes in cognition, gait and balance in abstinent and relapse alcoholic men: Relationships to changes in brain structure. *Neuropsychology, 14*, 178–188.

Sullivan, E. V., Rosenbloom, M. J., & Pfefferbaum, A. (2000). Pattern of motor and cognitive deficits in detoxified alcoholic men. *Alcoholism: Clinical and Experimental Research, 24*, 611–621.

Sullivan, E. V., Shear, P. K., Zipursky, R. B., Sager, H. J., & Pfefferbaum, A. (1997) Patterns of content, contextual and working memory impairments in schizophrenia and nonamnetic alcoholism. *Neuropsychology, 11*(2), 195–206.

Tarter, R. E., & Butters, M. (2001). Neuropsychological dysfunction due to liver disease. In R. E. Tarter, M. Butters, & S. R. Beers (Eds.), *Medical neuropsychology* (2nd ed., pp. 85–105). Dordrecht, The Netherlands: Kluwer Academic Publishers.

Tarter, R. E., & Edwards, K. L. (1986). Multifactorial etiology of neuropsychological impairment in alcoholics. *Alcoholism: Clinical and Experimental Research, 10*, 128–135.

Tata, P. R., Rollings, J., Collins, M., Pickering, A., & Jacobson, R. R. (1994). Lack of cognitive recovery following withdrawal from long-term benzodiazepine use. *Psychological Medicine, 24*, 203–213.

Testa, M., Livingston, J. A., & Leonard, K. E. (2003). Women's substance use and experiences of intimate partner violence: A longitudinal investigation among a community sample. *Addictive Behaviors, 28*, 1649–1664.

Thoma, R. J., Hanlon, F. M., Miller, G. A., Huang, M. X., Weisend, M. P., Sanchez, F. P., et al. (2006). Neuropsychological and sensory gating deficits related to remote alcohol abuse history in schizophrenia. *Journal of the International Neuropsychological Society, 12*, 34–44.

Thompson, P. M., Hayashi, K. M., Simon, S. L., Geaga, J. A., Hong, M. S., Sui, Y., et al. (2004). Structural abnormalities in the brains of human subjects who use methamphetamine. *Journal of Neuroscience, 24*, 6028–6036.

Toomey, R., Lyons, M. J., Eisen, S. A., Hong, X., Sunanta, C., Seidman, L. J., et al. (2003). A twin study of the neuropsychological consequences of stimulant abuse. *Archives of General Psychiatry, 60*, 303–310.

Tramullas, M., Martínez-Cué, C., & Hurlé, M. A. (2008). Chronic administration of heroin to mice produces up-regulation of brain apoptosis-related proteins and impairs spatial learning and memory. *Neuropharmacology, 54*, 640–652.

Tune, L. E., & Bylsma, F. W. (1991). Benzodiazepine-induced and anticholinergic-induced delirium in the elderly. *International Psychogeriatrics, 3*, 397–408.

U.S. Department of Health and Human Services Substance Abuse and Mental Health Services Administration. (2000). *1999 National household survey on drug abuse.* Rockville, MD: U.S. Department of Health and Human Services.

Van Gorp, W. G., Wilkins, J. N., Hinkin, C. H., Moore, L. H., Hull, J., Horner, M. D., et al. (1999). Declarative and procedural memory functioning in abstinent cocaine abusers. *Archives of General Psychiatry, 56*, 85–89.

Victor, M., Adams, R. D., & Collins, G. A. (Eds.). (1989). *The Wernicke-Korsakoff Syndrome and related neurological disorders due to alcoholism.* Philadephia: F. A. Davis.

Volkow, N. D., Hitzemann, R., Wang, G. J., Fowler, J. S., Wolf, A. P., Dewey, S. L., et al. (1992). Long-term frontal metabolic changes in cocaine abusers. *Synapse, 11*, 184–190.

Weber, D., Franceschi, D., Ivanovic, M., Atkins, H., Cabahug, C., Wong, C., et al. (1993). SPECT planar brain imaging in crack abuse: Iodine-123-iodoamphetamine uptake and localization. *Journal of Nuclear Medicine, 34*, 899–907.

Winick, C. (1962). Maturing out of narcotic addiction. *Bulletin on Narcotics, 14,* 1–7.

Woods, S. P., Rippeth, J. D., Conover, E., Gonzalez, R., Cherner, M., Heaton, R. K., et al. (2005). Deficient strategic control of verbal encoding and retrieval in individuals with methamphetamine dependence. *Neuropsychology, 19,* 35–43.

Young, N. K., Boles, S. M., & Otero, C. (2007). Parental substance use disorders and child maltreatment: Overlap, gaps, and opportunities. *Child Maltreatment, 12,* 137–149.

Neurotoxicology 25

Raymond Singer

Introduction

Neurotoxicity describes the harmful effects of toxic substances on the nervous system. All parts and aspects of the nervous system are susceptible to neurotoxicity, including the central and peripheral nerves, the brain, sensory organs, autonomic and motor functions, neurochemical processes, cognition, emotion, conation, perception, executive function, and personality. Neuropsychologists are the best qualified professionals to assess functional effects of neurotoxic substances, due in part to their comprehensive background in understanding the function of the entire nervous system, and their specialized training and experience in assessment.

Most cases of neurotoxicity that come to the attention of neuropsychologists involve exposure to notorious neurotoxic substances: solvents, pesticides, carbon monoxide, metals such as lead, mercury, and arsenic, and products of repeated water intrusion (mold). (See Singer 2005a, 2005b, and Singer & Gray, 2007, for examples of neuropsychological techniques applied to the evaluation of mold neurotoxicity.) However, be forewarned that mold neurotoxicity has been dismissed as imaginary by some neuropsychologists, and will be discussed at the end of this chapter.

Exceedingly few commercial products have been adequately tested prior to marketing for their potential to cause neurotoxic injuries, particularly mild cognitive impairment, and particularly for susceptible individuals and groups (Singer, 1990a; Kilburn, 1998).[1] In 1976, it was estimated that more than 1,000 new compounds were being developed each year and added to the approximately 40,000 chemicals and 2,000,000 mixtures already in industrial use (Environmental Protection Agency, 1976). Regarding substances permitted prior to 1987, most commercial substances had not even been examined for neurotoxicity (Williams et al., 1987).

More than 850 chemicals have been identified as producers of neurobehavioral disorders (Anger & Johnson, 1985). Most of these chemicals fall into the categories of solvents, pesticides, and metals. Workplace regulations were established for 200 chemicals in part because of neurotoxicity. Regulations may underestimate the risk from exposure to neurotoxic chemicals, for reasons including the lack of appreciation of the cumulative effects of chronic exposure to low levels of neurotoxicants, the risk to sensitive individuals, and multiple exposures at the same work site.

Irrespective of the efforts of our government to protect its citizens, the scientific literature is replete with reports of the neurotoxicity of common substances, such as carbon monoxide and other asphyxiants, pesticides, some herbicides (Singer, Moses, Valciukas, Lilis, & Selikoff, 1982), fumigants, solvents, and some metals. These reports rely on data drawn from clinical experience, case reports, epidemiologic studies, experiments using laboratory animals, and in-vitro testing.

The number of people with significant neurotoxic chemical exposures and potential chemical brain injuries remains very high and uncharted. Factors affecting neurotoxic outcomes include variable and sometimes intermittent exposure levels; duration of exposure over levels of exposure; synergistic effects of multiple exposures; chronic versus acute effects; susceptibility factors such as gender, age, race, constitution, and condition; DNA susceptibility factors; prior function of the immune, hepatic, and renal systems; prior neurotoxic chemical exposures; concomitant exposures in various settings; possible additive or synergistic effects of all of these factors; and other variables. In the final analysis, the clinical judgment of the neuropsychologist must be relied upon to reach an accurate diagnosis, who collates data from attending physicians, expert reports from industrial hygienists and other experts on the case, and integration of the medical and toxicology literature.

Every person touched by modern civilization is at risk of significant chemical exposure and neurotoxicity. Significant neurotoxic injury may result from occupational exposures in such diverse occupations as automobile sales managers (Singer, 1997a), being an office worker in a building undergoing renovations (Singer, 1997b), dentists (Singer, 1995), electrical products (transformer) salvage workers (Singer, 1994), herbicide workers (Singer et al., 1982), and postal workers (Singer, 1985).

Even if a person does not work, they may suffer neurotoxicity from use of consumer products (Singer, 1996), prescription drugs (Singer, 1997c), drinking water at home (Singer, 1990b), or drinking beverages at a restaurant (Singer, 2000).

Simply going to school can be hazardous for both students and teachers (Singer, 1999a), if your school district is repairing the roof of your school while school is in session. Or, when trying to get away from the pressures of modern life and building a life in a beautiful rural county, one can be exposed to a witches' brew of human and industrial waste called sewage sludge. Municipalities can pay your neighbor to accept sewage sludge, thus creating a hazardous dump for your own neighborhood (Singer, 1999b).

Pesticides are especially promiscuous in their targets. Even if a person does not work or consume, he or she may live or enter a structure with pesticide over-application, or drizzled by pesticide drift when walking down a country lane or sitting in his/her rocking chair on his/her front porch, or sleeping in his/her bed in an agricultural area (Singer, 1999c, 2002b, 2003).

A product as seemingly innocuous as carbonless copy paper can cause relentless neurotoxicity, when it is amassed in large quantities in an office, under poor ventilation conditions, and with lengthy exposure (Singer, 1998).

Living very far from industrialization may not always provide protection from hazardous chemical products: the highest blood levels of the neurotoxic polychlorinated biphenyl (PCB) have been found among the Inuit (Eskimo) people of Baffin Island, near the Arctic Circle, thousands of miles from where PCB is used. As a result of various atmospheric processes, industrial effluent discharged into the air in the tropics can collect in polar regions (Lean, 1996).

Once neurotoxic chemicals have been used in the manufacture and production of consumer goods, and the product is stabilized, this does not mean that we are forever safe from its reach. For example, neurotoxic substances can be released by fire, as found in the wake of the World Trade Center attack, with significant levels of neurotoxic substances such as benzene, dioxin, metals, and other substances being discharged at Ground Zero into the air and water (Gonzales, 2001). Currently, a number of people exposed at the site, including First Responders and other emergency workers, are reporting nervous system symptoms.

When people are hurt by neurotoxic products, they have the judicial right of compensation for their injuries. These matters are often brought to court for adjudication. The forensic neurotoxicologist and neuropsychologist will be called upon to help the judge and jury understand the nature and extent of possible nervous system injury.

With that in mind, let us now examine the common symptoms of neurotoxicity.

Symptoms of Neurotoxicity

The residual neurobehavioral symptoms of neurotoxicity from various substances are similar (Singer, 1990a). They include:

1. Cognitive changes
    (a) Attentional dysfunction, concentration difficulties: The affected person reports difficulty with keeping his mind in focus. His thoughts may drift and seem fuzzy, with increased susceptibility to distraction.
    (b) Cognitive and psychomotor slowing, which may be described by the patient as confusion or "brain fog."

(c) Memory dysfunction: Probably combination of attentional and memory encoding/storage dysfunction.

(d) Disturbance of executive function: Difficulty with planning, multi-tasking, organizing, assessing outcomes, and changing plans accordingly.

e) Learning dysfunction, due to the above factors, often with sparing of memory prior to exposure and onset of illness. People with this condition may be inappropriately diagnosed with attention-deficit/hyperactivity disorder (ADHD)–adult onset, or in children, inappropriately diagnosed as ADHD, mental retardation, slow learning, or other diagnostic labels.

2. Personality changes

(a) Irritability: Reduction of cognitive and emotional capacities from neurotoxicity can be frustrating and perplexing. The subject may report frequent strife with family members, friends, and co-workers, or difficulty with conformity. Irritability could also be a primary effect of the neurotoxicant autonomic processes that mediate or cause emotion, which are often affected in patients with diagnosed neurotoxicity.

(b) Increased sadness, depression, crying. Helplessness and hopelessness can develop from neurotoxic injuries.

(c) Social withdrawal occurs as the person becomes increasingly frustrated with his disabilities. He may feel that people are staring at or scrutinizing him. Word dysfluency often is present. Upon personality testing, the examiner might find avoidant personality disorder, which is common among patients with diagnosed neurotoxicity.

3. Autonomic and sensory dysfunction

(a) Sleep disturbance, often with choppy sleep patterns and frequent awakening. Disruption of sleep-controlling autonomic, endocrine[2] and hormonal systems can occur with neurotoxicity. Sleep disturbance contributes to learning dysfunction and chronic fatigue. Patients may carry a diagnosis of sleep apnea, which in some patients, may result from, or be exacerbated by, neurotoxicity.

(b) Chronic fatigue: Subjects may report that they are always tired, with reduced ability to lift, carry, climb stairs, walk distances, or stay awake.

(c) Headache, which may be diagnosed as migraine, tension, or cluster headaches.

(d) Sexual dysfunction: Males may have difficulty maintaining an erection. In both genders, there is usually reduced desire for sexual activities, perhaps secondary to fatigue, emotional dysfunction (i.e., irritability), pain disorders from neurotoxicity or self-concept issues.

(e) Chronic pain disorders.

(f) Photophobia: unusual eye pain in moderately bright light.

(g) Difficulty with body temperature sensing and regulation.

(h) Color vision decline.

(i) Multiple chemical sensitivity: This can occur as a "silent symptom," without the patient's awareness that this is a reportable symptom. Careful questioning of the patient is recommended when neurotoxicity is suspected. (See Singer, in press, for a further description of multiple chemical sensitivity, also known as chemical hyper-reactivity syndrome, as a symptom of neurotoxicity. For a recent appeals court decision admitting chemical sensitivity as a compensable illness within the context of neurotoxicity, see Vaughn, 2009.)

4. Peripheral neuropathy, including numbness in the hands or feet (depends upon the substance): Some neurotoxic agents damage peripheral nerves. Nerves with very long axons, such as nerves that serve the feet (and the hands to a lesser extent) are more susceptible to damage from neurotoxic agents. Disruption of the peripheral nervous system may be described by the patient as numbness, tingling, "pins and needles" sensation, or a feeling that the limb "falls asleep."

The aforementioned symptoms form the core of the "Neurotoxicity Syndrome" (Singer, in press).

Because neurotoxic agents generally can affect any area or function of the brain, it is likely that any psychiatric or neurological disease could have its origin in neurotoxicity, depending to a considerable extent upon pre-morbid constitution and conditions.

Parkinson's disease (PD),[3] senile dementia–Alzheimer's type,[4] and other commonly diagnosed neurobehavioral conditions could result from, or be exacerbated by, neurotoxicity. As opined in the *American Psychologist* (Koger, Schettler, & Weiss, 2005), "Developmental, learning, and behavioral disabilities are a significant public health problem. Environmental chemicals can interfere with brain development during critical periods, thereby impacting sensory, motor, and cognitive function. Because regulation in the United States is based on limited testing protocols and essentially requires proof of harm rather than proof of lack of harm, some undefined fraction of these disabilities may reflect adverse impacts of this 'vast toxicological experiment'" (H. L. Needleman, as quoted in Weiss & Landrigan, 2000, p. 373).

Other neurotoxicity symptoms/diseases, depending upon various susceptibility factors, could include:

1. Neurological conditions may include motor dysfunction (tremor, reduced dexterity, etc.). This symptom may be expressed as difficulty in walking or handling tools, and can progress to severe motor loss. Neurotoxicity may be misdiagnosed as multiple sclerosis (Singer, 1997a); "MS-like" disease (Singer, 1990b), amyotrophic lateral sclerosis, opsoclonos-myoclonos, seizures, and other diseases affecting the neuromotor system.

2. Sensory-perceptual disturbances: Blindness, hearing loss, pain, burning sensations, and kinesthetic dysfunction are examples of sensory disturbance that can occur with neurotoxicity. If the peripheral and central nervous system (CNS) degenerate, the nerves have reduced ability to transmit accurate information to the CNS. Any sensory system can be affected, to the point of system failure.

3. Emotional and thought disorders, including anxiety, panic attacks (Singer, 2002a), depression (Singer, 2008), and psychosis (Singer, 2006), depending upon a number of factors, including the patient's prior susceptibility to these disorders.

Scope of Neurotoxicity

Important classes of neurotoxic substances include pesticides, solvents, some metals, and gases, such as carbon monoxide. A full discussion of this topic is beyond the scope of this chapter. Pesticides are egregious neurotoxic offenders and will be discussed briefly here for illustration purposes. For further exploration, see Singer, 1990a.

Exposure of Agricultural Workers to Pesticides

Approximately 1 billion pounds of pesticides are used annually in agriculture in the United States, costing over $5 billion. Agricultural workers exposed to pesticides include field workers, pesticide applicators, food transporters, and storage personnel (Office of Technology Assessment, 1990).

An estimated 5 million Americans farm as a primary source of income. Children under the age of 16 are often involved in agriculture. About 3 million workers in the United States are migrant and seasonal agricultural workers, and there are an estimated 1 million pesticide handlers who are certified (Office of Technology Assessment, 1990). Unfortunately, nondocumented migrant workers will not have access to judicial compensation for their injuries, as well as often lacking medical care for these conditions.

The estimated prevalence of pesticide poisoning in the United States is 300,000 cases, only 1–2% of which are reported (Office of Technology Assessment, 1990). Estimated prevalence rates need to account for the low rate of identification of pesticide neurotoxicity, as few clinicians are trained to diagnose neurotoxicity. Cases of neurotoxicity: (a) may not come to the attention of health care workers, (b) may be dismissed without a diagnosis, (c) may be diagnosed as psychiatric or neurologic disorders, without awareness of cause of the illness. For example, residential exposure to the pesticides Maneb and Paraquat from agricultural applications in the central valley of California within 500 meters of the home increased PD risk by 75% (Costello, Cockburn, Bronstein, Zhang, & Ritz, 2009).

Examples of Neurotoxic Pesticides

Organophosphate and carbamate pesticides are widely used. Because of their rapid toxicity, they are the most common cause of acute pesticide poisoning. These pesticides affect insects and humans by interfering with the biochemistry of nerve transmission. Acute symptoms can include hyperactivity, breathing difficulties, sweating, tearing, urinary frequency, abnormal heartbeat, anxiety, gastrointestinal disturbance, weakness, dizziness, convulsions, coma, and death. Typical organophosphorus pesticides include Parathion, Thimet, EPN, Chlorpyrifos, Dursban,

DDVP, and Vapona. Carbamate pesticides include Aldicarb, Temik, Carbaryl, and Sevin (Office of Technology Assessment, 1990).

Organochlorine pesticides are less acutely toxic than organophosphate and carbamate pesticides, but they have a greater potential for chronic toxicity, due to their persistence in the environment and in the affected person's body. From 1940 through the 1970s, several organochlorine pesticides were widely used, including DDT, aldrin, mirex, lindane, chlordane, and heptachlor. Chlordane, introduced in 1947, was banned in 1978 for most uses except termite control (Office of Technology Assessment, 1990). Chlordane is highly persistent, and has an estimated half-life of 20 years.

Pyrethroids are a group of insecticides that are highly toxic to insects but less toxic to humans than the organophosphate and organochlorine pesticides. They are replacing the more toxic pesticides.

Fumigants are gases used to kill insects (including termites) and their eggs, and are the most acutely toxic pesticides used in agriculture. Methyl bromide is a particularly problematic pesticide, as it is colorless, almost odorless, and relatively inexpensive, so widely used. It has caused death and severe neurotoxic effects in fumigators, applicators, and structural pest-control workers (exterminators) (Office of Technology Assessment, 1990).

The notoriously toxic herbicide, 2,4,5-T, infamous from its use in Vietnam, is contaminated with neurotoxic dioxins. In 1970, the United States Department of Agriculture halted the use of 2,4,5-T on all food crops except rice, and in 1985, the EPA terminated all remaining uses in the United States of this herbicide.[5]

Nonagricultural Exposure to Pesticides

Two billion dollars is spent annually on nonagricultural pesticide products (Office of Technology Assessment, 1990). Neurotoxic pesticides are used to control termites, cockroaches, and other household insects. The elderly, adults, and children are exposed to these substances in environments including the home, school, public and private offices, restaurants and other public stores, and public parks. Usually, the person being exposed is not aware that an exposure is occurring, nor is there awareness of the potential for both acute and cumulative neurotoxicity. Additional exposures to pesticides and herbicides can occur during chemical treatment of lawns, golf courses, and sports fields.

Pesticide Residue in Foods

An estimated 17% of the preschool population in the United States are exposed to neurotoxic pesticides above levels the Federal government has declared as safe (National Resources Defense Council, 1989; Office of Technology Assessment, 1990). This analysis was based upon raw fruits and vegetables alone, and does not consider other sources of pesticide exposure. Children are considered to be more at risk of neurotoxicity than adults, because they absorb more pesticides per pound of body weight, their immature development makes them less able to detoxify substances, and their nervous system is developing and may be more vulnerable to permanent disruption (Office of Technology Assessment, 1990). Of course, chronic pesticide exposure creates the risk of reducing overall cognitive function, which ironically, schools are attempting to improve.

Pesticides banned for use in the United States can return to the food supply via produce from other countries with fewer regulations. For example, DDT, which was banned in the United States years prior, was still found in the U.S. food supply (National Resources Defense Council, 1984; U.S. General Accounting Office, 1989a). This phenomenon has been termed "banned pesticide rebound." Pesticides may be over-applied by applicators who have difficulty reading the manufacturer's instructions, which may only be available in English. The U.S. Food and Drug Administration is too short-staffed to adequately monitor the pesticide status of imported food (U.S. General Accounting Office, 1989b).

Pesticides can also contaminate water supplies. Highly persistent pesticides, such as aldicarb, have been found in groundwater supplies (Barrette, 1988).

Of course, pesticides are only one class of neurotoxic substances. There are many more (Singer 1990a), and it is likely that the total effects will be additive or synergistic.

What will result from chronic low-level pesticide ingestion? To the extent that this exposure harms brain cells, it is likely that the result will be cumulative. The decline of neurologic integrity associated with the aging process might be linked with the cumulative effects of endogenous or exogenous poisons (Butler, 1985; Williams et al., 1987). Chronic subclinical effects may make those affected especially prone to the consequences of age-related neuronal attrition (Lewin, 1987). Arezzo and Schaumburg (1989) suggested that neurotoxic damage early in life can enhance CNS dysfunction that occurs late in life, such as PD. Therefore, it would be prudent to limit all exposure to pesticides, including those in food.

Elements of the Forensic Evaluation for Neurotoxicity

For a more complete discussion, see Singer (in press), specifically, the section on "Neuropsychological Examination of The Neurotoxicity Syndrome."

Symptoms

Perhaps the most important element of this evaluation is the detection and assessment of symptoms. The examiner should assess for the presence of a constellation of symptoms characteristic of neurotoxicity. An instrument that I have found helpful is *The Neurotoxicity Screening Survey* (Singer, 1990c),[6] which helps quantify the frequency and severity of neurotoxicity symptoms in 10 factors. This instrument also aids in record keeping, as it assesses the extent to which the subject may have had similar symptoms prior to exposure. It also has a measure of distortion, so that the examiner can determine the extent of symptom over-reporting.

Interview

The subject's overall condition can be assessed during the interview, and useful information regarding the degree of the subject's veracity can emerge. To help keep a record of the interview, behavioral observations can be recorded on an extended checklist, such as that provided by Zuckerman (2005). A head-and-shoulder photograph for the case records can help refresh the expert's memory if testimony is needed. It is often helpful to interview members of the family or household to obtain their perspective on any disabilities the subject may have, and to help determine the impact of the illness on family members. Collateral interviews can help an examiner determine the consistency of his and other's observations of the case, with regard to the subject's self-report, which may be useful for detecting malingering (Sbordone, Seyranian, & Ruff, 2000). Statements or interviews of employers, clergy, and long-time friends of the case can also be very helpful, particularly for assessing premorbid function.

Past Mental and Emotional Function

To develop a pre-exposure criteria of cognitive function, pre-exposure record examination may include records of all educational and scholastic activities, any standardized tests, military service, or evidence of intellectual achievement, such as papers, patents, and so on. These materials can be used to quantify overall prior mental function, and determine specific levels of cognitive function in various cognitive, perceptual, and emotional domains.

In addition, demographic equations to predict pre-morbid intellectual function are available (e.g., Vanderploeg & Schinka, 1995). Because crystallized cognitive function is more resistant to recent insults than more fluid cognitive functions, this differential can be helpful in estimating overall pre-morbid intellectual function and determining possible declines. A percentile rank differential equivalent to a four scaled scores decline (see Singer, in press, for more details) provides useful guideline for determining deficits. Collateral and family interviews as described previously may also be helpful.

Psychometric Tests

Cognitive function can be assessed using the numerous commercially available tests for intellectual, memory, and other cognitive functions. The overall intelligence quotient may be a misleading indicator of a person's actual ability, due to disabling deficits in specific domains forming the quotient. For the analysis of the onset of neurotoxicity, it is important to analyze the results with regard to the possible discrepancy between crystalized and fluid cognitive functions. Crystalized functions are more resistant to neurotoxic effects. Perceptual distortions are common with neurotoxicity. Interpretation of test results must account for prior cognitive ability. The person should not be compared with the hypothetical average.

Emotional Function

It is often helpful to quantify emotional function. Tests such as depression and anxiety scales can help assess the extent of emotional factors in the cases's pathology. Disruption of emotional function may result from the actual neurotoxic injury, or may be secondary to loss of cognitive and physical function. In addition, these measures may help in differential diagnosis. Yet, even if depression is found, the responses should be checked to determine whether the depression shows the classic stigmata of feelings of guilt, low self-worth, or whether responses are more weighted toward psychomotor slowing and hopelessness, which often accompanies neurotoxicity.

Personality Function

Many neuropsychologists routinely use the *MMPI-2 (Minnesota Multiphasic Personality Inventory-2)* to identify personality pathology. However, the *MMPI-2* has not been normed on patients with neurotoxicity or other neurological disorders, so it is not valid for differentiating between neurotoxicity and personality disorders. Interpretation of the *MMPI-2* test results can be misleading to a jury, in part due to the antiquated names that had been applied to the scales. More modern tests, such as the NEO Personality Inventory, may offer clearer evidence to help juries adjudicate cases.

General Well-Being

Instruments such as the Human Activity Profile or the General Well-Being Schedule help quantify the impact of the sickness on general functioning.

Malingering and Distortion

These issues are covered in separate chapters.

Neurophysiological Tests

Many neurotoxic substances also affect the peripheral nervous system. Nerve conduction-velocity tests offer a reliable and inexpensive way to evaluate peripheral nerve function (Kimura, 1989; Singer, 1990a). Choose to measure nerves that are most susceptible to neurotoxicity, such as the median sensory and sural nerves, and measure both sides of the body.

Other techniques that may provide helpful information include the various brain potential tests (somatosensory, etc.), evoked potential measures of attentional processes, and quantitative electroencephalogram (EEG).

Because sleep is so often disrupted, laboratory sleep studies might provide helpful information to the examiner. Note that most neurophysiological test results are not specific to neurotoxicity.

CNS Imaging

Typically, routine computer-assisted tomography (CAT) and magnetic resonance imaging (MRI) brain imaging may be helpful to rule out other causes of pathology. Findings, if any, are usually non-specific for neurotoxicity. PET (positron emission tomography), SPECT (single photon emission computed tomography), and functional MRI (fMRI) scans are more sensitive, but their specificity for neurotoxicity has been questioned. Although these results may be useful to the diagnostician, they may or may not be accepted as probative in court.

Testing for Traces, Metabolites, or Other Indications of Exposure in Blood and Urine

Although these measures might be valuable when assessing acute exposures, in general, these tests are of little value for assessing the effects of a substance months or years after exposure. Exceptions may include urine testing for mycotoxins or metals. Some testing may be valuable, but this topic is beyond the scope of this chapter. Antimyelin antibody measures are often elevated in neurotoxic conditions.

New Frontiers of Forensic Neurotoxicology

Criminal Litigation

Neurotoxicity can be a factor in a criminal defendant's ability to be competent to commit a crime. It can affect executive function, ability to plan, decide, judge, comprehend, control impulses, and so on. In many jurisdictions, an impaired cognitive or executive ability can affect the possibility of a guilty verdict, or can mitigate the severity of a punishment. In cases in which an accused faces the death penalty, the jury may find that neurotoxic injury can be a factor mitigating against execution.

Neuropsychologists have been called upon to opine whether toxic chemicals contributed to a defendant's ability to prevent themselves from committing various crimes, including multiple homicide (Singer, 2002c). It is remarkable that when neurotoxicological investigations are performed in cases of many offenders, including those accused of multiple murders (upon request by lawyers who prescreen the cases for neurotoxicity, prior to being evaluated by the neuropsychologist), neurotoxicity has often been determined to be a factor in horrific crimes. Increased awareness of the potential for neurotoxicity to increase criminality may spur society to reduce its citizens' exposure to neurotoxicants.

Civil Litigation

In addition to precedent-setting criminal cases, neuropsychology and neurotoxicology have been at the center of some pivotal court decisions.

The Agent Orange Settlement Fund was created by the resolution of the Agent Orange Product Liability Litigation, a class-action lawsuit brought by Vietnam veterans and their families regarding injuries allegedly incurred as a result of the exposure of Vietnam veterans to chemical herbicides used during the Vietnam war. The suit was brought against the major manufacturers of these herbicides. The class action case was settled out-of-court in 1984 for $180 million dollars, reportedly the largest settlement of its kind at that time.[7] Integral to the settlement was the testimony of a neuropsychologist/neurotoxicologist, one of approximately five medical experts, who examined the approximately six test plaintiffs, and opined that some of the plaintiffs suffered significant neuropsychological injuries from Agent Orange.

In 1992, the Supreme Court of Ohio[8, 9] heard a case regarding the admissibility of plaintiff's neuropsychologist's testimony in neurotoxicity litigation. The case involved a family who developed an MS-like illness following gasoline ingestion from a contaminated well on their property.

After the trial court and the appeals court rejected the causation testimony of a non-physician that gasoline ingestion caused the illnesses, the plaintiffs took the case to the Supreme Court of Ohio. In support of the defense were briefs filed by the Ohio State Medical Association, and in support of the plaintiffs were briefs filed by the Association of Trial Lawyers of America (now the American Association for Justice).

The judges' decision in this case was unanimous. They wrote that, "The issue presented is whether an expert witness who is not a physician, but a Ph.D. who specializes in neurotoxicology, is qualified to render an opinion that the ingestion of gasoline caused injury to the brain and nervous system. For the reasons that follow, we hold that such an expert can be so qualified."

The Court examined the witnesses' "knowledge, skill, experience, training, or education" to determine that in the instant case, he was indeed qualified to render such an opinion.

Darnell v. Eastman (1970), 23 Ohio St.2d 13, 52 O.O.2d 76, 261 N.E.2d 114, was cited by the defense as precedent to indicate that only a medical doctor can testify as to the causal connection between an injury and a subsequent physical disability. The syllabus in Darnell states as follows: "......the issue of causal connection between an injury and a specific subsequent physical disability involves a scientific inquiry and must be established by the opinion of medical witnesses competent to express such opinion."

However, the Court ruled that "the somewhat ambiguous term 'medical witnesses' does not require that such witnesses be medical doctors," and permitted the testimony of an otherwise qualified nonmedical doctor witness, further stating that "the trial court erred in granting summary judgment, as there remain material issues of fact for a jury to determine."

Neuropsychology has also been at the forefront in precedent-setting Daubert rulings of admissibility.[10]

The case involved a substance, gamma-Butyrolactone,[11] on which there were relatively few clinical or research reports concerning its toxicity at the time of trial. The defense argued that too little was known about the substance for the plaintiff to prove his/her case. The neuropsychologist/neurotoxicologist presented evidence (in part) that the substance was a solvent, and that much is known about solvent effects on the CNS.

In this Federal Appeals Court case,[12] the plaintiff alleged that workplace exposures to defendant's organic solvent caused (a) psychological problems, caused both by initial exposure and subsequent health problems, (b) cognitive impairments and personality disorders, caused by brain damage, and (c) Parkinsonian symptoms caused by brain damage. The plaintiff offered two causation experts: a pharmacologist/toxicologist, and a neuropsychologist/neurotoxicologist. The defendant moved to exclude their testimony under Daubert.

The court affirmed the trial court's admission of the neuropsychologist/neurotoxicologist's testimony. They stated that in general toxic tort, plaintiffs must prove both that the toxic substance is capable of causing injuries like the plaintiff's in human beings, and that it did in fact cause plaintiff's injuries. However, several victims of new toxic tort should not be barred from suit simply because medical literature, which will eventually support causal connection, has not yet been completed.

The plaintiffs need not produce mathematically precise tables equating levels of exposure with levels of harm, but need merely offer evidence from which jurors can reasonably conclude that exposure probably caused injuries.

There is no requirement that plaintiff's expert must always cite published studies on general causation, nor that pertinent epidemiological studies supporting plaintiff's position exist. Even if the trial judge believes there are better grounds for some alternative conclusion, and that there are some flaws in the expert's methods, the expert's opinion should be admitted if there exist good grounds to support it. The only question is whether the testimony is sufficiently reliable and relevant to assist a jury. Factual basis of expert opinion generally goes to credibility, not admissibility.

The neuropsychologist/neurotoxicologist testified that exposures to solvent caused the plaintiff to suffer permanent organic brain dysfunction manifesting itself in Parkinsonian physical symptoms, cognitive impairments, and personality disorders. He also testified that inhalation was a more potent exposure mechanism than ingestion, and that he followed normal procedures for evaluating patients with potential toxic exposure.

The defendant stated that his expert witness's theory was developed for litigation, not subjected to peer review, had not been published in the scientific literature, and was unsupported by epidemiology. Further, the defendant also stated that he did not quantify the plaintiff's exposure, did not opine on threshold exposure necessary for injury, failed to rule out other potential causes, and did not follow established guidelines for evaluating brain injury. But the district court's role was not to determine whether his theory was correct, and the appellate court's role is not to duplicate the district court's analysis, which correctly held after exacting scrutiny that his testimony was based on sufficiently good science to go to jury.

The court also opined that the defendant offered no studies indicating its solvent was incapable of causing permanent damage:

Our role is not to determine whether Dr. Singer's opinion was correct; that was for the jury to decide....We perform only the comparatively narrow analysis of whether the district court's determination that the opinion was sufficiently grounded in "good science" to assist the jury constituted an abuse of that court's discretion....ISP's attacks on Dr. Singer's testimony indicate no more than that his conclusion is not yet established as fact in the scientific community. ISP has not indicated that any scientific theory or studies indicate that BLO is incapable of causing permanent damage....The district court conducted an exacting review of the science involved and correctly concluded that, because Dr. Singer's methodology was scientifically valid, the scientific questions were best addressed by allowing each side to present *its experts and then submitting their opinions to the jury....ISP's final contention is that the district court abused its discretion when it denied ISP's motion for a new trial based on an excessive verdict. A verdict should be set aside as excessive only when it is so excessive that it shocks the conscience....In this case, the jury heard evidence that Bonner's past and future earnings losses were expected to total some $600,000, and that she could be expected to suffer from disabling physical and psychological problems for the remainder of her 25-year life expectancy. In light of this evidence, we agree with the district court's determination that an award of $2.2 million[13] does not shock the conscience.*

The judgment is affirmed.

These two cited cases provide precedent for a qualified neuropsychologist to offer causation opinion regarding both psychiatric and neurological diseases.

A New Frontier of Neurobehavioral Toxicology

Mold litigation is being compared with asbestos litigation, in that the number of cases is mushrooming, as awareness increases of the potential of mold to cause neurotoxicity. Neuropsychologists have testified in a number of mold cases. For example, see Singer (2005a, 2005b) and Singer and Gray (2007).

Although some neuropsychologists believe that mold and the products of repeated water intrusions can cause neurotoxicity, other neuropsychologists disagree, some quite vehemently.

Repeated indoor water intrusions produce a very complex indoor biological environment, including mold, mold spores, mold parts, such as glucans, volatile organic compounds, and most notably, mycotoxins, the naturally occurring highly toxic by-products of mold metabolism. In addition, the moldy environment causes the proliferation of various bacteria, some of which also produce toxins. The levels of exposure will vary, depending upon moisture and ventilation levels, and a number of other factors. The genera *Penicillium* and *Aspergillus* are often present in contaminated indoor environments, so in this witches' brew, you may find ergotomines, as ergot alkaloids can be produced by fungi of the genera *Penicillium* and *Aspergillus*, notably by some isolates of the human pathogen *Aspergillus fumigatus*. (*Aspergillus fumigatus* is a fungus of the genus *Aspergillus*, and is one of the most common *Aspergillus* species to cause disease in immuno-compromised individuals[14]). Ergotamine is used to synthesize lysergic acid, an analog of and precursor of LSD. Moreover, ergot sclerotia naturally contain some amounts of lysergic acid.[15]

What will be the effect of these substances on a person's acute or chronic mental health? Many of these substances, and combinations thereof, have not been fully characterized as to their potential for neurotoxicity, though some have.

The evidence for neurotoxicity from by-products of repeated indoor water intrusions (mold) is drawn from a multitude of sources, including case reports and group analyses of human mold neurotoxicity cases, naturalistic studies of mold poisoning in animals, experimental animal studies, and other sources and methods of scientific inquiry. In my opinion, the evidence of mold neurotoxicity is reasonably convincing.

There are three minimal requirements of a neuropsychologist asked to evaluate a case in which mold is suspected of causing neuropsychological dysfunction:

(a) examine each individual case with an open mind, using the standard techniques developed in neuropsychology for detecting brain dysfunction, (b) either become familiar and current with the toxicological literature on this topic, or consult a suitable specialist in this area, and (c) study the temporal relationship between the onset of symptoms and the onset of exposure.

Unfortunately, some patients and plaintiffs presenting with this condition are ridiculed as hysterics, some are treated as if they had a purely psychological disorder, and probably most are ignored. This iatrogenic approach does not promote human welfare and justice.

Notes

1. For current EPA Neurotoxicity Risk Assessment guidelines, see http://oas pub.epa.gov/eims/eimscomm.getfile?p_download_id=4555
2. Researchers are studying endocrine effects of neurotoxic substances, such as lead, mercury, and arsenic. It is likely that neurotoxicity and endocrine disruption occur in tandem in neurotoxicity patients (see Iavicoli, Fontana, & Bergamaschi, 2009).
3. Residential exposure to the pesticides Maneb and Paraquat from agricultural applications in the central valley of California within 500 m of the home increased PD risk by 75% (Costello, Cockburn, Bronstein, Zhang, & Ritz, 2009).
4. History of exposure to one or more solvent groups (benzene and toluene, phenols and alcohols, ketones, other solvents) yielded an adjusted Alzheimer's disease odds ratio of 2.3 (95% confidence interval 1.1–4.7); among males only, it increased to 6.0 (95% confidence interval 2.1–17.2). Thus, past exposure to organic solvents may be associated with onset of Alzheimer's disease (Kukull et al., 1995).
5. Retrieved May 22, 2009, from http://en.wikipedia.org/wiki/2,4,5 Trichlorophenoxyacetic_acid
6. Available for your clients to self-administer on-line at www.neurotox.com/ survey
7. Retrieved May 28, 2009, from http://www.vba.va.gov/bln/21/Benefits/ Herbicide/AOno2.htm
8. *Shilling v. Mobile Analytical Servs., Inc.*, 602 N.E.2d 1154 (Ohio 1992)
9. According to the plaintiff's lawyer, the Ohio State Supreme Court is considered to be one of the most influential courts in the United States of America (Blumenstiel, personal communication).
10. Retrieved May 26, 2009, from http://www.daubertontheweb.com/ toxicologists.htm
11. Retrieved May 26, 2009, from http://en.wikipedia.org/wiki/ Gamma-Butyrolactone
12. *Bonner v. ISP Techs., Inc.*, 259 F.3d 924 (8th Cir. 2001) and ibid note 9.
13. According to the plaintiff's lawyer, this verdict was the largest amount ever awarded to a plaintiff in that jurisdiction to that date (Ponder, personal communication)
14. Retrieved May 27, 2009, from http://en.wikipedia.org/wiki/ Aspergillus_fumigatus

15. Retrieved May 27, 2009, from http://en.wikipedia.org/wiki/
    Aspergillus_fumigatus

References

Anger, W. K., & Johnson, B. (1985). Chemicals affecting behavior. In J. O'Donoghue (Ed.), *Neurotoxicity of industrial and commercial chemicals* (Vol. 1). Boca Raton, FL: CRC Press.

Arezzo, J. C., & Schaumburg, H. H. (1989). Screening for neurotoxic disease in humans. *American College of Toxicology, 8,* 147–155.

Barrette, B. (1988). The Rhode Island Department of Health (DOH) private well surveillance program. *Northeast Regional Environmental Public Health Center Newsletter, 2,* 1–2.

Butler, R. (1985). Keynote address, workshop on environmental toxicity and the aging process. In S. R. Baker & M. Rogul (Eds.), *Environmental toxicity and the aging process* (1st ed., Vol. 1, pp. 11–18). New York: Alan R. Liss.

Costello, S., Cockburn, M., Bronstein, J., Zhang, X., & Ritz, B. (2009). Parkinson's disease and residential exposure to maneb and paraquat from agricultural applications in the central valley of California. *American Journal of Epidemiology, 169*(8), 919–926.

Ecobichon, D., & Joy, R. (1982). *Pesticides and neurological disease* (1st ed.). Boca Raton, FL: CRC Press.

Environmental Protection Agency. (1976). *Core activities of the office of toxic substances (draft program plan),* EPA publication 560/4-76-005. Washington, DC: Author.

Iavicoli, I., Fontana, L., & Bergamaschi, A. (2009). The effects of metals as endocrine disruptors. *Journal of Toxicology and Environmental Health,* Part B, *12*(3), 206–223.

Kilburn, K. (1998). *Chemical brain injury.* New York: Van Nostrand Reinhold.

Kimura, J. (1989). *Electrodiagnosis in diseases of nerve and muscle: Principles and practice* (2nd ed.). Philadelphia: F.A. Davis.

Koger, S. M., Schettler, T., & Weiss, B. (2005). Environmental toxicants and developmental disabilities: A challenge for psychologists. *American Psychologist, 60,* 243–255.

Kukull, W. A., Larson, E. B., Bowen, J. D., McCormick, W. C., Teri, L., & Pfanschmidt, M. L. (1995). Solvent exposure as a risk factor for Alzheimers' disease: A case-control study. *American Journal of Epidemiology, 141*(11), 1059–1071.

Lean, G. (1996, December 15). World industry poisons Arctic purity. *Independent on Sunday,* p. 15.

Lewin, R. (1987). Environmental hypothesis for brain diseases strengthened by new data. *Science,* 583–584.

National Resources Defense Council. (1984). *Pesticides in food: What the public needs to know.* San Francisco: Author.

National Resources Defense Council. (1989). *Intolerable risk: Pesticides in our children's food.* Washington, DC: Author.

Office of Technology Assessment. (1990). *Neurotoxicity. Identifying and controlling poisons of the nervous system* (OTA-BA-436). Washington, DC: Author.

Sbordone, R. J., Seyranian, G. D., & Ruff, R. M. (2000). The use of significant others to enhance the detection of malingerers from traumatically brain-injured patients. *Archives of Clinical Neuropsychology, 15*(6), 465–477.

Singer, R. (1985, August). Neuropsychological evaluation of neurotoxicity. In *Neurobehavioural methods in occupational and environmental health: Document 3. Environmental health* (pp. 86–90). Copenhagen, Denmark: World Health Organization Regional Office for Europe.

Singer, R. (1990a). *Neurotoxicity guidebook.* New York: Van Nostrand Reinhold.

Singer, R. (1990b). Neurotoxicity can produce "MS-like" symptoms. *Journal of Clinical and Experimental Neuropsychology, 12*(1), 68.

Singer, R. (1990c). *The Neurotoxicity Screening Survey.* Available from the author, Santa Fe, NM.

Singer, R. (1990d). Formaldehyde neurotoxicity. *Archives of Clinical Neuropsychology, 5*(2), 214.

Singer, R. (1994). Chronic polychlorinated biphenyl exposure and neurobehavioral effects. *Toxicologist, 14,* 1.

Singer, R. (1995). Neuropsychological assessment of a practicing dentist with elevated urinary mercury. *Fundamental and Applied Toxicology, 151*(Suppl.).

Singer, R. (1996). Neurotoxicity from outdoor, consumer exposure to a methylene chloride product. *Fundamental and Applied Toxicology: Supplement: The Toxicologist, Pt. 2, 30*(1).

Singer, R. (1997a). Wood-preserving chemicals, multiple sclerosis, and neuropsychological function. *Archives of Clinical Neuropsychology, 12*(4), 404.

Singer, R. (1997b). Sick building syndrome: Neuropsychological study. *Fundamental and Applied Toxicology* (Suppl.), *Toxicologist* (Part 2), *36*(1), 59.

Singer, R. (1997c). Neuropsychological evaluation of desipramine toxicity. *Journal of Neuropsychiatry and Clinical Neurosciences, 9,* 1, 167.

Singer, R. (1998). Evaluating a carbonless copy paper neurotoxicity case. *Archives of Clinical Neuropsychology, 13*(1), 127.

Singer, R. (1999a). Neurobehavioral screening of child and adult bystander exposure to toluene diisocyanate application. *Fundamental and Applied Toxicology* (Suppl.), *Toxicologist, 48*(1-S), 359.

Singer, R. (1999b). Neurotoxicity from municipal sewage sludge. *Archives of Clinical Neuropsychology, 14,* 160.

Singer, R. (1999c). Neuropsychological evaluation of bystander exposure to pesticides. *Journal of Neuropsychiatry and Clinical Neurosciences, 11*(1), 161–162.

Singer, R. (2000). Neurobehavioral evaluation of residual effects of acute chlorine ingestion. *Fundamental and Applied Toxicology* (Suppl.), *Toxicologist, 54*(1), 181.

Singer, R (2002a). Panic disorder can be caused by neurotoxicity. *Archives of Clinical Neuropsychology, 17*(8), 813–814.

Singer, R. (2002b). Neurobehavioral evaluation of residual effects of low-level bystander organophosphate pesticide exposure. *Fundamental and Applied Toxicology* (Suppl.), *Toxicologist, 55*(1).

Singer, R. (2002c, April). *Death penalty mitigation factors: Neurotoxicity.* Paper presented at the 18th Annual Symposium of the American College of Forensic Psychology, San Francisco.

Singer, R. (2003). Neurobehavioral evaluation of household exposure to Dursban. *Toxicological Sciences, 72*(S-1), 311.

Singer, R. (2005a). *Clinical evaluation of suspected mold neurotoxicity.* Proceedings of the Fifth International Conference on Bioaerosols, Fungi, Bacteria, Mycotoxins and Human Health. Albany, NY: Boyd Printing.

Singer, R. (2005b). Forensic evaluation of a mold (repeated water intrusions) neurotoxicity case. *Archives of Clinical Neuropsychology, 20*(7), 808.

Singer, R. (2006). Forensic neuropsychological autopsy of a suicide following occupational solvent exposure. *Archives of Clinical Neuropsychology, 21*(6), 606.

Singer, R. (2008). Forensic evaluation of neuropsychological decline following solvent exposure. *Archives of Clinical Neuropsychology, 23*(6), 746.

Singer, R. (in press). The neurotoxicity syndrome. In M. R. Schoenberg & J. G. Scott (Eds.), *The black book of neuropsychology: A syndrome-based approach.* New York: Springer Publishing Company.

Singer, R., & Gray, M. (2007). Neuropsychological evaluation of a practicing physician with mold exposure. *Archives of Clinical Neuropsychology, 22*(7), 892.

Singer, R., Moses, M., Valciukas, J., Lilis, R., & Selikoff, I. J. (1982). Nerve conduction velocity studies of workers employed in the manufacture of phenoxy herbicides. *Environmental Research, 29,* 297–311.

U.S. General Accounting Office. (1989a). *Pesticides: Export of unregistered pesticides is not adequately monitored by EPA* (GRD/HRD-89-128). Washington, DC: Author.

U.S. General Accounting Office. (1989b). *Imported foods: Opportunities to improve FDA's inspection program* (GAO/HRD-89-128). Washington, DC: Author.

Vanderploeg, R. D., & Schinka, J. A. (1995). Predicting WAIS-R IQ premorbid ability: Combining subtest performance and demographic variable predictors. *Archives of Clinical Neuropsychology, 10,* 225–239.

Vaughn, S. R., (2009). Before the Board of Industrial Insurance Appeals, State of Washington, in Re: Steven R. Vaughn, Docket No. 07 13382, Claim No. Y-965493, Proposed Decision and Order, Industrial Appeals Judge: Nancy E. Curington, Jan. 6, 2009.

Williams, J. R., Spencer, P. S., Stahl, S. M., Borzelleca, J. F., Nichols, W., Pfitzer, E., et al. (1987). Interactions of aging and environmental agents: The toxicological perspective. In *Environmental toxicity and the aging process* (pp. 81–135). New York: Alan L. Liss.

Zuckerman, E. (2005). *Clinician's thesaurus* (6th ed.). New York: Guilford Press.

Part V
Conclusion

Conclusion

Forensic Neuropsychology in the Future

26

Arthur MacNeill Horton, Jr.

The preceding chapters have described the history and current status of forensic neuropsychology (Purish & Sbordone, 1997). Chapters in previous sections have dealt with foundations of forensic neuropsychology, ethical/legal issues, practice issues, and special areas and populations in forensic neuropsychology. This chapter, however, looks to the future, rather than the past and present. The intent of this chapter is to suggest future directions in forensic neuropsychology. The focus is upon projected future developments in forensic neuropsychology (Ruff, 2004; Zillmer, 2004; Zillmer & Green, 2006). The future possible developments in forensic neuropsychology are organized under the headings of new problems, new procedures, and new populations to facilitate communication.

New Problems

In this section, the problems of reimbursement for services, the Internet, and credentialing will be addressed.

Reimbursement for Services and Forensic Neuropsychology

It is fairly clear that reimbursement for all types of neuropsychological services will be strongly influenced by changes in the United States health care system (Sbordone & Saul, 2000). Simply put, the history of health care in recent years has been one of drastic change (Cummings, 1986). Although in earlier decades, there was concern regarding the quality of health care services, there have been changes. In more recent decades, the concern in health care has been cost containment. In the United States, national health care costs have been increasing at a rate both greater than the inflation rate and the production of other goods and services for the country (Strosahi, 1994). At the same time, the productivity of the American workers in the United States has leveled off. The result is inflation has continued to rise, and there is continued pressure from employees to have health care benefits. Unfortunately, the amount of new productivity necessary to pay for health care benefits has not been available in the United States economic system. Therefore, the United States has had greater demands for health care with fewer resources to pay for it.

Health care costs have greatly increased in recent years. Reasons for the increases include greater use of expensive technological procedures, efforts to keep terminally ill patients alive through artificial means, and extremely inefficient managed care systems with excessive administrative costs. The public perception has been that there is little accountability with respect to the excessive costs of health care procedures (Armenti, 1993). Managed care organizations have arisen in the United States promising to reduce costs of health care. In theory, managed care applies a cost metric to health care, and allocates it on the most efficient basis (Armenti, 1993). In other words, there is review of health care services prior to delivery, and denial of services not deemed "medically necessary." As noted by Ruff (2004), "not medically necessary" can be seen as including all clinical neuropsychological services. Managed care organizations have required massive amounts of paperwork, frequently deny or excessively limit neuropsychological services, and reimburse poorly (Kanauss, Schatz & Puente, 2005).

As managed care has reduced the incomes of psychologists, they appear to be moving into the forensic area in order to gain income (Kanauss, Schatz & Puente, 2005; Otto & Heilbrun, 2002). Managed care organizations may disavow services that have, in many cases, been delivered without a research base upon which to base these decisions. As noted by Peterson and Harbeck (1988), the development of a research base is critical to the maturing of any field. Managed care organizations are disliked by a majority of clinical neuropsychologists (Kanauss et al., 2003). As far as forensic neuropsychologists are concerned, however, the extant research findings regarding managed care influences on neuropsychology are gloomy, at best, and disastrous, at worst (Sweet, Westergaard, & Moberg, 1995).

Federal budget deficits have produced a need to reduce health care costs, so efforts have been made to apply rigid cost-containment strategies. Unfortunately, the efforts have been based on the need to reduce health care costs, and there has been a dearth of planning as to how to best reduce those costs (Cummings, 1986).

In many cases, the effect of managed care appears to have been to reduce the quality of health care. The denial of adequate health care can have horrible consequences to ill and impaired individuals. The likely impact of the increasing influence of managed care is to drive many clinical neuropsychologists to become forensic neuropsychologists.

The Internet and Forensic Neuropsychology

Technological influences on forensic neuropsychology are likely to be enormous in the coming years. The Internet has changed the way that human beings in the whole world approach information processing, transfer, and storage. The citizens of the world can trade information with others halfway around the world, with international contributions from individuals in South American, Australia, England, and Canada, as well as the United States and other countries. In addition to communication advantages, the technological revolution can facilitate the development of assessment applications and expert systems in forensic neuropsychology (Schatz & Browndyke, 2002). Computer programs in a computer network could be developed to provide forensic neuropsychologists with guidance. Software has already been developed for administration and scoring applications. There are a number of computer programs, for instance, for making neuropsychological interpretations in terms of patients' neuropsychological test data (Russell, 1995). These appear to be most capable of making a simple diagnosis of presence or absence of brain damage, and are less capable for making decisions regarding laterality, etiology, localization, or process of cerebral injury. Nonetheless, the potential for further development of expert systems in forensic neuropsychology is available. There are already ubiquitous computer interpretations of psychological tests, such as the *Minnesota Multiphasic Personality Inventory, Second Edition* (MMPI-2), and the use of these computer interpretations over decades has definitely established the MMPI-2 computer interpretations as significant aids to clinical psychologists.

Credentialing and Forensic Neuropsychology

In clinical neuropsychology, there are two major Diplomate boards offering board certification credentials. These are the American Board of Clinical Psychology (ABCN), which is affiliated with the American Board of Professional Psychology (ABPP), and the American Board of Professional Neuropsychology (ABN). In the interests of appropriate disclosure, it might be mentioned the chapter author is a past president of ABN and has written on the history of board certification elsewhere (Horton, 1997a). Both ABCN and ABPN have similar application processes that include the following: work sample review, objective multiple-choice examination, and oral examination procedures.

Available literature suggests there is a preference by attorneys to hire forensic neuropsychologists who are board certified, but no clear preference for either ABN or ABCN (Essig, Mittenberg, Peterson, Strauman, & Cooper, 2001).

In addition, there has also been a new board devoted to pediatric neuropsychology; the American Board of Pediatric Neuropsychology (ABPN) has similar procedures to ABCN and ABN. Recently, ABPN has offered advance qualifications in a number of specialty areas, which have included forensic neuropsychology. The expectation is that professional practice standards in forensic neuropsychology will show continual development. Others have noted the need for additional training guidelines in neuropsychology (Johnstone & Farmer, 1997).

New Procedures

The Daubert decision (*Daubert vs. Merril Dow Pharmaceuticals*, 1993) has imposed new standards for forensic neuropsychological evaluation. The Daubert decision has set standards for assisting trial judges in evaluating the value of scientific evidence offered in the context of litigation (Project on Scientific Knowledge and Public Policy, 2003, June). The purpose of the Daubert decision was to remove "junk science" from the courtroom. Forensic neuropsychologists are concerned about the application of scientific standards in the hands of individuals such as trial judges who, although highly intelligent, are not always trained in science. Clarification of the Daubert decision in actual court decisions is ongoing.

Neuropsychology Assessment Measures and Forensic Neuropsychology

Clinical neuropsychological assessment tests are noteworthy for their careful external validation, relative to explicit neurological criteria (Reitan & Davison, 1974; Reitan & Wolfson, 1993). The impressive empirical validity of neuropsychological tests to determine the presence of brain damage and lateralization of the brain damage has been well demonstrated (Horton, 1997b). Unfortunately, there has not been the same amount of research with neuropsychological tests addressing questions related to ecological validity issues.

Although there is a research evidence basis for making decisions regarding day-to-day functioning and vocational abilities (Horton & Wedding, 1984), there is also a clear need for additional empirical evidence to further improve the ecological validity of neuropsychological tests (Sbordone & Saul, 2000).

Neuroimaging and Forensic Neuropsychology

Neuroimaging measures such as magnetic resonance imaging (MRI), functional magnetic resonance imaging (fMRI), positron emission topography (PET) scanning, and other neuroimaging measures have provided windows through which to see the human brain (Bigler, Lowry, & Porter, 1997). Increased use of neuroimaging brain-imaging techniques is expected in forensic neuropsychology. The combining of neuropsychological testing and neuroimaging evidence is expected to further develop the empirical basis for forensic neuropsychology. Moreover, the elucidation of controversial diagnostic entities, such as post-concussion disorder, may be clarified by neuroimaging (Bigler, 2008).

Effort Measures and Forensic Neuropsychology

In the 21st century, forensic neuropsychology has demonstrated explosive growth of effort test measures (Franzen & Iverson, 1997; Iverson, 2003; Reynolds, 1998).

The development of new specialized effort measures is expected in the future, as problems with psychometric dilemmas (i.e., validity and reliability) and generalizability across samples (i.e., base rate variability related to different settings, diagnoses and demographic variables) are successfully addressed (Rohling & Boone, 2007). Moreover, the development of better embedded effort measures based on standard neuropsychological tests is expected (Larrabee, 2003; Meyers & Volbrecht, 2003). Similarly, it will be important to have additional comparative research that investigates the sensitivity and specificity of the large array of specialized and embedded effort tests (Gervais, Rohling Green, & Ford, 2004). An important challenge to the development of effort testing is prevention of the effects of coaching by attorneys (Essig et al., 2001, Gervais, Allen, & Green, 2001; Youngjohn, 1995). Information, for example, is available on the Internet, by which non-forensic neuropsychologists can learn means of passing effort testing (Bauer & McCaffery, 2006). Similarly, more attention to the development of better normative data and empirically based cut-off scores is expected in the future (Iverson, 2003).

New Populations

New populations for forensic neuropsychology might include the following.

Medical/Health Care Patients and Forensic Neuropsychology

Medical specialties are fertile areas for forensic neuropsychologists (Johnstone, Coppel, & Townes, 1997). Patients with systemic illnesses that have secondary brain effects, such as lung disease, cardiovascular disorders, liver disease, and selected ontological disorders, among many others, as well as cases in which the effects of pharmaceuticals are in question, or in which health care may have been inappropriate and brain damage is a possible consequence, are areas for forensic neuropsychological assessment. Similarly, cases in which medical complications/treatment may have an effect (direct or indirect) on brain functioning, and in which neurotoxic effects of chemicals/substances/toxins are in question, are within the ambit of forensic neuropsychology (Hartman, 1995). In addition, the increased proportion of elderly individuals in the United States suggests many future issues, with respect to determination of capacities to make various types of decisions or activities (i.e., make a will, refuse medical treatment, live independently, handle one's legal/fiscal affairs, participate in research studies, drive a motor vehicle, etc.). All of these decisions have legal ramifications, and are potential areas in which forensic neuropsychologists can practice. Medical/health neuropsychology (Horton, 1997a) will provide many opportunities for forensic neuropsychologists to make important contributions to society.

Minority Groups and Forensic Neuropsychology

The population of the United States has grown much more diverse in the last few decades. Given that there are many new individuals with different ethnic backgrounds in the United States, increased attention to the neuropsychological evaluation of these newly arrived individuals is essential, in terms of providing appropriate services. There is a famous story (possibly true) concerning Ray Corsini, PhD, a famous psychologist. Corsini, on arriving from Italy as a young boy, was tested at Ellis Island in the New York City Harbor to determine his intelligence. Dr. Corsini was labeled mentally retarded with an IQ of 50. Of course, after 1 year in the New York City Public Schools, Dr. Corsini was given an IQ test and earned an IQ score of 150 or in the very superior range, or an increase of 100 IQ points. The major difference was not due to the educational program in the New York City Public Schools, but rather to the fact that Dr. Corsini learned to speak the English language in the ensuing year, as previously, he only spoke his native language, Italian. As one might expect, both IQ tests were administered in the English language. Dr. Corsini went on to a very successful career in psychology and wrote many books in the English language. The implications for forensic neuropsychological evaluation of minority group members, and particularly, recent immigrants to the United States, are straightforward and clear.

Appropriate neuropsychological assessment should be tailored to the cultural context of new immigrants to the United States, as well as persons who maintain a different cultural identity than the majority culture (Ponton & Ardila, 1999).

Interestingly, Ralph M. Reitan, PhD, ABPP, ABN (1974), a famous neuropsychologist (the father of American neuropsychology) was born in the United States, but early in life, lived in Lutheran communities in the Midwest (Reitan's father was a Lutheran minister) and grew up speaking the Norwegian language. Dr. Reitan only learned the English language, as a second language, when he had to attend elementary school. Interestingly, Dr. Reitan noted that his later acceptance into the University of Chicago for doctoral studies in psychology was facilitated by his ability to speak Norwegian to Professor Thurstone, the famous psychometrician (Reitan & Davison, 1974; Reitan & Wolfson, 1993).

There is great need for additional research on forensic neuropsychological assessment in a multicultural context (Horton, Carrington, & Lewis-Jack, 2001). Clearly, a firm empirical basis for forensic neuropsychology decision making with minority group members is needed. For example, recent attention with respect to death penalty decisions made based on forensic neuropsychology evaluations of the intelligence of minority group members has demonstrated the importance of this issue. Much additional work will be needed with respect to forensic neuropsychological services within a multicultural context.

Summary

The future of forensic neuropsychology practices is still to be determined, but is likely to be rewarding and exciting (Zillmer & Green, 2006). It is possible that managed care will drive many clinical neuropsychologists to move into forensic neuropsychology (Ruff, 2004). Health care service availability may be as influential as legal developments in shaping the future of forensic neuropsychology (Sweet, King, Malina, Bergman, & Simmons, 2002). The potential value of computer technology advances will likely improve forensic neuropsychology practices. Credentialing and training issues are likely to persist. Also, there is need for greater ecological validity for neuropsychological tests and the future uses of MRI and PET scans (Bigler, 2008) and need for measures to assess biased responding. The new populations of medical/health care patients (Hall & Cope, 1995) and minority group members were proposed as areas in great need of future forensic neuropsychological assessments. The hope and expectation is that this chapter will serve to expedite the future progress of forensic neuropsychology. It should be stated that the above speculations are the judgments of the chapter author, and the veracity of the above speculations is not guaranteed. Similar to all scientific matters, the future remains to be experienced, and the only likely constant is that new developments will be surprising.

References

Armenti, N. (1993). Managed health care and the behaviorally trained professional. *Behavior Therapist, 14*, 13–15.

Bauer, L., & McCaffery, R. J. (2006). Coverage of the test of malingered memory, Victoria symptom validity test and word memory test on the internet: Is test security threatened? *Archives of Clinical Neuropsychology, 21*, 121–126.

Bigler, E. D. (2008). Neuropsychology and clinical neuroscience of persistent post-concussive syndrome. *Journal of the International Neuropsychological Society, 14*(1), 1–22.

Bigler, E. D., Lowry, C. M., & Porter, S. S. (1997). Neuroimaging in forensic neuropsychology. In A. M. Horton, Jr., D. Wedding, & J. S. Webster (Eds.), *The neuropsychology handbook* (2nd ed., Vol. 1, pp. 171–220). New York: Springer Publishing Company.

Cummings, N. (1986). The dismantling of our health care systems: Strategies for the survival of psychological practice. *American Psychologist, 41*, 426–431.

Daubert vs. Merril Dow Pharmaceuticals, 113 S. Ct. 2786 (1993).

Essig, S. M., Mittenberg, W. Peterson, R. S., Strauman, S., & Cooper, J. T. (2001). Practices in forensic neuropsychology: Perspectives of neuropsychologists and trial attorneys. *Archives of Clinical Neuropsychology, 16*(3), 271–291.

Franzen, M. D., & Iverson, G. L. (1997). Detection of biased responding in neuropsychological assessment. In A. M. Horton, Jr., D. Wedding, & J. S. Webster (Eds.), *The neuropsychology handbook* (2nd ed., Vol. 2, pp. 393–423). New York: Springer Publishing Company.

Gervais, R. O., Allen, L. M., & Green, P. (2001). Effects of coaching on symptom validity testing in chronic pain patients presenting for disability assessments. *Journal of Forensic Neuropsychology, 2*, 1–19.

Gervais, R. O., Rohling, M. L., Green, P., & Ford, W. (2004). A comparison of the WMT, CARB and TOMM failure rates in non-head injury disability claimants. *Archives of Clinical Neuropsychology, 19*, 475–488.

Hall, K. M., & Cope, D. N. (1995). The benefits of rehabilitation in traumatic brain injury: A literature review. *Journal of Head Trauma Rehabilitation, 10*(1), 1–13.

Hartman, D. (1995). *Neuropsychological toxicology* (2nd ed.). New York: Plenum Press.

Horton, A. M., Jr. (1997a). Human neuropsychology: Current status. In A. M. Horton, Jr., D. Wedding, & J. S. Webster (Eds.), *The neuropsychology handbook* (2nd ed., Vol. 1, pp. 3–29). New York: Springer Publishing Company.

Horton, A. M., Jr. (1997b). Halstead-Reitan neuropsychological test battery: Problems and prospects. In A. M. Horton, Jr., D. Wedding, & J. S. Webster (Eds.), *The neuropsychology handbook* (2nd ed., Vol. 1, pp. 221–254). New York: Springer Publishing Company.

Horton, A. M., Jr., & Wedding, D. (1984). *Clinical and behavioral neuropsychology*. New York: Praeger.

Horton, A. M., Jr., Carrington, C. H., & Lewis-Jack, O. (2001) Neuropsychological assessment in a multicultural context. In L. A. Suzuki, J. G. Ponterotto, & P. J. Meller (Eds.), *Handbook of multicultural assessment* (2nd ed., pp. 233–260). San Francisco: Jossey-Bass.

Iverson, G. L. (2003). Detecting malingering in civil forensic evaluations. In A. M. Horton, Jr., & L. C. Hartlage (Eds.), *Handbook of forensic neuropsychology* (pp. 137–177). New York: Springer Publishing Company.

Johnstone, B., Coppel, D., & Townes, B. D. (1997). The future of neuropsychology in medical specialties. *Journal of Clinical Psychology in Medical Settings, 4*(2), 219–229.

Johnstone, D., & Farmer, J. E. (1997). Preparing neuropsychologists for the future: The need for additional training guidelines. *Archives of Clinical Neuropsychology, 12*(6), 523–530.

Kanauss, K., Schatz, P., & Puente, A. E. (2005). Current trends in the reimbursement of professional neuropsychological services. *Archives of Clinical Neuropsychology, 20*(3), 341–353.

Larrabee, G. (2003). Detection of malingering using atypical performance on standard neuropsychological tests. *Clinical Neuropsychologist, 17*, 410–442.

Meyers, J. E., & Volbrecht, M. E. (2003). A validation of multiple malingering detection measures in a large clinical sample. *Archives of Clinical Neuropsychology, 18*(3), 261–276.

Otto, R. K., & Heilbrun, K. (2002). The practice of forensic psychology. *American Psychologist, 57*(1), 5–18.

Peterson, L., & Harbeck, C. (1988). *The pediatric psychologist.* Champaign, IL: Research Press.

Ponton, M. O., & Ardila, A. (1999). The future of neuropsychology with Hispanic populations in the United States. *Archives of Clinical Neuropsychology, 14*(7), 565–580.

Project on Scientific Knowledge and Public Policy. (2003, June). *Daubert: The most influential Supreme Court ruling you've never heard of.* Retrieved January 15, 2007, from http://www.defending science.org/courts/Daubert-report-excerpt.cfm

Purish, A. D., & Sbordone, R. J. (1997). Forensic neuropsychology: Forensic issues and practice. In A. M. Horton, Jr., D. Wedding, & J. S. Webster (Eds.), *The neuropsychology handbook* (2nd ed., Vol. 2, pp. 309–373). New York: Springer Publishing Company.

Reitan, R. M. (1974). Psychological effects of cerebral lesions in children of early school age. In R. M. Reitan & L. A. Davison (Eds.), *Forensic neuropsychology: Current status and applications* (pp. 53–90). New York: John Wiley.

Reitan, R. M., & Davison, L. A. (Eds.). (1974). *Forensic neuropsychology: Current status and applications.* New York: John Wiley.

Reitan, R. M., & Wolfson, D. (1993). *Halstead-Reitan neuropsychological test battery.* Tucson, AZ: Neuropsychology Press.

Reynolds, C. R. (1998). *Detection of malingering during head injury litigation.* New York: Plenum Press.

Rohling, M. L., & Boone, K. B. (2007). Future directions in effort assessment. In K. B. Boone (Ed.), *Assessment of feigned cognitive impairment* (pp. 453–469). New York: Guilford Press.

Ruff, R. M. (2004). A friendly critique of neuropsychology: Facing the challenges of our future. *Archives of Clinical Neuropsychology, 18*(8), 847–864.

Russell, E. W. (1995). The accuracy of automated and clinical detection of brain damage and lateralization in neuropsychology. *Neuropsychology Review, 5*(1), 1–68.

Sbordone, R. J., & Saul, R. E. (2000). *Neuropsychology for health care professionals and attorneys* (2nd ed.). Boca Raton, FL: CRC Press.

Schatz, P., & Browndyke, J. (2002). Applications of computer-based neuropsychological assessment. *Journal of Head Trauma Rehabilitation, 17*(5), 395–410.

Strosahi, K. (1994). Entering the new frontier of managed mental health care: Gold mines and land mines. *Cognitive and Behavioral Practice, 1*, 5–23.

Sweet, J. J., King, J. H., Malina, A. C., Bergman, M. A., & Simmons, A. (2002). Documenting the prominence of forensic neuropsychology at professional meetings and in relevant professional journals. *Clinical Neuropsychologist, 16*(4), 481–494.

Sweet, J. J., Westergaard, C. K., & Moberg, P. J. (1995). Managed care experiences of forensic neuropsychologists. *Forensic Neuropsychologist, 9*(3), 214–218.

Youngjohn, J. R. (1995). Confirmed attorney coaching prior to neuropsychological evaluation. *Assessment, 2*, 279–283.

Zillmer, E. A. (2004). The future of neuropsychology. *Archives of Clinical Neuropsychology, 19*, 713–724.

Zillmer, E. A., & Green, H. K. (2006). Neuropsychological assessment in the forensic setting. In R. P. Archer (Ed.), *Forensic uses of clinical assessment instruments* (pp. 209–227). Mahwah, NJ: Lawrence Erlbaum.

Index